INSIGHT AND CONTROL OF INFECTIOUS DISEASE IN GLOBAL SCENARIO

Edited by **Priti Kumar Roy**

Insight and Control of Infectious Disease in Global Scenario
Edited by Priti Kumar Roy

Published by InTech

Janeza Trdine 9, 51000 Rijeka, Croatia

Publishing Process Manager Petra Nenadic

Technical Editor Teodora Smiljanic

Cover Designer InTech Design Team

Additional hard copies can be obtained from orders@intechopen.com

Insight and Control of Infectious Disease in Global Scenario, Edited by Priti Kumar Roy
p. cm.
ISBN 978-953-51-0319-6

For EU product safety concerns:
IN TECH d.o.o., Prolaz Marije Krucifikse Kozulić 3, 51000 Rijeka, Croatia,
info@intechopen.com or visit our website at intechopen.com.

Meet the editor

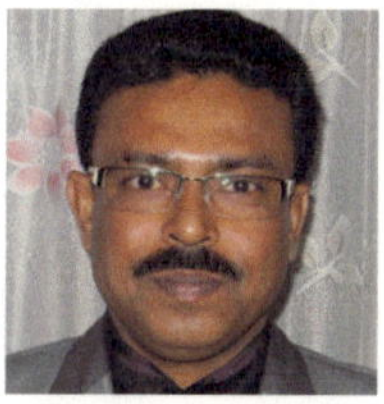

Dr. Priti Kumar Roy has been rewarded Ph.D. degree from Jadavpur University. Scientific publications in international height inaugurated before this and at this moment a lots of his publications have occurred. Eight Ph.D. students are perusing their research work under his esteemed guidance. Dr. Roy has performed as reviewer in International and National Journals. He has served in Government colleges in different parts of West Bengal, India. Now, he is engaged at teaching in the Faculty of Science, Jadavpur University since 2008. Dr. Roy was also invited to deliver his impressive lectures in a variety of Indian Universities, Institutes and abroad also. He has been selected as an eminent member in different National and International Societies like Bio mathematical Society of India and IAENG. He has completed some Research Projects and three major Research Projects are continuing under his pioneer supervision, sponsored by various India Government agencies. Dr. Roy has received Best Paper Award in World Congress on Engineering 2010 which was held in London, UK. He has been selected as an Indian Scientist for nomination under International Collaboration/Exchange Programme2011-2012 by INSA. He is served as an organizing secretary in different National and International Conference. He is now working the research on the chronic disease Psoriasis, HIV Infection and Control Therapeutic Approach and Host Pathogen Interaction very progressively.

Contents

Preface

In a Global scenario, economically progressive nations have developed medical sciences. But still it lacks precise information during the enhancement of potent drugs to combat ailment, which is the legacy of the organisms that generate diseases. Rising countries had long been perceived the threat, which at times, down the lane has been the major factor for magnanimous economic disaster and human poverty. Lot of resources was put into force by the world community to abscond the microbial fauna and genetically inherited diseases to contain them within the safe limits. However, endemics, epidemics and pandemics occur in recent situation due to various host-pathogen interactions. Bioscience has been the buzz of the 21st century but mathematical science has been the leader behind empowering the biologists to formulate laws and theories to combat diseases with precise and accurate information. Biomathematics and Epidemics has joined hands together to emerge as a novel strategic tie up that lead to prognosis, diagnose and formulate effective combat schedule to emerge and re-emerge as a winner against the dreadful infectious diseases. Diseases like HIV, Mycobacterium and Diphtherias are the most feared and live threatening fast communicable infection that can roam from one place to the other within very short period. Over the years drug resistance has also contributed severe efficacy loss to the conventional disease therapy. Mathematical models can contribute and map the lagging information to the biologists to solve the puzzle and challenge infectious disease effectively. This book has been a step forward in the modern era to understand, analyze and fight infectious disease in an effective and accurate manner through the language of biomathematics. The authors find great research potential in combining the two fundamental branches of science to the most lucid detail that serves the researchers, scholars, and medical professionals. The most crucial information about the pathways of control theoretical approach is to be encroached about the infectious diseases that are the menace in the world. As the pride editor of this introspecting research compendium, I am privileged to account some modern and interesting research topics in the prized volume of the book. I hope that this literature serves as a lee forward in understanding the basic host-pathogen interaction in a more coherent and scientific fashion and its *modus operandi* in relation to the various biotic and abiotic modules. This book introspect the major thrust areas of infectious diseases both in anthropogenic and zoonotic domains and as the editor; I include the research articles in most prudent manner. I wish that this volume in its present format will serve the nourishing and nurturing delicacy to the bio-mathematician, drug modelers and clinical researchers in a novel flavor. Pieces of writings have been preferred with scrupulous concern; so that a few of them may imitate and include a huge number of apparently oscillate looking ones, thus reducing the quantum of recurrence. My intention in writing the book is not to talk about the infectious disease, but to let the readers to be familiar with such manifestation as would them to undertake any question in the mind.

I expect this book may have an immense impact on our socio-economical environment. My endeavor is to enlighten the shady features of infectious disease to surroundings, such that the humanity may emerge from blind superstitions.

It is too incongruous to cover the complete topics, based on infectious disease, but I have performed my level best workings to include a big portion of the curriculum. Analyses, information, gathered in this book, have been integrated from a variety of national and international journals, to institute this text. My wholehearted effort will be successful, if societal advantage may be achieved to the civilization.

I extend my heartfelt salute to the contributors of the volume for their articles and christening me the honor as being the editor of the volume. I am grateful to Dr. Sumit Nandi of Narula Institute of Technology, Dr. Joydeep Mukharjee of Jadavpur University, Dr. Sutapa Biswas Majee of NSHM College of Pharmaceutical Technology, Mr. Joydeep Pal of Indian Statistical Institute, my scholars specially Mr. Abhirup Datta and all colleagues of my Department, for their incessant encouragement and motivation. Without their hard strained efforts and impulsive collaboration, it is too impossible for me to edit this book. I thank to the mighty god, my friends, well wishers and family for keeping the energy live in me in finishing the job and present this book to the society for a better knowledge to combat disease. Lastly, I obtain the capacity of extending my heartfelt thanks to all the members of "Intech Open Science" for their kind assistance in bringing out this book. With all the constrictions concerning power, paper and time, I have tried to optimize the accessible benefit to the readers with supreme concern. The ultimate responsibility for inaccuracy or misprints is mine and notices will be auspiciously cherished for improvement of the book, if they are pointed out.

Dr. Priti Kumar Roy,
Jadavpur University
Kolkata,
India

Part 1

General Epidemics and Its Control Through Mathematical Approach

1

Biomedical Importance of Host Genetic Factors in Infectious Diseases

Farrukh Jamal[1], Tabish Qidwai[2] and Sangram Singh[1]
[1]*Department of Biochemistry, Dr. Ram Manohar Lohia Avadh University, Faizabad, U.P.*
[2]*Department of Biotechnology, Faculty of Engineering and Technology, R.B.S. College, Agra, U.P., India*

1. Introduction

Tuberculosis, human immunodeficiency virus/acquired immunodeficiency syndrome and malaria are the three most profound cause of death worldwide. In developing country tuberculosis is a serious problem. It is estimated that one third of the world's population is infected with *M. tuberculosis*; however, only a minority (10%) of those infected ever develop clinical disease (Corbett et al., 2003). Such clinical diversity suggests that factors other than bacterial infection alone determine disease development. Tuberculosis (TB) is a significant disease affecting both humans and animals. Susceptibility to *Mycobacterium tuberculosis* is relatively higher in humans than other primates and guinea pigs. Cattle, rabbits and cats are susceptible to *M. bovis* and are quite resistant to *M. tuberculosis*.

Each year, 8.8 million patients are newly diagnosed with active TB and 1.6 million patients die of TB. The rapid spread of the human immunodeficiency virus has fueled the TB epidemic, especially in sub-Saharan Africa, where 28% of TB patients are HIV positive (WHO 2007). The current first-line treatment for TB is a multidrug regimen consisting of rifampin, isoniazid, pyrazinamide, and ethambutol (RIZE). Several major problems are associated with the currently available TB treatment. There is an increasing incidence of multidrug-resistant (MDR; resistance to at least rifampin and isoniazid) and extensively drug-resistant (XDR; MDR resistance plus resistance to a fluoroquinolone and an aminoglycoside) which is creating an alarming situation as far as treatment of the disease is concerned.

1.1 Causes of drug resistance

The emergence of drug resistance in *M. tuberculosis* in India has been associated with a variety of management, health provider and patient-related factors. These include, deficient or deteriorating TB control programs resulting in inadequate administration of effective treatment; poor case holding, administration of sub-standard drugs, inadequate or irregular drug supply and lack of supervision; ignorance of health care workers in epidemiology, treatment and control; improper prescription of regimens; interruption of chemotherapy due to side effects; non-adherence of patients to the prescribed drug therapy; availability of anti-TB drugs across the counter, without prescription; massive bacillary load; illiteracy and low socio-economic status of the patients; the epidemic of HIV infection; laboratory delays in identification and susceptibility testing of *M. tuberculosis* isolates; use of non-standardized laboratory techniques, poor quality drug powders and lack of quality control measures; use of anti-TB drugs for indications other than tuberculosis.

1.2 Initial drug resistance in India

Indian Council of Medical Research (ICMR) undertook drug resistance studies during 1965-67 in nine urban areas of the country. However, this exercise was not a surveillance study and did not use strict sampling techniques, the centres being selected more for logistic considerations than for epidemiological reasons. Sputum specimens collected from all patients attending chest clinics were tested for drug susceptibility to streptomycin, Isoniazid, para amino salicyctic acid (PAS) and thioacetazone. The first study was on patients who had denied any history of previous treatment, while in the second study, patients with and without previous chemotherapy was included. The results showed that in the first study resistance to Isoniazid ranged from 11-20 per cent, to streptomycin from 8-20 per cent and to both drugs from 4-11 per cent. The second study showed resistance to Isoniazid to range from 15-69 per cent, to streptomycin from 12-63 per cent and to both drugs from 5-58 per cent. Further, the level of drug resistance was proportional to the duration of previous treatment.

1.3 Multi drug resistance in other countries

Resistance towards the responsible pathogens are also seen in developed countries. The situation has worsened often due to limited resource available to investigate and provide reliable susceptibility data on which rational treatments can be based as well as means to optimize the use of antimicrobial agents. The emergence of multi-drug-resistant isolates in tuberculosis, acute respiratory infections and diarrhea, often referred to as diseases of poverty, has had its greatest toll in developing countries. The epidemic of HIV/AIDS, with over 30 million cases in developing countries, has greatly enlarged the population of immuno compromised patients. The disease has left these patients at great risk of numerous infections and even greater risks of acquiring highly resistant organisms during long periods of hospitalization. This article discusses antimicrobial resistance in developing countries and the associated risk factors. Magnitude of resistance by regions Africa, America, Eastern Mediterranean, European, South East Asian, Western Pacific region has shown greater diversity in TB.

2. Symptoms

Symptoms of tuberculosis include: a bad cough that lasts 3 weeks or longer, pain in the chest, coughing up blood or sputum (phlegm from deep inside the lungs). Other symptoms of active TB disease are weakness or fatigue, weight loss, no appetite, chills, fever and sweating at night.

3. Spread

TB spreads through the air from one person to another. The bacteria are put into the air when a person with active TB disease of the lungs or throat coughs or sneezes. People nearby may breathe in these bacteria and get infected. When a person breathes in TB bacteria, which may settle in the lungs and begin to grow. From there, they can move through the blood to other parts of the body, such as the kidney, spine, and brain. TB in the lungs or throat can be infectious. This means that the bacteria can spread to other people. TB in other parts of the body, such as the kidney or spine, is usually not infectious.People with active TB disease are most likely to spread it to people they spend time with every day. This includes family members, friends, and coworkers.

4. Diagnoses

4.1 Molecular diagnosis of *Mycobacterium*

During the past several years, many molecular methods have been developed for direct detection, species identification, and drug susceptibility testing of mycobacteria.

4.1.1 Direct detection of mycobacteria from specimens

Many mycobacterial species, including *M. tuberculosis,* grow extremely slowly in the laboratory and require 3–8 weeks of incubation on solid medium or at least 2 weeks in a radiometric liquid culture system (BACTEC). This slow growth often leads to delay in TB diagnosis. Nucleic acid amplification (NAA) methods allow for detection of mycobacterial DNA or RNA directly from the specimens before the culture results are available. The Food and Drug Administration (FDA) has approved two NAA tests for direct detection of *M. tuberculosis* from clinical specimens. These are the Enhanced *Mycobacterium tuberculosis* Direct Test (E-MTD; Gen-Probe, San Diego, CA) and the Amplicor *Mycobacterium tuberculosis* Test (Amplicor; Roche Diagnostic Systems, Inc., Branchburg, NJ).

4.1.2 Amplicor test

Based on PCR assay, Mycobacterium is amplified. After amplification, the amplicons are denatured to form single strands and added to a microtiter plate containing a bound, *M. tuberculosis* complex-specific oligonucleotide probe. An avidin-horseradish peroxidase conjugate then binds to the bound, biotin-labeled amplicons. The conjugate reacts with peroxide and 3, 39, 5, 59-tetramethylbenzidine in dimethylformamide to form a color complex. The results are measured with a photometer.

4.1.3 E-MTD

The E-MTD test is based on the transcription-mediated amplification system developed by Kwoh et al. (1989). In this assay, rRNA is released from the target cells by sonication, and a promoter-primer binds to the rRNA target. Reverse transcriptase is then used to copy rRNA to a cDNA-RNA hybrid. The initial RNA strand is degraded, and a second primer binds to the cDNA and is extended, leading to the formation of double-stranded cDNA, which is then transcribed by DNA-directed RNA polymerase to produce more rRNA molecules. The new transcripts serve as templates for reverse transcription and further amplification. The

RNA amplicons are detected with an acridinium ester-labeled DNA probe in a solution hybridization assay.

4.1.4 DNA probes

Commercial DNA probes are available for detection of mycobacterium. These are based on species-specific DNA probes that hybridize with rRNA released from bacteria. The probes are labeled with acridinium ester, and results are measured with a luminometer.

4.1.5 Line-probe assay

The Line Probe assay (LiPA; Inno-Genetics N.V., Zwijndrecht, Belgium) has been developed for rapid detection of RIF resistance. The test is based on the reverse hybridization method, and it consists of PCR amplification of a segment of the *rpoB* gene and denaturation and hybridization of the biotinylated PCR amplicons to capture probes bound to a nitrocellulose strip. The bound amplicons are then detected with alkaline phosphatase-conjugated streptavidin and BCIP/NBT chromogen, producing a color reaction.

4.2 TB skin test

The TB skin test may be used to find out if you have TB infection. You can get a skin test at any pathology laboratory. A technician will inject a small amount of testing fluid (called tuberculin or PPD) just under the skin on the under side of the forearm. After 48 hours, you must return to have your skin test read by the laboratory technician. You may have a swelling where the tuberculin was injected. The technician will measure this swelling and tell you if your reaction to the test is positive or negative. A positive reaction usually means that you have been infected by someone with active TB.

5. National and international status

Tuberculosis (TB) is a major, global public health problem, particularly in sub-Saharan Africa, where the prevalence of TB is increasing dramatically with the rise of the HIV pandemic. One third of the world is infected by Mtb (*Mycobacterium tuberculosis*). (Raviglione et al., 1995). According to the World Health Organization, almost 8 million new cases of TB occur annually, with 2 million deaths attributed to the disease each year. There were globally an estimated 9.27 million new cases of tuberculosis (TB) and 1.3 million deaths in 2007 (WHO, 2009).

Uganda is one of the world's 22 highest burden countries with TB, with an estimated annual risk of tuberculosis infection of 3% and an annual incidence of new smear positive TB cases of 9.2 per 1000 in an urban setting (Guwatudde et al., 2003). Pakistan ranks 7th globally in terms of tuberculosis (TB) disease burden (Ansari et al., 2009).

TB is one of the leading causes of mortality in India killing more than 300,000 people every year. The Human Immunodeficiency Virus (HIV, the virus that causes AIDS) is the strongest risk factor for tuberculosis among adults. Tuberculosis is one of the earliest opportunistic diseases to develop amongst persons infected with HIV. HIV debilitates the immune system increasing the vulnerability to TB and enhancing the risk of progression from TB infection to TB disease. An HIV positive person is six times (50-60% life time risk) more likely of developing TB disease once infected with TB bacilli, as compared to an HIV negative person, who has a 10% life-time risk. Since 1993, the Government of India has been implementing the WHO-recommended DOTS strategy via the Revised National Tuberculosis Control Programme (RNTCP). The revised strategy was pilot-tested in 1993 and launched as a national programme in 1997. By March 2006, the programme was implemented nationwide in 633 districts, covering 1114 million (100%) population.

India accounts for one fifth of the world's incident TB cases. The reported incidence in 2003 was 168 per 100,000 and in 2006 is nearly 175 per 100,000. Every year, nearly 2 million people die in India, and nearly 1 million cases are smear positive; An estimated 40% of the Indian population is latently infected with *M. tuberculosis*. A number of factors - cultural, social, political, economic and technical - have determined the nature of society's response to TB. It has been shown that most of the infectious TB cases in a rural community in South India. About three-fourths of them are worried about their sickness; and, about half of them actively seek treatment for their symptoms at rural medical hospital. The existing facilities deal with only a very small fraction of even these patients who are actively seeking treatment. The various study report carried out in India has shown increase in TB and MDR-TB . India is classified along with the sub-Saharan African countries to be among those with a high burden of TB.

5.1 Epidemiology

The aim of epidemiology is the determination of natural history of disease and measurement of its frequency.

5.1.1 Aims of epidemiology

- Describe the trends of disease.
- Evaluation of intervention
- Define the risk group
- Frequency, distribution, time, place and person

6. Available drugs

6.1 Fluoroquinolone- fluoroquinolone is a promising class of drugs for the treatment of TB

6.1.1 Moxifloxacin- Moxifloxacin is a broad-spectrum 8-methoxy fluoroquinolone with activity against both gram-positive and gram-negative bacteria, including anaerobes. It inhibits bacterial DNA gyrase, an enzyme that is essential for the maintenance of DNA supercoils.

6.1.2 Gatifloxacin: Like the other fluoroquinolones, gatifloxacin blocks the bacterial DNA gyrase, thereby preventing chromosomal replication.

6.2 Diarylquinolines. Diarylquinolines have been identified in a process of screening various compounds for potential anti-TB activity.

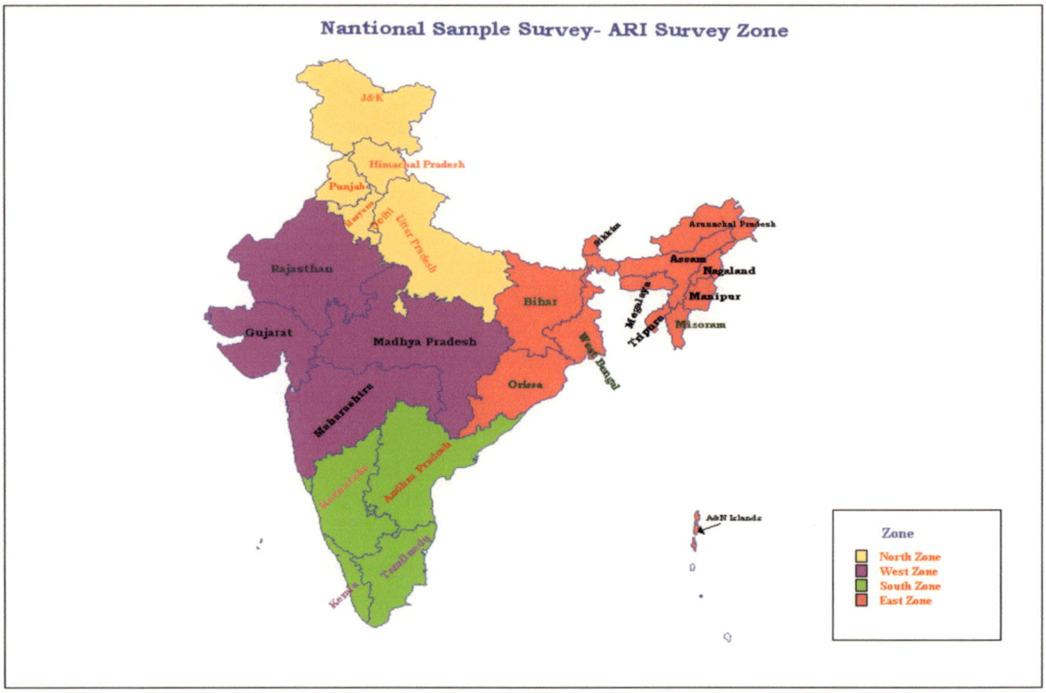

Fig. 1. Estimation of annual risk of Tuberculosis in different regions of India 2000-2003 (From National TB Institute Bangalore).

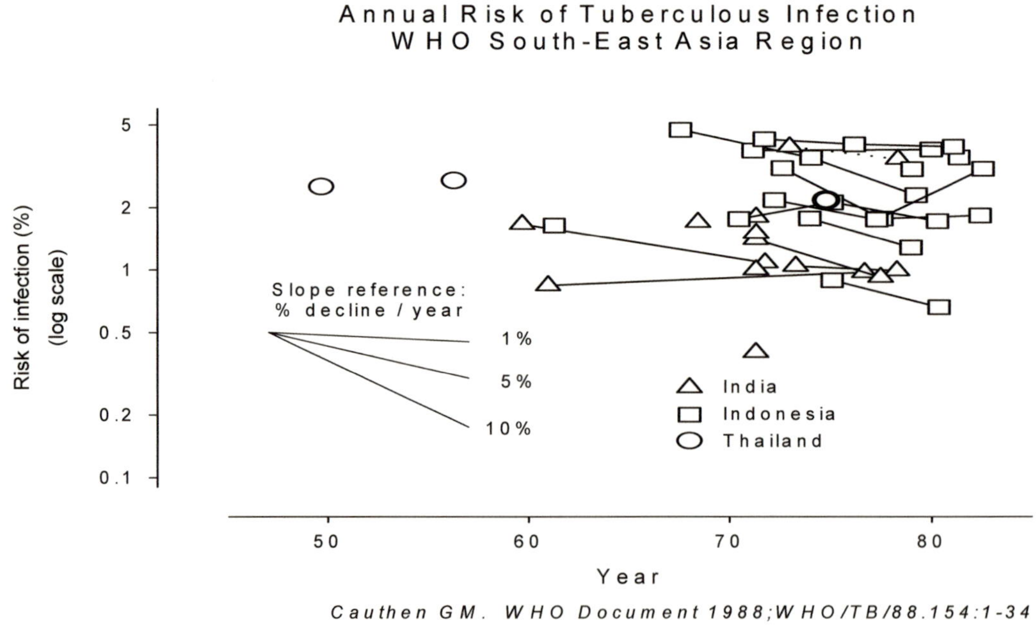

Fig. 2. Annual risk of Tuberculosis infection in South East Asia region.

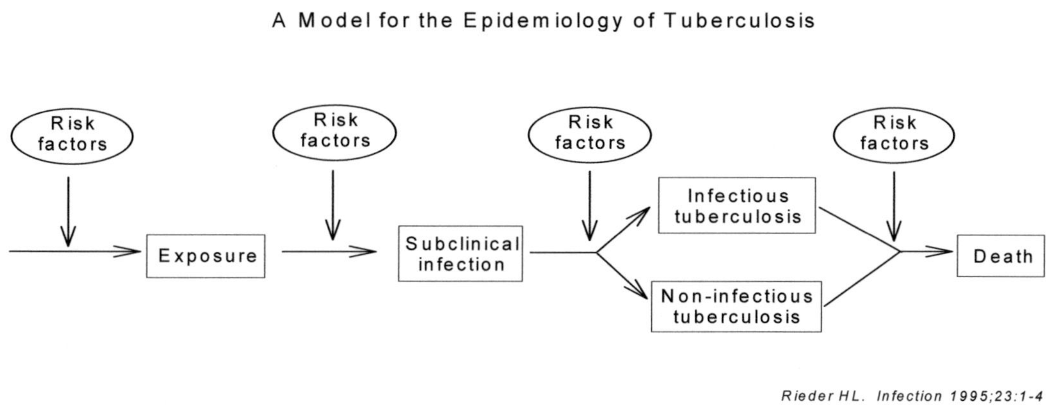

Fig. 3. Model of epidemiology of Tuberculosis.

6.2.1 TMC207: it inhibits the mycobacterial ATP synthase enzyme

6.2.2 PA-824. Activated: PA-824 inhibits the synthesis of proteins and cell wall lipids.

6.3 Nitroimidazopyrans: Nitroimidazopyrans have been derived from the bicyclic nitroimidazofurans that were originally developed for cancer chemotherapy but also exhibited activity against tuberculosis.

6.3.1 OPC-67683: OPC-67683 is a mycolic acid biosynthesis inhibitor.

6.4 Diamines

6.4.1 SQ109: SQ109 inhibits mycobacterial cell wall synthesis.

6.5 Pyrroles: In the search for compounds with activity against mycobacteria and fungi, several pyrrole derivatives have been developed.

7. Genetic polymorphisms and tuberculosis

The genetic contribution of the host plays a significant role in determining susceptibility to developing the active form of tuberculosis and severity of infection (Comstock, 1978; Schurr, 2007). Several genes of host immune response appear to play role in tuberculosis. Genetic polymorphisms and tuberculosis have been identified in several genes of host. A number of genes have been identified that play important role in tuberculosis (Fernando & Britton, 2006; Hoal, 2002). Several candidate gene studies and genome-wide linkage association studies (Bellamy et al., 2000; Jamieson et al., 2004; Miller et al., 2004; Cooke et al., 2008; Berrington & Hawn, 2007) have been performed for investigation of their role in disease risk.

Infectious disease has profound impact on human evolution. Tuberculosis is a multifactorial disorder in which the environment interacts with host-related factors, contributing to the overall phenotype. Improved understanding of the individuals balance between degrees of exposure and inherited genetic susceptibility to infection, as well as the respective effects of environmental and host-related factors will improve the understanding in the development of disease. Several host genes have been proven to contribute to active tuberculosis (TB) (Pesut, 2009). In human genome different types of variations are reported such as copy number variations (CNV), microsatellite repeats (SSR) and single nucleotide polymorphisms (SNP). Among these SNPs is the most common type of variations. Presence of polymorphisms affects either structure or level of gene products.

SNP description alone will not be sufficient to describe susceptibility to tuberculosis in a broad diverse population, and thus, functional gene studies need to be done. A real challenge is to associate candidate genes with a biologically plausible mechanism that explains the epidemiological data for tuberculosis in which only 10% of the infected individuals will develop tuberculosis. Lienhardt et al., (2002) stated that host-related and environmental factors for tuberculosis have usually been investigated separately using different study designs. Joint investigation of the genetic, immunologic, and environmental factors at play in susceptibility to tuberculosis represents an innovative goal for obtaining a better understanding of the pathogenesis of the disease. Host genetic susceptibility has been suggested as one of the most important explanations for inter-individual differences in tuberculosis (TB) risk. Multi-drug-resistant tuberculosis (MDR TB) is caused by strains of the tuberculosis bacteria resistant to the two most effective anti-tuberculosis drugs available-isoniazid and rifampicin. MDR TB can only be diagnosed in a specialized laboratory.

8. Genetic polymorphisms in tuberculosis pathogenesis

8.1 Tumor necrosis factor-alpha (TNF-α) polymorphisms

The host genetic factor plays a significant role in determining susceptibility to developing the active form of tuberculosis (Schurr, 2007). Several host immune response genes appear to play role in tuberculosis. Tumor necrosis factor-α (TNF-α) and lymphotoxin-α (LT-α), genes located within the MHC III region of chromosome 6, shows close linkage to the HLA class I (HLA-B) and class II (HLA-DR) genes (Nedwin et al., 1985) and play role in the pathogenesis of tuberculosis due to its role in the formation and maintenance of granulomas. It also plays a major role in host defense to *M. tuberculosis* by its synergistic action with interferon-γ (IFN-γ) to activate macrophages and thereby affects disease perpetuation (Mohan et al., 2001). Elevated serum TNF-α (sTNF-α) levels have been reported in advanced tuberculosis patients compared to those with mild tuberculosis and healthy controls. Several promoter polymorphisms region of TNF-α and the intron-1 polymorphism of LT-α, have been associated with altered levels of TNF-α (Sharma et al., 2008; 2010). Some of these polymorphisms have also been studied in several ethnic groups. Correa Paula et al. (2005) detected TNF-α gene polymorphisms (-308 and -238) in controls and patients of several diseases [systemic lupus erythematosus (SLE), rheumatoid arthritis (RA), primary Sjogren's syndrome (SS), and tuberculosis (TB)]. TNF -308G was associated with TB and -308 GG genotype was protective for autoimmunity. TNF-238A allele was protective for autoimmunity but a susceptibility factor for TB. Haplotype -308A-238G have been reported as a protective factor for TB, but susceptibility factor for RA, SLE, and primary SS; opposite association of TNF polymorphism with autoimmunity and TB, suggested that autoimmune diseases are a consequence of natural selection for enhanced TB resistance. Ates et al., (2008), detected TNF-α (-308 G/A, -238 G/A, -376 G/A) and IL10 (-1,082 G/A, -819 C/T, -592 C/A) polymorphisms in patients with TB and healthy controls. A significant association was found between TB and -1,082 G allele. Significant difference was observed in IL10 GCC and ACC haplotypes distribution between TB and controls. No significant association was found between IL-10 -819 C/T, TNF-α, 308 G/A, -238 G/A, -376 G/A polymorphisms and Tuberculosis. Sharma et al. 2010, performed a case control study including TNF-α gene (-1031, -863, -857, -308,-238) and LT-α gene (+252) polymorphisms in North-Indian population. No significant differences of the allele frequencies between the tuberculosis patients and controls have been reported. All the polymorphisms included in this study did not give a significant association with any of the patient sub-groups but a significant difference in the serum TNF-α level in the patients and the controls have been reported.

8.2 ALOX5 polymorphisms

ALOX5 gene encodes 5-lipoxygenase (5-LO) that play a key role in the biosynthesis of LTs and LXs from arachidonic acid. Leukotrienes (LTs) and lipoxins (LXs) are play a role in the generation of appropriate responses to inflammatory disease (Parkinson, 2006) and are involved in the regulation of immune cells and cytokine release. Phagocytosis of microorganisms by alveolar macrophages and polymorphonuclear leukocytes PMN was shown to be dependent on LTB_4, class of LXs (Bailie, 1996; Mancuso et al., 2001). A T-helper cell type 1 immune response is supported by enhanced production of interferon (IFN)- γ and interleukin (IL)-12 (Aliberti et al., 2002). The anti-inflammatory properties of LXs antagonize those of LTs in innate immunity by inhibiting PMN and NK cell functions, suppressing IL-12 release and modulating the immune response by stimulation of IL-4 production (Hachicha et al., 1999), while blocking IL-5 and IL-13 and inhibiting eosinophil effector functions (Bandeira-Melo et al., 2000). A case control study was performed by Herb et al. 2008 including a variable number of tandem repeats (VNTR) in promoter and an exonic non-synonymous variant g.760G>A polymorphisms in TB patients and controls from Ghana. Carriers of one variant and one wild-type VNTR allele ($n = 5$) or of the exonic allele g.760A had a higher risk of TB. The strongest association with TB was for the 'non-5/760A' haplotype as compared to the 'non-5/760G' haplotype.

8.3 CD209 polymorphism

CD209 on chromosome 19p13.3, encodes dendritic Cell-Specific ICAM3-Grabbing Non-integrin (DC-SIGN), is a C-type lectin, expressed on subsets of dendritic cells (DCs) and alveolar macrophages (Soilleux, 2000; Tailleux, 2003). DC-SIGN has ability to bind a variety of ligands (Gordon, 2002), endogenous ligands include endothelial cells through ICAM-2, T-lymphocytes through ICAM-3, neutrophils through MAC-1 and various endogenous glycosylated structures (Gordon, 2002; Van Kyook et al., 2003), exogenous ligands such as glycosylated moieties on *M. leprae, M. tuberculosis,* Bacillus Calmette-Guérin (BCG), *H. pylori, K. pneumoniae, S. pneumoniae,* HIV-1, HIV-2, SIV-1, Dengue virus, Ebola Virus, Cytomegalovirus, Hepatitis C virus, *S. mansoni, L. pifanoi and C. albicans* (Alvarez et al., 2002;

Tassaneetrithep et al., 2003). The contribution of *CD209* polymorphisms in human susceptibility to infectious diseases including *M. tuberculosis* and *M. leprae,* HIV-1, and Dengue is important (Barreiro et al., 2006). CD209 -336A/G (rs4804803) promoter polymorphism have shown an association with infectious disease susceptibility or protection in *M. leprae* case-control study. Martin et al. (2004) demonstrated that the -336G allele was associated with susceptibility to parenteral but not mucosal HIV-1 infection, although this was not replicated in individuals of recent African descent. Vannberg et al. (2008), investigated the role of the *CD209* -336A/G polymorphism and susceptibility to tuberculosis in sub-Saharan Africans. Significant protection was observed with *CD209* -336G variant allele in individuals from sub-Saharan Africa and, cases with -336GG were significantly less likely to develop tuberculosis-induced lung cavitation. Therefore it has been suggested, that decreased levels of the DC-SIGN receptor may be protective against both clinical tuberculosis and cavitory tuberculosis disease.

8.4 SP110 polymorphisms

Ipr1 gene is attributed to tuberculosis susceptibility gene in mice. Polymorphisms in the human homologue, SP110, have been investigated in various populations and only one study reports an association with TB susceptibility. Eight SP110 polymorphisms in a South African population, including two novel polymorphisms had been investigated. No significant association was found with any of the polymorphisms investigated, including two polymorphisms that were previously found to be associated with TB susceptibility in West African populations (Babb et al., 2007).

8.5 CARD15 polymorphisms

Caspase recruitment domain-containing protein 15 genes (*CARD15*) encodes the nucleotide-binding oligomerization domain 2 proteins (NOD2) and is considered as a susceptibility gene for Crohn's disease (CD). *CARD15* gene was investigated as a candidate gene in Tuberculosis and its product (NOD2) have been recognized as a non-redundant recognition mechanism of *M. tuberculosis*. Moller et al. 2007, genotyped the R702W, G908R and 1007fs variants, in TB cases and controls from the admixed South African Coloured population. No statistically significant differences between cases and controls were observed for these variants. Previously these polymorphisms have been reported to be associated with CD. The CD-associated mutations occur at very low frequencies in this population. The *CARD15* is not a major susceptibility gene for TB in the South African Coloureds.

8.6 BTNL2 polymorphisms

Butyrophilin-like2 gene (*BTNL2)* gene, a MHC class II gene-linked butyrophilin family member, has been recently associated with the inflammatory autoimmune diseases, such as tuberculosis, sarcoidosis, and leprosy. *BTNL2* was investigated as a candidate gene for tuberculosis in the South African Coloured population. Moller et al. (2007) genotyped 18 SNPs in *BTNL2* gene in pulmonary tuberculosis cases and controls. No significant association was detected between the truncating rs2076530 SNP, previously associated with sarcoidosis, and tuberculosis. No other studied SNPs have shown an association with disease and none of the predicted haplotypes showed any association with TB. Comparative analyses of the data from South African, German and American populations revealed that, for a segment of *BTNL2*, the admixed, but not stratified, South African population resembles the African-Americans more than white populations. Six SNPs of *BTNL2* gene in tuberculosis cases and controls in Chinese Han population was investigated by Lian et al. 2010. No significant association was detected between any of the polymorphisms investigated and TB, including rs2076530 SNP that was previously found to be associated with sarcoidosis. Genetic study revealed a significant association between the rs3763313, rs9268494, rs9268492 SNPs in the *BTNL2* gene and tuberculosis. Haplotypes 1–5, and 8 (C/A/G/T/G/A, C/A/G/T/G/G, C/A/T/G/C/A, C/A/T/G/C/G, and C/G/T/G/C/G, T/A/T/G/C/A) presented a significant association with susceptibility to tuberculosis.

8.7 IL1 B, IL4, IL10, IL12B, IL12RB, IL12RB2, IL18, IFN-γ WNT5A, FZD5 gene polymorphisms

Genes involved in the regulation of inflammatory cytokine, interferon gamma, may influence tuberculosis susceptibility, as interferon gamma is a major macrophage-activating cytokine, during *M. tuberculosis* infection. Cytokine gene polymorphisms and cytokine levels in pulmonary tuberculosis were detected (Selvaraj et al., 2008). Moller et al. (2010), investigated fifty-four polymorphisms in eight candidate genes [Interleukin 4 (*IL4*), interleukin 10 (*IL10*), interleukin 12B (*IL12B*), interleukin 12 receptor beta 1 (*IL12RB1*), interleukin 12 receptor beta 2 (*IL12RB2*), interleukin 18 (*IL18*), wingless-type MMTV integration site family, member 5A (*WNT5A*) and frizzled homolog 5 (*FZD5*)] in tuberculosis cases and healthy controls in South African population. A functional SNP (rs2243250, IL-4 -C590T), has been associated with increased promoter strength, stronger binding of transcription factors and with different levels of IL-4 activity (Luoni et al., 2001; Rosenwasser et al., 1995) but was not associated with TB in study population. The CC genotype of this polymorphism was previously associated with protection against pulmonary TB in south India and Russia (Naslednikova et al., 2009; Vidyarani et al., 2006) but not in Gambia (Bellamy et al., 1998). Two polymorphisms -511 and +3953 in *IL1B* and one in the *IL1RN*, 86 bp VNTR in smear positive TB patients, and control in Gambian individuals (all HIV negative) was investigated. Decreased risk of pulmonary TB was associated with both heterozygosity and homozygosity for the *IL1B* -511-C allele. There was no association between the *IL1B*+3953-T/C polymorphism or the 86 bp *IL1RN* pentallelic repeat and TB in this population. Using an *ex-vivo* whole blood assay, healthy Gambian individuals who are homozygous for the *IL1B* -511-T allele failed to exhibit a significant increase in IL-1β production in response to LPS after IFN-γ priming.

IFN-γ play a central role in the modulation of Tuberculosis disease severity as it is involved in host immune response against *M. tuberculosis* infection. The 12 CA repeat microsatellite allele in the non coding region of the first intron is associated with a high level of *in vitro* cytokine production (Pravica et al., 1999). Recently, it has been reported that, polymorphism at position +874 is associated with risk of tuberculosis in different populations (Rossouw et al., 2003; Lopez-Maderuelo et al., 2003). Ansari et al. (2009) have reported that the ratio of two key cytokines (IFN-γ and IL10) show significant correlation with the severity spectrum of tuberculosis in Pakistani population. In this study frequency of cytokine gene polymorphisms linked to high and low responder phenotypes (IFNγ +874 T/A and IL10 -

1082 G/A) in tuberculosis patients was analyzed. These findings are consistent with the role of IL10 in reducing collateral tissue damage and the protective role of IFNγ in limiting disease in the lung.

A+874T polymorphism on the intron 1 of IFNγ gene, which is associated with the secretory capacity of IFNγ, was reported to be associated with the development of TB among Sicilians, South Africans, Hong Kong Chinese and Spanish, although this association was not found in Malawians54 and in other populations from Houston, West Africa, South India and China. A recent study of 77 TB patients from Japan revealed that the *IFNG* + 874 AA genotype were strongly and independently predictive of a lower likelihood of sputum conversion. Indeed, IL-12, a heterodimeric pro-inflammatory cytokine produced by monocytes, macrophages, DCs and B lymphocytes and SNP in the gene responsible in the expression of this subunit was first described by Hall et al. (2000). Several polymorphisms in promoter, introns and 3'UTR in the IL-12B gene have been reported to be associated with TB in various populations, with inconsistent results. Polymorphisms in the coding sequence of the IL-12 receptor b1 gene have been reported to be associated with TB in Moroccan and Japanese populations, but, again, not in Koreans. Reports indicate that, the *IL-12B* polymorphism is not correlated with susceptibility to tuberculosis in black and white North American populations. Four SNPs, 641 A-G, 684 C-T, 1094 T-C, and 1132 G-C causing three mis-sense variants (Q214R, M365T and G378R) and one synonymous substitution in the extracellular domain of the *IL-12Rβ1* genes have been detected. Investigators have reported that the association of R214-T365-R378 allele (allele 2) is over-expressed in Japanese tuberculosis patients with the homozygosis for R214 - T365 - R378 (the 2/2 allele) being significantly associated with tuberculosis.

8.8 IFNγR1 polymorphisms

Interferon-γ Receptor-1 plays a role in host immune response. Several SNPs in IFNγR1 have been studied in falciparum malaria cases and controls. The frequencies of interferon-γ (IFN-γ) receptor-1 (IFNγR1) promoter polymorphisms (G-611A, T-56C) in tuberculosis patients and controls were not significantly different. Because of these studied SNP affect transcription, the expression of the IFNγR1 gene does not confer susceptibility to disease in patients from Croatia (Bulat-Kardum et al., 2006). A significant association between the protective (CA) n polymorphism (22 repeats, 192 FA1), located in intron five of the IFNγR1 gene and GT promoter haplotype (-611; -56) that showed the strongest expression capacity have been reported. In addition to this cis relationship, the (CA) 22 allele was correlated in trans with an IFN-γ SNP (IFNγ Gþ2109A), which might affect the transcription of the IFNγ gene. These results suggest that a particular combination of IFNγ and IFNγR1 SNP (gene-gene) interaction might provide a better protection against tuberculosis in this population. Several families with Mendelian susceptibility to mycobacterial disease that has mutations in one of two subunits of the *IFN-γ* receptor gene (*IFN-γR1* and *IFN-γR2*) (Ottenhoff et al., 2002) have been discovered.

8.9 NOS2A polymorphisms

Nitric oxide (NO) act as is a free radical and second messenger and has been shown to be important in the development of several diseases, including tuberculosis. NO, produced by NOS2A, plays a major role in the pulmonary host-defense mechanism in response to infections, and is implicated in bacteriostatic as well as bactericidal processes. The cytokines like, TNF-α, IL-1β along with IFN-γ produced by T-cells can induce NO via action of NOS2A. It has been proposed that NO produced by tuberculosis-infected human macrophages and by epithelial cells is anti mycobacterial against *M. tuberculosis* (Liu et al., 2006). A report indicates that the alveolar macrophages from the lungs of patients with tuberculosis express NOS2A in potentially mycobactericidal amounts and this NOS2A can kill mycobacterium *in vitro* (Qidwai & Jamal, 2010). We have review the role of three SNPs (-954G/C, -1173C/T, -1659 A/T), one microsatellite repeat in promoter and one SNP in exon 16 of gene in several case control studies (Qidwai & Jamal, 2010). The promoter polymorphisms (-954G/C, -1173C/T, -1659 A/T) have been shown to increase NO synthesis (Hobbs et al., 2002). This region in the human gene is situated from -0.7 to -2.6 kb upstream of the transcription start and contains important DNA motifs for binding of NF-κB, activator protein 1, signal transducer, and activator of transcription protein 1, and NF-κB repressing factor (Coia et al., 2005). The -954G/C variant is believed to have originated as a consequence of selective pressure of *Plasmodium* in endemic area of Africa. The G allele has been shown to be absent from Caucasian populations (Kun et al., 1998) as well as from the Peruvian population (Martin et al., 1999). In Mexicans, the G allele was not associated with tuberculosis (Flores-Villanueva et al., 2005). Two chromosome 17 genes NOS2A and CCL2 plays a role in susceptibility to tuberculosis in South African population (Moller et al., 2009). Haplotype of two functional (rs9282799 and rs8078340) SNPs in the NOS2A promoter have been significantly associated with tuberculosis. Presence of T allele decreases the DNA-protein complex formation and decreases the duration of DNA-protein interaction, which leads to decrease NO production. The T allele of SNP rs8078340 is over represented in the patients. As NO possess potent antimicrobial effects, having ability to inhibit the growth of many infectious organisms *in vitro*, polymorphism in the promoter alters the level of NOS2A, decreasing the level of NO and thereby increases the susceptibility to tuberculosis.

A case-control association study of TB, patients and controls was performed in African-Americans and Caucasians by Velez et al. (2009). Thirty-nine SNPs were selected from the NOS2A gene, for single SNP, haplotype, and multilocus interaction analyses with other typed candidate genes. In African-Americans, ten NOS2A SNPs were associated with TB. The strongest associations were observed at rs2274894 and rs7215373. The strongest gene-gene interactions were observed between NOS2A rs2248814 and IFNGR1 rs1327474 and NOS2A rs944722 and IFNGR1 rs1327474. Three other SNPs in NOS2A interacted with TLR4 rs5030729 and five other NOS2A SNPs interacted with IFNGR1 rs1327474. No significant associations were observed in Caucasians. These results suggest that NOS2A variants may contribute to TB susceptibility, particularly in individuals of African descent, and may act synergistically with SNPs in TLR4 and IFNGR1.

9. Vitamin D receptor (VDR) polymorphisms

The investigation of the genetic polymorphisms of vitamin D, VDBP, TLR, NOS2A and IFN-γ genes and resistance or susceptibility to *M. tuberculosis* infection was summarized by (Preto, 2009). The vitamin D receptor (VDR) gene is one of the most important candidate genes that play role in susceptibility to tuberculosis. Polymorphisms that affects the activity of the receptor have profound impact. Genetic variants of the natural resistance-associated macrophage protein (*NRAMP1*) and vitamin D receptor (*VDR*) genes are associated with smear-positive pulmonary tuberculosis in Gambian populations (Bellamy et al., 1998a,b;

1999). Vitamin D receptor (VDR) genotypes have been shown to be associated with differential susceptibility or resistance to tuberculosis. The influence of FokI, BsmI, ApaI and TaqI variants of VDR gene on 1, 25(OH)(2) D(3) modulated granzyme A expression of cytotoxic lymphocytes induced by culture filtrate antigen (CFA) of Mycobacterium tuberculosis (Vidyarani et al., 2009). The ApaI aa genotype and bbaaTT extended genotype were associated with a significantly decreased percentage of granzyme A positive cells in normal healthy controls. The study suggest that 1, 25(OH)(2) D(3) suppresses granzyme A probably by down-regulating Th1 cytokine response. Gao et al. (2010), has reviewed published studies on VDR polymorphisms and TB susceptibility and quantitatively summarized associations of the polymorphisms (*Fok*I, *Taq*I, *Apa*I and *Bsm*I). Among Asians, the *Fok*I ff genotype showed a pronounced positive association, a significant inverse association was observed for the *Bsm*I bb genotype, and marginal significant associations were found for *Taq*I and *Apa*I polymorphisms. None of the studied polymorphisms have shown a significant association to TB among Africans or South Americans.

9.1 Vitamin D-binding protein

VDBP is a multifunctional, highly expressed, polymorphic serum protein encoded by Gc gene and is the major plasma carrier of vitamin D_3 and its metabolites and ensures that vitamin D is transported to the liver, $25(OH)_2D_3$ to the kidney, and 1, $25(OH)_2D_3$ to target cells and organs. A multi gene cluster at chromosome 4q11-q13 includes albumin, α-fetoprotein and *Gc* gene. Variations in exon 11 of the *Gc* gene at codons 416 and 420 give rise to electrophoretic variants of VDBP, called Gc1 fast (Gc1F), Gc1 slow (Gc1S) and Gc2 differing by amino-acid sequence, as well as by attached polysaccharides. Combinations of the three VDBP or Gc variants result in six common circulating phenotypes: Gc1F/Gc1F, Gc1F/Gc1S, Gc1S/Gc1S, Gc1F/Gc2, Gc1S/Gc2, and Gc2/Gc2 (23). *DBP* polymorphism (Gc phenotype) is related to the VDBP concentration and vitamin D status (Lauridsen et al., 2005). The authors showed a strong correlation between higher, intermediate and lower circulating levels of $25(OH)_2D_3$ and $1,25(OH)_2D_3$ with Gc1-1, Gc1-2 and Gc2-2 phenotypes, respectively, in Danish Caucasian postmenopausal women population. Variations in this property could affect the functioning of the immune system, as *DBP* knockout mice exhibited an impaired immune response to bacterial infections (White & Cook, 2000). A role of *DBP* polymorphism in autoimmune diabetes mellitus and infectious disease in Polynesia and Japan (Hirai et al., 2000) has been suggested. No differences in *DBP* phenotype were seen among patients and the control group. In that study, frequency of Gc2 in tuberculosis patients was slightly but not significantly higher than in the control group and this elevation was at the expense of both Gc1F and Gc1S alleles.

9.2 The Toll-like receptors

The TLRs represent a group of single-pass transmembrane receptors, are expressed on innate immune cells and works as sensors for pathogen-derived molecules, and play a role in host-pathogen interaction (Aderem et al., 2000). TNF-α and NO is induced mostly by macrophages soon after innate recognition of mycobacteria through TLRs (Underhill et al., 1999). The role of TLR in resistance to *M. tuberculosis* was suggested initially by the fact that MyD88-deficient mice are more susceptible to *M. tuberculosis* infection and by the observation that TRL2/TLR1 reduced the viability of intracellular *M. tuberculosis* in human monocytes and macrophages, but not in monocyte-derived DCs (Liu et al., 2006). They have also reported that TLR induces up-regulation of the *VDR*, 1α-vitamin D hydroxylase (enzyme that converts inactive to active vitamin D), and *CYP27B1* gene expression in monocytes and macrophages.

The human TLR2 gene is located on chromosome 4q32 and is composed of 2 non-coding exons and 1coding exon (Haehnel et al., 2002). In TLR2 gene, 89 SNPs have been reported, (26 in the 5'-untranslated region, 17 in the 3'-untranslated region, 29 located in intronic parts of the gene, and 17 modify bases of the third exon of TLR2). Six non-synonymous SNPs of the *TLR2* gene change amino acids in the cytosolic part of this receptor. Out of which, only two have been linked to reducing NF-κB activation and increasing risk of infection. The first SNP changes of C to T replacing arginine (Arg; R) with tryptophan (Trp, W) at position 677, abolishing the binding with MyD88 with TLR2. This specific polymorphism located within the *bb* loop of *TLR2* (Arg677Trp) abolishes activation of NF-κB in response to *M. tuberculosis*, resulting in decreased IL-12 serum level production by 677W carriers. The second *TLR2* SNP changes G to A, which substitutes an arginine for glutamine at position 753. The *TLR2* 753Q seems to be associated with an increased risk of developing tuberculosis for carriers the AA and AG genotypes (Ogus et al., 2004). Thuong et al. (2007) described a strong association of SNP T597C *TLR2* with susceptibility to military tuberculosis patients from Vietnam. Further association was described among Koreans regarding the microsatellite polymorphisms in intron II or *TLR2* (Yim et al., 2006). In addition, *TLR1* polymorphism in a non-synonymous region (I602S) could be associated with TLR1/2 heterodimer binding sites to mycobacterial lipopeptide, since individuals with 602II genotype produced substantially more IL-6 than those with the 602SS variant. Currently, the polymorphism in *TLR2* might be an important risk factor for disease progression. The G to A (Arg753Gln) polymorphism at position 2258 in exon 3 and the guanine-thymine (GT) microsatellite repeat polymorphism (100 bp upstream of the translational start site) in intron 2, have been associated with susceptibility to clinical tuberculosis (TB) disease in Turkish and Korean patients, respectively (Ogus et al., 2004; Yim et al., 2006). TLR2 promoter region, namely, -16934 A>T and -196 to -174 insertion (Ins) >deletion (Del), polymorphisms have been associated with asthma and gastric cancer, respectively (Eder et al., 2004; Tahara et al., 2007).

Patients with pulmonary TB and healthy controls, were examined for TLR2 polymorphisms over locus -100 (microsatellite guanine-thymine repeats), -16934 (T>A), -15607 (A>G), -196 to -174 (insertion>deletion), and 1350 (T>C) (Chen et al., 2010). An association exists between the haplotype [A-G-(insertion)-T] and susceptibility to pulmonary tuberculosis. Patients with systemic symptoms of tuberculosis had a lower -196 to -174 deletion/deletion genotype frequency than those without systemic symptoms. TB patients with the deletion/deletion genotype had higher blood NK cell counts than those carrying the insertion allele whereas patients with pleuritis had a higher 1350 CC genotype frequency than those without pleuritis. Patients of tuberculosis with the 1350 CC genotype had higher blood NK cell counts than those carrying the T allele. TB patients carrying homozygous short alleles for GT repeats had higher blood NK cell counts than those carrying one or no short allele. Thus, an association between the specific TLR2 haplotype and susceptibility to pulmonary TB have been reported. In patients with pulmonary TB, both the -196 to -174 Del/ Del and 1350 CC genotypes were associated with an increased blood absolute NK cell counts.

9.3 TLR4 polymorphism

Toll-like receptor (TLR) 4 has been described to play a main role in the innate immunity against TB. The association between two particular SNPs in human TLR4 (Asp299Gly and Thr399Ile) and active TB has been studied in non-HIV Africans with contradictory results. However, studies focusing on the effect of these TLR4 SNPs in active TB within a Caucasian HIV population are lacking. The association between TLR4 Asp299Gly and Thr399Ile SNPs and active TB, in Caucasian Mediterranean HIV-infected individuals were analyzed by Ildefonso et al. (2010). Asp299Gly were independently associated with active TB and inversely with latent TB prophylaxis. An independent association between TLR4 Asp299Gly SNP and active TB in Caucasian Mediterranean HIV-infected patients was detected.

9.4 Toll-like receptor 8 polymorphisms

Davila et al. (2008) studied TB association and expression of 18 genes involved in the Toll-like receptor (TLR) pathways. The polymorphisms in pulmonary TB patients and controls from Indonesia was genotyped. The four polymorphisms in the TLR8 gene on chromosome X showed evidence of association with TB susceptibility in males, including a non-synonymous polymorphism rs3764880 (Met1Val).They have also genotyped these four TLR8 polymorphisms in an independent collection of pulmonary TB patients and controls from Russia and again found evidence of association in males (for rs3764880). A marked increase in TLR8 protein expression was also observed directly in differentiated macrophages upon infection with *M. bovis*, bacille Calmette-Gue´rin (BCG). A role for the TLR8 gene in susceptibility to pulmonary TB across different populations have been reported. Polymorphisms (1805 G/T in TLR1, 2258 A/G in TLR2, -857 C/T and -863 A/C in TNF-α and -819 C/T in IL-10) was genotyped in tuberculosis patients and controls by Mai Juan et al. 2010. Multivariate logistic regression analysis revealed that the TT genotype of -857 C/T in TNF-α gene was significantly associated with lower risk of PTB, in comparison with other genotypes. The genetic variant of -863 A/C in TNF-α gene was associated with susceptibility to PTB and clinical severity of disease. The results of the study suggest that the variants in TNF-α gene were associated with susceptibility to PTB and clinical severity of disease, while no significant association have been reported for TLRs and IL-10 genes polymorphisms and tuberculosis.

9.5 PTPN22 gene polymorphism

The PTPN22 gene encodes the lymphoid tyrosine phosphatase that has an important regulatory effect on T- and B-cell activation in immune response. Lamsyah et al. (2009) reported an association of PTPN22 gene functional variants with development of pulmonary tuberculosis in Moroccan population. The two missense polymorphisms of the PTPN22 gene (R620W and R263Q) and susceptibility to TB in the Moroccan population was investigated. A statistically significant difference exists in the distribution of the PTPN22 1885T allele between pulmonary TB patients and healthy controls. In case of PTPN22 R263Q (G788A) SNP, there is an increase of 788A allele frequencies in TB patients compared with those in healthy individuals. These results suggest that PTPN22 gene variants may affect susceptibility to TB in the Moroccan population.

9.6 Human V-ATPase polymorphism

Capparelli et al. (2009) tested for polymorphisms in the intron 15 and the 5′-untranslated region of the gene coding for the a3 isoform of the human ATPase gene in pulmonary tuberculosis patients and controls. Alleles (two at each site) segregated in the form of four haplotype pairs. The double heterozygous patients were protected against tuberculosis and the double homozygous patients were susceptible to the disease.

9.7 MIF, FCGR2A, and FCGR3A gene polymorphisms

The polymorphisms of macrophage migration inhibitory factor (MIF), Fcg receptors CD16A (FCGR3A) and CD32A (FCGR2A) genes and susceptibility to pulmonary tuberculosis (PTB) in the Moroccan population, was analyzed (Sadki et al., 2010). The genotyping for MIF-173 (G/C) (rs755622), FCGR2A-131 H/R (rs1801274), and FCGR3A-158V/F (rs396991) have been done. A statistically significant increase of the MIF -173CC homozygote genotype and MIF -173*C allele frequencies in PTB patients compared with healthy controls was detected. In contrast, no association was observed between FCGR2A-131H/R and FCGR3A-158V/F polymorphisms and tuberculosis disease. The finding suggests that MIF -173*C variant may play an important role in the development of active tuberculosis.

9.8 CCR2, MCP-1, SDF-1a & DC-SIGN gene polymorphisms

Investigation showed that chemokine, chemokine receptor and DC-SIGN gene polymorphisms were associated with susceptibility/resistance to HIV and HIV-TB in south India (Alagarasu et al., 2009). CCR2 V64I (G/A), monocyte chemoattractant protein-1 (MCP-1) -2518 A/G, stromal cell derived factor-1alpha; (SDF-1alpha) 3'UTR G/A and DC-SIGN gene polymorphisms were studied in HIV-1 infected patients without TB, with pulmonary TB (PTB) and extrapulmonary TB, PTB patients without HIV and healthy controls. No significant difference was detected in the genotype frequencies of CCR2 V64I, MCP-1 -2518 and DC-SIGN polymorphisms between the study groups. A significantly increased frequency of GG genotype of SDF-1alpha polymorphism was observed among positive for HIV and PTB patients compared to healthy controls. The GG genotype of SDF-1alpha 3'UTR polymorphism may be associated with susceptibility to PTB in HIV-1 infected patients. Raghavan et al. (2009) have detected the HLA-DR2 subtypes and the possible HLA-A/-B/-DRB1 haplotype combinations that are associated with susceptibility or resistance to HIV and HIV with pulmonary tuberculosis (HIV^+PTB^+). Overrepresentation of HLA-DRB1*1501 in HIV^+PTB^- patients and DRB1*1502 in HIV^+PTB^+ patients as compared to healthy controls was detected. An increased frequency of HLA-A2-DRB1*1501 haplotype in HIV^+PTB^- patients and HLA-A2-DRB1*1502 among HIV^+PTB^+ patients compared to healthy controls have been identified. The study suggests that HLA-A2-DRB1*1501 haplotype may be associated with HIV infection while HLA-A2-DRB1*1502 haplotype might be associated with susceptibility to PTB in HIV patients. HLA-B40-DRB1*1501 and HLA-B40-DRB1*04 haplotypes may be associated with susceptibility to HIV infection and to PTB in HIV patients (Raghvan et al., 2009).

9.9 TIRAP polymorphisms and susceptibility to childhood TB

The adaptor protein TIRAP mediates downstream signaling of TLR2 and TLR 4. TIRAP gene polymorphisms have been associated with susceptibility and resistance to tuberculosis

(TB) in adults in South Africa. Dissanayeke et al. (2009), identified 13 SNPs, and found significant differences in frequency of the variants between the two ethnic groups. The frequency of individual polymorphisms or combinations did not vary between TB cases and controls in either cohort. The 558C→T polymorphism previously associated with TB meningitis (TBM) in a Vietnamese population was found to be associated with TBM in the mixed ancestry group. The study suggests that, polymorphisms in TIRAP do not appear to be involved in childhood TB susceptibility in South Africa.

10. Mannose-binding lectin (MBL) polymorphisms

Mannose-binding lectin (MBL) is considered an important component of innate immunity. Four functional MBL2 alterations in codons 52, 54, 57 and in the promoter at position c.1-290 are correlated with significantly lowered MBL serum levels. These variants have been associated with susceptibility to a variety of infectious agents as well as with various immunologic disorders. The gene encoding MBL is located on chromosome 10 and is designated as MBL2. MBL elicits complement activation by binding to mannose- and N-acetylglucosamine sugar groups on various microorganisms. Variations in the serum MBL levels are mainly due to the presence of three common point mutations in exon1 of MBL2 gene at the codons 52 (rs5030737), 54 (rs1800451) and 57 (rs1800450). MBL deficiency is an example of evolutionary selection, as MBL deficiency reduces the capacity of mycobacteria to invade macrophages, thus provide resistance to TB (Garred et al., 1994). Variations at codons 52, 54 and 57 lead to low or near absent serum MBL. A study from South African suggested that hetrozygotes for MBL54 have protection against tuberculosis meningitis (Hoal-Van Helden et al., 1999). TB patients as compared to controls have an increased genotype frequencies for mutant homozygotes at codons 52, 54 and 57in South Indians but no such association have been reported in China, Poland, Turkey, Malawi, Tanzania and Gambia.

10.1 Complement receptor polymorphisms

The complement receptor-1(CR1) present on the surface of the macrophages is associated with phagocytosis of various microorganisms, including *M. tuberculosis*. Homozygotes in one of five CR1polymorphisms (Q1022H) are associated with increased TB risk in Malawi.

10.2 Purinergic P2X7 receptor

Purinergic P2X7 receptors are cationic channels present on the cells in the blood and immune systems. A polymorphism with a 1513 A-C (rs3751143) that replaces the glutamic acid at residue 496 by alanine, was not associated with pulmonary TB in Gambia (Li et al., 2002). No link of 1513 SNP with pulmonary TB was found in Southeast Asian refugees from Australia but a strong association existed between the C polymorphism and extrapulmonary TB (Fernando et al., 2006).

10.3 Association analysis of susceptibility region on chromosome 5q31 for tuberculosis

In the Asian population the chromosome 5q23.2–31.3 has been identified as a region with linkage to tuberculosis (Ridruechai et al., 2010). A putative tuberculosis susceptibility locus was investigated, in a family-based association test between the dense SNP markers within chromosome 5q31 and tuberculosis in Thai trio families. Seventy-five SNPs located within candidate genes covering SLC22A4, SLC22A5, IRF1, IL5, RAD50, IL13, IL4, KIF3A and SEPT8 were genotyped. Association analysis revealed the most significant association with tuberculosis in haplotypes comprising SNPs rs274559, rs274554, and rs274553 of SLC22A5 gene, which remained significant after multiple testing corrections. The two haplotypes within the SLC22A4 and KIF3A region were associated with tuberculosis. Haplotypes of SLC22A5 were significantly associated with the expression levels of RAD50 and IL13. The variants carried by the haplotypes of SLC22A4, SLC22A5, and KIF3A region potentially contribute to tuberculosis susceptibility among the Thai population.

10.4 Genome-wide analysis of genetic susceptibility to tuberculosis

Bellamy et al. (1998b), performed genome-wide analysis of genetic susceptibility to tuberculosis in Africans. A two-stage genome-wide linkage study to search for regions of the human genome containing tuberculosis-susceptibility genes was carried out. Sibpair families that contain two full siblings, affected by clinical tuberculosis were used. 299 highly informative genetic markers, spanning the entire human genome, were typed in 92 sibpairs ffrom Gambia and South Africa in the first round. To identify whether any of these regions contained a potential tuberculosis-susceptibility gene, 22 markers from these regions were genotyped in a second set of 81 sibpairs from the same countries. Markers on chromosomes 15q and Xq showed suggestive evidence of linkage to tuberculosis. These results indicate that genome-wide linkage analysis can contribute to the mapping and identification of major genes for multifactorial infectious diseases of humans. Thye et al. (2009) have identified a genetic variant, which increases susceptibility to tuberculosis (TB) in African populations using genome-wide association (GWA) study. The studies involve analysing hundreds of thousands of genetic markers across the human genomes in search of variants found in patients but not in healthy controls.

Control of the TB epidemic requires more than developing new drugs. The diagnostic and therapeutic facilities of health care centers in developing countries must be improved, and the socioeconomic status and general welfare of patients (including nutritional and HIV status) should be addressed to help eradicate TB. The development of tuberculosis or other mycobacterial diseases is the result of a complex interaction between the host and pathogen influenced by environmental factors. Numerous host genes are likely to be involved in this process. A variety of study methods, have contributed to substantial progress in advancing our understanding of genetic susceptibility to tuberculosis.

11. References

Aderem, A. & Ulevitch, R.J. (2000) Toll-like receptors in the induction of the innate immune response. Nature, 406, 782-787.

Alagarasu, K., Selvaraj, P., Swaminathan, S., Narendran, G. & Narayanan, P. R. (2009). 5' regulatory and 3' untranslated region polymorphisms of vitamin D receptor gene in south Indian HIV and HIV-TB patients. *J. Clin. Immunol.* 29, 196–204.

Aliberti, J., Serhan, C. & Sher, A. (2002). Parasite-induced lipoxin A4 is an endogenous regulator of IL-12 production and immunopathology in *Toxoplasma gondii* infection. *J. Exp. Med,* 196,1253–1262.

Alvarez, C.P., Lasala, F., Carrillo, J., Muñiz, O., Corbi, A.L. & Delgado, R. (2002). C-type lectins DC-SIGN and L-SIGN mediate cellular entry by Ebola virus in cis and in trans. *J. Virol,* 76, 6841–6844.

Ansari, A., Talat, N., Jamil, B., Hasan, Z., Razzaki, T., Dawood, G. & Hussain R. (2009). Cytokine Gene Polymorphisms across Tuberculosis Clinical Spectrum in Pakistani Patients. *PLos One,* 4,1-7.

Ates, O., Musellim, B., Ongen, G. & Topal-Sarikaya, A. (2008). Interleukin-10 and tumor necrosis factor-alpha gene polymorphisms in tuberculosis. *J. Clin. Immunol,* 28, 232-236.

Babb, C., Keet, E.H., Van Helden, P.D. & Hoal, E.G. (2007). SP110 polymorphisms are not associated with pulmonary tuberculosis in a South African population. *Hum. Genet,* 121,521-522.

Bailie, M.B., Standiford, T.J., Laichalk, L.L., Coffey, M.J., Strieter, R. & Peters-Golden, M. (1996). Leukotriene-deficient mice manifest enhanced lethality from Klebsiella pneumoniae in association with decreased alveolar macrophage phagocytic and bactericidal activities. *J. Immunol,* 157, 5221–5224.

Bandeira-Melo, C., Bozza, P.T., Diaz, B.L., Cordeiro, R.S., Jose, P.J., Martins, M.A. & Serhan, C.N. (2000) Cutting edge: lipoxin (LX) A4 and aspirin-triggered 15-epi-LXA4 block allergen-induced eosinophil trafficking. *J. Immunol.* 164, 2267–2271.

Barreiro, L.B., Neyrolles, O., Babb, C.L. & et al. (2006). Promoter variation in the DC-SIGN-encoding gene CD209 is associated with tuberculosis. PLoS Med, 3:e20. *31.*

Bellamy, R., Ruwende, C., Corrah, T., McAdam, K.P., Whittle, H.C. & Hill, A.V. (1998b). Variations in the NRAMP1 gene and susceptibility to tuberculosis in West Africans. *N. Engl. J. Med,* 338, 640-644.

Bellamy, R., Ruwende, C., Corrah, T., McAdam, K.P., Whittle, H.C. & Hill, A.V. (1998a). Assessment of the interleukin 1 gene cluster and other candidate gene polymorphisms in host susceptibility to tuberculosis. *Tuberi. Lung Dis,* 79, 83–89.

Bellamy, R., Ruwende, C., Corrah, T., McAdam, K.P., Thursz, M., Whittle, H.C. & Hill, A.V. (1999). Tuberculosis and chronic hepatitis B virus infection in Africans and variation in the vitamin D receptor gene. J. Infect. Dis, 179, 721–724.

Bergmann, J.S., Yuoh, G., Fish, G. & Woods, G.L. (1999). Clinical evaluation of the enhanced Gen-Probe amplified Mycobacterium tuberculosis direct test for rapid diagnosis of tuberculosis in prison inmates. *J. Clin. Microbiol,* 37, 1419–1425.

Berrington, W.R. & Hawn, T.R. (2007). Mycobacterium tuberculosis, macrophages, and the innate immune response: does common variation matter? *Immunol. Rev,* 219, 167–186.

Boogaard, J., Kibiki, G.S., Kisanga, E.R. & *et. al.* (2009). New Drugs against Tuberculosis: Problems, Progress, and Evaluation of Agents in Clinical Development. Antimicrobial agents and chemotherapy, pp. 849–862

Bulat-Kardum, L., Etokebe, G.E., Knezevic, J. & et al. (2006). Interferon-g Receptor-1 Gene Promoter Polymorphisms (G-611A; T-56C) and Susceptibility to Tuberculosis. *Scand. J. of Immuno,* 63, 142–150.

Capparelli, R., Palumbo, D., Iannaccone, M. & Iannelli, D. (2009). Human V-ATPase gene can protect or predispose the host to pulmonary tuberculosis. *Genes Immun,* 10, 641-646.

Chen, Y.C., Hsiao, C.C., Chen, C.J. & et al. (2010). Toll-like receptor 2 gene polymorphisms, pulmonary tuberculosis, and natural killer cell counts. *BMC Medical Genetics,* 11:17.

Coia, V., Jüliger, S., Mordmüller, B. & et al. (2005). Analysis of polymorphic sites in the promoter of the nitric oxide synthase 2 gene. *Biochem. Biophys. Res. Commun,* 335, 1123-1131.

Comstock, G.W. (1978). Tuberculosis in twins: a re-analysis of the Prophit survey. *Am. Rev. Respir. Dis,* 117, 621-624.

Cooke, G.S., Campbell, S.J., Bennett, S., Lienhardt, C., McAdam, K.P. & et al. (2008). Mapping of a Novel Susceptibility Locus Suggests a Role for MC3R and CTSZ in Human Tuberculosis. *Am. J. Respir. Crit. Care Med,* 178, 203–207.

Corbett, E.L., Watt, C.J., Walker, N. & et al. (2003). The growing burden of tuberculosis: global trends and interactions with the HIV epidemic. *Arch. Intern. Med,* 163: 1009–1021.

Correa, P.A., Gomez, L.M., Cadena, J. & Anaya, J.M. (2005). Autoimmunity and tuberculosis. Opposite association with TNF polymorphism. *J. Rheumatol,* 32, 219-224.

Davila, S., Hibberd, M.L., Hari Dass, R. & et al. (2008). Genetic Association and Expression Studies Indicate a Role of Toll-Like Receptor 8 in Pulmonary Tuberculosis. *PLoS Genet,* 4(10): e1000218.

Dissanayeke, S.R., Levin, S., Pienaar, S., Wood, K., Eley, B., Beatty, D., Henderson, H., Anderson, S. & Levin, M. (2009). Variation in TIRAP is not associated with susceptibility to childhood TB but may determine susceptibility to TBM in some ethnic groups. *PLoS One,* 4(8): e6698.

Eder, W., Klimecki, W., Yu, L., von Mutius, E., Riedler, J., Braun-Fahrländer, C., Nowak, D. & Martinez FD (2004). ALEX Study Team. Toll-like receptor 2 as a major gene for asthma in children of European farmers. *J. Allergy Clin. Immunol,* 113, 482-488.

Fernando, S.L. & Britton, W.J. (2006). Genetic susceptibility to mycobacterial disease in humans. Immunol. *Cell Biol,* 84, 125-137.

Flores-Villanueva, P.O., Ruiz-Morales, J.A., Song, C.H., et al. (2005). Functional promoter polymorphism in monocytchemo attractant protein-1 is associated with increased susceptibility to pulmonary tuberculosis. *J. Exp. Med,* 202, 1649-1658.

Gao, L., Tao, Y., Zhang, L. & Jin, Q. (2010). Vitamin D receptor genetic polymorphisms and tuberculosis: updated systematic review and meta-analysis. The Int. J. Tuberc. and Lung Dis, 14, 15-23.

Garred, P., Harboe, M., Oettinger, T. & et al. (1994). Dual role of mannan binding protein in infections: another case of heterosis? *Eur. J.Immunogenet,* 21, 125–131.

Gordon, S. (2002). Pattern recognition receptors doubling up for the innate immune response. *Cell,* 111, 927–930.

Guwatudde, D., Zalwango, S., Kamya, M.R., Debanne, S.M., Diaz, M.I. & et al. (2003). Burden of tuberculosis in Kampala, Uganda. Bull. *World Health Organ,* 81, 799–805.

Hachicha, M., Pouliot, M., Petasis, N.A. & Serhan, C.N. (1999). Lipoxin (LX) A4, and aspirin-triggered 15-epi-LXA4 inhibit tumor necrosis factor 1 alpha-initiated neutrophil responses and trafficking: regulators of a cytokine-chemokine axis. *J. Exp. Med,* 189, 1923–1930.

Haehnel, V., Schwarzfischer, L., Fenton, M.J. & Rehli, M. (2002). Transcriptional regulation of the human toll-like receptor 2 gene in monocytes and macrophages. J. Immunol, 168, 5629-5637.

Hanna, S. & James, M. M. (2001). Molecular Diagnosis of Mycobacteria. *Clinical Chem,* 47, 809–814.

Hirai, M., Suzuki, S., Hinokio, Y., Hirai, A., Chiba, M., Akai, H., Suzuki, C. & Toyota, T. (2000). Variations in vitamin D-binding protein (group-specific component protein) are associated with fasting plasma insulin levels in Japanese with normal glucose tolerance. *J. Clin. Endocrinol. Metab,* 85, 1951-1953.

Hoal-Van Helden, E.G., Epstein, J., Victor, T.C. & et al. (1999). Mannose binding protein B allele confers protection against tuberculosis meningitis. *Pediatr. Res,* 45, 459–464.

Hobbs, M.R., Udhayakumar, V., Levesque, M.C., Booth, J., Roberts, J.M. & Tkachuk, A.N. (2002). A new NOS2 promoter polymorphism associated with increased nitric oxide production and protection from severe malaria in Tanzanian and Kenyan children. *Lancet,* 360, 1468-1475.

Ildefonso, P., Manuel, L., Miguel, G., Yolanda, P.M., Maria, E.S. & Sarabia, N.S. (2010). The TLR4 ASP299GLY Polymorphism is a Risk Factor for Active Tuberculosis in Caucasian HIV-Infected Patients. *Cur. HIV Res,* 8, 253-258.

Jamieson, S., Miller, E., Black, G., Peacock, C., Cordell, H. & et al. (2004). Evidence for a cluster of genes on chromosome 17q11-q21 controlling susceptibility to tuberculosis and leprosy in Brazilians. Genes and Immunity, 5, 46–57.

Kwoh, D.Y., Davis, G.R., Whitefield, K.M., Chapelle, H.L., DiMichele, L.J., Gingeras, T.R. (1989). Transcription-based amplification system and detection of amplified human immunodeficiency virus type 1 with a bead-based sandwich hybridization format. *Proc. Natl. Acad. Sci. U S A,* 86,1173–1177.

Krishnamurthy, M.S. (2001). Problems in estimating the burden of pulmonary tuberculosis in India: a review C.N. Paramasivan & P. Venkataraman (2003). Drug resistance in tuberculosis in India pp 377-386

Kun, J.F., Mordmuller, B., Lell, B., Lehman, L.G., Luckner, D. & Kremsner, P.G. (1998). Polymorphism in promoter region of inducible nitric oxide synthase gene and protection against malaria. *Lanc,* 351, 265-266.

Lamsyah, H., Rueda, B., Baassi, L., Elaouad, R., Bottini, N., Sadki, K. & Martin, J. (2009). Association of PTPN22 gene functional variants with development of pulmonary tuberculosis in Moroccan population. *Tissue Antigens,* 74, 228-232.

Lauridsen, A.L., Vestergaard, P., Hermann, A.P., et al. (2005). Plasma concentrations of 25-hydroxy-vitamin D and 1,25-dihydroxy-vitamin D are related to the phenotype of Gc (vitamin D-binding protein): a cross-sectional study on 595 early postmenopausal women. *Calcif. Tissue Int,* 77, 15-22.

Lienhardt, C., Bennett, S., Del Prete, G., et al. (2002). Investigation of Environmental and Host-related Risk Factors for Tuberculosis in Africa. I. Methodological Aspects of a Combined Design. American Journal of Epidemiology, 155, 1066-1073.

Li, C.M., Campbell, S.J., Kumararatne, D.S., et al. (2002). Association of a polymorphism in the P2X7 gene with tuberculosis in a Gambian population. *J. Infect. Dis.* 186, 1458-1462.

Liu, P.T., Stenger, S., Li, H., et al. (2006). Toll-like receptor triggering of a vitamin D-mediated human antimicrobial response. Science, 311, 1770-1773.

Liu, W., Zhang, F., Xin, Z.T., et al. (2006). Sequence variations in the MBL gene and their relationship to pulmonary tuberculosis in the Chinese Han population. *Int. J. Tuberc. Lung Dis.* 10, 1098–1103.

Lopez-Maderuelo, D., Arnalich, F., Serantes, R., Gonzalez, A., Codoceo, R., Madero, R., Vazquez, J.J. & Montiel, C. (2003). Interferon gamma and interleukin-10 gene polymorphisms in pulmonary tuberculosis. Am. J. Respir. Crit. Care Med, 167, 970–975.

Luoni, G., Verra, F., Arca, B., et al. (2001). Antimalarial antibody levels and IL4 polymorphism in the Fulani of West Africa. *Genes Immun*, 2, 411–414.

Mancuso, P., Nana-Sinkam, P., Peters-Golden, M. (2001). Leukotriene B4 augments neutrophil phagocytosis of Klebsiella pneumoniae. *Infect. Immun*, 69, 2011–2016.

Martin, J., Calzada, J.E., Nieto, A. (1999). Inducible nitric oxide synthase (NOS2) gene polymorphism and parasitic diseases. Lanc, 353: 72.

Martin, M.P., Lederman, M.M., Hutcheson, H.B. & et al. (2004). Association of DC-SIGN promoter polymorphism with increased risk for parenteral, but not mucosal, acquisition of human immunodeficiency virus type 1 infection. *J. Virol*, 78,14053–14056.

Miller, E., Jamieson, S., Joberty, C., Fakiola, M., Hudson, D., et al. (2004). Genome wide scans for leprosy and tuberculosis susceptibility genes in Brazilians. *Genes Immun,* 5, 63–67.

Mohan, V.P., Scanga, C.A., Yu, K. et al. (2001). Effects of tumor necrosis factor alpha on host immune response in chronic persistent tuberculosis: possible role for limiting pathology. *Infect. Immun,* 69, 1847-1855.

Moller, M., Nebel, A., Valentonyte, R., van Helden, P.D., Schreiber, S., Hoal, E.G. (2009). Investigation of chromosome 17 candidate genes in susceptibility to TB in a South African population. *Tuberculosis*, 89,189-194.

Moller, M., Nebel, A., Kwiatkowski, R., Van Helden, P.D., Hoal, E.G. & Schreiber, S. (2007). Host susceptibility to tuberculosis: CARD15 polymorphisms in a South African population. *Human and Cellular Probes*, 21, 148-151.

Moller, M., Nebel, A., Van Helden, P.D., Schreiber, S. & Hoal, E.G. (2010). Analysis of eight genes modulating interferon gamma and human genetic susceptibility to tuberculosis: a case-control association study. *BMC Infect. Dis,* 10: 154.

Naslednikova, I.O., Urazova, O.I., Voronkova, O.V., et al. (2009). Allelic polymorphism of cytokine genes during pulmonary tuberculosis. *Bull. Exp. Biol. Med.* 148, 175–180.

Nedwin, G.E., Naylor, S.L., Sakaguchi, A.Y. et al. (1985). Human lymphotoxin and tumor necrosis factor genes: structure, homology and chromosomal localization. Nucleic Acids Res, 13, 6361-6373.

Nicholson, S., Bonecini-Almeida, M.G., Lapa de Silva, J.R., Nathan, C., Xie, Q.W. (1996). Mumford R Inducible nitric oxide synthase in pulmonary alveolar macrophages from patients with tuberculosis. J. Exp. Med, 183, 2293-2302.

Ogus, A.C., Yoldas, B., Ozdemir, T., et al. (2004). The Arg753Gln polymorphism of the human toll-like receptor 2 gene in tuberculosis disease. *Eur. Respir. J*, 23, 219-223.

Ottenhoff, T.H., Verreck, F.A., Lichtenauer-Kaligis, E.G., Hoeve, M.A., Sanal, O., van Dissel, J.T. (2002). Genetics, cytokines and human infectious disease: lessons from weakly pathogenic mycobacteria and salmonellae. *Nat. Genet*, 32, 97-105.

Parkinson, J.F. (2006). Lipoxin and synthetic lipoxin analogs: an overview of anti-inflammatory functions and new concepts in immunomodulation. *Inflamm. Aller. Drug Tar.* 5, 91–106.

Pesut, D.P. (2009). Marinkovic Lung cancer and pulmonary tuberculosis –a comparative population-genetic study. British J. Med. Genetics, 12/2, 45-52.

Pravica, V., Asderakis, A., Perrey, C., Hajeer, A., Sinnott, P.J. & Hutchinson, I.V. (1999). In vitro production of IFN-gamma correlates with CA repeat polymorphism in the human IFN-gamma gene. Eur. J. Immunogenet, 26, 1-3.

Preto, R. (2009). Genetic polymorphisms in vitamin D receptor, vitamin D-binding protein, Toll-like receptor 2, nitric oxide synthase 2, and interferon-γ genes and its association with susceptibility to tuberculosis. Braz. J. Med. Biol. Res, 42, 312-322.

Qidwai, T. & Jamal, F. (2010). Inducible Nitric Oxide Synthase (iNOS) Gene Polymorphism and Disease Prevalence. Scandinavian Journal of Immunology, 72, 375–387.

Raghavan, S., Selvaraj, P., Swaminathan, S., Alagarasu, K., Narendran, G. & Narayanan, P.R. (2009). Haplotype analysis of HLA-A, -B antigens and -DRB1 alleles in south Indian HIV-1-infected patients with and without pulmonary tuberculosis. Int. J. Immunog, 36, 129–133.

Raviglione, M., Snider, D. & Kochi, A. (1995). Global epidemiology of tuberculosis: Morbidity and mortality of a worldwide epidemic. JAMA, 273, 220– 226.

Ridruechai, C., Mahasirimongkol, S., Phromjai, J. & et al. (2010). Association analysis of susceptibility candidate region on chromosome 5q31 for tuberculosis Genes and Immunity, 11, 416-422.

Rosenwasser, LJ, Klemm DJ, Dresback JK, Inamura H, Mascali JJ, Klinnert M. & Borish L. (1995). Promoter polymorphisms in the chromosome 5 gene cluster in asthma and atopy. Clin. Exp. Allergy, 25, 74–78.

Rossouw, M., Nel, H.J., Cooke, G.S., Van Helden, P.D. & Hoal, E.G. (2003). Association between tuberculosis, and a polymorphic NFkappaB binding site in the interferon gamma gene. *Lancet*, 361,1871-1872.

Sadki, K,, Lamsyah, H., Rueda, B., Akil, E., Sadak, A., Martin, J., El Aouad, R. (2010). Analysis of MIF, FCGR2A and FCGR3A gene polymorphisms with susceptibility to pulmonary tuberculosis in Moroccan population. J. Gent. and Geno, 37, 257-264.

Sakuntabhai, A., Turbpaiboon, C., Casademont, I. & et al. (2005). A variant in the CD209 promoter is associated with severity of dengue disease. Nat. Genet, 37, 507–513.

Schurr, E. (2007). Is susceptibility to tuberculosis acquired or inherited? *J. Intern. Med,* 261,106-111.

Selvaraj, P., Alagarasu, K., Harishankar, M. & et al. (2008). Cytokine gene polymorphisms and cytokine levels in pulmonary tuberculosis. *Cytokine,* 43, 26–33.

Sharma, S., Ghosh, B., Sharma, S.K. (2008). Association of TNF polymorphisms with sarcoidosis, its prognosis and tumour necrosis factor (TNF)-alpha levels in Asian Indians. *Clin. Exp. Immunol,* 151, 251-259.

Sharma, S., Rathored, J., Ghosh, B. & et al. (2010). Genetic polymorphisms in *TNF* genes and tuberculosis in North Indians. BMC Infectious Diseases, 10,165.

Soilleux, E.J., Barten, R., Trowsdale, J. (2000). DC-SIGN; a related gene, DC-SIGNR; and CD23 form a cluster on 19p13. J. Immunol, 165, 2937–2942.

Tahara, T., Arisawa, T., Wang, F. & et al. (2007). Toll-like receptor 2 -196 to 174del polymorphism influences the susceptibility of Japanese people to gastric cancer. Cancer Sci, 98, 1790-1794.

Tailleux, L., Schwartz, O., Herrmann, J.L. & et al. (2003). DC-SIGN is the major Mycobacterium tuberculosis receptor on human dendritic cells. *J Exp Med,* 197, 121–127.

Tassaneetrithep, B., Burgess, T.H., Granelli-Piperno, A., & et al. (2003). DC-SIGN (CD209) mediates dengue virus infection of human dendritic cells. *J. Exp. Med.* 197, 823–829.

Thuong, N.T., Hawn, T.R., Thwaites, G.E. & et al. (2007). A polymorphism in human TLR2 is associated with increased susceptibility to tuberculous meningitis. *Genes Immun.* 8, 422-428.

Thye, T., Nejentsev, S., Intemann, C.D., et al. (2009). MCP-1 promoter variant -362C associated with protection from pulmonary tuberculosis in Ghana, West Africa. *Hum. Mol. Genet,* 18, 381-388.

Underhill, D.M., Ozinsky, A., Smith, K.D. & Aderem, A. (1999). Toll-like receptor-2 mediates mycobacteria-induced proinflammatory signaling in macrophages. Proc. Natl. Acad. Sci. USA, 96, 14459-14463.

Vannberg, F.O., Chapman, S.J., Khor, C.C. & et al. (2008). CD209 genetic polymorphism and tuberculosis disease. *PLoS One,* 3(1):e1388.

Van Kooyk, Y., Appelmelk, B. & Geijtenbeek, T.B. (2003). A fatal attraction: Mycobacterium tuberculosis and HIV-1 target DC-SIGN to escape immune surveillance. *Trends Mol. Med,* 9, 153–159.

Velez, D.R., Hulme, W.F., Myers, J.L., Weinberg, J.B., Levesque, M.C., Stryjewski, M.E., Abbate, E., Estevan, R., Patillo, S.G., Gilbert, J.R. *& et al. (2009).* NOS2A, TLR4, and IFNGR1 interactions influence pulmonary tuberculosis susceptibility in African-Americans. *Hum. Gene,* 126, 643-653.

Vidyarani, M., Selvaraj, P., Raghavan, S., Narayanan, P.R. (2009). Regulatory role of 1, 25-dihydroxyvitamin D3 and vitamin D receptor gene variants on intracellular granzyme A expression in pulmonary tuberculosis. *Exp. Mol. Pathol,* 86, 69–73.

Vidyarani, M., Selvaraj, P., Prabhu, A.S., Jawahar, M.S., Adhilakshmi, A.R., Narayanan, P.R. (2006). Interferon gamma (IFN-γ) & interleukin-4 (IL-4) gene variants & cytokine levels in pulmonary tuberculosis. Indian J. Med. Res, 124, 403–410.

White, P. & Cooke, N. (2000). The multifunctional properties and characteristics of vitamin D-binding protein. *Trends Endocrinol. Metab.* 11, 320-327.

World Health Organization. (2009). Global Tuberculosis Control - Surveillance, Planning, Financing. URL: http://www.who.int. Accessed in 15/11/2009.

W.H.O. Report 2007. Global tuberculosis control. Surveillance, planning and financing. World Health Organization, Geneva, Switzerland.

Yim, J.J., Lee, H.W., Lee, H.S., Kim, Y.W., Han, S.K., Shim, Y.S. & Holland, S.M. (2006). The association between microsatellite polymorphisms in intron II of the human toll-like receptor 2 gene and tuberculosis among Koreans. *Genes Immun,* 7, 150-155.

2

Development of Therapeutic Interventions for Emerging Diseases

Nigel J. Silman
Research & Development, Health Protection Agency Porton, Porton Down, Salisbury, UK

1. Introduction

New infectious diseases emerge with a high regularity; it has recently been estimated that a novel infectious disease agent either emerges or re-emerges approximately every 8 months. This latter statistic is supported by the observation that there have been over 335 emerging infectious disease (EID) events between 1940 and 2004 (Jones *et al.*, 2008). Of course, not all of these EID events represent a threat to human health, indeed many of these are infections of animals, although approximately 60% are also zoonotic infections (which by definition can be transmitted between animals and humans); another additional proportion also have the potential to cross the species barrier. Since 1970 there have been approximately 30 new species of pathogen emerge which cause human infection. Table 1 lists these pathogens (taken from World Health Organisation, 1999).

Year	Pathogen	Year	Pathogen
1972	Small Round Structured Viruses	1989	Hepatitis C virus
1973	Rotavirus	1990	Human herpesvirus-7
1975	Astrovirus	1990	Hepatitis E virus
1975	Parvovirus B-19	1991	Hepatitis F virus
1976	*Crytosporidium parvum*	1992	*Vibrio cholerae* 0139:H7
1977	Ebola virus	1992	*Bartonella henselae*
1977	*Legionella pneumophila*	1993	Sin Nombre virus
1977	Hantaan virus	1993	Hepatitis G virus
1977	*Cambylobacter jejuni*	1994	Sabia virus
1980	HTLV-1	1994	Human herpesvirus-8
1981	Toxigenic *Staphylococcus aureus*	1995	Hendra virus
1982	HTLV-II	1996	Prion (BSE/vCJD)
1982	*Borrelia burgdorferii*	1997	Influenza A virus (H5N1)
1983	*E.coli* 0157:H7	1997	Transfusion-transmitted virus
1983	HIV	1997	Enterovirus 71
1983	*Helicobacter pylori*	1998	Nipah virus
1988	Human herpesvirus-6	1999	Influenza A virus (Hong Kong 'flu)
1989	*Ehrlichia* spp.	1999	West Nile virus

Table 1. Emerging Infectious Disease Pathogens, 1972-1999.

An emerging infectious disease may be defined as one that has appeared in a population for the first time, or that may have existed previously but is rapidly increasing in incidence or geographic range (World Health Organisation [WHO]). This definition is quite generic and many consider EID's as those which are either genuinely novel infectious disease pathogens (examples include the SARS coronavirus which emerged in 2003) or those where there has been a paradigm shift in their genotype or phenotype such that it poses a new threat to health (examples include the appearance of multi-drug resistant *Mycobacterium tuberculosis* and other bacterial pathogens). These latter pathogens are frequently referred to as re-emerging infectious diseases, to discriminate them from completely novel disease agents. Because of the apparent rise in the incidence of EIDs during the 1980's and 90's (HIV/AIDS, vCJD *etc.*), factors involved in the process of emergence were analysed by a number of workers. One such study (Taylor *et al.*, 2001), concluded that although over half of EIDs were zoonotic in origin, the route of transmission had no effect on the likelihood of emergence, rather it was the taxonomy of the organism that was the root cause. They concluded that viruses and bacteria were of much higher likelihood of emergence, whereas parasites such as Helminths, were very unlikely to ever emerge.

Despite the advances in medical science, infectious diseases still constitute a threat to human survival, health and well-being and have done since human life began. Immediately following the discovery of penicillin, there was a mood of optimism that felt that the conquest of infectious diseases was a war that had been won; rather it seems it was merely the first skirmish in a very long-lasting battle. In the first decade of the 21st century, we know that infectious diseases represent a major global threat, accounting for some 41% of the global disease burden and in the UK alone, infectious diseases now account for approximately 70,000 deaths per annum and 40% of the population in the country consult a medical practitioner each year because of infection (Donaldson, 2001). It is clear, therefore, that infectious diseases remain a major global threat and that the burden of disease with an infectious aetiology is very high. There are a large number of interventions that can be applied to the control of infectious disease and for health protection. Interventions include simple public health control measures (hand-washing, quarantine, supply of clean water *etc.*), diagnostic tests, therapeutic treatments and vaccines. These different aspects will be discussed in greater depth in the following sections.

2. Vaccination

Vaccination is the process by which the adaptive immune system is stimulated to produce a deliberate response. Typically, vaccines comprise an antigenic component (or components) which are administered by a variety of routes and mimic the infection against which protection is sought. Modern vaccination was probably first described by Edward Jenner (there are reports that a similar approach had been used some years earlier) in 1796; indeed it was Jenner who coined the phrase vaccination. The term is derived from the Latin word *vacca* meaning "cow", so derived since the first "vaccination" used material from cowpox viral lesions on a milk-maids hands as protection against Smallpox infection (reviewed in Lombard *et al.*, 2007). Strictly, vaccination may be considered to be the process of introducing a foreign antigen into the body for the purpose of protection against infectious disease, whereas, immunisation is the process by which a vaccine induces an immune response against a foreign antigen – a subtle difference in meaning, although in practice the two terms are often used interchangeably. From these early beginnings, there are 26 currently licensed vaccines widely available and administered as components of vaccination programmes. These 26 vaccines are shown in Table 2 below.

Vaccine	Vaccine
Anthrax	Pertussis
Cervical cancer (papilloma virus)	Pneumococcal infection
Chicken pox virus	Poliomyelitis
Cholera	Rabies
Diphtheria	Rotavirus
Group A & C Meningococcal infections	Rubella
Hib infection	Shingles
Hepatitis A	Smallpox
Hepatitis B	Tetanus
Japanese encephalitis	Tuberculosis
Influenza	Typhoid Fever
Measles	Varicella
Mumps	Yellow Fever

Table 2. Licensed Vaccines Currently Available for Use.

The table above illustrates that there are available vaccines for many of the "common" infectious diseases, yet despite this availability, there still exists a considerable disease burden for many of the diseases shown in Table 2. One might reasonably question why this is so, and the answer is multi-fold. Firstly the aspect of vaccine efficacy needs to be considered; the availability of a licensed vaccine does not, of course, indicate that use will result in 100% protection of the recipient. Due to the very different immune profiles observed within the human population, there will be a response curve which at one end results in next to no (or at least very low) levels of protection, whereas at the other end of the scale, recipients will show good protection. Taken on a population level, this means that there will always be a proportion of the population which are unprotected and thus the disease is still able to circulate. The above reasoning also assumes that take-up (and indeed availability) of any vaccine is 100% within a population; it is not due both to the cost involved in vaccinating entire populations and the choice which some make not to receive vaccination when offered. This latter point is very well illustrated by the recent issues surrounding the MMR (Measles, Mumps & Rubella) tri-valent vaccine within the UK. Adverse scientific publications (for an update on the current scientific evidence and lack of any link between these events see DeStefano & Williams, 2004), indicating a link between receipt of the vaccine and autism in children has meant that many parents decided not to allow their children to receive the vaccine and the UK now has a considerable measles outbreak due to much higher levels of susceptibility within the population (see ECDC measles Surveillance Report, 2011). It is of note, though, that the risk of real adverse events with the MMR vaccine are very low; the risk of brain damage due to receipt of the vaccine is calculated to be approximately 1/100,000 (this is due to the measles component of the vaccine), whereas the risk of brain damage if a child catches measles is approximately 1/1000, a figure which is considerably higher.

2.1 Types of vaccine

There are basically three ways of making vaccines against infectious diseases, all rely on a level of knowledge about the pathogenesis of the disease and ideally about the virulence factors which the pathogen employs. That vaccination is an effective method to protect the health of a population is well known and documented; the figure below illustrates the reduction in numbers of ill and in numbers of deaths for a fictitious respiratory disease, spreading with a population of approximately 60 million people (Fig. 1). A large number of assumptions have been made in running this very simple Susceptible, Infected, Recovered (SIR) model, one of which was that a new vaccine had to be developed and that the time taken to both produce a crude, whole-cell vaccine, plus manufacture enough to be used widely, resulted in an approximately 50% reduction in the overall numbers of fatalities (C. Norris & N J Silman, Unpublished). Of course, modelling the same disease, but making the assumption that a vaccine already exists can reduce the impact of the disease even more than that shown in Fig.1.

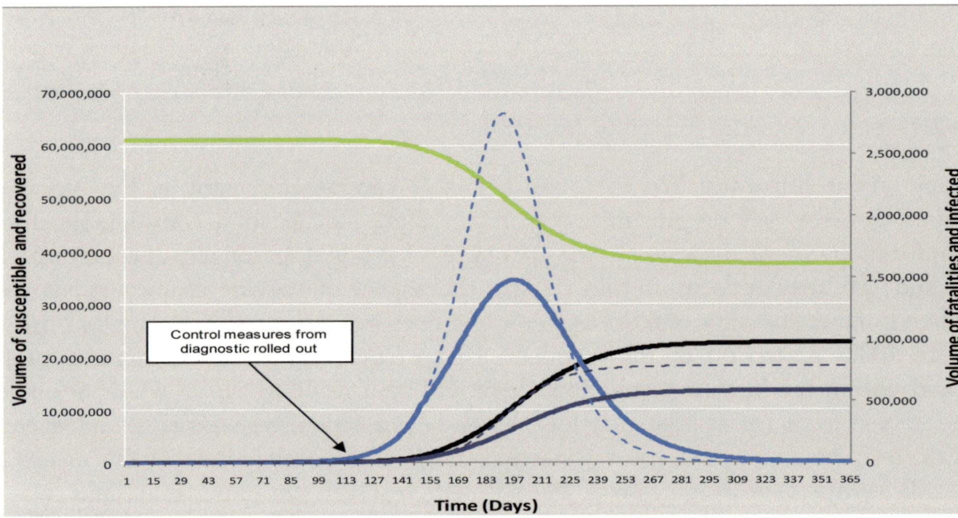

Fig. 1. SIR Model of the Impact of Vaccine Introduction on the Course of Infectious Disease. Key: ____ Susceptible population; _ _ _ Infected population; ___ Infected population after vaccine introduced; _ _ _ Fatalities if vaccine not used; ______ Fatalities when vaccine used; ___ Numbers Recovered

This figure is shown merely to illustrate the point that development of a new vaccine in the event of an emerging disease can have a very profound effect on the outcome of the disease (this point was well made during the recent H1N1 influenza pandemic). The illustration also includes an element of diagnostic roll-out, where we made the assumption that in the early stages of a newly emerged pathogen, simple public health control measures would be invoked to control person to person transmission and that these measures would be supported by a diagnostic test.

The three different approaches to vaccine development will be discussed in greater detail in the sections which follow, and their potential for use in producing vaccines against rapidly emerging pathogens will be discussed further.

2.1.1 Whole-cell vaccines

The simplest vaccines comprise growing up the pathogen and inactivating a crude, unfractionated preparation. This is an approach which has been used for a considerable length of time and vaccines made using this relatively simple rationale are still widely used. Examples taken from table 2 include Anthrax, Japanese encephalitis, influenza, yellow fever and typhoid fever; the reader will note that both bacterial and viral vaccines are made using the same approach and both types can show good efficacy in use. There are, of course, a number of examples where such an approach is not successful; examples here include vaccines that were produced against Cholera, Plague, meningitis and Smallpox. These vaccines failed because of a paucity of understanding of the mechanisms of virulence (*e.g.* the major virulence factor for Cholera is a toxin and thus a crude whole-cell preparation would not contain this secreted component). However, it is still considered that this method of rapidly producing a vaccine could be used in the event of a newly emerging infectious disease that had a high mortality rate and was highly transmissible within the population. Although there are examples of vaccines for both bacteria and viruses produced by this method, it is generally considered that the approach is probably more suited to production of viral vaccines due to their lower complexity. Probably the most commonly used vaccine of this type which is still produced and updated year on year is the split virion influenza vaccine that is produced seasonally. This vaccine comprises an unpurified preparation of virus typically grown in egg-culture (although there are notable examples of cell-culture grown influenza virus vaccines which are licensed for use or in clinical trial) and inactivated. The rationale is that the major antigenic components of the influenza virus are the haemagglutinin and neuraminidase, both of which are surface proteins against which considerable immune responses are mounted. Interestingly, despite the longevity of use of this vaccine and the considerable number of clinical trials and research work that has been conducted, the correlates of protection for influenza are still unknown (Montomoli *et al.*, 2011).

Looking at the list of recently emerged pathogens shown in Table 1, it is interesting to note that this approach has been used to develop vaccine candidates for a number of the pathogens. The most notable example is HIV/AIDS, for which there is still no effective vaccine and that an inactivated viral preparation did not exhibit high protective efficacy. Thus, for this method of vaccine development to be of value for an emergent pathogen a number of criteria need to be fulfilled, some of which will not be obvious when the disease first emerges. Firstly, the disease needs to have a high mortality rate, such that use of a vaccine is absolutely required. Secondly, it must be highly transmissible, since an infection with a low rate of transmission (R_0) can be controlled by other public health measures, a good example of such a pathogen was the SARS coronavirus, which was transmissible but had a relatively low R_0 and thus was adequately controlled by quarantine. Thirdly, natural infection should induce a protective immunity, otherwise an inactivated preparation is unlikely to induce immunity if the natural infection is incapable of so doing. This last consideration is very unlikely to be understood at the point when the pathogen emerges and will only be fully understood after a considerable length of time, most probably once an epidemic or pandemic situation has passed. The speed that a vaccine must be deployed is illustrated in Fig.2, which shows the effect on the numbers of infectious people within a population as the reproduction rate of the infectious disease pathogen is varied.

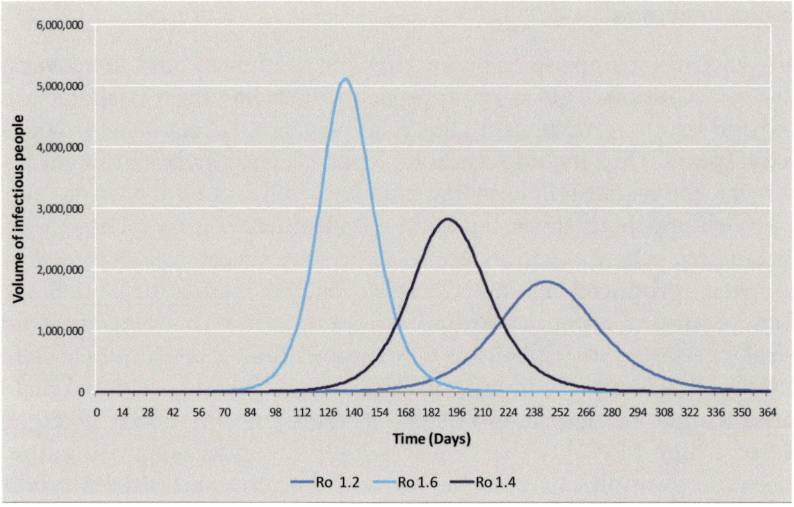

Fig. 2. Effect of Varying R_0 on the Number of Infectious People within a Population.

This figure illustrates a modest range of R_0 values between 1.2 and 1.6, the point to note is that even with small variations in the R_0 value, large differences in the numbers of infected people are observed and the time that maximum numbers of people are infected varies between approximately 130 and 240 days. This should be compared with the reproduction rate of typical influenza viruses which may be up to $R_0 = 3$ (that is, 3 uninfected people are infected by each infectious member of the population). The lower values used in this illustration were seen with the SARS coronavirus and perhaps illustrate why a vaccine was not developed against this pathogen during the epidemic phase.

2.1.2 Attenuated vaccines

Another approach to the rational design of vaccines for existing or emerging pathogens is the attenuation of virulent strains. Here, a strain is used which is not able to produce fulminant infection as a result of its' attenuation. In contrast to the inactivated vaccines described in section 2.1.1, these vaccines comprise live micro-organisms. Historically, attenuated strains were first obtained by serendipity often following prolonged sub-culture or passage (for example see Barrett *et al.,* 1990). Good examples of this occurrence are the Yellow fever 17D strain which was naturally attenuated by repeated passage and has been used as a vaccine against this disease since the 1950's. Interestingly, the mechanism of attenuation is still not known, although the vaccine has a long history of safe use, except in those members of the population with an egg allergy (the virus is propagated in egg culture). Another well-known example of an attenuated vaccine strain is the Polio virus vaccine, of which there are two vaccines in use. The first, the Salk vaccine is an inactivated viral preparation whilst the second, called the Sabin strain is an attenuated Polio virus (see Pearce, 2004). The Sabin vaccine was trialled between 1957 and 1962, when it was licensed for widespread use. The vaccine is taken orally and was attenuated by repeated passage in the brains of mice. By the seventh passage the virus was found to be no longer capable of infecting mice via the neurological route. A further 2 to 3 passages through rats confirmed the attenuation and the strain was considered safe for human inoculation. The development of polio vaccines in the 1950's was a response to the large burden of disease caused by this virus and delivery of the Salk and Sabin vaccines constitutes the first mass-immunisation programmes. At the current date, Polio is still yet to be eradicated, despite efforts which began in 1988 between the WHO, UNICEF and the Rotary Foundation, however the hope is that this virus will soon be committed to history.

As the above example illustrates, the process of attenuation is not one which can be undertaken rapidly. There is no rational way of determining whether a strain may be attenuated by simple repeated passage or not and therefore the utility of such an approach is of limited value in responding to emergence of new infectious diseases. There are, of course, alternative ways of attenuating pathogenic strains of microorganism. For example, in the time between isolation of the Sabin strain and the present day, the mutations which are responsible for this strains lack of neuro-infectivity have been mapped to the internal ribosome entry site (IRES) of the virus in the currently used strain, a derivative of the original Sabin isolate. Extensive characterisation of the series of viruses that have been used as live-attenuated Polio vaccines has indicated that there are fifty-seven nucleotide substitutions which distinguish the attenuated Sabin 1 strain from its virulent parent (the Mahoney serotype), with a two further nucleotide substitutions between the Sabin 2 and parent strain, and ten more substitutions are involved in further attenuating the Sabin 3 strain (Kew *et al.*, 2005).

An alternative to repeated passage is the rational deletion of one or more genes from the genome of the organism. This approach requires in-depth knowledge of the virulence or pathogenicity factors which the infectious micro-organism uses to achieve infection in the human host. There are a number of examples where this approach has been successfully used. In view of the subject within this chapter to look at prospects for emerging infectious diseases, the live attenuated influenza vaccine (LAIV) will be used as a discussion example to illustrate this approach. There is currently only one licensed influenza vaccine based upon this LAIV technology, although, like other influenza vaccines, the virus backbone is used to construct vaccines against currently circulating strains by recombination with the genomic segments encoding the haemagglutinin and neuraminidase genes from the currently circulating strains. The LAIV is licensed in the USA by FDA and sold under the trade name of FluMist™. The backbone strain used for this vaccine is a cold-adapted strain which is attenuated since it is not able to complete the cycle of replication at normal human body temperatures. The relatively small genome of the influenza virus has been completely sequenced from this strain and many nucleotide substitutions have been made to ensure that the strain cannot revert and also to improve its growth properties in cell, rather than egg culture as this is a more scalable technology for rapid vaccine manufacture than is egg culture.

A similar approach may be envisioned for viral groups such as the Flaviviruses. This is an important group of viruses, whose members have been responsible for several infectious disease outbreaks during the last two decades. Their members include Yellow fever virus, West Nile virus and Dengue virus and they are viruses with segmented RNA genomes. One of the key factors in the emergence of new pathogens is the presence of an RNA genome as this allows rapid recombination, mutation and hence evolution and adaptation. This group is therefore of great importance when horizon scanning for the next emergent viral disease and only one flavivirus already has a licensed vaccine (Yellow fever). There are vaccines against Dengue virus in clinical trial, since this is a disease with a worldwide distribution and serious complications can be observed if re-infection with a different serotype occurs (Dengue haemorrhagic fever). West Nile virus is a classic example of an emergent viral infection; it arose in the West Nile delta in North Africa and was transported by cervid birds into North America where, as it is a mosquito vector-transmitted disease, it has caused seasonal outbreaks in every subsequent year (see Campbell *et al.,* 2002). Chikungunya virus has similarly spread across the Indian Ocean and has also been imported into Europe where it caused a limited outbreak in Italy during 2009 (Beltrame *et al.,* 2007). It is likely that infection with one flavivirus induces an immunity against some other viruses within the group, based on the observation that antibodies against many of these viruses cross-react with flaviviral antigens in ELISA assays and thus make clinical infection with a particular virus impossible to diagnose by serology alone. By comparing different flaviviruses with the Yellow fever 17D vaccine, it should be possible to produce vaccines against this range of viruses by using the same approach to attenuate different viruses. What is unknown, once again, are the correlates of immunity for not only Yellow fever infection but for any of the other flavivirus infections. Care will also be needed to avoid any complications by priming the immune system as are seen in Dengue virus infection. As a method of rapidly producing a vaccine strain, attenuation by repeated passage is not useful due to the extensive length of time that it may take to produce an attenuated virus and the additional time required to demonstrate irreversible attenuation.

2.1.3 Sub-unit vaccines

Probably the most rapid way to make a vaccine against a newly emerging pathogen is to use a recombinant technology approach and identify a single immunogenic antigen, clone out and express the gene encoding that particular antigen. A common theme that we have observed whilst discussing vaccinology, is that rational vaccine design has an absolute requirement for good understanding of both the factors which affect pathogen virulence as well as those which contribute to immunity in the host. Although this has been discussed previously, it bears repeating that in the event of a newly emerging pathogen, these data will not be available and that the second best approach is to fall back to an inactivated whole pathogen preparation. Assuming, however, that we are aiming to develop a vaccine against a pathogen which is similar to one about which we have considerable knowledge, then a rational sub-unit approach is likely to be used. Once again the caveat is that a single sub-unit(s) may not induce complete protective immunity, as there may well be multiple components involved in protection following natural infection. There are numerous examples where single sub-unit vaccine candidates fail to provide complete or even any protection, a good illustration of this observation is the lack of complete protection afforded by single sub-unit vaccines in HIV infection (inactivated virus also fails to induce protection though).

Yersinia pestis, the bacterial causative agent of plague, is a re-emergent infection as it has caused recent outbreaks in geographical areas that have previously not experienced infections caused by this organism. Fig. 3 below illustrates that although there are a large number of surface antigens, against which an immune response is induced (as determined by the presence of human antibody response), only two are associated with protective immunity, these are the F1 and V antigens and both are virulence factors encoded by transferrable plasmids. A vaccine containing the F1 and V-antigens is being developed, although because of the low prevalence of disease, it is unlikely to be widely used. As an exemplar of the approach that can be taken with emerging and re-emerging diseases, it illustrates perfectly the requirement for a thorough understanding of the pathogenesis of the organisms as well as understanding the host immune response.

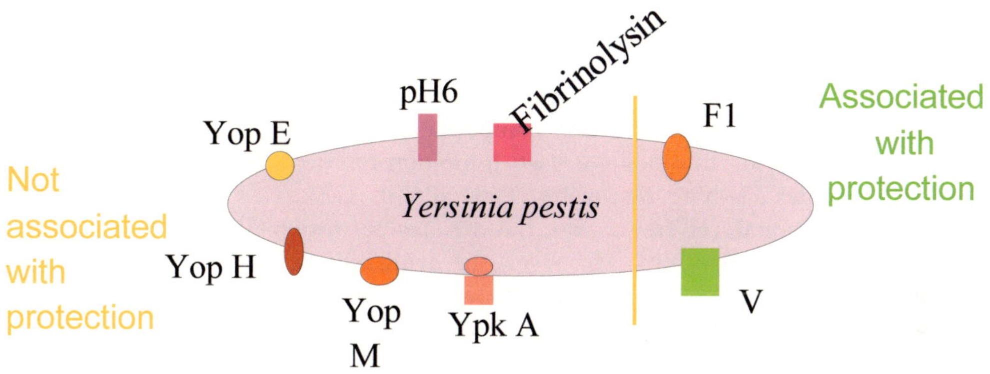

Fig. 3. Identification of Protective Antigens in *Yersinia pestis.*

3. Therapeutic interventions

There are a great number of therapeutic interventions that can be applied to the control of infectious diseases. The key type of interventions are discussed in greater detail below, and as a general trend, we have observed a move towards more targeted approaches to design of therapeutic compounds. During the last 30 years, the period under discussion when considering emerging infectious diseases, there has been a marked change in the scientific approaches to discovery of therapeutic molecules. There were a great many researchers using natural product libraries during the 1970's and 80's to discover compounds with activity against a wide range of biological activities; of relevance to infectious diseases are those which exhibited antimicrobial activity. A consequence of these high-throughput screening programmes was that several new classes of antibiotic were discovered during this time, but subsequently there have been very few new discoveries and there is now a real shortage of new antimicrobial compound groups to counteract the rise of antimicrobial resistance. Future research to meet clinical unmet needs, must incorporate the rational design and discovery of new ways of combating antimicrobial resistance, be it new antibiotics or other therapeutic approaches.

3.1 Antimicrobial compounds

The majority of currently licensed antibiotics were discovered between 40 and 60 years ago and modern drugs are mostly derivatives of existing classes of drug. Despite the increased need to treat expanding populations against micro-organisms exhibiting increasing levels of resistance, there has been a reduction in the effort by the major pharmaceutical companies to discover new antibiotics (Marinelli, 2009). There have been a number of high, but unrealised expectations driven by high-throughput screening, combinatorial chemistry and microbial genome sequencing that have failed to deliver the new compounds required. It is interesting to note that during the "Golden Age" of antibiotic discovery (1940-1960) approximately 12,000 compounds were screened and resulted in 160 licensed products (0.01%). This statistic played a major part in the evolution of antibiotics where research effort was directed towards the improvement of existing chemotypes (increased potency, stability and pharmokinetics, reduced side-effects) rather than discovery of novel compound classes. Those that did continue to invest research funds into discovery rather than improvement were rewarded by the discovery of some new chemotypes such as thienamycin, daptomycin and echinocandins. One of the main confounders to the discovery of new compounds was the high rate of re-isolation of existing compounds, requiring a different approach to screening assays from the traditionally used inhibition of bacterial growth that has been used since Alexander Fleming discovered Penicillin in 1928. This need has led to the introduction of functional, cell-free assays, but this has not resulted in the desired increase in discovery of novel compounds. Moreover, the availability of whole genome sequence data for a wide range of pathogenic bacteria and viruses similarly has not resulted in discovery of novel chemotypes, despite high investment by the pharmaceutical companies.

There are, however, several prospects for the discovery of new classes of chemotype. The first of these is to harness the wealth of structural data that are now available, but this approach requires an in-depth knowledge of the biology of the target micro-organism. There are a number of documented examples of this approach being coupled with virtual high-throughput screening (VHTS) against virtual compound libraries. One example is that described by Reddy *et al.* (2006) for the rational discovery of small molecule inhibitors of prion protein, a key emergent disease. Here a virtual compound library was screened for molecules that would theoretically bind and inhibit prion protein from entering cells. A similar approach has been taken to the design of inhibitors of the Anthrax toxin cell-binding component (protective antigen; PA) which combines with two further toxin components to exert the toxic effects, which typically result in death of the animal or human host. The protein crystallography data were used for the PA molecule and the cell-receptor binding site was identified from published research (Bradley *et al.*, 2001). This crystal structure was screened using VHTS and small-molecule inhibitors of this binding reaction were identified and then synthesised and screened *in vitro* using functional assays for one of the two Anthrax toxins (lethal toxin, a combination of PA and lethal factor). Many of the molecules screened using this approach were subsequently found to have significant activity in the *in vitro* assays; approximately 3% of the compounds screened were found to possess activity, compared with the 0.01% that are typically obtained by high-throughput screening of compound libraries (B. Chen, personal communication). This approach clearly holds much promise for the rational design of novel chemotypes of antimicrobial compound and the approach works irrespective of whether the pathogen is a virus or bacteria. This is therefore, an attractive approach for the development of targeted inhibitors of a range of processes involved in the pathogenesis of disease. The main caveat, though, is that a thorough understanding of the virulence factors and pathogenesis of the disease are needed, along with suitable structural data to enable this approach to be used to combat emerging diseases. Clearly, when a pathogen first emerges, it is completely uncharacterised and such a directed approach is not possible.

Other approaches to the discovery of new chemotypes are the screening of compound libraries derived from different sources. This approach somewhat mimics the approach used during the "Golden Age", in that compound libraries are screened using high-throughput methods and inhibition of microbial growth at this stage is a precursor to further characterisation. The libraries from which most antibiotics were derived are soil organisms, but there are also untapped resources in the oceans, where there is a large number and range of micro-organisms and from plant extracts where a number of compounds have already been shown to possess antibacterial and/or antiviral activity. Examples are the extracts from the garlic and clove plants (Arora & Kaur, 1999). A range of spice plants were screened for activity and only these two extracts exhibited antimicrobial activity, however, they were active against a range of Gram positive and Gram negative bacteria and yeasts.

As an adjunct to antimicrobial compounds, we should also consider those compounds which modify activity of existing drugs. Such examples include ß-lactamase inhibitors such as clavulanic acid (used as a proprietary preparation in conjunction with amoxicillin and other ß-lactam antibiotics) and efflux inhibitors which maintain an elevated drug concentration within cells and hence improve antimicrobial efficacy.

3.2 Therapeutic antibodies

An alternative therapeutic approach to emerging infectious diseases is the use of antibodies to treat disease. This is a concept which has existed for a considerable time, however, only relatively recently have therapeutic antibodies really been used against infectious diseases. As of 2006, there were 20 therapeutic antibodies approved as therapeutics by the FDA (Das, 2006), but they offer considerable potential for the rapid treatment of emerging infectious diseases. One may question why this should be; the answer is straightforward, since protection from infection by pathogenic micro-organisms may be either active, and induced by immunization using prophylactic vaccines (see section 2.1), or passive. One of the issues discussed in section 2 was that prophylactic vaccines take a considerable time to make and formulate and these can be too slow for a pathogen with a high rate of reproduction (R_0) in a susceptible population. Passive immunity, where specific antibodies are administered, is a viable alternative here and also for the treatment of diseases where antimicrobial therapy may exacerbate the disease symptoms and also result in higher transmissibility (*e.g.* ulcerative colitis caused by *Clostridium difficile* infection and toxin). Many advances have been seen over the past decade which has allowed improved antibody engineering technologies along with improvements in safety and efficacy. These developments, along with a greater understanding of the immunomodulatory properties of antibodies, have paved the way for the next generation of new and improved antibody-based drugs for the treatment of human diseases. One major factor that makes this an attractive technology is that antibody "factories" can be rapidly turned around to produce a stock of antibodies for therapeutic use. This approach was recently described by Rogers *et al.* (2008) where they developed a panel of neutralising antibodies against the SARS coronavirus, a recently emerged pathogen, using a novel DNA display method. They describe their approach which involved panning the library using whole SARS virus rather than just the spike protein (which had been used by others, being a primary virulence factor for cell binding and entry). Other therapeutic antibody approaches in development include those to treat toxigenic effects following bacterial infection (*Clostridium difficile,* verotoxigenic *E.coli,* Anthrax toxin).

The use of therapeutic antibodies certainly holds much promise for the treatment of infectious diseases and is particularly attractive due to the rapidity that recombinant antibodies may be selected, produced and manufactured at scale.

3.3 Other therapeutics

There are a considerable number of other therapeutic approaches in development or at the research stage, far too many to comprehensively review here. Instead, we will concentrate on some of the key areas where there are noteworthy developments.

3.3.1 Therapeutic vaccines

Firstly, we will consider therapeutic vaccines. In section 2 previously, we have considered the use of vaccines for induction of prophylactic immunity. There is an alternative use of some vaccines, however, and this is for prophylaxis following exposure to an infectious disease micro-organism. A good example is the AIDS virus, HIV, which emerged in 1983 and for which, despite many attempts, there is no prophylactic vaccine. The Norwegian biotech company, Bionor Pharma recently released results from a study of its therapeutic HIV vaccine, Vacc-4x. There are recent data showing that the vaccine lowered patients' viral loads and negated the need for antiretroviral therapy (Fierce Vaccines, 2011).

3.3.2 Phage therapy

Phage therapy entails the use of bacteriophage viruses that infect bacteria for the treatment of bacterial infections. Phages are ubiquitously found in bacterial populations and control the growth of bacteria in many environments, including in the intestine, the oceans, and the soil. Phage therapy was in used in the 1920s and 1930s in the USA, Western & Eastern Europe, however, success rates of this therapy have never been firmly established, because only a limited number of clinical trials testing the efficacy of phage therapy have ever been conducted. These studies were performed mainly in the former Soviet Union. The development of antibacterial-resistant bacteria has once again sparked renewed interest in phage therapy with several companies, universities and foundations across the world now focusing on phage therapeutics. One of the main difficulties is that of delivery of the phage to the site of infection, making them potentially more suitable for treatment of respiratory or skin diseases than for deep-seated infections. There is also the safety concern about giving live viruses to human subjects.

3.3.3 Bacteriocins

Bacteriocins are peptides that can potentially be more readily engineered than small combinatorial chemistry generated molecules and are potential alternatives to conventional antibacterial compounds. Different classes of bacteriocins have different potential as therapeutic agents. Small-molecule bacteriocins (*e.g.* microcins and lantibiotics) are similar to the classic broad-spectrum antibiotics whereas colicin-like bacteriocins possess a much narrower activity spectrum, and require pathogen identification (and susceptibility testing) prior to therapy. Limitations of large-molecule antibacterials include reduced transport across membranes and within the human body. For this reason, they are usually used topically or gastrointestinally.

3.3.4 Chelation

A novel approach relies on the removal of essential nutrients for bacterial growth within the host by chelation. These compounds are not suitable for use alone, but may have utility in combination with conventional antibacterial compounds. A similar approach forms the basis of a treatment for lymphoblastic leukaemia, where bacterially-derived L-asparaginase is used as a therapeutic to remove L-asparagine, an essential amino acid for leukaemia cells to grow and divide, from the circulating blood stream and hence effectively "starving" the cancer cells.

3.3.5 Probiotics

Probiotics consist of live cultures of bacteria, which may become established as competing commensal organisms and thus inhibit or interfere with colonization by microbial pathogens. This approach has been used to reduce nasal carriage with Methicillin-resistant *Staphylococcus aureus* (MRSA) by replacement therapy using a skin commensal *Corynebacterium* sp. (Uehara *et al.* 2000).

4. Diagnostic tests

Diagnostic testing is not a therapeutic intervention, of course, but like other public health control measures, this chapter would be incomplete without mention of its use. In the early stages of an outbreak caused by any infectious disease pathogen, the public health control measures are inevitably supported by diagnostic testing. When a new disease emerges, the only factor that can be used for diagnosis is the clinical presentation. This is frequently compounded by the observation that many diseases present at the early stage with non-specific symptoms that are common with many less severe diseases. For example, the early symptoms of the SARS virus are very similar to many other respiratory infections caused by a range of viral pathogens, most of which do not require any intervention. Thus the power and value of a good diagnostic is in the differentiation of a pathogen causing severe infection from seasonally circulating infections of much lower consequence. Recently the Health Protection Agency undertook a study to model the value of rapid diagnostics development in the control of an outbreak caused by an emerging infectious disease (C. Noris & N. J. Silman, unpublished). The conclusion was that the diagnostic was of value only early in an outbreak when differential diagnosis was used to drive a policy of "containment" of the disease, that is, preventing onward transmission by preventing non-infected persons coming into contact with those who were infectious. Of course, quarantine cannot be enforced, but it was an effective tool used in controlling the spread of the H1N1 "swine" influenza pandemic during 2009. At the stage of the outbreak where containment is no longer possible, *i.e.* there are sufficiently high numbers of cases, then laboratory diagnosis ceases to have any real value in the CONTROL of the pandemic. That is not to say that it is of no value at all though.

5. Public health control measures

Although this chapter is focussing on the different therapeutic interventions that may be used to tackle the problems of emerging infectious diseases, it would be incomplete without mention of non-therapeutic means of controlling spread of infectious disease. In the initial stages of responding to an emergent infectious disease, the only tools available to limit spread of the disease and prevent nosocomial infection of clinical staff are non-therapeutic public health interventions. Perhaps the earliest described successful approach was in 1854 when John Snow removed the handle from a water pump in Broad Street, Soho, London. Before the discovery of pathogenic micro-organisms, Snow, a physician, was sceptical about the "miasma" theories that surrounded what we know to be infectious disease outbreaks. Miasma theory suggested that the cause of disease was a form of pollution or bad air. Snow carefully pieced together the evidence surrounding the distribution of the Cholera cases in the Soho area of London and concluded that the water pump in Broad Street was the common denominator; he removed the pump handle to prevent people from drawing and hence consuming water contaminated by *Vibrio cholerae* and very effectively curtailed the outbreak.

The same general, non-therapeutic approach may be taken with newly emerging diseases. For example, many of the diseases that have emerged in the last 30 years have an insect vector involved in the dissemination of the infectious disease pathogen (Jones *et al.*, 2008). The most effective intervention for vector-borne diseases is the eradication or reduction in the numbers of the insect vector using pesticides, rather than prophylaxis (not generally available) or therapeutics (Rose, 2001). Another recent example is the reduction in the numbers of cases of hospital acquired infection (HCAI). A contribution to this reduction is the reminder that good hand hygiene is vital and re-education of medical and nursing staff in the UK on good hand-washing practice, as well as the introduction of hand sanitizer gels (Grayson *et al.*, 2009). Thus these important interventions, although mostly quite simple can have very pronounced outcomes in the control of infectious diseases.

6. Conclusion

There are a number of therapeutic interventions that can be used to combat emerging infectious diseases. When a new pathogen emerges and subsequently causes a widespread outbreak, the interventions that can be applied differ during the course of the outbreak. At the early stage, recognition of the disease is heavily reliant upon clinical case definition, as was used in differentiating the new variant H1N1 influenza virus in 2009, prior to the development of a molecular diagnostic assay. We have seen that the development of a diagnostic assay is used in support of clinical case definition. The most effective interventions are therapeutic or prophylactic ones, however, since they are able to either treat those infected or protect onward spread by inducing herd immunity within a population. The downside of a therapeutic approach against a newly emerging disease is the length of time that is required to develop an effective vaccine or therapeutic against any specific pathogen. Here we require more generic, broad-spectrum interventions such as antimicrobials. What is evident is that more investment in R&D to discover new therapeutic molecules that can be used against newly emerging pathogens. Currently we are relatively well-served by the availability of broad-spectrum antibiotics, but increasingly widespread multi-drug resistance is a major problem and new chemotypes are urgently required. Perhaps the greatest hope is available by using recombinant antibody technology, where using the high-throughput genome sequencing approaches now available, we can rapidly sequence newly emerged pathogens, clone out and express surface antigens for rapid development of therapeutic antibody preparations. Many countries have invested heavily in infrastructure to build rapid vaccine facilities that can be turned around quickly in the event of the emergence of a new highly infectious pathogen and these sorts of adaptable facilities are of potentially great value in combating emerging infectious diseases.

7. References

Arora, D, S, & Kaur, J. (1999). Antimicrobial activity of spices. *Int. J. Antimicrob. Agents.* 12, pp. 257-262.

Barrett, A, D, T, Monath, T, P, Cropp, C, B, Adkins, J, A, Ledger, T, N, Gould, E, A, Schlesinger, J, J, Kinney, R, M, & Trent, D, W. (1990). Attenuation of wild-type yellow fever virus by passage in HeLa cells. *J. gen. Virol.* 71, pp. 2301-2306.

Beltrame, A, Angheben, A, Bisoffi, Z, Monteiro, G, Marocco, S, Calleri, G, Lipani, F, Gobbi, F, Canta, F, Castelli, F, Gulletta, M, Bigoni, S, Del Punta, V, Iacovazzi, T, Romi, R, Nicoletti, L, Grazia Ciufolini, M, Rorato, G, Negri, C, & Viale, P. (2007). Imported Chikungunya Infection, Italy. *Emerg. Inf. Dis.* 13, pp. 1264-1266.

Bradley, K, A, Mogridge, J, Mourez, M, Collier, R, J, & Young, J, A, T. (2001). Identification of the cellular receptor for anthrax toxin. *Nature* 414, pp. 225-229.

Campbell, G, L, Marfin, A, A, Lanciotti, R, L, & Duane J Gubler, D, J. (2002). West Nile Virus. *Lancet Inf. Dis.* 2, pp. 519-529.

Das, R, C. (2006). Antibody Therapeutics: Product Development, Market Trends, and Strategic Issues, Revised Edition. *Drug and Market Development Publishing*. Available from: http://www.researchandmarkets.com/reports/354677

DeStefano, F, & Thompson, W, W. (2004). MMR vaccine and autism: an update of the scientific evidence. *Ex. Rev. Vaccines* 3, pp. 19-22.

Donaldson, L. (2001). Getting Ahead of the Curve: A strategy for combating infectious diseases. *A Report by the Chief Medical Officer, Dept. of Health.* Available from: http://www.dh.gov.uk/en/Publicationsandstatistics/Publications/PublicationsPolicyAndGuidance/DH_4007697

ECDC Measles Surveillance Report. (2011). Eurpoean Monthly Measles Monitoring (EMMO). Available from: http://ecdc.europa.eu/en/publications/Publications/2011_June_measles_montly.pdf

Fierce Vaccines. (2011). Results From Phase IIB Placebo Controlled Study of Bionor Pharma's Vacc-4x Show Excellent Safety Profile. Available from: http://www.fiercebiotech.com/press-releases/results-phase-iib-placebo-controlled-study-bionor-pharmas-vacc-4x-show-exce

Grayson, M, L, Melvani, S, Druce, J, Barr, I, G, Ballard, S, A, Johnson, P, D, R, Mastorakos, T, & Birch, C. (2009). Efficacy of Soap and Water and Alcohol-Based Hand-Rub Preparations against Live H1N1 Influenza Virus on the Hands of Human Volunteers. *Clin. Inf. Dis.* 48, pp. 285-291.

Jones, K E, , Patel, N G, Levy, M A, Storeygard, A, Balk, D, Gittleman, J L, & Daszak, P. (2008). Global trends in emerging infectious diseases. *Nature,* 451, pp. 990-994, doi:10.1038/nature06536.

Kew, O, Sutter R, de Gourville, E, Dowdle, W, & Pallansch, M (2005). Vaccine-derived polioviruses and the endgame strategy for global polio eradication. *Annu Rev Microbiol.* 59, pp. 587–635. PMID 16153180

Lombard, M, Pastoret, P P, & Moulin A M. (2007). A brief history of vaccines and vaccination. *Rev Sci Tech.* 26, pp. 29-48. PMID: 17633292

Marinelli, F. (2009). Antibiotics and *Streptomyces:* the future of antibiotic discovery. *Microbiology Today* February 2009. Available from: http://www.sgm.ac.uk/pubs/micro_today/pdf/020903.pdf

Montomoli, E, Capecchi, B, & Hoschler, K. (2011). Correlates of protection against influenza. In *Influenza Vaccines for the Future.* Eds: Rappuoli, R & Del Giudice, G. pp. 199-222. Springer. Retrieved from http://www.springerlink.com/content/p2l4v614p282h828/

Pearce, J (2004). Salk and Sabin: poliomyelitis immunisation. *J Neurol Neurosurg Psychiatry* 75, pp. 1552. PMID 15489385

Reddy, T, R, K, Mutter, R, Heal, W, Guo, K, Gillet, V,J, Pratt, S & Chen, B. (2006). Library Design, Synthesis, and Screening: Pyridine Dicarbonitriles as Potential Prion Disease Therapeutics. *J. Med. Chem.* 49, pp. 607-615.

Rogers, J, Schoepp, R, J, Schröder, O, Clements, T, L, Holland, T, F, Li, J, Q, Lewis, L, M, Dirmeier, R, P, Frey, G, J, Tan, X, Wong, K, Woddnutt, G, Keller, M, Reed, D, S, Kimmel, B, E, & Tozer, E, C. (2008) rapid discovery and optimization of therapeutic antibodies against emerging infectious diseases. *Prot. Eng. Des. Sel.* 21, pp. 495-505.

Rose, R, I. (2001). Pesticides and public health: integrated methods of mosquito management. *Emerg. Inf. Dis.* 7, pp. 7-23.

Taylor, L H, Latham, S M, & Woolhouse, M E J. (2001). Risk factors for human disease emergence. *Phil. Trans. R. Soc. Lond.*, 356, pp. 983-989.

Uehara, Y, Nakama, H, Agematsu, K, Uchida, M, Kawakami, Y, Abdul Fattah, A, S, M, & Maruchi, N. (2000). Bacterial interference among nasal inhabitants: eradication of *Staphylococcus aureus* from nasal cavities by artificial implantation of *Corynebacterium* sp. *J. Hosp. Inf.* 44, pp. 127-133.

World Health Organisation. (1999). Emerging issues in water and infectious diseases. *A Report by the World Health Organisation.* Available from: http://www.who.int/water_sanitation_health/emerging/emergingissues/en/

3

Human Immunodeficiency Virus, Hepatitis B and Hepatitis C Virus Infections Among Injecting and Non-Injecting Drug Users in Inner City Neighborhoods

Lu-Yu Hwang and Carolyn Z. Grimes
Center for Infectious Diseases,
Division of Epidemiology and Center For Infectious Diseases,
School of Public Health,
University of Texas Health Science Center at Houston,
Houston, Texas,
USA

1. Introduction

Substance abuse is a continuing problem in the United States (US), impacting the individual and their social networks, and impacting society, economically and through public health programs. According to the 2004 National Household Survey on Drug Abuse (NHSDA), there were 19.1 million illicit drug users in the US. Drug use is directly and indirectly related to three blood-borne diseases, HIV, HBV and HCV. Direct exposure occurs through needle sharing and sharing other paraphernalia used to prepare and inject drugs [1-5]. The probability of direct exposure to HIV varies in relation to the procurement, preparation, and injection practices of drug users [6-10]. Frequency of injection and duration of injection are major factors for acquisition of HBV or HCV infections [11-13]. IDU is the primary mode of transmission of HCV in the US [14].

Drug use indirectly contributes to HIV exposure by decreasing inhibitions to engage in high-risk sexual activities and/or increased inhibitory effects on achieving sexual satisfaction [8, 15]. The use of cocaine has been shown to affect biological and behavioral processes related to HIV infection [16-19]. Engaging in risky sexual behaviors associated with drug use remains a significant risk factor for the acquisition of HBV, also, by men having sex with men (MSM) or heterosexual transmission. This interrelationship between drug use and high-risk sexual behavior makes it crucial to understanding the drug user population in order to develop appropriate interventions [20].

Houston is the fourth largest city and has the eighth highest AIDS caseload in the US. The number of African American and Hispanic Houstonians diagnosed with AIDS are increasing. The reason for the change in focus of the epidemic in Houston, from MSM to persons of color, may be related to the use of crack cocaine [4, 5]. Smoking crack cocaine, which became widespread in many poor, African American neighborhoods in the mid-1980s, continues to dominate the inner city drug use scene, and crack smokers, in addition to injection drug users, are at elevated risk for HIV infection. HBV and HCV were endemic among injecting drug users, even before HIV was introduced into this population. Common risk factors for these blood-borne viral agents, such as multi-person use of injecting equipment and sexual behaviors, have resulted in a high prevalence of infection of all three viruses among drug users. However, a significant proportion does remain at risk, as our previous studies in Houston have shown [4, 5] and should be targeted for vaccine prevention.

The purpose of this study was to estimate the prevalence of HIV, HBV and HCV infections and associated socio-demographic, drug use and sexual risk factors in a sample of predominantly African American injecting and non-injecting drug users who were recruited for a HBV vaccination study in Houston, Texas.

2. Material and methods

2.1 Study population

A sample of 2,779 injecting and non-injecting drug users was recruited for a community-based HBV vaccine study from February 2004 to October 2007. Participants were recruited from targeted congregation sites such as copping areas, street corners, and crack houses from predominantly two inner city neighborhood communities of Houston, Texas, by using outreach and chain referral recruiting methods. Target neighborhoods were selected based on previous studies [4, 5]. Potential study participants were asked to go to the designated field site in the area where they were recruited. The eligibility criteria for the study were 1) ages 18 and over, 2) local residence, 3) self-report and confirmed urine drug screen, 4) competent and willing to sign an informed consent form for HIV, HBV, and HCV antibody testing. This study had Institutional Review Board (IRB) approval through the University of Texas Health Science Center Committee for the Protection of Human Subjects.

2.1 Data collection

Data collectors received extensive training in obtaining informed consent, keeping participant information confidential, and administering the questionnaire. The interview was conducted confidentially in a private office and was identified only by a unique study identification number. Socio-demographic measures such as age, gender, race/ethnicity, living arrangement, jail history of >24 hours; drug use history including lifetime injection drug use (IDU), times injected drugs in past 7 and 30 days, lifetime and number of times shared needles in past 30 days, duration of IDU, types and frequency of drugs used in past 48 hours, 7 and 30 days, and drug treatment history; sexual behaviors such as number of sexual partners in the past 30 days, sexual orientation, condom use, history of sexually transmitted diseases, and trading sex for money or drugs in the past 30 days; history of blood transfusion and occupational exposure to blood. All interviews were verbally administered and recorded electronically via computer administered personal interview (CAPI, QDS, Bethesda, Maryland).

After the interview was completed, drug use was confirmed via urine drug screen, using OnTrak TesTstik, (Varian Inc,. Palo Alto, CA) to test for the presence of cocaine, opiates, and/or methamphetamines. Participants with a positive drug screen were asked to provide 10 ml of peripheral venous blood. Participants received a gratuity of $10.

2.2 Laboratory methods

Specimens were screened for HIV 1/2 antibodies, hepatitis B surface antigen (HBsAg), and antibodies to HCV (anti-HCV) by Core Combo HIV-HBsAg-HCV (Core Diagnostics, United Kingdom). Verification of HIV occurred by enzyme immunoassay (EIA), anti-HIV, using Abbott PPC Commander system, third generation HIV antibody test (Abbott Laboratories, Chicago, IL) , to HCV (Anti-HCV), hepatitis B surface antigen (anti-HBs) and antibody to hepatitis B core antigen (anti-HBc), by the Abbott AxSYM system, using microparticle enzyme immunoassay (MEIA) (Abbott Laboratories, Chicago, IL).

Case definition for HIV infection was repeatedly reactive specimen by EIA. The detection of HBsAg or anti-HBc, with or without anti-HBs was the definition of HBV infection. HCV infection definition was based on the presence of antibody to HCV. We have 2,779 observations for the HIV analysis, 1,712 for HBV analysis and 1,867 for HCV analysis at the time of manuscript preparation.

2.3 Statistics

Data from the questionnaire was imported into SAS 9.1 (Cary, NC) and laboratory results were entered into a Microsoft Access database. Data analysis was performed using STATA 9.0 (College Station, TX) software. Prevalence of HIV, HBV and HCV infections were estimated for the overall population and stratified by injecting status. Univariate and multivariable logistic analyses were performed. Any variable demonstrating a p-value of 0.2 or less or was biologically plausible was carried forward from univariate to multivariable analyses. Variables in the multivariable analyses that had a p-value of 0.05 or less were retained as the final model. Asian and other race were combined with Hispanic race because of small numbers. Variables with more than 10% missing responses from participants were not considered reliable enough to be examined.

3. Results

3.1 Demographic characteristics of the participants

Out of the 2,779, 85% of participants were African American, 11% White, and 4% Hispanic or other race with the majority (76%) being male. The median age was 43 and ranged from 18 to 76 years. About 3% reported having received a transfusion and the majority (78%) had a history of being in jail > 24 hours. Twelve percent were currently living in a shelter, and 62% had a history of being in a drug treatment program.

Almost 98% of the study participants had smoked crack in the past 7 days, 5% used methamphetamines and 5% were heroin users. About one-third (32%) had a history of injection drug use and 13% had a history of sharing needles. Almost half (43%) reported less than 50% condom use in the past 30 days. Nearly two-thirds (68%) reported a history of STD, with syphilis (42%) and gonorrhea (50%) being the two most prevalent. About one-fifth (19%) of the study population included MSM, more than one-third had traded sex for money/drugs in the past 30 days, and 23% reported having >3 male sexual partners and 40% had >3 female sexual partners in past 30 days.

3.2 Prevalence and risk factors associated with HIV infection

The prevalence of HIV infection in this population was 8.7%. Variables that had a significant association with being HIV infected in the univariate analysis were gender, shelter status, sexual orientation, condom use, MSM, trading sex for money or drugs in the past 30 days, and number of sex partners in the past 30 days (Tables 1 and 2). The drug-related variables explored in this analysis did not demonstrate any significant associations. After adjustment, HIV positive participants were more likely to be African American {OR= 2.8 (95% CI 1.6, 4.9)}, Hispanic and other race {OR= 2.5 (95% CI 1.1, 5.7)}, men having sex with men {OR= 2.5 (95% CI 1.7, 3.5)}, consistent condom users {OR= 2.9 (95% CI 2.0, 4.2)}, and be a male or female that had more than three male partners in the past 30 days {OR= 1.6 (95% CI 1.0, 2.4)} (Table 3). Study participants that lived in a shelter {OR= 0.5 (95% CI 0.3, 0.9)} or a male or female participant that had more than three female partners in the past 30 days {OR= 0.4 (95% CI 0.2, 0.5)} were less likely to be HIV positive (Table 3).

Variables	Total Number (%)	HIV Positive (%)	HBV Positive (%)	HCV Positive (%)
Total	2779 (100%)	8.7%	44.8%	36.1%
Gender				
Male	2111 (76%)	7.8%*	43.7% ∆	37.5%*
Female	668 (24%)	11.7%	48.8%	30.8%
Age (years)				
≤29	341 (12%)	7.7%	22.5%*	10.3%*
30-39	682 (25%)	10.7%	34.4%	20.7%
40-49	1177 (42%)	9.1%	50.1%	44.2%
>=50	579 (21%)	6.4%	57.5%	54.6%
Race/ethnicity				
Caucasian	302 (11%)	6.0%	37.9%*	53.4%*
Blacks	2354 (85%)	9.0%	46.3%	32.9%
Others	123 (4%)	10.6%	32.9%	55.7%
Currently living in a shelter				
No	2458 (88%)	9.2%*	45.0%	35.6%
Yes	321 (12%)	4.7%	43.3%	39.5%
Ever in drug treatment				
No	1070 (38%)	9.3%	43.3%	30.1%*
Yes	1709 (62%)	8.3%	45.7%	39.7%
Ever received a transfusion				
No	2692 (97%)	8.7%	43.8%*	34.1*
Yes	87 (3%)	8.0%	53.1%	54.0
Ever in Jail >24 hours				
No	613 (22%)	9.5%	41.3%	27.5%*
Yes	2166 (78%)	8.5%	45.6%	38.3%

*P value <0.05

Table 1. Prevalence of HIV, HBV and HCV infections among demographic characteristics in drug users, Houston, Texas.

Variables	Total	HIV positive N(%)	HBV positive N(%)	HCV positive N(%)
Drugs use in past 7 days				
No	16 (1%)	0%	46.2%	23.1%
Yes	2763 (99%)	8.8%	45.0%	36.2%
Marijuana				
No	1289 (46%)	8.5%	45.8%	38.3%
Yes	1490 (54%)	8.9%	43.8%	34.2%
Methamphetamines				
No	2632 (95%)	8.9%	45.1%	35.5%*
Yes	147 (5%)	6.1%	39.0%	47.2%
Cocaine				
No	62 (2%)	11.3%	48.0%	48.2%
Yes	2717 (98%)	8.6%	44.7%	36.0%
Heroin				
No	2636 (95%)	8.8%	43.9%*	34.8%*
Yes	143 (5%)	7.0%	59.8%	61.6%
Ever injected drugs				
No	1829 (66%)	8.6%	36.6%*	17.9%*
Yes	950 (34%)	8.8%	59.6%	70.0%
Duration of Injecting				
≤5 years	2218 (80%)	8.5%	36.0%*	26.5%*
>5 years	561 (20%)	9.4%	63.9%	78.3%
Ever shared needle/work				
No	2407 (87%)	8.7%	43.0%*	30.2%*
Yes	369 (13%)	8.4%	55.1%	72.1%
History of STD				
No	875 (32%)	7.9%	37.0%*	30.1%*
Yes	1904 (68%)	9.1%	48.9%	39.3%
History of Syphilis				
No	1597(58%)	8.5%	41.4%	34.5%*
Yes	1182(42%)	9.1%	51.1%	39.3%
What % of use a condom:				
Never	1095 (41%)	5.7%*	40.9%	35.5%
Sometimes	1137 (43%)	9.2%	40.5%	36.5%
Always	445 (16%)	14.2%	40.3%	33.1%
Sexuality				
Homosexual	112 (4%)	32.1%*	50.0%	32.0%*
Heterosexual	2137 (77%)	7.1%	44.7%	34.7%
Bisexual	530 (19%)	10.2%	44.2%	42.1%
Men had sex with men				
No	2248 (81%)	7.3%*	45.4%	36.1%
Yes	531 (19%)	14.7%	44.7%	36.2%

Variables	Total	HIV positive N(%)	HBV positive N(%)	HCV positive N(%)
Traded sex for money/drugs past 30 days				
No	1832 (66%)	7.3%*	45.1%	36.1%
Yes	947 (34%)	11.4%	44.0%	36.2%
Number of male sex partners in the past 30 days				
0	1732 (63%)	6.0%*	43.9%	37.3%
1-2	401 (14%)	10.2%	45.9%	33.2%
>=3	630 (23%)	15.2%	47.4%	34.4%
Number of female sex partners in the past 30 days				
0	919 (33%)	14.0%*	50.0%*	37.0%
1-2	759 (27%)	6.9%	41.6%	37.7%
>=3	1091 (40%)	5.5%	43.5%	33.9%

*P value <0.05

Table 2. Prevalence of HIV, HBV and HCV Infections by Drug Use and Sexual Behavior Variables in Past 30 Days among Drug Users in DASH Project.

	HIV	HBV	HCV
Risk Factors	OR (95% CI)	OR (95% CI)	OR (95% CI)
Race/Ethnicity			
White	1.00		
African American	2.8 (1.6-4.9) *	1.7 (1.2-2.4)*	0.4(0.3-0.6)*
Other	2.5 (1.1-5.7) *	0.9(0.5-1.6)	1.5(0.8-2.8)*
Age (per year)	1.00 (0.98-1.02)	1.05 (1.04-1.06)*	1.10(1.08-1.12)*
Injecting Drug use			
Yes	1.11 (0.8-1.5)	2.7 (2.27-3.5)*	9.4 (7.4-12.1)*
Shelter			
Yes	0.5(0.3-0.9)*	-----	------
History of blood transfusions			
Yes	------	------	1.6 (1.1-2.3)*
Condom use			
Always	2.9 (2.0-4.2) *	------	------
Sometimes	1.5(1.1-2.2)*		
History of syphilis diagnosis			
Yes	------	1.30(1.05-1.61)*	------
Men had sex with men			
Yes	2.5 (1.7-3.5) *	------	------
No. of male sex partners last 30 days			

	HIV	HBV	HCV
Risk Factors	**OR (95% CI)**	**OR (95% CI)**	**OR (95% CI)**
>3	1.6 (1.0-2.4)*	------	------
No. of female sex partners last 30 days			
>3	0.4(0.2-0.5)*	0.6(0.5-0.8)*	------
1-2	0.5(0.4-0.8)*		

*P value <0.05

Table 3. Multivariable Analyses of Risk Factors for HIV, HBV, HCV Infections Among Drug Users, Houston, TX.

To determine if associations differed between females and males and IDUs and non-IDUs, stratification by gender and injecting status were explored. The male study population analysis did not differ from the results from the total study population above (data not shown). Among the 668 female participants, African American race {OR 3.64 (95% CI 1.07-12.36)} and always using condoms in the past 30 days {OR 2.18, (95% CI, 1.10-4.33)} were found to be independently associated with HIV infection. Among non-injectors and injectors, the results from the multivariable analyses were fairly consistent with what was found in the total study population (Table 5).

Stratification also occurred by MSM status (Table 5) to determine if MSM status masked IDU as a risk factor for HIV. IDU status was not a significant risk factor for HIV in either the non-MSM or MSM analyses (Table 5).

3.3 Prevalence and risk factors associated with Hepatitis B virus infection

The prevalence of HBV in this study was 44.8%. Seropositivity for HBsAg (carrier) was 2.0% and for anti-HBc (previous or current infection), 38.5%. Of those with HBV infection, 412 (53.7%) out of 766 were co-infected with HCV. In Table 1 and 2, significant differences were observed between HBV positive and negative participants in variables representing gender, age, race, transfusion history, use of heroin in the past 30 days, number of sex partners in the past 30 days, history of STD, history of injection drug use, and history of sharing needles or works. After adjustment in the multivariable analysis, African American race {OR= 1.7 (95% CI 1.2, 2.4)}, increasing age per year {OR= 1.05 (95% CI 1.04, 1.06)}, history of injection drug use {OR= 2.7 (95% CI 2.3, 3.5)}, and having a history of being diagnosed with syphilis {OR= 1.3 (95% CI 1.05, 1.61)} remained independently associated with HBV infection, while having more than 3 female partners in 30 days, whether male or female, was inversely related to HBV infection {OR= 0.6 (95% CI 0.5, 0.8)} (Table 3).

To determine if non-IDUs shared the same risk characteristics as IDUs for HBV infection, stratification by injection status occurred. After adjusting for confounders in the multivariable analysis, two risk factors for HBV infection remained significant among non-injectors, increasing age and history of STD, while females or males with more than three female partners were less likely to have HBV infection (Table 4). Injectors that had increasing age, of African American race, female and had injected drugs for more than 5 years were all at risk for HBV infection after adjustment (Table 4).

	HBV		HCV	
Risk Factors	**NIDU OR (95%CI)**	**IDU OR (95%CI)**	**NIDU OR (95%CI)**	**IDU OR (95%CI)**
Gender				
Male	1.0(0.7-1.4)	1.8(1.1-2.9)*	0.9(0.6-1.3)	1.5(0.9-2.5)
Race/Ethnicity				
White				
African American	1.1(0.6-2.1)	1.7(1.1-2.9)*	0.5(0.2-097)*	0.4(0.2-0.7)*
Others	0.4(0.1-1.4)	1.0(0.5-2.2)	1.5(0.5-4.5)	1.3(0.5-3.0)
Age (per year)	1.03(1.01-1.04)*	1.09(1.07-1.12)*	1.09(1.07-1.12)*	1.10(1.07-1.13)*
Transfusion History				
Yes	-----	-----	1.8(1.1-2.93)	-----
History in jail >24 hours				
Yes	-----	-----	2.5 (1.5-4.1)*	-----
Duration of IDU				
>6 years	-----	2.1(1.4-3.1)*	2.0(1.4-3.0)*	-----
Men sex with men				
Yes	-----		-----	-----
History of STDs				
Yes	1.5(1.1-1.9)*		-----	-----
Number male sex partners				
>3 partners	-----		-----	-----
Number female sex partners				
>3 partners	0.6(0.4-0.9)*		-----	-----

*P value <0.05

Table 4. Multivariable Analyses of Risk Factors for HIV Infection Stratified by Injecting Status Among Drug Users, Houston, Texas.

	HIV		HIV	
Risk Factors	**NIDU OR (95%CI)**	**IDU OR (95%CI)**	**Not MSM OR (95%CI)**	**MSM OR (95%CI)**
Gender				
Male			0.52(0.07-3.84)	-----
Race/Ethnicity				
White	1.00		1.00	1.00
African American	1.9(0.8-4.4)	2.5(1.1-5.5)*	4.93(1.53-15.87)*	2.27(1.04-4.93)*
Others	1.2(0.3-5.0)	3.1(1.2-8.3)*	5.97(1.42-25.07)*	1.71(0.54-5.35)
Age (per year)	1.0(0.98-1.02)	1.0(0.97-1.03)	1.00(0.98-1.02)	1.01(0.98-1.04)
Shelter				
Yes	0.3(0.1-0.9)*		-----	0.39 (0.15-1.00)*
Ever IDU				
Yes	-----		-----	0.61(0.34-1.10)
Men sex with men				
Yes	2.5(1.6-3.9)*	1.8(1.0-3.3)*	-----	-----
History of Chlamydia				
Yes	-----		-----	0.11(0.03-0.38)*
History of genital warts				
Yes	-----		-----	3.28(1.00-10.77)*
Condom				
Never			1.00	1.00
Always	2.1(1.3-3.4)*	5.6(2.8-11.4)*	2.85 (1.81-4.48)*	3.51(1.56-7.88)*
Sometimes		2.7(1.4-5.1)*	1.45(0.95-2.21)*	2.14(1.12-4.09)*
Number male sex partners				
0			1.00	
1-3 partners			4.38(0.58-33.32)	
>3 partners	2.6(1.5-4.5)*		6.92(0.92-52.12)	
Number female sex partners				
0				1.00
1-3 partners				0.26(0.13-0.53)*
>3 partners	0.4(0.3-0.7)*	0.4(0.2-0.7)*		0.16(0.08-0.31)*

IDU stratification adjusted for history in jail for >24 hours, duration of IDU, history of STDs

MSM stratification adjusted for alcohol use, methamphetamine, cocaine use in the past 30 days, crack use in the past 48 hours, duration of IDU, trading for sex/money past 30 days, history of syphilis or genital herpes

*p value<0.05

Table 5. Multivariable Analyses of Risk Factors for HIV Infection Stratified by Injecting Status and MSM Status Among Drug Users, Houston, Texas.

3.4 Prevalence and risk factors associated with Hepatitis C virus infection

The prevalence of HCV infection in this population was 36.1%. Of 668 participants infected with HCV, 61.7% were coinfected with HBV. In Tables 1 and 2, gender, age, race, history of drug treatment, history of transfusion, history of being in jail for >24 hours, sexuality, methamphetamine use, heroin use, history of injecting drugs, history of sharing needles or works, sexuality, history of STD, and history of diagnosis or treatment for syphilis all showed significant differences between HCV positive and negative participants univariately. After adjustment in the multivariable analysis, increasing age {OR= 1.10 (95% CI 1.08, 1.12)}, history of injection drug use {OR= 9.4 (95% CI 7.4, 12.1)}, and having a history of a transfusion {OR= 1.6 (95% CI 1.1, 2.3)}were all still independently associated with HCV infection, while African American race was inversely related to HCV infection {OR= 0.4 (95% CI 0.3, 0.6)} (Table 3).

Because of the striking difference between injectors (70%) and non-injectors (17.9%) in HCV positive study participants, and the overwhelming magnitude of association between injection drug use status and HCV positivity, stratification by injection status was performed to uncover risk characteristics of non-IDUs that may have been masked. In the multivariable analysis, increasing age and having a history of transfusion were found to be independently associated with HCV infection among non-IDUs. African American race was inversely related with HCV infection (Table 4). The significant variables associated with HCV infection among injectors after adjustment were increasing age, having been in jail for more than 24 hours, and injecting drugs for more than 5 years, while African American race remained inversely associated with HCV infection (Table 4).

4. Discussion

This is the first study to evaluate both IDUs and non-IDUs for HIV, HBV and HCV infections in not-in-treatment urban community settings. In this study, prevalence of HIV, HBV, and HCV was 9%, 45% and 36% respectively. The predominant risk characteristics associated with HIV infection in drug users are sexual behaviors, especially MSM, while the predominant risk characteristic associated with HBV and HCV infections is injection drug use. African American race among IDUs is positively associated with HIV and HBV infections and inversely associated with HCV infection. Increasing age is significantly associated with HBV and HCV infections, but not with HIV infection. Duration of injection drug use is also significantly associated with HBV and HCV infections.

Sexual behaviors are the most prevalent risk factors associated with HIV in this study of primarily African American crack cocaine users, which we have found in our previous studies [4, 5]. Any altering substance, such as crack cocaine and methamphetamines, can influence a person to engage in higher frequencies of risky sexual acts, which increases the total number of exposure events, resulting in a higher likelihood of being infected with HIV [17, 21-23]. Crack cocaine is the drug of choice in this study, as 98% of the participants used this drug, with very few using other drugs, such as methamphetamines. Several studies have shown that crack cocaine users engage in more unprotected sexual acts, trade sex for money or drugs and have more sexually transmitted diseases, all factors contributing to greater risk for HIV infection [17, 21, 23-26]. One third of the study participants had a history of injection drug use, but no associations were identified between IDU and HIV infection in males or females in this study, a conflicting finding from other studies [27-31]. Therefore, crack cocaine use and resulting sexual behaviors from its use infer the most likely way HIV is transmitted amongst drug users in this population.

Study participants that had more than 3 male partners were more likely to have HIV than study participants with less male partners in the past 30 days, emphasizing the point of higher frequencies of sexual acts increases exposure. This result remains significant for non-IDU HIV infected study participants and non-MSM female study participants. Non-IDU and IDU HIV infected MSMs show greater likelihood of infection, adding credence to this finding. Two variables to help explain these risky sexual acts, condom use and trading sex for money or drugs, failed to show a significant association in this study, after adjustment for other variables. Men traded sex for money or drugs more often than women in this study, but neither group showed a significant association. However, 40% of the men that traded sex had at least one male sexual partner in their lifetime, clouding the association between HIV infection and trading sex due to the collinearity of "trading sex" and "MSM" variables. Frequency of partners may have also been collinear with trading sex, and they really point to the same issue, whether being male or female, heterosexual or homosexual, the more partners and unprotected acts one has, the increase in likelihood for exposure to HIV. Of note, the measurement tool captured sexual activity in the past 30 days, not lifetime risk, and prevalent data does not necessarily reflect the risk profile of the study participant at the time of HIV acquisition. This is the case with condom use. Study participants were more likely to be HIV infected and always use a condom.

The majority of study participants in this study are African American. It is important to note that studies on African American male sexual behaviors show incongruity between reported sexual identity and actual behavior, greater in African American MSM, but other races as well [32]. Williams et al. [33] conducted qualitative analyses of HIV positive gay identifying and non-gay identifying African Americans, and revealed consequences of alienation, low self-esteem, unsupportive networks, a need to protect their HIV status, and inconsistent condom use after acknowledgement of the importance of condom use due to race and sexual orientation status. The higher prevalence of HIV in African American MSM and their higher level of bisexual activity can put African American women at risk, therefore identifying two high risk groups where sensitive interventions need to be developed and delivered in supportive surroundings. Our study also alludes to the importance of African American MSM and their risk for HIV infection. In the MSM stratification analysis, minority races were significantly more at risk for HIV infection versus Caucasians. Most of our MSM were African American, 69%, followed by Caucasian, 24%, further heightening the urgency to reach this very high risk group. In this group of drug users, having a male partner, whether bisexual or homosexual, is an overwhelming risk factor for HIV infection, and may be interrelated with injection drug use. IDU does not show to be a significant risk factor in this study for HIV infection, however, the correlation between MSM status and IDU status may be masking the true association. It is logical to assume that an MSM-IDU has the greatest risk for HIV infection.

While sexual practices were associated with HIV infection, injecting practices were significant factors associated with HBV or HCV infection in this same population. This study supports previous work that risky injection drug use practices result in the transmission of HBV or HCV [4, 7, 11, 13, 34-36], and the longer one injects, in regards to age and duration, in a high risk population, the more likely the person will be infected [11-13, 37, 38]. However, sharing needles was not associated with HBV or HCV in this study, contrasting a previous study by our principal investigator [4], and others [13]. This most likely reflects the strong correlation between history of injection drug use and sharing paraphernalia occurring in this study.

African American IDUs in this study were less likely to have HCV infection, but were more likely to have HBV infection, a conclusion supported by two other studies that did not stratify by injection drug use [4, 39]. One last finding associated with HCV infection among IDUs is history of being in jail for at least 24 hours or more. Possible explanations that were not explored in this study but were found in other studies are sharing needles in jail, and/or receiving a tattoo in jail, but all consistently found a high prevalence of HCV in the prison/jail systems, heightening the risk for HCV infection [13, 40, 41].

Non-injecting drug users with HBV infection were more likely to have reported a history of STD and be older, but less likely to have more than 3 female sex partners. Non-injectors with HCV infection were associated with transfusion history, increasing age, but less likely to be African American. The median age of the study participants in this study is 43, and documented to be participating in risky drug and sexual behaviors, plus vulnerable to infection, therefore, increasing age is an understandable risk. Sexual behavior in non-injecting drug users may be influenced by stimulant drug activity, especially crack cocaine [17, 21, 23-26], influencing the drug user to participate in risky sexual behaviors, resulting in increased risk for HIV, hepatitis B, and STDs. From our previous studies and others, there was no significant association found between HCV infection and sexual risk behaviors [4, 34]. Transfusion-associated HCV has been documented [42].

HIV, HBV, and HCV infections, drug use behaviors, and social network dynamics vary widely between populations, even at the neighborhood level. This analysis applies directly only to drug users in the urban neighborhoods in Houston, although generalizations about urban drug users may be used to guide further research in other communities. Every attempt to limit recall bias by limiting the reference period for recall of events and reporting bias through using discretion in interviewing and questions deemed appropriate throughout the pilot study was made, but some bias inevitably exists in the data. High-risk activity may have changed with time, either independent of or dependent on, one's HIV or HBV/HCV serostatus, masking true associations that were not covered by the timeframe in question or creating the appearance of spurious associations between HIV or HBV/HCV and current behaviors that had not been expressed at the time of infection.

Characterizing determinants of risk for HIV, HBV, or HCV infection among drug users will improve targeting of health services and prevention education. The greatest association between HIV and drug users in this study was sexual practices, while injecting drug use was the greatest factor associated with HBV and HCV infections. African American drug users are disproportionately affected by these three blood-borne diseases. The vaccine for HBV is being underutilized in high risk drug users, and outreach efforts to understand the barriers to accepting HBV vaccination need to be explored to prevent further HBV transmission. Studies targeting young drug users to prevent initiation into injecting or curb injecting soon after initiation combined with using social networks for counseling about prevention of these three diseases will impact and interrupt transmission cycles.

5. Acknowledgements

We would like to thank the efforts of our field data collection staff, Lawrence Duncan, Madelyn Randle, Janice Robinson, and Edward Johnson, as well as our Field Coordinators, Sandra Timpson, Jay Johnson and Janel Dennison. For supportive data analysis, we would like to thank Shenying Fang and Rui Xia. This study was funded by The National Institute of Drug Abuse (NIDA# 1R01DA017505).

6. References

[1] Shah S.M., Shapshak P., Rivers J. E., Stewart R. V., Weatherby N. L., Xin K. Q. *et al.* Detection of HIV-1 DNA in needles/syringes, paraphernalia, and washes from shooting galleries in Miami: a preliminary laboratory report. *J Acquir Immune Defic Syndr Hum Retrovirol* 1996; 11: 301-6.

[2] Bradshaw C. S., Pierce L. I., Tabrizi S. N., Fairley C. K., Garland S. M. Screening injecting drug users for sexually transmitted infections and blood borne viruses using street outreach and self collected sampling. *Sex Transm Infect* 2005; 81: 53-8.

[3] Mehta S. H., Galai N., Astemborski J., Celentano D. D., Strathdee S. A., Vlahov D. *et al.* HIV incidence among injection drug users in Baltimore, Maryland (1988-2004). *J Acquir Immune Defic Syndr* 2006; 43: 368-72.

[4] Hwang L. Y., Ross M. W., Zack C., Bull L., Rickman K., Holleman M. Prevalence of sexually transmitted infections and associated risk factors among populations of drug abusers. *Clin Infect Dis* 2000; 31: 920-26.

[5] Ross M. W., Hwang L. Y., Leonard L., Teng M., Duncan L. Sexual behaviour, STDs and drug use in a crack house population. *Int J STD AIDS* 1999; 10: 224-30.

[6] Gold R., Skinner M., Ross M. Unprotected anal intercourse in HIV-infected and non-HIV-infected gay men. *J Sex Res* 1994; 31: 59-77.

[7] Koester S., Hoffer L. "Indirect Sharing:" Additional HIV risks associated with drug injection. *AIDS Public Policy J* 1994; 9: 100-05.

[8] McCoy C., Inciardi J. *Sex, Drugs, and Continuing Spread of AIDS*. Los Angeles: Roxbury Publishing Company, 1995.

[9] Kippax S., Campbell D., Van de Ven P., Crawford J., Prestage G., Knox S. *et al.* Cultures of sexual adventurism as markers of HIV seroconversion: A case control study in a cohort of Sydney gay men. *AIDS Care* 1998; 10: 677-88.

[10] Clatts M. C., Heimer R., Abdala N., Goldsamt L. A., Sotheran J. L., Anderson K. T. *et al.* HIV-1 transmission in injection paraphernalia: heating drug solutions may inactivate HIV-1. *J Acquir Immune Defic Syndr* 1999; 22: 194-99.

[11] Gyarmathy V. A., Neaigus A., Miller M., Friedman S. R., Des Jarlais D. C. Risk correlates of prevalent HIV, hepatitis B virus, and hepatitis C virus infections among noninjecting heroin users. *J Acquir Immune Defic Syndr* 2002; 30: 448-56.

[12] Garten R. J., Lai S., Zhang J., Liu W., Chen J., Vlahov D. *et al.* Rapid transmission of hepatitis C virus among young injecting heroin users in Southern China. *Int J Epidemiol* 2004; 33: 182-88.

[13] Samuel M. C., Doherty P. M., Bulterys M., Jenison S. A. Association between heroin use, needle sharing and tattoos received in prison with hepatitis B and C positivity among street-recruited injecting drug users in New Mexico, USA. *Epidemiol Infect* 2001; 127: 475-84.

[14] Daniels D., Grytdal S., Wasley A. Surveillance for acute viral hepatitis-United States, 2007. *MMWR Surveill Summ* 2009; 58: 1-27.

[15] Gordon C.M., Carey M., Carey K.B. Effects of a drinking event on behavioral skills and condom attitudes in men: implications for HIV risk from a controlled experiment. *Health Psychol* 1997; 16: 490-95.

[16] Booth R.E., Watters J. How effective are risk-reduction interventions targeting injecting drug users? *AIDS* 1994; 8: 1515-24.

[17] Edlin B. R., Irwin K. L., Faruque S., McCoy C. B., Word C., Serrano Y. *et al.* Intersecting Epidemics--Crack Cocaine Use and HIV Infection among Inner-City Young Adults. *N Engl J Med* 1994; 331: 1422-27.

[18] Wilson T., DeHovitz J. A. STDs, HIV, and crack cocaine: a review. *AIDS Patient Care STDS* 1997; 11: 62-6.

[19] Petry N. M. Alcohol use in HIV patients: What we don't know may hurt us. *Int J STD AIDS* 1999; 10: 561-70.

[20] Siegal H. A., Falck R. S., Wang J., Carlson R. G. History of sexually transmitted diseases infection, drug-sex behaviors, and the use of condoms among midwestern users of injection drugs and crack cocaine. *Sex Transm Dis* 1996; 23: 277-82.

[21] Jones D. L., Irwin K. L., Inciardi J., Bowser B., Schilling R., Word C. *et al.* The High-Risk Sexual Practices of Crack-Smoking Sex Workers Recruited From the Streets of Three American Cities. *Sex Transm Dis* 1998; 25: 187-93.

[22] Campsmith M. L., Nakashima A. K., Jones J. L. Association between crack cocaine use and high-risk sexual behaviors after HIV diagnosis. *J Acquir Immune Defic Syndr* 2000; 25: 192-98.

[23] Booth R. E., Watters J. K., Chitwood D. D. HIV Risk-Related Sex Behaviors among Injection Drug Users, Crack Smokers, and Injection Drug Users Who Smoke Crack. *Am J Public Health* 1993; 83: 1144-48.

[24. McCoy C. B., Lai S., Metsch L. R., Messiah S. E., Zhao W. Injection Drug Use and Crack Cocaine Smoking: Independent and Dual Risk Behaviors for HIV Infection. *Ann Epidemiol* 2004; 14: 535-42.

[25] Kral A. H., Bluthenthal R. N., Booth R. E., Watters J. K. HIV Seroprevalence among Street-Recruited Injection Drug and Crack Cocaine Users in 16 US Municipalities. *Am J Public Health* 1998; 88: 108-12.

[26] Hudgins R., McCusker J., Stoddard A. Cocaine use and risky injection and sexual behaviors. *Drug Alcohol Depend* 1995; 37: 7-14.

[27] Nguyen T. A., Hoang L. T., Pham V. Q., Detels R. Risk factors for HIV-1 seropositivity in drug users under 30 years old in Haiphong, Vietnam. *Addiction* 2001; 96: 405-13.

[28] Kozlov A. P., Shaboltas A. V., Toussova O. V., Verevochkin S. V., Masse B. R., Perdue T. *et al.* HIV incidence and factors associated with HIV acquisition among injection drug users in St Petersburg, Russia. *AIDS* 2006; 20: 901-6.

[29] Ruan Y., Qin G., Liu S., Qian H., Zhang L., Zhou F. *et al.* HIV incidence and factors contributed to retention in a 12-month follow-up study of injection drug users in Sichuan Province, China. *J Acquir Immune Defic Syndr* 2005; 39: 459-63.

[30] Kawichai S., Celentano D. D., Vongchak T., Beyrer C., Suriyanon V., Razak M. H. *et al.* HIV voluntary counseling and testing and HIV incidence in male injecting drug users in northern Thailand: evidence of an urgent need for HIV prevention. *J Acquir Immune Defic Syndr* 2006; 41: 186-93.

[31] Barrio G., De La Fuente L., Toro C., Brugal T. M., Soriano V., Gonzalez F. *et al.* Prevalence of HIV infection among young adult injecting and non-injecting heroin users in Spain in the era of harm reduction programmes: gender differences and other related factors. *Epidemiol Infect* 2007; 135: 592-603.

[32] Millett G., Malebranche D., Mason B., Spikes P. Focusing "down low": bisexual black men, HIV risk and heterosexual transmission. *J Natl Med Assoc* 2005; 97(7Suppl): 52S-59S.

[33] Williams J. K., Wyatt G. E., Resell J., Peterson J., Asuan-O'Brien A. Psychosocial issues among gay- and non-gay-identifying HIV-seropositive African American and Latino MSM. *Cultur Divers Ethnic Minor Psychol* 2004; 10: 268-86.

[34] Hammer G. P., Kellogg T. A., McFarland W. C., Wong E., Louie B., Williams I. *et al.* Low incidence and prevalence of hepatitis C virus infection among sexually active non-intravenous drug-using adults, San Francisco, 1997-2000. *Sex Transm Dis* 2003; 30: 919-24.

[35] Bialek S. R., Bower W. A., Mottram K., Purchase D., Nakano T., Nainan O. *et al.* Risk factors for hepatitis B in an outbreak of hepatitis B and D among injection drug users. *J Urban Health* 2005; 82: 468-78.

[36] Hagan H., McGough J. P., Thiede H., Weiss N. S., Hopkins S., Alexander E. R. Syringe exchange and risk of infection with hepatitis B and C viruses. *Am J Epidemiol* 1999; 149: 203-13.

[37] Nyamathi A. M., Dixon E. L., Robbins W., Smith C., Wiley D., Leake B. *et al.* Risk factors for hepatitis C virus infection among homeless adults. *J Gen Intern Med* 2002; 17: 134-43.

[38] Garfein R. S., Vlahov D., Galai N., Doherty M. C., Nelson K. E. Viral infections in short-term injection drug users: the prevalence of the hepatitis C, hepatitis B, human immunodeficiency, and human T-lymphotropic viruses. *Am J Public Health* 1996; 86: 655-61.

[39] Butterfield M. I., Bosworth H. B., Stechuchak K. M., Frothingham R., Bastian L. A., Meador K. G. *et al.* Racial differences in hepatitis B and hepatitis C and associated risk behaviors in veterans with severe mental illness. *J Natl Med Assoc* 2004; 96: 43-52.

[40] Babudieri S., Longo B., Sarmati L., Starnini G., Dori L., Suligoi B. *et al.* Correlates of HIV, HBV, and HCV infections in a prison inmate population: results from a multicentre study in Italy. *J Med Virol* 2005; 76: 311-17.

[41] Hennessey K. A., Kim A. A., Griffin V., Collins N. T., Weinbaum C. M., Sabin K. Prevalence of infection with hepatitis B and C viruses and co-infection with HIV in three jails: a case for viral hepatitis prevention in jails in the United States. *J Urban Health* 2009; 86: 93-105.

[42] Armstrong G. L., Wasley A., Simard E. P., McQuillan G. M., Kuhnert W. L., Alter M. J. The prevalence of hepatitis C virus infection in the United States, 1999 through 2002. *Ann Intern Med* 2006; 144: 705-14.

4

Isolator System For Laboratory Infectious Animals

Xin Pan
Animal Biosafety Level 3 Laboratory, Second Military Medical University, Shanghai, China

1. Introduction

The international mutual acceptance of safety data in certification and accreditation system have led to high-level bio-safety laboratories becoming an irreplaceable hardware in peacetime for the study of pathogen in emerging and re-emerging infectious disease, and in important international activities for detection and identification high-risk pathogen in antiterrorism security.

In an effort to minimize the risks for scientists exposure to the infectious environment and avoiding infectious incident, high-level bio-safety laboratories are designed and constructed to improve experimental safety by preventing laboratory infectious waste causing harm to people or the environment. The possibility of high-risk pathogens spread to the public environment with flow of people and materials and water and air is strictly controlled by improvement physical protection to reduce human infection rates and incidence of environment contamination to zero. The air flow safety, including interior mechanical ventilations and the suction and exhaust process in large working process equipments, is ensured by installing air conditioning system, air filter system, one working and one on standby extraction blowers, constant or variable air volume damper in pipes, automation and monitoring system, and power supply system (including dual power supply system and online emergency power supply) to maintain suitable directional negative filtering air flow with constant temperature and humidity working conditions for the operators. The materials flow safety, including experimental materials, laboratory animals and laboratory infectious waste, is mastered by installing transfer system (including delivery window and double port transfer exchange system) and sterilization system (double-doored autoclave). The liquid flow safety, including launching and softened water, is controlled by reverse osmosis disinfection system and independent sewage discharge system (including high temperature and high pressure sterilizer and chemical disinfection tank). The people flow safety, including walking around in the laboratory, carrying out experimental procedures, changing protective clothing, and physiological activity such as respiration, is protected by primary barriers (including biological safety cabinet and negative-pressure isolator), secondary barriers (building envelope and facility construction), third barriers (personal protective equipment, PPE), communication systems between the lab and outside, visual monitoring devices and alarm system.

In high-level bio-safety laboratories, animals infected with Risk Group 3 pathogens (as defined by the World Health Organization) must be housed in isolation chambers (World Health Organization, 2004). Animal isolation system is used broadly in laboratory research, pharmaceuticals and medical areas, gene modified animals, and gnotobiotic animals. Isolators were developed for studying the disease of scrub typhus in 1940 during the Second World War (Bantin, 2004). Today, the isolators are much more advanced, especially the commercial rodent isolator systems (Wathes & Johnson, 1991). But for infectious medium-sized animal (sheep, pigs, goats, nonhuman primates, dogs, cats, rabbits and chickens) research, the market normally supplied semi-open negative pressure cabinet. This kind of cabinet can not provide completely physical barrier for safeguarding animal and occupational health and the odors and allergens environment, because the directly face-to-face manipulation exist between animal and operator in the research procedure. The Class III biological safety cabinet (glove box) was mainly used for experiment operation (Kruse et al., 1991), its internal work area was maintained negative pressure during running state, it was able to provide security, even in the physical prevent contamination system failure. The requirements for wind speed and pressure were relatively higher to maintain the glove box internal laminar flow, but were not conducive to animal care, the occupants had to suffer high stress and uncomfortable environment under the high velocity air flow. If the glove box was simply expanded to an isolator, large area filtration equipment was easy to plug, animal welfare was difficult to achieve in insufficient space (limited height) (Huang, 2005). Recently we developed a set of automatic multi-functional isolation system for feeding (Pan et al., 2010) and dissection and micrurgy laboratory animals carrying infectious diseases. The isolation system, including the transfer chain, disinfection chain, negative air pressure isolation system, animal welfare system and the automated system, are designed to meet all biological safety standards.

Isolator was mainly designed to separate the internal controlled environment from external environment, and the operator from the experimental process and products. The primary aim was to prevent the leakage of the contaminated products within the internal environment to the external environment, or the penetration of substances of the external environment into the internal environment, or both simultaneously (Tattershall, 2006). Isolators were used to improve operators and process safety, avoid operator wearing too many protective suits, improve operator comfort and flexibility and personnel availability, improve safety level against operator errors, completely control the contaminated material and minimize the contaminated area (Sawyer et al., 2007).

There are many types of isolators, mainly included positive pressure isolators and negative pressure isolators. Specified-pathogen-free (SPF) laboratory animals housed in positive pressure isolators for the protection of any animals inside the isolator from outside contaminants (Clough et al., 1995). Infectious animal housed in negative pressure isolators to prevent migration of hazardous contaminants to the outside (Wathes & Johnson, 1991).

In general, the commonly used physical separation mainly included rigid and soft barriers (ISO 14644-7:2004). Rigid barriers can be made of many different materials, and the more rigid the material, the more reliable the physical barrier. Construction of these rigid barriers usually makes of plastic enclosures, metal profile enclosures or hot-worked metal enclosures (ISO 10648-1:1997). The isolation chamber is designed to house a living animal, and therefore continuous airflow inside the enclosure is needed to drive out heat and moisture generated by the animal's metabolism and to decrease the concentration of odor, dust, and infectious substances (Hillman et al., 1992). The resulting exhaust gas is subject to a filtering system designed to prevent pathogen contamination of the external environment (Institute of Laboratory Animal Resources Commission on Life Sciences, National Research Council, 1996). The aerodynamic is joined in the physical separation cabinet to allow for one-way flow or turbulence of the airflow inside the isolation chamber, negative pressure relative to the environment. Supply and exhaust air can be passed through high-efficiency particulate air filters (HEPA) to prevent the formation of aerosols that could potentially escape into the environment (Runkle et al., 1969).

Double port transfer exchange (DPTE) system is used in the isolator to allow the transfer of experiment materials from one container to another without exposing the experiment material to the outside environment (Allen et al., 2009). The technology was developed in the early 1960s by a French company for the French nuclear industry to greatly reduce Alpha and Beta exposures and Gamma dose. The acronym DPTE was originally derived from the French phrase 'double porte de transfert etanche', meaning double door sealed transfer or double door transfer port. A newly validated rapid transfer port boasts bi-directional transfer as one of its features, a system also known as an Alpha-Beta transfer port or rapid transfer port (RTP) (Michael et al., 2004). The biological sciences involving dangerously toxic or infectious materials (such as poisons, bacteria or viruses) also need to use DPTE system as the transfer tool to enclose the dangerous materials without escaping into the surroundings.

Laboratory animal models are often susceptible to a number of diseases and parasites found in humans or economic animals (Tauraso et al., 1969). The similarities of genetic, physiological, and behavioral characteristics between research objects and laboratory animal models, and the occurrence of similar pathological changes upon infection, have led to laboratory animal models becoming an irreplaceable experimental materials for the study of pathogen infection, the screening of anti-pathogen drugs, and vaccine evaluation (Pan & Sun, 2004; Conly & Johnston, 2008). Because of the critical role that laboratory animal models play in the study of these pathogens, it is critical to find safe and reliable methods for their physical containment.

2. Isolator system composition and structure

The structure of stainless-steel medium-sized animal breeding isolator and acrylic mice breeding isolator and acrylic anatomy isolator and acrylic micrurgy isolator include top ventilation unit, isolator working zone, lower part of control system and isolator support frame (Fig. 1).

The isolation chamber is supported by type 304 stainless-steel isolation chamber support stand. The ventilation unit is on the top of the isolation chamber. Stainless-steel slideways are mounted on the top of the isolation chamber box. The pipes, air blower, valve, and adjustable illumination lamp are fastened to the reserved mounting holes or mounting plates of the slideways by a fixing screw.

Two extraction blowers share one exhaust port in which an anemometer is installed. Each of the extraction blowers is connected with its own coupling clamp to the outlet ventilation pipe, exhaust ventilation pipe and exhaust electronic control ball valve to form an exhaust channel. The two exhaust channels have a parallel connection. Two sets of sterilizing agent bypass tubes have a series connection with an ipsilateral sterilizing agent bypass electronic control ball valve, and a parallel connection with the same side of the exhaust ventilation pipe on two ends of the exhaust electronic control ball valve. All of the valves are automatically controlled by the programmable logic controller (PLC).

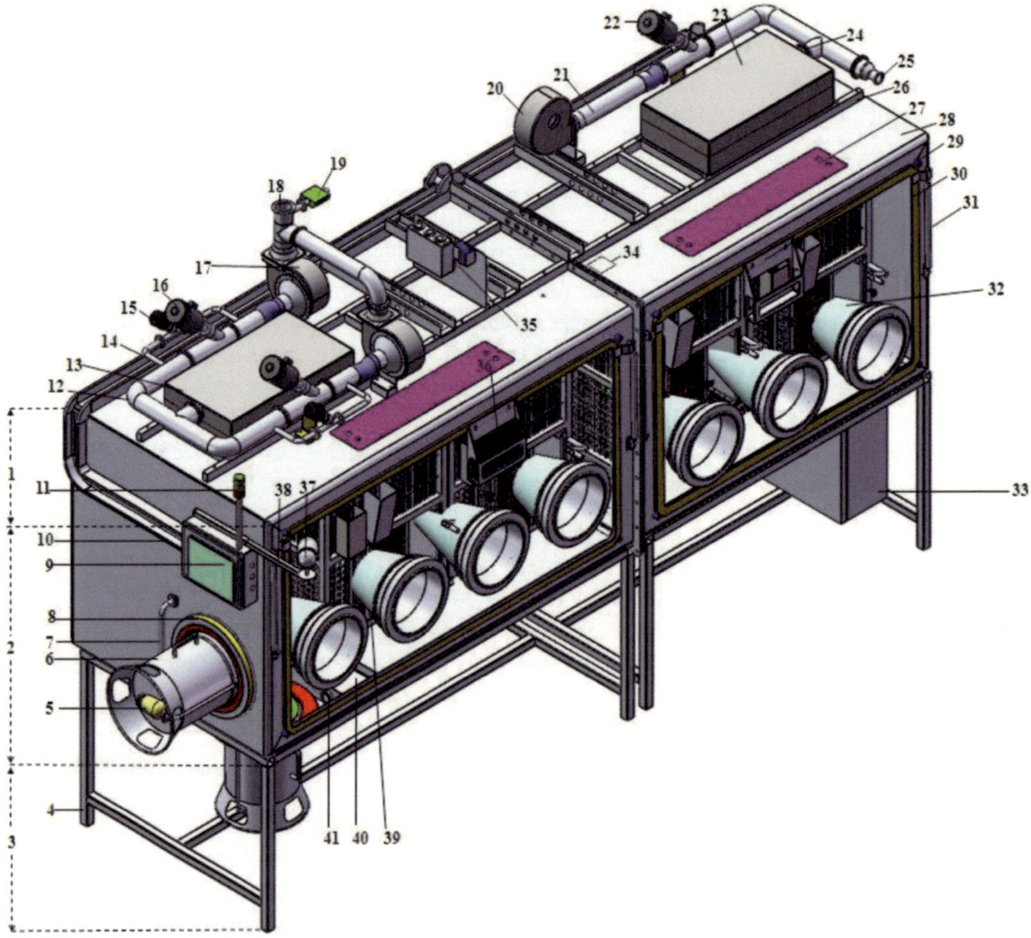

Fig. 1. Structure diagram of stainless-steel medium-sized animal breeding isolator. 1. top ventilation unit; 2. isolation chamber working zone; 3. lower part of the control system; 4. isolation chamber support stand; 5. transfer bin container HEPA filter; 6. DPTE 270 transfer bin container; 7. water inlet pipe; 8. DPTE 270 α door; 9. control touch panel; 10. cable duct; 11. alarm indicator light tower; 12. exhaust ventilation pipe; 13. Two in series HEPA exhaust filters; 14. sterilization bypass pipe; 15. sterilization bypass electric control ball valve; 16. exhaust electronic control ball valve; 17. extraction blower; 18. exhaust export; 19. anemometer; 20. inlet air blower; 21. inlet ventilation pipe; 22. inlet air electronic control ball valve; 23. inlet HEPA filter; 24. coupling clamp for inlet ventilation pipe; 25. sterilization reagent import; 26. top installation slideway; 27. adjustable illumination lamp; 28. stainless-steel box; 29. television-installed box; 30. front door; 31. damping-brace for the front door; 32. glove and sleeve system; 33. control cabinet; 34. temperature humidity sensor; 35. micro-differential pressure sensor; 36. flat television; 37. rotatable camera; 38. installed camera base; 39. animal cage; 40. disinfection pool; 41. drain valve.

The airflow direction through the isolation chamber via the air inlet and outlet is shown in Figure 1. Room air is drawn into the interior of the isolation chamber through the inlet pre-filter, inlet air blower, inlet ventilation pipe, inlet air electronic control ball valve, and inlet HEPA filter in the animal breeding mode. The air from the isolation chamber is drawn out of the exhaust export through two exhaust HEPA filters arranged in series, exhaust ventilation pipe and exhaust electronic control ball valve via an extraction blower. The HEPA filters are arranged in series to ensure that if one fails, the other can still ensure exhaust security and prevent pathogens from being discharged into the atmosphere.

The isolation chamber interior pressure is controlled by automated instrumentation that is connected to the supply and exhaust ventilation system. The automatic pressure regulation system is capable of maintaining the relative pressure inside the isolation chamber via the exhaust ventilation system, which can account for transient volume changes such as glove entry or withdrawal.

The isolation chamber working zone is composed of chamber, doors, glove-sleeve system and DPTE system. The welded box of medium-sized animal breeding isolator is manufactured using dumb-gloss stainless-steel 316L with a thickness of 3 mm. The adhesion acrylic isolator is manufactured with 10mm polymethylmethacrylate (PMMA).

The stainless-steel isolation chamber front door includes damping braces on each front side with dual-pistons mechanism for holding the front door securely open to let the animal cages in, operation panels with stainless-steel 316L framework and the door hinges connected to the stainless steel box. The operation panel is made of transparent PMMA. The transparent front door allows for visualization of the contents of the isolation chamber. Silicone seals around the PMMA panel ensure that the system is air tight. The front door is manually fastened onto the box framework with a hammer bolt. One gas-tight water service valve with a serrated hose is mounted on one side interior. A spray gun is connected to the serrated hose for cleaning the isolator. Animal cages can be placed on the stainless steel cage slideways in the isolator. The slideways are attached to the isolator bottom in a manner that allows cage movement in a direction along the axis perpendicular to the axis of the isolator front door. The type of animal cages can be changed, but each time just only one kind of animal species cages can be inside. In a breeding isolator all the cages share the same air space so the same microbiologically or genetically must be assure.

One door is used as a sidewall in the acrylic isolator. It allows the internal equipments and frames entry. The door can be fixed on the PMMA panel by compressing the gasket and pressure ring around the edge of the door until all the screws are tightened.

There are circular polyethylene (PE)-machined glove ports on the operation panels. The glove-sleeve port inner diameter is 300 mm and the center-to-center spacing of each port is 450 mm. The glove port assembly includes a glove port ring, glove port gasket, pressure ring and glove port inner-securing ring. The glove port ring and glove port inner-securing ring are jointed with a thread connection. The glove port ring edges are fixed on the PMMA panel by compressing the glove port gasket and pressure ring on each side of the PMMA panel by tightening a fixing screw.

The changeable sleeve and glove combination is mounted on the glove port through a sleeve fixing ring that secures the elastic Hypalon sleeve onto the glove port inner-securing ring. A glove port bung connects the glove and sleeve. Neoprene glove shapes are ambidextrous.

The transfer system for the isolation chamber is composed of DPTE systems. The DPTE system with an alpha transfer door is built into one wall of the isolation chamber using a transfer port assembly kit. The transfer port assembly kit includes the DPTE transfer port external flange, DPTE transfer port external flange sealing ring and DPTE transfer port internal flange. The DPTE transfer port external flange is fixed onto the inside isolation chamber wall by compressing the DPTE transfer port external flange sealing ring on the outside of the isolation chamber wall with a tightening fixing screw.

The transfer container is autoclavable and contains a beta door that can be manually docked to the port. The depth of the transfer container can be changed according to the research projects, its volume is enough to transfer the animal or material into the isolator. The transfer container can be autoclaved without compromising its containment and can be opened with a specialized tool to remove the sterilized waste. It also can be opened with the specialized tool in the negative pressure exhaust hood, the samples (such as animal blood samples) can be moved out for further analysis (e.g. centrifugation), while the transfer container is closed and put into a sterilizable plastic bag for autoclaving. This system works very well for rapidly and safely transferring experimental materials and animals and waste.

A videotape system mounted on the control touch panel stainless-steel box on the side of the medium-sized animal breeding isolator includes a rotatable camera and camera-installation base. The camera installation base is fastened to the control touch panel stainless-steel box by fixing screws. The position of the rotation camera can be adjusted by using the telescopic locking nut and rotating locking nut. This system enables recording of both the scientist's experimental procedures and the status of animals living in the isolation chamber. The video is displayed on the personal computer (PC) screen and saved automatically in the central control room through the control interface connected to the videotape system.

To ensure the comfort and welfare of animals in the isolation chamber, chambers are equipped with an automatic light control system and a television entertainment system. The automatic light control system includes adjustable illumination lamps and a lampshade. The adjustable illumination lamps are composed of three cold light lamps and their conditioners. The illumination system can be used to meet the needs of the animal's physiology, as well as experimental requirements.

The television entertainment system consists of a flat television and the transparent television installation box fastened to the front door by fixing screws. The animal can watch the appropriate television program to reduce depression associated with the space constraints faced by the animals and to ensure the ethical treatment of the animals.

The videotape system and lamps and television do not mount on the acrylic isolators. The videotape system and lamps in the laboratory can provide related services for transparent acrylic isolators.

The composition of the isolation control system includes an alarm indicator light tower, liquid crystal display (LCD) touch screen and control cabinet. The liquid crystal display touch screen is fastened on the outside of the isolation chamber by a fixing screw.

The PLC is built into the control cabinet. The control cabinet, which has a fan and a filter cover, is mounted onto the stainless steel shelf of isolator support stand through fasteners and fixing screw.

3. Intelligent control of isolator system

Simatic Manager Step 7 software installed in the PLC central processing unit (CPU), and through the LCD touch screen enables users to automatically control a variety of options. The animal breeding mode program, leakage test program, sterilization program, auto/manual control mode, maintenance mode, and custom procedure can all be automatically controlled by the PLC CPU and associated touch screen (Pan et al., 2010).

The management system for isolator touch screen is developed by Simatic Wincc flexible software. The operation and any system failures can be recorded and printed. The data interchange between PLC and touch screen is made possible through an industrial trunk Profibus decentralized periphery (DP).

The temperature, humidity, illumination, atmospheric pressure and air flow velocity are measured by appropriate sensors, and the values are imported to the PLC through control lines. Normal value ranges for each parameter can be programmed into the PLC, and if the parameter values deviate from the set upper and lower limits, the PLC automatically adjusts the interior environment of the isolator to match the programmed values. For example, the levels of humidity, illumination and ventilation can all be controlled by the PLC to adjust values back to pre-determined normal levels. If the PLC is unable to bring the parameter back into a normal range, the digital output module in the PLC lights an alarm bulb and sounds a buzzer, as all alarms are indicated with both a warning light and sound.

The control system controls alarms for a variety of isolation chamber problems including major equipment error alarms (such as the air blower or HEPA), major parameter alarms when values are out of the desirable ranges (such as temperature, humidity, illumination, atmospheric pressure, air exchange rate and air flow velocity), an alarm when switching to the uninterruptible power supply (UPS) / emergency power supply (EPS) and alarms for experimental failure or error (such as negative pressure breeding mode procedures or pressure test procedures).

To control pressure, a micro-differential pressure sensor is mounted on the side of the first exhaust filter. The analog module in the PLC compares the values of program settings with the values collected from the micro-differential pressure sensor, and automatically conducts proportional-integral-differential (PID) regulation. The adjusted output values are used to control blower velocity through the output module of the PLC, regulating the isolation chamber internal pressure. If a plug or leak occurs, the micro-differential pressure sensor transmits the detected signal to the PLC. If the detected values are beyond the scope of the pre-loaded high and low pressure settings, the exhaust electronic control ball valve and inlet air electronic control ball valve automatically shut down to maintain the isolation chamber as a fully-contained environment and to prevent the escape of pathogens into the outside environment. At the same time an alarm indicator light tower would start to sound an Alarm, and the touch-screen would display information on the alarm. The alarm information would then be transmitted to the lab server through the industrial Ethernet module in the PLC. The alarm message displayed is recorded onto the lab server for analysis at a later date.

The blower rotation rate and frequency are automatically controlled by the PLC system to ensure that the airflow velocity, air exchange rate, and atmospheric pressure match the set values. If one exhaust blower fails, the PLC system responds by switching to another backup exhaust blower to ensure ventilation safety and the internal negative pressure state of the isolation chamber.

The cold light lamp regulator is controlled by the PLC digital output module to automatically adjust the illumination time according to animal behavior. The illumination time and intensity can be set from the touch screen by the operator and automatically executed. The lamps also can be switched on or off manually to meet different lighting requirements during an experimental operation.

Temperature and humidity sensors are equipped within the isolator. The isolator internal temperature is maintained within 18～29°C, and relative humidity is kept within 40～70%. The isolator internal temperature and humidity electrical signals are collected by the PLC analog module, visualized as the project value (actual values of temperature and humidity), and automatically displayed and recorded on the touch screen. The values also recorded on the lab server.

4. Installation isolator system in high-level biosafety laboratory

The design of isolator system in high-level biosafety laboratory must consider about types and groups of laboratory animals, shape and actual area of the experiment field in order to the effective utilization of the independent negative-pressure ventilation system of the robust isolator offering maximizing population density and the welfare of animals. The isolator support frames and box bodies can be assembled after laboratory partitions and self-leveling floors and cable ducts on the sidewall all being in the right place. Once the large-scale isolators have been installation, the movements are quite difficult.

The vent thread hose mounted on the exhaust export of the isolator is connected to laboratory heating, ventilation and air conditioning (HVAC) exhaust main pipe via constant volume venturi valve and dynamoelectric airtight valve. The airflow velocity through each open glove port can be regulated using the external venturi valve. The air from the type 304 stainless-steel main pipe is drawn out of the exhaust export through the exhaust in-place scan testable HEPA filter combination unit via the laboratory extraction blower. This connection can reduce the exhaust exports of the building and comply with environmental protection requirements.

The isolator locating leaks may be detected by placing a dish of ammonia and using compressed air to pressurize with a positive pressure of up to 1000 Pa. Suspected areas will turn blue for the leaked ammonia reacts with bromine on the covered yellow bromide developing cloth. Leaks are commonly in soft and hard junction. The gel has to be removed and the sealing ring has to be cleaned or replaced and resealed with gel.

5. Detection the technology performance parameters of isolator system

The technology performance parameters of isolator system are established according with related China national standards and European standards and international standards (Table 1).

TSI8386A-M-GB multi-parameter ventilation meter is used to detect airflow differential pressure, vertical section airflow velocity and air velocity into open glove port. BCJ-1 airborne particle counter is used to measure air cleanliness. TES-1350A sound level meter is used to monitor noise. Testo540 luxmeter illumination tester is used to measure illumination. MARK-Ⅱ micro manometer was used to test alarm function. TSI8386A-M-GB and HM34C humidty / temperature meter are used to checkout pressure integrity. Test procedures are carried out according to the protocol as GB50591-2010, GB19489-2008 and ISO10648-2:1994 described.

Apply power and clean compressed air to the isolator before testing. The main power on the control cabinet is first turned on. Turn on the lock-controlled switch. The experimental personnel exit the lab to start and run the high-level biosafety laboratory HVAC in central control room. Personal protective clothing should be worn when entering the running normally lab to perform testing work. Detecting equipments are transferred into isolation chamber by DPTE container. The starting and stopping control and the setup of operating parameters of isolator can be controlled by staff to adopt computer technology to remote control in central control room, or to implement on-the-spot control with control touch panel of the isolator. The current operating parameters are displayed on the touch screen interface and can be adjusted by the operator following the interface prompts.

The room lamps are turned off in order to measure the independent illumination system of the stainless-steel isolator. The illumination of acrylic isolator without independent lamp is detected by using the lab illumination system.

The accuracy temperature control of air-conditioning system with all fresh air in the lab is 0.5°C. The HVAC has to be turned off when using pressure change method to test the isolator leak tightness. The leak rate test data are obtained by detecting in relatively stable room temperature. The glove-sleeve systems need to be changed by blind plates. Each overexpansion glove-sleeve in 1000Pa can create tiny deformation to change volume during the pressure changing and the air volume changes can result in significant pressure attenuation during the multi-glove-sleeve system detection stage. Flexible film windows of micrurgy isolator also have to be changed by blind plates.

The glove-sleeve system must be in place during operation and a breach in glove integrity can be serious consequence. The multi-glove-sleeve system cannot complete extension into the isolator in -250 Pa. The guideline for ABSL-4 building enclosure integrity test on GB19489-2008 is selected for measurement the isolator with the multi-glove-sleeve system or flexible film windows or both in place. The natural attenuation of pressure is less than 250 Pa in 20 min when the isolator internal air pressure down to -500Pa. This test is also a good

Testing Items	Parameters	Reference
Temperature, ℃	18～29	Architectural and technical code for laboratory animal facility. GB50447-2008
Diurnal temperature, ℃ ≤	4	
Relative humidity, %	40～70	
Vertical section airflow velocity, m/s ≤	0.2	
Air changes per hour, ACH	8～50	Laboratory animal- requirements of environment and housing facilities. GB14925-2001
Airflow differential pressure, Pa	20～150	
Air cleanliness, class	100～10000	
Settling microbe, cfu/(Φ90mm • 0.5h)	0	
Light / dark rhythms, h	12/12 or 10/14	
Animal illumination, lux	5～200	
Working illumination, lux ≥	150	
Noise, dB ≤	68	Architectural and technical code for biosafety laboratories. GB50346- 2004
Air velocity into open glove port, m/s ≥	0.7	Biotechnology-Performance criteria for microbiological safety cabinets. EN 12469:2000
-1000 Pa hourly leak rate (rateacceptance test), h^{-1} <	2.5×10^{-3}	Containment enclosures - Part 2: Classification according to leak tightness and associated checking methods. ISO10648-2:1994
-500 Pa pressure attenuation in 20 min (glove- sleeve in place), Pa ≤	250	Laboratories-General equirements for biosafety. GB19489-2008

Table 1. The technology performance parameters of isolator.

way to perform to be sure the leak rate is in the tolerable range before starting the experiment. This kind of periodic testing should be established and recorded for comparison preventative maintenance requirements.

The test results of isolator system have been compiled together in table 2 and they all meet technology criterion. The isolator internal dust concentration test indicate that the result for particle size ≥0.5μm is ≤3.5 particles/L, for particle size ≥5.0μm is 0 particles/L. It is supposed that the air cleanliness in isolator internal is Class 100. The temperature of the isolator internal is 0.1-0.5°C below room temperature. The relative humidity of the isolator internal is determined by the lab atmosphere.

Isolator -1000 Pa pressure decay test results show in figure 2. During the acceptance test, inlet air blower, inlet air electronic control ball valve, sterilizing agent by-pass electronic control ball valve, exhaust electronic control ball valve and extraction blower are all closed. Part of the inlet ventilation pipes, an inlet HEPA filter, two exhaust HEPA filters arranged in series, part of exhaust ventilation pipes and part of sterilizing agent bypass tubes are all in the range of pressure integrity testing. If leakage present in the installed HEPA filters, the negative or positive pressure tests will be failure. Anyway the isolators pass through the

Type of isolator	Vertical section airflow velocity (m/s)	-1000Pa hourly leak rate(h^{-1})	-500Pa pressure attenuation in 20min (Pa)	Air velocity into open glove port (m/s)	Airflow differential pressure ΔP(pa)	Interior dust concentration (Particles/L)				Noise	Illumination (average values)	
						Maximum average values of measuring points		Statistical mean values in isolator working zone		[dB(A)]	(lux)	
						≥0.5μm	≥5.0μm	≥0.5μm	≥5.0 μm		Animal illumination	Working illumination
medium-sized arimal breeding isolator	0.03	$1.54x10^{-3}$	76.1	0.72	-55.9	0	0	0	0	60.8	17	162
mice breeding isolator	0.06	$1.59x10^{-3}$	31.4	0.72	-65.8	0	0	0	0	67.3		282
anatomy isolator	0.04	$1.03x10^{-3}$	132.6	0.71	-62.5	0.24	0	0.15	0	64.7		349
micrurgy isolator	0.02	$0.96x10^{-3}$	101.4	0.70	-51.6	0.47	0	1.10	0	67.1		367

Table 2. Measuring results of isolators.

leakage rates tests in both positive and negative states. During normal operation, the directional air flow from the isolation chamber to the exhaust export and into the attached thread chimney should pass through two exhaust HEPA filters arranged in series. Airborne contaminants in the isolator are removed by the two HEPA filters, so the vent thread hose and the part of the exhaust ventilation pipes installed behind the electronic control ball valves need not do the leak rate test with the isolator. Even the leakage present among the hoses, the laboratory is in the negative pressure atmospheric conditions, the emitted particles can be mechanical captured by the lab filters. The exhaust in-place scan testable

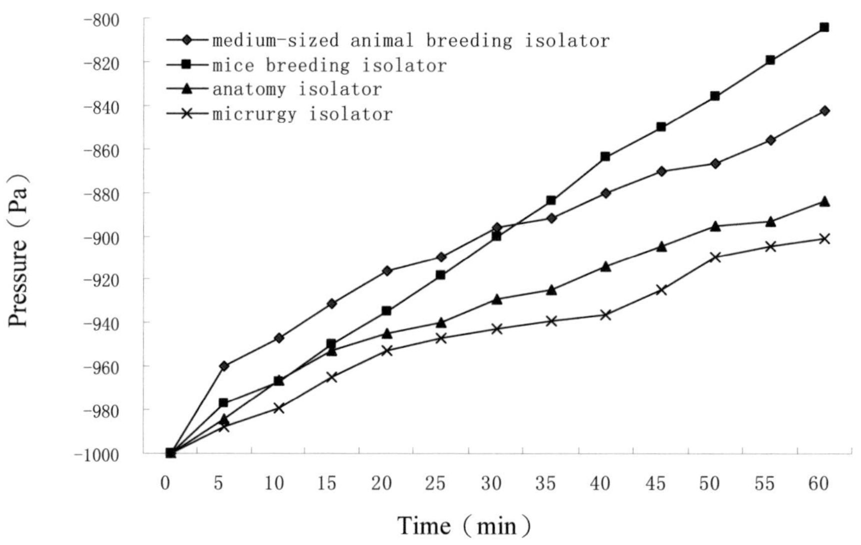

Fig. 2. Negative 1000Pa pressure decay test of isolator.

HEPA filter combination housing assembly is another important downstream exhaust filter devices of isolators and the lab before the air flow can disperse to the environment. The airborne contaminants can be detected by the leakage detection device of the unit if the leaks occur in-service. The actual test results of the exhaust filter units downstream are zero particles/L.

The maximum airflow rate of the isolator is 180 m^3/h and the maximum air exchange rates is 36 ACH. The airflow rates of the laboratory are 740 ~ 3900 m^3/h and are excessively greater than the airflow rate of the isolator. The isolators are turned on or off one by one via remote control by the dedicated computer in the central control room, and the lab pressure changes being observed actually have no significant effect.

Testing of the alarm system of isolator is essential to ensure proper function. The value of negative pressure is reduced by manually exposing the glove port when the isolation chamber running normally. Buzzer alarm of the isolator alarms as loss of pressure when the negative pressure absolute value of the isolator internal is less than 20Pa. The resistance of exhaust HEPA filter is increased artificially covering the isolator filter with plastic membrane. Buzzer alarms as filter blocking.

6. Operation method of isolator system

The isolation chamber should be monitored for 48 hours to ensure that it is running normally in a Class 10000 high-level bio-safety laboratory. This includes supplying filtered air to the isolator and ensuring that the exhaust air is cleaned by the double in-line HEPA filters and passed through the exhaust air system into the open air. Fresh air exchanges should be conducted at a rate of about 36 air changes per hour. Following 48 hours of monitoring, the inside temperature is 22~23 °C, the relative humidity is 60%, the working negative pressure in the isolation chamber is adjusted to -50 Pa with respect to the laboratory. Healthy animals should be passed through the quarantine system and transferred into the isolation chamber via the DPTE system.

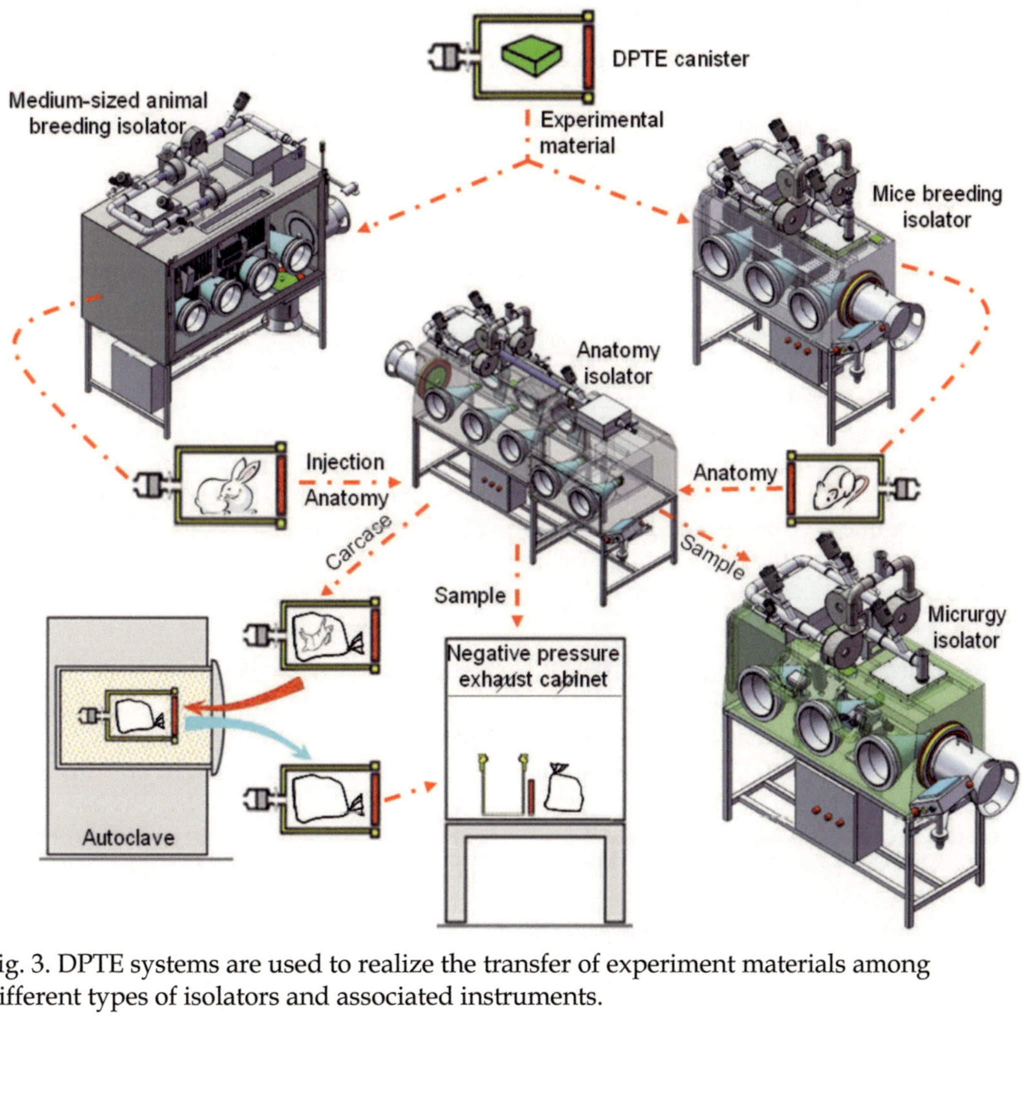

Fig. 3. DPTE systems are used to realize the transfer of experiment materials among different types of isolators and associated instruments.

The experiment in isolator systems can be carried out according to the protocol showing in figure 3.

The feeds and aseptic water can be kept enough in the isolator to minimize disturbances to breeding animals. The glove-sleeve systems allow direct complete animal feeding operations without compromising the health status or contamination of the animals within the isolator. Rapid pressure changes when operating under transient volume changes such as glove entry or withdrawal are adjusted via a variable frequency drive inlet air blower and extraction blower.

Non-human primates breeding need special approval by government, so New Zealand white rabbits are the first residents in the medium-sized animal breeding isolators. The animal excrement and other waste materials are cleaned out by DPTE container and sent to sterilize by autoclave every week. The rabbits selected for immunity with inactive pathogen are moved to the anatomy isolator with large space in an independence room by DPTE system to perform the operation of injection. The animal is sent back to the breeding isolator in the breeding room by transfer container after injection.

The ventilation performance of mice breeding isolator in mice breeding room allows using ordinary transparent mice cages and water bottles, and an extended cage-changing period up to one month (6 mice per cage,~15g/mice). The changed cages without mice are transferred to autoclave by DPTE system.

The operation of animal anatomy can be performed in the anatomy isolator. Blood of immunity rabbit can be transferred to negative pressure exhaust cabinet by transfer canister. The β-door of the canister can be opened with a specialized tool, and the blood samples can then be removed to the biological safety cabinet for further stages of analysis (e.g., centrifugation), while the transfer canister is closed and sent into autoclave. The Leica CM1100 cryostat in the anatomy isolator can be used to rapid freezing and manual sectioning of animal tissue specimens. The frozen section slides of mice infected by attenuated strain of pathogen are packaged and transferred to micrurgy isolator for immunostaining assays and observing under a fluorescence microscope in the micrurgy isolator. It is determined by the fluorescence microscopy that the attenuated strain of pathogen in mice tissues is specific binding with its strain-specific rabbit antiserum. The image data are sent out from the lab local area network. The dead animal and experimental waste materials in the isolator are collected respectively into plastic bags for autoclaving by DPTE canister.

The animal experiment should be performed according to bio-safety operation standard procedures. If the gloves are removed during the operation, a low pressure audible/visual alarm system is activated, and a minimum velocity value of 0.7 m/s in the center of the glove port is maintained. If a glove is damaged by a needle, the blowers are capable of maintaining the isolation chamber pressure at -50 Pa but the alarm system would not be activated because the micro-differential pressure sensor is not sensitive enough for a leak of this size. Proper procedure dictates that the small hole be labeled by the operator and a new glove exchanged. All of the feeds, experimental material, waste, feces and other materials can be transferred into or out of the isolation chamber by the DPTE system. There are several breeding isolation chambers in one room, and the autoclave does not connect with any of them. Instead, DPTE beta canisters are filled with items and are then sterilized in the autoclave. After sterilization, the sterile items are removed after opening the beta door with specialized tools. The sterile items are then sent to a centralized disposal center for medical waste. Following the completion of studies with single animals, each animal is treated as dictated by bio-safety operation standards and general animal welfare. The cadavers are autoclaved in beta canisters and sent to animal carcass disposal sites.

7. Isolator system decontamination

The isolator systems need biodecontamination after finishing the breeding program and experiment. The choice of sterilant depends on what kind of devices in the isolator. If only the cages are in the isolator, or there is nothing in the isolator, the stainless-steel or acrylic isolation chamber can be connected to the peracetic acid sterilizer to sterilize the interior of the isolation chamber. During the sterilization process, inlet air blower, inlet air electronic control ball valve, exhaust electronic control ball valve and extraction blower are all closed. Raven Labs offered *Bacillus atrophaeus* spore strips can be used for sterility testing by Soproper in isolator sterilization environments. Amount (A) of Soproper in the evaporation reservoir of peracetic acid sterilizer can be calculated with the formula: A (mL) = T×70mL/h+150mL, where T = sterilization time (h). The sterilizing agent by-pass electronic control ball valve is opened. The sterilizing agent in the peracetic acid sterilizer evaporation tank is heated and its vapors are pushed by compressed air into the volume to be sterilized by a sterile connecting hose, a sterilization reagent import, a coupling clamp for the inlet ventilation pipe and an inlet HEPA filter. The sterilizing vapors escape from the interior of the isolator through two in series HEPA filters, a sterilizing agent by-pass tube, a sterilizing agent by-pass electronic control ball valve and an extraction blower to the exhaust export. The sterilization time using Soproper vapor is 12h for the interior chamber with 400cm(*L*)×120cm (*W*)×120cm(*H*) dimensions sterilization. *B. atrophaeus* spore strips placed in 13 critical locations of the isolator internal surface (such as DPTE α door, stainless-steel cages, glove-sleeve systems, the end of HEPA filter) were all destroyed.

Minncare dry fog system is also a good disinfection device for breeding isolator. This system can be transferred into the isolator with 30% hydrogen peroxide in the reservoir. The nozzle allows for rapid vapor dispersion and ensures that the entire isolator space is exposed to dry fog when compressed air source connected with the dry fog system. The isolator is maintained under positive 750 Pa for 5 min, and then the isolator internal pressure allows natural attenuation to zero. All *Bacillus atrophaeus* spore strips placed in the isolator were inactive. Anyway the system always sprays out some large droplets at the beginning, then stride forward to 7.5 μm normal droplets. So it is still not be used for decontaminating equipments.

Hydrogen peroxide vapor technology used by BioQuell Z system has been developed to be the effective system available for rapid and secure biodecontamination of equipment and facilities. The anatomy isolator and micrurgy isolator and their internal equipments can be decontaminated simultaneity with the laboratory terminal disinfection. There are conditioning, gassing, dwell and aeration four phases as described by the Z manufacturers. The gassing time (T) can be calculated with the experience formula: T= V×5 (g/m^3) /20 (g/min), where V = room volume (m^3). Apex Laboratories offered *Geobacillus stearothermophilus* spore stainless steel discs can be used for sterility testing by 30% hydrogen peroxide in isolator and its located room sterilization environments. The anatomy isolator and micrurgy isolator are in the independent 63 m^3 room respectively. The isolator negative pressure sets as -20 Pa. The lab ventilation is off, four desktop fans are on. The room temperature is 16°C, relative humidity is 40%~70%. Connected the Z well, and check area to be bio-decontaminated no people or animal. All doors and windows are shut and secured, and seal the door with tape. The gassing time sets as 15 min, dwell time sets as 25 min. The injection rate of hydrogen peroxide during dwell phase is 5g/min as to maintain the concentration necessary for decontamination. At the end of aeration, the concentration of hydrogen peroxide within the room is reduced down to zero, and the Z can be stopped. The total time is 8h for the isolator and its interior equipment and the room sterilization. *G. stearothermophilus* spore discs placed in 13 critical locations of the isolator internal surface (such as DPTE α door, stainless-steel frame of equipment, glove-sleeve systems, the bottom and surface of equipment, the end of HEPA filter) were all inactive. The black paint on the microscopy are disappear after 20 times of this kind of disinfection, but the other paints still keep well, and the optical system of microscope is also not affected.

8. Conclusions

The isolator systems achieve multiple technical improvements: (1) By using variable frequency drive blowers as the inlet air and extraction blowers, adjustments for rapid pressure changes (e.g., insertion of gloves) can occur automatically without breaching the inert atmosphere. The extraction blowers contain an integrated backup system with one blower running at full strength and another on standby to act as a backup. Negative or positive pressure states are kept stable and at a safe level through the automatic control system. The pressure is adjusted depending on different requirements for different animals and/or experimental conditions. (2) The control cabinet installation is comprised mainly of the programmable logic controller, electric element (which includes the voltage transformer, secure alternating current contactor, circuit breaker, electric cable, indicating lamp and button), network port (for data output) and industrial Ethernet interface (which allows for the remote data control of multiple isolation chambers by the WINCC 6.0 program system). Automatic control and monitoring of the isolation chamber and sterilization system are achieved by the exchange of data between the touch screen and control cabinet through the industrial bus Profibus DP to meet different laboratory animal research project parameter requirements such as pressure, humidity, temperature, illumination and disinfection. A human operator can set the isolation chamber environment parameters according to the requirements of the infectious animals or for cleaning animals, allowing for the acquisition of adequate and authentic data. (3) Animal welfare is ensured by installing adjustable illumination lamps, a rotatable camera, a flat television, a micro-differential pressure sensor and temperature humidity sensor to maintain comfortable living conditions for the animal.

9. Acknowledgements

This work was supported by the Natuional Natural Science Foundation of China (30972633).

10. References

World Health Organization, (2004). Laboratory biosafety manual, 3rd ed. World Health Organization, Geneva.

Bantin GC. (2004). A comparison between the application of flexible film isolators and individual ventilated cages. Shanghai Laboratory Animal Science. 24(1):3-6.

Wathes CM, Johnson HE. (1991). Physical protection against airborne pathogens and pollutants by a novel animal isolator in a level 3 containment laboratory. Epidemiol Infect. 107(1):157-170.

Kruse RH, Puckett WH, Richardson JH. (1991). Biological safety cabinetry. Clin Microbiol Rev. 4(2):207-241.

Huang R. (2005). Isolator of using negative prcssure for big animals. CN Patent Publication number 1625942A.

Pan X, Long M, Liang H, Chen X, Li H, Li GB, Zhao ZY. (2010). Development of a multifunction isolator system for the care of medium-sized laboratory animals harboring infectious diseases. J Med Devices. 4(4): 041004.

Tattershall SF. 2006. Enclosure for handling hazardous material. US Patent No.: US7077486 B2.

Sawyer J, Bennett A, Haines V, Elton E, Crago K, Speight S. (2007). The effect of microbiological containment systems on dexterity. J Occup Environ Hyg, 4(3):166-173.

Clough G, Wallace J, Gamble MR, Merryweather ER, Bailey E. (1995). A positive, individually ventilated caging system: a local barrier system to protect both animals and personnel. Lab Anim. 29(2):139-151.

Wathes CM, Johnson HE. (1991). Physical protection against airborne pathogens and pollutants by a novel animal isolator in a level 3 containment laboratory. Epidemiol Infect. 1991;107(1):157-70.

ISO 14664-7:2004，Cleanrooms and associated controlled environments —Part 7: Separative devices (clean air hoods,gloveboxes, isolators and minienvironments). International Organization for Standardization, Geneva.

ISO 10648-1:1997, Containment enclosures – Part 1: Design principles. International Organization for Standardization, Geneva.

Hillman P, Gebremedhin K, Warner R. (1992). Ventilation system to minimize airborne bacteria, dust, humidity, and ammonia in calf nurseries. J Dairy Sci. 75(5):1305-1312

Institute of laboratory animal resources commission on life sciences, National research council. (1996). Guide for the care and use of laboratory animals. Washington,D.C: National Academy Press.

Runkle RS, Allendale NJ, Marsh RC, Albuquerque NM. (1969). Unit for providing environmental control of animals. US Patent No.: 3630174.

Allen JR, Burgess M, Aiken SC. (2009). Container lid gasket protective strip for double door transfer system. US Patent Pub.No.: US2009/0212054 A1.

Michael A, Szatmary FT, Worth TX. (2004). Rapid transfer port. US Patent No.: US6779567 B1.

Tauraso NM, Norris GF, Sorg TJ, Cook RO, Myers ML, Trimmer R. (1969). Negative-pressure isolator for work with hazardous infectious agents in monkeys. Appl Microbiol. 18(2):294-297.

Pan X, Sun Y. (2004). Expression of SARS-CoV spike protein functional receptor ACE2 in human cornea and conjunctiva tissues. High Technology Letters. 10 (supplement): 273-277.

Conly J, Johnston B. (2008). The infectious diseases consequences of monkey business. Can J Infect Dis Med Microbiol. 19(1):12-14.

Pan X, Qi JC, Long M, Liang H, Chen X, Li H, Li GB, Zheng H. (2010). New technique: Development of a large-scale isolation chamber system for the safe and humane care of medium-sized laboratory animals harboring infectious diseases. J Zhejiang Univ Sci B. 11 (10): 771-778.

GB50447-2008, Architectural and technical code for laboratory animal facility. National Standard. China.

GB14925-2001, Laboratory animal- requirements of environment and housing facilities. National Standard. China.

GB50346-2004, Architectural and technical code for biosafety laboratories. National Standard. China.

EN 12469:2000, Biotechnology-Performance criteria for microbiological safety cabinets. European Standard. European Committee for Standardization.

ISO10648-2:1994, Containment enclosures - Part 2: Classification according to leak tightness and associated checking methods. International Organization for Standardization, Geneva.

GB19489-2008, Laboratories-General equirements for biosafety. National Standard. China.

GB50591-2010, Code for construction and acceptance of cleanroom. National Standard. China.

5

Mathematical Modeling of IL-2 Based Immune Therapy on T Cell Homeostasis in HIV

Priti Kumar Roy[1,*], Sonia Chowdhury[1],
Amarnath Chatterjee[1] and Sutapa Biswas Majee[2]
[1]Centre for Mathematical Biology and Ecology, Department of Mathematics,
Jadavpur University, Kolkata,
[2]NSHM College of Pharmaceutical Technology,
NSHM Knowledge Campus, Kolkata
India

1. Introduction

The past few years there have been witnessed the initiation of new or more effective therapies for the treatment of HIV disease. But it is the established reality for the treatment procedure of HIV disease; mathematical modeling is very essential and supportive, in accepting the dynamics of HIV infection and also for the purpose of specific antiviral treatment strategies. Mathematical models have been constructed to explore the co- relation between disease progression, generation of HIV specific immune response in primary stage, depletion of $CD4^+$ T cell population, leading to severe impairment and dysregulation of host immune system and emergence of numerous opportunistic infection. Mathematical model accompanied with definite biological interpretation and relevance can provide a clear representation of host-pathogen interaction dynamics. Human Immunodeficiency Virus (HIV) targets the immune cells mainly CD4 positive T lymphocytes ($CD4^+$T, a type of white blood cells), which is the main component of immune system. $CD4^+$T cells or " helper" T cells also send signals to the second group of immune response cells ($CD8^+$T cell or CTL) in the body, the precursor Cytotoxic T Lymphocytes (CTL_p) to induce HIV-specific CTL response through the generation of functionally active effector CTL (CTL_e). HIV infection can be finally eradicated through co-ordinated interplay between $CD4^+$T cells and CTLs when infected $CD4^+$T cells are killed by CTLs. Thus, if CTL population can be maintained at a high level, the HIV-infected individuals can remain healthy for a longer period of time due to slower disease progression. The safest and cheapest therapeutic intervention aims to keep the $CD4^+$T cell population together with CTL count at a positive value, both of which will bring down the viremia to very low levels.

From an immunological standpoint, progression of HIV can be characterized by continual reduction of $CD4^+$T lymphocyte subset levels in peripheral compartment and lymphoid tissue as well, with greater reduction being observed in the former. Dysfunctional lymphocytes with high propensity for apoptosis and loss of proper cell cycle control account

*Research is supported by the Government of India, Ministry of Science and Technology, Mathematical Science office, No. SR/S4/MS: 558/08.

for deviation from T cell homeostasis in an HIV-infected individual. HIV antigen activates immune system, increases cell turnover and induces apoptosis of uninfected $CD4^+T$ and $CD8^+T$ cells leading to complete impairment of immune system (Sereti et al., 2004).

Immune activation and subsequent sensitivity to apoptotic stimuli can be reverted back by introduction of potent antiretroviral agents. Successful therapy with Highly Active Anti Retroviral Therapy (HAART) efficiently suppresses viral replication but with only partial immune reconstitution. Moreover, complete eradication of viral population from the system is practically not feasible with HAART alone, even if continued for a long time. Viral relapse is known to occur as soon as the therapy is discontinued (Roy & Chatterjee, 2011). Thus arises the need of addition of new therapeutic modalities in the form of administration of immunomodulatory agent, IL-2, to the armamentarium of antiretroviral agents promoting complete immune reconstitution.

IL-2 is a very well characterized T-cell growth factor determining proliferation and differentiation of whole T cell compartment. Following antigen-activation, IL-2 is produced by both $CD4^+$ and $CD8^+T$ (in comparatively lesser quantities) cell subsets, in the peripheral lymphoid tissues of spleen and lymph nodes, in an autocrine and paracrine fashion respectively (Smith, 2001), (Banerjee, 2008).

Infection by HIV affects $CD4^+T$ and $CD8^+T$ cells in a differential manner with selective depletion of the $CD4^+T$ cells whereas expansion of $CD8^+T$ cells is maintained till late stages of infection (Marchettia et al., 2004). Though IL-2 is produced by $CD4^+$ and $CD8^+T$ cells, it exerts differential effects on $CD4^+T$ cells, with preferential expansion and prolonged survival of peripheral naïve and recall subsets, but not effector and memory phenotype (Sereti et al., 2004), (Marchettia et al., 2004). IL-2 does not target progenitor cells of the bone marrow or thymus (Smith, 2001), (De, 2001). Net outcome of IL-2 therapy is rejuvenation of T cell pool marked by decreases in T cell turnover, proliferation and activation. IL-2 therapy also increases T cell responsiveness to suboptimal levels of endogenous IL-2 by increasing expression of its receptor, CD25, on $CD4^+$ T cells (Sklar et al., 2007). $CD8^+$ cells seem to follow different homeostatic dynamics, more or less independent of immunoregulatory activity of IL-2. Apart from its regulatory activity on specific cellular populations, IL-2 can also augment the production of IL-2 itself (Bortolin et al., 2001). In contrast, HAART alone results in selective rescue of $CD4^+$ memory cells, with no change in naïve compartment (Franzetti et al., 2005). Thus, IL-2 immunotherapy broadens HAART-induced immune recovery.

The degree of $CD4^+T$ cell recuperation after IL-2 administration depends on the nadir $CD4^+$ T cell count and the dose and duration of IL-2 therapy (Paredes et al., 2002). IL-2 can be given either intravenously or subcutaneously at a low dose intermittently but it is recommended that it should never be given alone. It should always be administered as an adjuvant to HAART for maximum biological and clinical benefits. It may be stopped as soon as $CD4^+T$ cell count is "normalized" to pre-infection levels and immune activation is reduced (De, 2001). Improvement in immunological parameters of the host such as expansion of $CD4^+T$ cells may continue for several months even after IL-2 administration has been interrupted (Bortolin et al., 2001). The potential of IL-2 to reverse the HIV-mediated T cell homeostasis imbalances by altering the in vivo dynamics of T-lymphocytes and regulatory cytokines, with transient or almost no change in HIV viral load, offers the appealing prospect of obtaining major immune reconstitution in the treatment of HIV disease.

Several mathematical models have been developed to describe the behavior of the HIV, when it interacts with the human immune system and causes a decline in the $CD4^{+}T$ cells count (Bonhoeffer et al., 1997), (Perelson & Nelson, 1999), (Wodarz et al., 2000), (Gumel et al., 2002), (Roy & Chatterjee, 2010). In their research they expand a innovative thinking, impact of drag in a HIV individual integrating with their model dynamics. Perelson et al. utilized clinical data from HIV infected patients and fitted them to their mathematical model and subsequent numerical simulations to prove the clinical manifestations of AIDS such as long latency period, depletion of $CD4^{+}T$ cells and low level of free virus in the whole body.

Now a days most of the authors developed their work by including various aspects of HIV specific antiviral immune response dominated by CTLs because of its significant role in controlling virus replication and disease progression. A simple mathematical model was developed by Wodarz et al. (Wodarz et al., 1999) to study the co-relation between HIV and immune system during the natural course of infection and in the background of different antiviral treatment regimes. They have suggested the need for an efficient CTL memory response for effective containment of viral replication. CTL memory is adversely affected during long-term infection due to depletion of $CD4^{+}T$ cell pool in the system. From analytical and numerical analysis in their mathematical model, (Roy & Chatterjee, 2011) has been shown that when the immune response are high, less medication is needed to control and regulate infection. Their mathematical model also reflect that optimal treatment is reduces the period of time while the immune response of the uninfected T cell takes over.

Discrete and continuous time delay or time lag is assumed to exist in the various stages of HIV progression (Herz et al., 1996), (Calshaw et al., 2000), (Roy & Chatterjee, 2011), and (Roy & Chatterjee, 2010) which have been incorporated into the mathematical model with firm biological explanations. It is well known that, delay differential equations cause a stable steady state to lose its stability and cause oscillations. For avoiding the side effects due to chemotherapy, various mathematical models have been formulated in control therapeutic approach (Fleming et al., 1975), (Gumel et al., 2002).

In the present paper, the reconstitution dynamics of $CD4^{+}T$ cells and effect on CTLs in HIV-infected individuals has been studied in presence of HAART and IL-2, where the basic model as proposed by Wodarz and Nowak has been modified (Wodarz and Nowak). They have suggested the need for an efficient CTL memory response for effective containment of viral replication. CTL memory is adversely affected during long-term infection due to depletion of $CD4^{+}T$ cell pool in the system. Mathematical modeling of such dynamics will help in delineating the interplay between T lymphocyte subsets in the course of HIV infection and thereby establishing optimum conditions for effective immune -based therapy associated with HAART. In this research article delay induced system in the same mathematical model of HIV has been investigated to understand the effect of combination therapy of HAART and IL-2. Attempts have also been made to apply the principles of optimal control theory to the proposed mathematical model for rational administration of IL-2 adjuvanated HAART in an effort to successfully eradicate the virus from the host system and cure the patient completely.

2. Presentation of the mathematical model

In this research article we develop a viral dynamical model of Wodarz et. al (Wodarz et al., 1999) by introducing IL-2 therapy in presence of HAART.

The model is given below,

$$\begin{aligned}\dot{x}(t) &= \lambda - \beta(1-\eta_1 u_1)x(t)y(t) - dx(t) + \gamma x(t)\\ \dot{y}(t) &= \beta(1-\eta_1 u_1)x(t)y(t) - ay(t) - py(t)z(t)\\ \dot{w}(t) &= cx(t)y(t)w(t) - cq_1 y(t)w(t) - bw(t) + \gamma_1 w(t)\\ \dot{z}(t) &= cq_2 y(t)w(t) - hz(t),\end{aligned} \tag{1}$$

with initial conditions: $x(0) > 0, y(0) > 0, w(0) > 0, z(0) > 0$.

Here x represents uninfected $CD4^{+}$T cells, and y, w, z are infected $CD4^{+}$T cells, Cytotoxic T lymphocyte precursors (CTL_p), CTL effector cells respectively. Here λ represents the rate of production of $CD4^{+}$T cells from bone marrow and these immature cells migrate to thymus and they are matured to immunocompetent T cells. The natural death rate of uninfected $CD4^{+}$T cell is d and β is the rate at which uninfected $CD4^{+}$T cell become infected. Natural death rate of infected cell is a. The clearance rate of infected cells by CTL effector is p. CTL_p are assumed to proliferate in response to antigenic stimulation and then differentiate into CTL memory. The rate of proliferation of CTL_p population is c and they decay at a rate b. Since the differentiation rate of precursor CTL (CTL_p) not at all same as the proliferation rate of effector CTL (CTL_e), thus we consider q_1 and q_2 as multiplicative capacity of differentiated precursor CTL and proliferated effector CTL respectively. We also assume that the removal rate of effector CTL is h.

Here we introduce IL-2 therapy in presence of HAART. We also consider that the RTI reduces the infection rate β by $(1 - \eta_1 u_1)$ where η_1 represents the drug efficacy parameter and u_1 is the control input doses of the drug RTI. By introducing interleukin protein it enhances the growth of uninfected T cell and also in a smaller quantity, increases growth of CTL_p. Here γ and γ_1 are the activation rates of uninfected T cell and CTL_p population respectively.

3. General analysis of the mathematical model

Figure 1 shows that, due to introducing of cocktail drug therapy (HAART and IL-2), uninfected $CD4^{+}$ T cell moves to its stable position. Further infected $CD4^{+}$ T cell population moves to a very lower levels, and ultimately goes towards extinction. Thus effector CTL population attains a lower steady state, where as CTL precursor enhanced due to effect of IL-2.

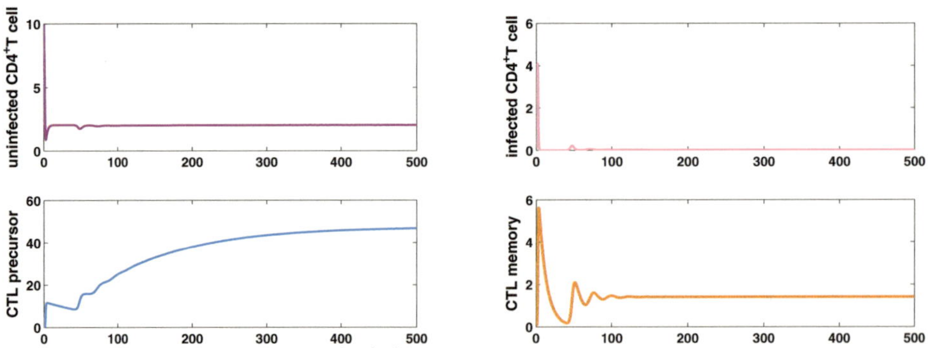

Fig. 1. Solution trajectory of the non-delayed system. All parameter values are taken from Table 1.

3.1 Equilibria and their existence

The system (1) with the initial condition possesses the following positive equilibrium $E_1(x_1, 0, 0, 0)$, $E_2(x_2, y_2, 0, 0)$ and $E^*(x^*, y^*, w^*, z^*)$.

Where, $x_1 = \frac{\lambda}{d-\gamma}$, $x_2 = \frac{a}{\beta(1-\eta_1 u_1)}$, $y_2 = \frac{\beta(1-\eta_1 u_1)\lambda + a(\gamma - d)}{a\beta(1-\eta_1 u_1)}$ and $x^* = \frac{\lambda}{d+\beta(1-\eta_1 u_1)y^* - \gamma}$,

$y^* = \frac{-\{(d-\gamma)cq_1+\beta(1-\eta_1 u_1)(b-\gamma_1)-c\lambda\}+\sqrt{\{(d-\gamma)cq_1+\beta(1-\eta_1 u_1)(b-\gamma_1)-c\lambda\}^2-4acq_1\beta(1-\eta_1 u_1)(b-\gamma_1)(d-\gamma)}}{2cq_1\beta(1-\eta_1 u_1)}$,

$w^* = \frac{h\beta(1-\eta_1 u_1)x^* - ha}{cpq_2 y^*}$, $z^* = \frac{\beta(1-\eta_1 u_1)x^* - a}{p}$.

During initial stages of infection when the virus enter in the system but not yet attack any CD4$^+$T cell, then infection free steady state E_1 exists, if $d > \gamma$, entail that death rate of uninfected CD4$^+$T cells is greater than the rate of production of uninfected cells under the influence of IL-2.

E_2 exists if $x_1 > x_2$, i.e at early stages of infection when T cells have become infected but CTL response is yet to develop and it indicates a very crucial situation. It exists when uninfected cell population at initial stage of infection is greater than steady state value of uninfected T cell population in presence of infection but without any immune response.

E^* exists if the following conditions holds, (i)$\frac{\gamma - d}{\beta(1-\eta_1 u_1)} < y^* < y_2$, (ii)$(b - \gamma_1)(d - \gamma) < 0$.

From the above two conditions we can say that (i) if infected cell population (y^*) at coexistence equilibrium point lies between these two threshold values and (ii) product of two terms $(b - \gamma_1)(d - \gamma)$, i.e. difference between death rate and production rate of CTL_p in presence of IL-2 $(b - \gamma_1)$ and difference between death rate and production rate of uninfected CD4$^+$T cell in presence of IL-2, $(d - \gamma)$ is negative.

3.2 Stability analysis of the system:

Here we study the nature of stability of the system (1) around different equilibrium points. From our mathematical study we have the following three propositions.

Proposition 1 : The system (1) is locally asymptotically stable around E_1 if the following condition holds,

$$(i)\gamma < d$$
$$(ii)\gamma_1 < b$$
$$(iii)\frac{\beta(1-\eta_1 u_1)\lambda + a(\gamma - d)}{a\beta(1-\eta_1 u_1)} < 0.$$

Proof :
The s/eigenvalues of the above upper triangular jacobian matrix are

$$\xi_1 = \gamma - d$$
$$\xi_2 = \frac{\beta(1-\eta_1 u_1)\lambda}{d-\gamma} - a$$
$$\xi_3 = \gamma_1 - b$$
$$\xi_4 = -h.$$

All the characteristic roots corresponding to E_1 will be negative if above proposed conditions are satisfied. Hence the system is locally asymptotically stable around E_1. Whenever E_1 is locally asymptotically stable E_2 does not exists.

Proposition 2: System (1) is locally asymptotically stable around E_2 if $y_2 < \frac{\beta(1-\eta_1 u_1)(b-\gamma_1)}{c(a-q_1\beta(1-\eta_1 u_1))}$ holds.

Proof :
By the same way we can prove this proposition.

Proposition 3: The system is locally asymptotically stable around E^* under R-H criterion for the following parameter values in Table 1.

Parameters	Definition	Values assigned
λ	Constant rate of production of$CD4^+T$ Cells	10.0 cells/ day
d	Death rate of Uninfected $CD4^+T$ cells	0.01 cells/ day
β	Rate of infection	0.001 cells/ day
a	Death rate of infected cells	0.24 cells/ day
p	Clearance rate of infected cells by CTL_e	0.002 / day
c	Rate of proliferation of CTL_p	0.6 /day
b	Decay rate of CTL_p	0.01 /day
h	Decay rate of CTL_e	0.02/day
γ	activation rate of uninfected CD4$^+$T cell by IL-2	0.5/day
γ_1	activation rate of CTL_p by IL-2	0.1/day
q_1	multiplication capacity of differentiated precursor CTL	0.5
q_2	multiplication capacity of proliferated effector CTL	0.3

Table 1. Variables and parameters used in the models (1), (2), (16, 17). All parameter values are taken from (Wodarz et al., 1999), (Calshaw et al., 2000), (Roy & Chatterjee, 2010), (Bonhoeffer et al., 1997), (Nowak and Bangham, 1996).

4. Delay induced system

In this section we proposed and analyzed the mathematical model (1), incorporating delay in activation of uninfected CD4$^+$T cell populations through IL-2 therapy. It should be mentioned here that delay-differential equations demonstrate in a complex dynamics rather than ordinary-differential equations in view of the fact that a time lag could cause a stable equilibrium to become unstable and hence the population may be fluctuated. For better understanding and also for realistic emulation of the delay induced system, we thus introduced a time delay in the production of CTL in our model (1). We also initiated another discrete time delay due to the account of the time lag in CTL_p activation. Thus we have the following delay differential equation model in the form of:

$$\begin{aligned}
\dot{x}(t) &= \lambda - \beta(1-\eta_1 u_1)x(t)y(t) - dx(t) + \gamma x(t-\tau_1) \\
\dot{y}(t) &= \beta(1-\eta_1 u_1)x(t)y(t) - ay(t) - py(t)z(t) \\
\dot{w}(t) &= cx(t)y(t)w(t) - cq_1 y(t)w(t) - bw(t) + \gamma_1 w(t-\tau_2) \\
\dot{z}(t) &= cq_2 y(t)w(t) - hz(t),
\end{aligned} \quad (2)$$

with initial conditions $x(\theta) = x_0 > 0, y(\theta) = 0, w(\theta) = 0, z(\theta) = 0$ for $\theta \in [-max\{\tau_1, \tau_2\}, 0]$.

4.1 Stability analysis of the delay induced system

We further paying our attention to investigate the local asymptomatic stability of the infected steady state E^* for the delay induced system (Equation 2). Now linearizing the system (2)

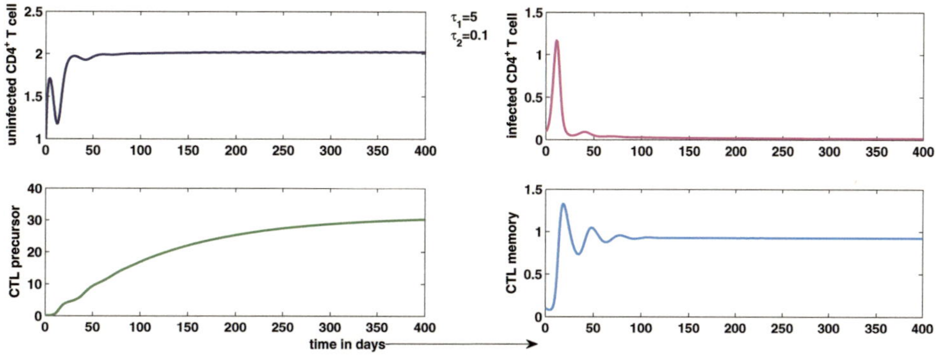

Fig. 2. Solution trajectory of the delayed system. Here $\tau_1 = 5, \tau_2 = 0.1$, and all other parameter values are same as Table 1.

about E^* we get,

$$\frac{dT}{dt} = FT(t) + GT(t - \tau_1) + HT(t - \tau_2). \tag{3}$$

Here F, G, H are 4x4 matrices given below,

$$F = \begin{pmatrix} -d - \beta(1-\eta_1 u_1)y^* & -\beta(1-\eta_1 u_1)x^* & 0 & 0 \\ \beta(1-\eta_1 u_1)y^* & \beta(1-\eta_1 u_1)x^* - a - pz^* & 0 & -py^* \\ cy^*w^* & cx^*w^* - cq_1 w^* & cx^*y^* - cq_1 y^* - b & 0 \\ 0 & cq_2 w^* & cq_2 y^* & -h \end{pmatrix}$$

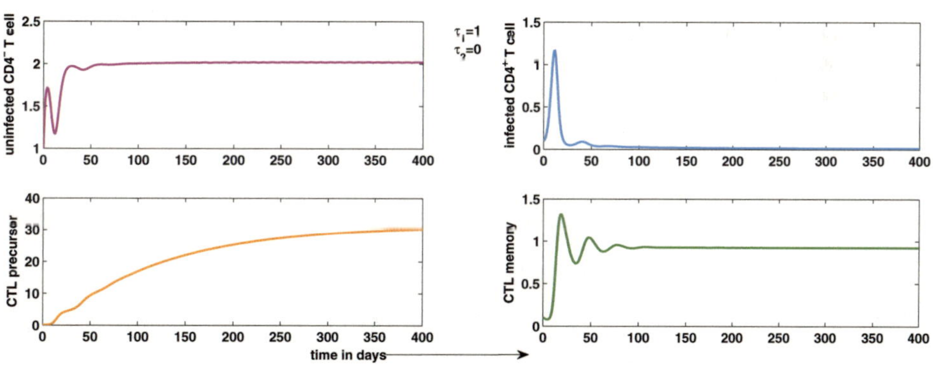

Fig. 3. Solution trajectory of the delayed system. Here $\tau_1 = 1, \tau_2 = 0$, and all other parameter values are same as Table 1.

$$G = \begin{pmatrix} \gamma & 0 & 0 & 0 \\ 0 & 0 & 0 & 0 \\ 0 & 0 & 0 & 0 \\ 0 & 0 & 0 & 0 \end{pmatrix}$$

$$H = \begin{pmatrix} 0 & 0 & 0 & 0 \\ 0 & 0 & 0 & 0 \\ 0 & 0 & \gamma_1 & 0 \\ 0 & 0 & 0 & 0 \end{pmatrix}$$

The characteristic equation of system (2) is given by,

$$\triangle(\xi) = \mid \xi I - F - e^{-\xi\tau_1} G - e^{-\xi\tau_2} H \mid = 0.$$

This equation can be written as,

$$\begin{aligned}\psi(\xi, \tau_1, \tau_2) &= \xi^4 + A_1\xi^3 + A_2\xi^2 + A_3\xi + A_4\xi + e^{-\xi\tau_1}[B_1\xi^3 + B_2\xi^2 + B_3\xi + B_4] \\ &e^{-\xi\tau_2}[C_1\xi^3 + C_2\xi^2 + C_3\xi + C_4] + e^{-\xi(\tau_1+\tau_2)}[D_1\xi^2 + D_2\xi + D_3] = 0. \qquad (4)\end{aligned}$$

The coefficients are given below,

$$\begin{aligned}&m_{11} = -d - \beta(1-\eta_1 u_1)y^*, \ m_{12} = -\beta(1-\eta_1 u_1)x^*, \ m_{21} = \beta(1-\eta_1 u_1)y^*, \\ &m_{22} = \beta(1-\eta_1 u_1)x^* - a - pz^*, \ m_{24} = py^*, \ m_{31} = cy^* w^*, \ m_{32} = cx^* w^* - cq_1 w^*, \\ &m_{33} = cx^* y^* - cq_1 y^* - b, \ m_{42} = cq_2 w^*, m_{43} = cq_2 y^*, m_{44} = -h,\end{aligned}$$

where,

$$\begin{aligned}A_1 &= m_{44} - m_{33} - m_{22} - m_{11}, \\ A_2 &= m_{33}m_{44} + m_{11}m_{44} + m_{22}m_{44} + m_{22}m_{33} + m_{11}m_{33} + m_{22}m_{11} - m_{12}m_{21} - m_{24}m_{42}, \\ A_3 &= -m_{11}m_{33}m_{44} - m_{22}m_{33}m_{44} - m_{11}m_{22}m_{44} + m_{12}m_{21}m_{44} - m_{24}m_{32}m_{43}, \\ &+ m_{24}m_{33}m_{42} + m_{11}m_{24}m_{42} + m_{11}m_{24}m_{42} - m_{11}m_{22}m_{33} + m_{12}m_{21}m_{33}, \\ A_4 &= m_{11}m_{22}m_{33}m_{44} - m_{12}m_{21}m_{33}m_{44} + m_{11}m_{24}m_{32}m_{43} - m_{12}m_{24}m_{31}m_{43} \\ &- m_{11}m_{24}m_{33}m_{42}, \\ B_1 &= -\gamma, \\ B_2 &= \gamma(m_{44} + m_{33}m_{22}), \\ B_3 &= \gamma(-m_{33}m_{44} - m_{22}m_{44} - m_{22}m_{33} + m_{24}m_{42}), \\ B_4 &= \gamma(m_{22}m_{33}m_{44} + m_{24}m_{32}m_{43} - m_{24}m_{33}m_{42}), \\ C_1 &= -\gamma_1, \\ C_2 &= \gamma_1(m_{44} + m_{22}m_{11}), \\ C_3 &= \gamma_1(-m_{22}m_{44} - m_{11}m_{44} - m_{22}m_{11} + m_{24}m_{42}), \\ C_4 &= \gamma_1(m_{11}m_{22}m_{44} - m_{12}m_{21}m_{44} - m_{11}m_{24}m_{42}), \\ D_1 &= \gamma\gamma_1, \\ D_2 &= \gamma\gamma_1(-m_{22}m_{44}), \\ D_3 &= \gamma\gamma_1(m_{22}m_{44}).\end{aligned}$$

The characteristic equation (4) is a transcendental equation in ξ. It is known that E^* is locally asymptotically stable if all the roots of the corresponding characteristic equation have negative real parts and unstable if purely imaginary roots are appears. As we know that the transcendental equation has infinitely many complex roots (Calshaw et al., 2000), so in presence of τ_1, τ_2, analysis of the sign of roots is very complicated. Thus, we begin our analysis by setting one delay which is equal to zero and then deduce the conditions for stability, when both time delays are non zero.

Case I :- When $\tau_1 = \tau_2 = 0$:
In absence of both the delays the characteristics equation (4) becomes,

$$\xi^4 + \xi^3(A_1 + B_1 + C_1) + \xi^2(A_2 + B_2 + C_2 + D_1) + \xi(A_3 + B_3 + C_3 + D_2) \\ +(A_4 + B_4 + C_4 + D_3) = 0. \quad (5)$$

Employing Routh Hurwitz criteria for sign of roots we have the same results as in non delayed system analysis.

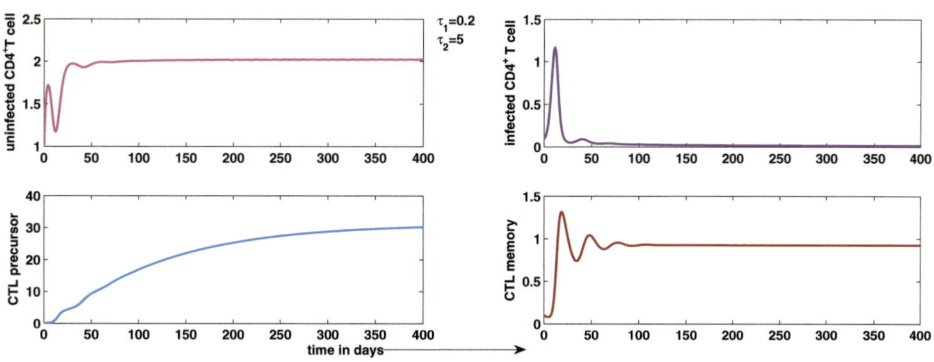

Fig. 4. Solution trajectory of the delayed system. Here $\tau_1 = 0.2, \tau_2 = 5$, and all other parameter values are same as Table 1.

Case II :- When $\tau_1 > 0, \tau_2 = 0$:

In this case we consider no delay in CTL precursor immune response i.e $\tau_2 = 0$, then the characteristic equation becomes,

$$\xi^4 + \xi^3(A_1 + C_1) + \xi^2(A_2 + C_2) + \xi(A_3 + C_3) + (A_4 + C_4) \\ +e^{-\xi\tau_1}[B_1\xi^3 + \xi^2(B_2 + D_1) + \xi(B_3 + D_2) + (B_4 + D_3)] = 0. \quad (6)$$

For $\tau_1 > 0$, (6) has infinitely many roots. Using Rouche's theorem and continuity of τ_1, the transcedental equation has roots with positive real parts if and only if it has purely imaginary roots. Let $i\theta$ be a root of equation (6) and hence we get,

$$\begin{aligned} \theta^4 - \theta^2(A_2 + C_2) + (A_4 + C_4) &= \cos\theta\tau_1[\theta^2(B_2 + D_1) - (B_4 + D_3)] \\ &\quad + \sin\theta\tau_1[\theta^3 D_1 - \theta(B_3 + D_2)] \\ \theta(A_3 + C_3) - \theta^3(A_1 + C_1) &= \cos\theta\tau_1[\theta^3 D_1 - \theta(B_3 + D_2)] \\ &\quad - \sin\theta\tau_1[\theta^2(B_2 + D_1) - (B_4 + D_3)]. \end{aligned} \quad (7)$$

Squaring and adding above two equations,

$$\theta^8 + \theta^6[(A_1 + C_1)^2 - 2(A_2 + C_2) - D_1^2] \\ +\theta^4[(A_2 + C_2)^2 + 2(A_4 + C_4) - 2(A_3 + C_3)(A_1 + C_1) - (B_2 + D_1)^2 \\ +2D_1(B_3 + D_2)] + \theta^2[(A_3 + C_3)^2 \\ -2(A_2 + C_2)(A_4 + C_4) + 2(B_2 + D_1)(B_4 + D_3) - (B_3 + D_2)^2] \\ +[(A_4 + C_4)^2 - (B_4 + D_3)^2] = 0. \quad (8)$$

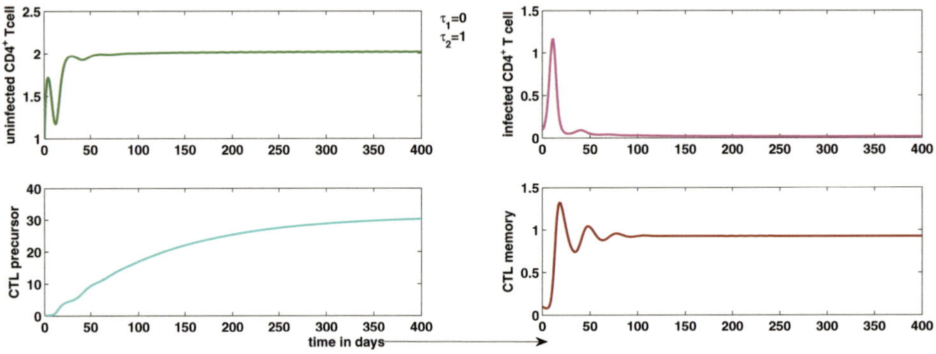

Fig. 5. Solution trajectory of the delayed system. Here $\tau_1 = 0, \tau_2 = 1$, and all other parameter values are same as Table 1.

Simplifying and substituting $\theta^2 = l$ in equation (8) we get the following equation,

$$l^4 + \alpha_1 l^3 + \alpha_2 l^2 + \alpha_3 l + \alpha_4 = 0. \tag{9}$$

Where,

$$\begin{aligned}
\alpha_1 &= (A_1 + C_1)^2 - 2(A_2 + C_2) - D_1^2, \\
\alpha_2 &= (A_2 + C_2)^2 + 2(A_4 + C_4) - 2(A_3 + C_3)(A_1 + C_1) - (B_2 + D_1)^2 + 2D_1(B_3 + D_2), \\
\alpha_3 &= (A_3 + C_3)^2 - 2(A_2 + C_2)(A_4 + C_4) + 2(B_2 + D_1)(B_4 + D_3) - (B_3 + D_2)^2, \\
\alpha_4 &= (A_4 + C_4)^2 - (B_4 + D_3)^2.
\end{aligned}$$

It may be noted that the equation (9) will have negative real part if and only if Routh-Hurwitz criterion is satisfied and hence equation (6) will have no purely imaginary root. From the above analysis we have the following proposition.

Proposition 4 : In the delay induced system (2), the infected steady state E^* will be locally asymptotically stable for all $\tau_1 > 0$ if the following conditions are satisfied:
$\alpha_1 > 0,\ \alpha_4 > 0,\ \psi = \alpha_1\alpha_2 - \alpha_3 > 0,\ \psi\alpha_3 - \alpha_1^2\alpha_4 > 0.$

Case III :- When $\tau_1 = 0, \tau_2 > 0$:
In absence of τ_1, the characteristic equation (4) have the following form,

$$\begin{aligned}
&\xi^4 + \xi^3(A_1 + B_1) + \xi^2(A_2 + B_2) + \xi(A_3 + B_3) + (A_4 + B_4) \\
&+ e^{-\xi\tau_2}[C_1\xi^3 + \xi^2(C_2 + D_1) + \xi(C_3 + D_2) + (C_4 + D_3)] = 0.
\end{aligned} \tag{10}$$

Similarly as in case II we substitute $\xi = i\theta$ and we get,

$$\begin{aligned}
\theta^4 - \theta^2(A_2 + B_2) + (A_4 + B_4) &= \cos\theta\tau_2[\theta^2(C_2 + D_1) - (C_4 + D_3)] \\
&\quad + \sin\theta\tau_2[\theta^3 C_1 - \theta(C_3 + D_2)].
\end{aligned} \tag{11}$$

$$\begin{aligned}
\theta(A_3 + B_3) - \theta^3(A_1 + B_1) &= \cos\theta\tau_2[\theta^3 C_1 - \theta(C_3 + D_2)] \\
&\quad - \sin\theta\tau_1[\theta^2(C_2 + D_1) - (C_4 + D_3)].
\end{aligned} \tag{12}$$

Squaring and adding, and then substituting $\theta^2 = s$ we have,

$$s^4 + \delta_1 s^3 + \delta_2 s^2 + \delta_3 s + \delta_4 = 0. \tag{13}$$

Where,

$$\begin{aligned}
\delta_1 &= (A_1+B_1)^2 - 2(A_2+B_2) - C_1^2 \\
\delta_2 &= (A_2+B_2)^2 + 2(A_4+B_4) - 2(A_3+B_3)(A_1+B_1) - (C_2+D_1)^2 + 2C_1(C_3+D_2) \\
\delta_3 &= (A_3+B_3)^2 - 2(A_2+B_2)(A_4+B_4) + 2(C_2+D_1)(C_4+D_3) - (C_3+D_2)^2 \\
\delta_4 &= (A_4+B_4)^2 - (C_4+D_3)^2.
\end{aligned}$$

From the above analysis we have the following proposition.
Proposition 5 : In the delay induced system (2), the infected steady state E^* will be locally asymptotically stable for all $\tau_2 > 0$ if the following conditions are satisfied
$\delta_1 > 0,\ \delta_4 > 0,\ \varphi = \delta_1\delta_2 - \delta_3 > 0,\ \varphi\delta_3 - \delta_1^2\delta_4 > 0$. If $\delta_4 < 0$ then we have the following proposition,

Proposition 6 : Equation (13) admits at least one positive root if $\delta_4 < 0$ is satisfied.

If θ_0 be a positive root of (13), then equation (10) will have a purely imaginary root $\pm i\theta_0$ corresponding to τ_2. Now we evaluate the critical value of τ_2 for which the deley induced system (2) remain stable. From equation (11,12),

$$\tau_2^* = \frac{acos\phi(\theta_0)}{\theta_0}. \tag{14}$$

Where,

$$\begin{aligned}
\phi(\theta_0) = {} & [\{\theta^2(C_2+D_1) - (C_4+D_3)\}\{\theta^4 - \theta^2(A_2+B_2) + (A_4+B_4)\} \\
& + \{\theta^3 C_1 - \theta(C_3+D_2)\}\{\theta(A_3+B_3) - \theta^3(A_1+B_1)\}] \\
& \div [\{\theta^2(C_2+D_1) - (C_4+D_3)\}^2 + \{\theta^3 C_1 - \theta(C_3+D_2)\}^2].
\end{aligned} \tag{15}$$

From the above analysis we construct the following theorem.

Theorem 1 :

If $\delta_4 < 0$ is satisfied, then the steady state E^* is locally asymptotically stable for $\tau_2 < \tau_2^*$ and becomes unstable for $\tau_2 > \tau_2^*$. When $\tau_2 = \tau_2^*$ a Hopf bifurcation occurs.

Case IV :- $\tau_1 > 0, \tau_2 > 0$

In this case we studied the stability of the steady state E^* in presence of both delays. If all the roots of equation (10) have negative real parts for $\tau > 0$ i.e when the system is locally asymptotically stable then there exists a τ_1^* depending upon τ_2 such that all roots of equation (4) have negative real parts whenever $\tau_1 < \tau_1^*$. Considering all the cases we have the following theorem .

Theorem 2 : Whenever $\delta_4 < 0$ holds then for $\tau_2 < \tau_2^*$, there exists a τ_1^* depending upon τ_2 the steady state E^* is locally asymptotically stable for $\tau_1 < \tau_1^*$ and $\tau_2 < \tau_2^*$.

Special Remarks of the Delay Induced System in view of Numerical Analysis:
Though it is eventually true from our analytical results that for a longer value of delay the

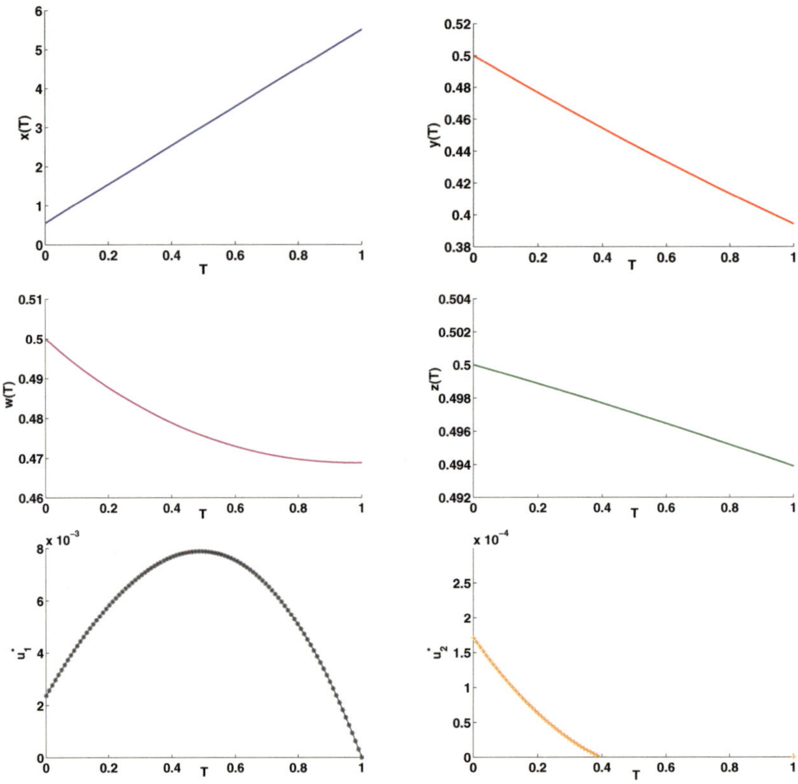

Fig. 6. This figure shows the system behavior for the Optimal treatment schedule of the control variable $u_1(t)$ and $u_2(t)$ for $R = 0.1$, $P = 0.5$, and $\eta_1 = 0.5$, $\eta_2 = 0.1$, $\eta_3 = 0.01$. All other parameter values are same as Table 1.

system become unstable (Theorem 1 and Theorem 2), however it is essential to mention here that in our delay induced system, numerical analysis reveal, when $\tau_1 = 0$ and $\tau_2 = 1$, its reflect from solution trajectory, there are no such oscillations in Figure, which may conclude that delay does affect the stability of the system.

Further we change the values of both delays τ_1, and τ_2, and varied them from 1 to 20, we also observe that no significant changes does arise in each case for which we can express that delay affect the stability of the system. Thus, in a nutshell we can say that incorporation of time delay into the existing model to account for time lag in activation of CTL_p did not exhibit any biologically significant interpretation.

5. The optimal control problem

In this section our main object is to minimize the infected $CD4^+T$ cells population as well as minimize the systemic cost of drug treatment. Here we formulate an optimal control problem. We also want to maximize the level of healthy $CD4^+T$ cells. So in our basic model (1), we use control variables $u_1(t), u_2(t)$ represents the drug dose satisfying $0 \leq u_1(t) \leq 1$ and $0 \leq u_2(t) \leq 1$. Here $u_1(t) = 1$, $u_2(t) = 1$ events are represents the maximal use of chemotherapy and $u_1(t) = 0$, $u_2(t) = 0$ represents no treatment.

Here we consider that the RTI reduces the infection rate by $(1-\eta_1 u_1)$, where η_1 represents the drug efficacy and u_1 is the control input doses of the drug RTI. We also consider the enrichment of uninfected T cell and CTL responses through IL-2 treatment is given by $\eta_2 u_2$, and $\eta_3 u_2$, where u_2 as a control input of IL-2 treatment and η_2, η_3 are the drug efficacy of IL-2 for uninfected T cell and precursor CTL responses.

In this section our main aim is to minimize the cost as well as minimize the infected CD4$^+$T cell and maximize the uninfected CD4$^+$T cell. Thus we construct the optimal control problem where the state system is

$$\begin{aligned}
\dot{x} &= \lambda - dx - \beta(1-\eta_1 u_1(t))xy + (1-\eta_2 u_2(t))\gamma x \\
\dot{y} &= \beta(1-\eta_1 u_1(t))xy - ay - pyz \\
\dot{w} &= cxyw - cq_1 yw - bw + (1-\eta_3 u_2(t))\gamma_1 w \\
\dot{z} &= cq_2 yw - hz,
\end{aligned} \tag{16}$$

and the control function is defined as

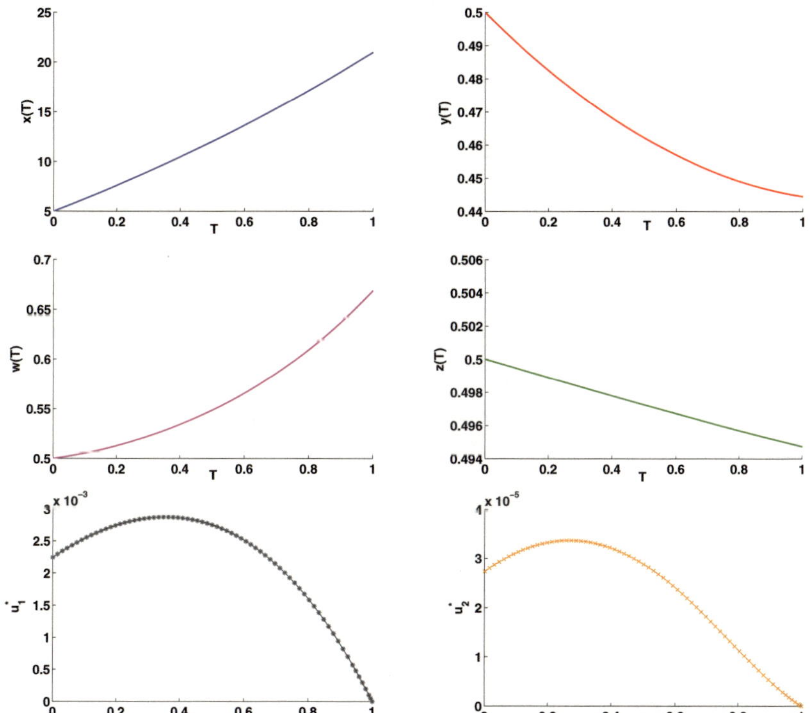

Fig. 7. This figure shows the system behavior for the Optimal treatment schedule of the control variable $u_1(t)$ and $u_2(t)$ for $R=10$, $P=50$, and $\eta_1 = 0.1$, $\eta_2 = 0.1$, $\eta_3 = 0.01$. All other parameter values are same as Table 1.

$$J(u_1, u_2) = \int_{t_0}^{t_f} [y(t) - x(t) - w(t) + Ru_1^2 + Pu_2^2]dt. \tag{17}$$

Where the parameter R and P respectively the weight on the benefit of the cost.

Here the control function $u_1(t)$ and $u_2(t)$ are bounded, Lebesgue integrable function (Swan, 1984).

In this problem we are seeking the optimal control pair $(u_1{}^*, u_2{}^*)$ such that
$J(u_1{}^*, u_2{}^*) = \min\{J(u_1, u_2) : (u_1, u_2) \in U\}$.

Here U is the control set defined by
$U = \{u = (u_1, u_2) : \; u_1, \, u_2 \text{ are the measurable}, \; 0 \leq u_1(t) \leq 1, \; 0 \leq u_2(t) \leq 1, \; t \in [t_0, t_f]\}$.

To determine the optimal control $u_1{}^*$ and $u_2{}^*$, we use the "Pontryagin Minimum Principle" (Pontryagin et al., 1986). To solve the problem we use the Hamiltonian given by

$$
\begin{aligned}
H = y(t) - x(t) - w(t) + Ru_1^2 + Pu_2^2 + \xi_1\{\lambda - dx - \beta(1 - \eta_1 u_1(t))xy + (1 - \eta_2 u_2(t))\gamma x\} \\
+\xi_2\{\beta(1 - \eta_1 u_1(t))xy - ay - pyz\} + \xi_3\{cxyw - cq_1 yw - bw + (1 - \eta_3 u_2(t))\gamma_1 w\} \\
+\xi_4\{cq_2 yw - hz\}. \qquad (18)
\end{aligned}
$$

By using the "Pontryagin Minimum Principle" and the existence condition for the optimal control theory (Fleming et al., 1975) we obtain the theorem.

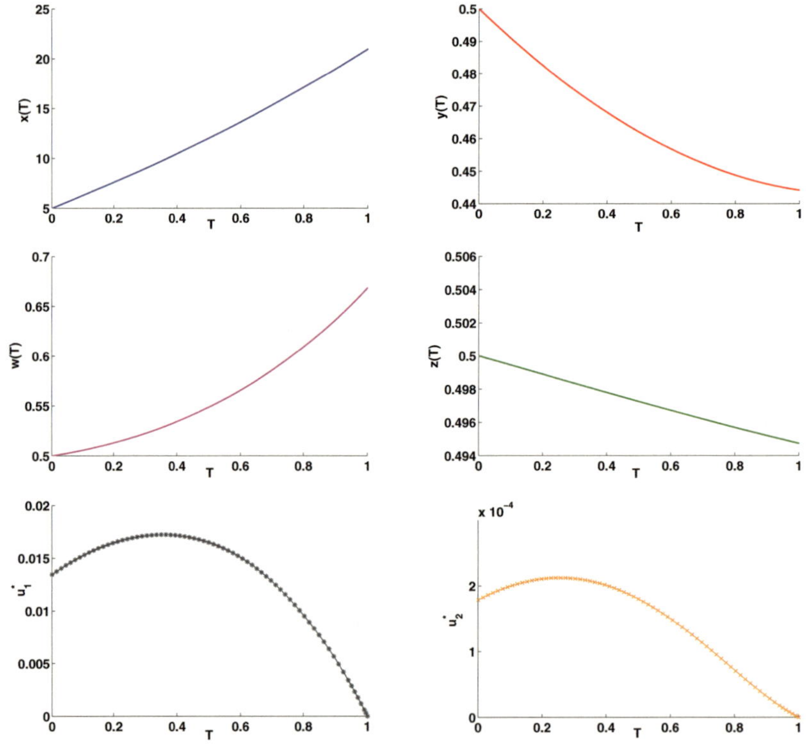

Fig. 8. This figure shows the system behavior for the Optimal treatment schedule of the control variable $u_1(t)$ and $u_2(t)$ for $R = 10$, $P = 50$, and $\eta_1 = 0.6$, $\eta_2 = 0.1$, $\eta_3 = 0.01$. All other parameter values are same as Table 1.

Theorem: The objective cost function $J(u_1, u_2)$ over U is minimum for the optimal control $u^* = (u_1{}^*, u_2{}^*)$ corresponding to the interior equilibrium (x^*, y^*, w^*, z^*). Also there exist adjoint function ξ_1, ξ_2, ξ_3, ξ_4 satisfying the equation (18) and (19).

Proof: By using Pontryagin Minimum principle (Fleming et al., 1975) the unconstrained optimal control variable $u_1{}^*$ and $u_2{}^*$ satisfy

$$\frac{\partial H}{\partial u_1{}^*} = \frac{\partial H}{\partial u_2{}^*} = 0. \tag{19}$$

Since

$$H = [Ru_1^2 - \xi_1(1-\eta_1 u_1(t))\beta xy + \xi_2(1-\eta_1 u_1(t))\beta xy] + [Pu_2^2 + \xi_1(1-\eta_2 u_2)\gamma x \\ + \xi_3(1-\eta_3 u_2)\gamma_1 w] + \text{other terms without } u_1 \text{ and } u_2, \tag{20}$$

then we obtain $\frac{\partial H}{\partial u_i{}^*}$ for $u_i{}^*$ where $(i = 1, 2)$, and hence equation with zero becomes,

$$\frac{\partial H}{\partial u_1{}^*} = 2Ru_1{}^* + \eta_1 \beta x^* y^* (\xi_1 - \xi_2) = 0$$
$$\frac{\partial H}{\partial u_2{}^*} = 2Pu_2{}^* - \xi_1 \eta_2 \gamma x^* - \xi_3 \eta_3 \gamma_1 z^* = 0.$$

Thus we obtain the optimal control $u_1{}^*$ and $u_2{}^*$ corresponding to the interior equilibrium (x^*, y^*, w^*, z^*) as,

$$u_1{}^* = \frac{\beta \eta_1 x^* y^* (\xi_2 - \xi_1)}{2R}$$
$$u_2{}^* = \frac{(\xi_1 \eta_2 \gamma x^* + \xi_3 \eta_3 \gamma_1 z^*)}{2P}. \tag{21}$$

According to Pontryagin minimum Principle (Pontryagin et al., 1986) we know that,

$$\frac{d\xi}{dt} = -\frac{\partial H}{\partial x}, \tag{22}$$

and

$$H(x(t), u^*(t), \xi(t), t) = \min_{u \in U} H(x(t), u(t), \xi(t), t). \tag{23}$$

The above equations are the necessary conditions satisfying the optimal control $u(t)$ and again for the system (16, 17) the adjoint equations are

$\frac{d\xi_1}{dt} = -\frac{\partial H}{\partial x}, \ \frac{d\xi_2}{dt} = -\frac{\partial H}{\partial y}, \ \frac{d\xi_3}{dt} = -\frac{\partial H}{\partial w}, \ \frac{d\xi_4}{dt} = -\frac{\partial H}{\partial z}.$

Taking the partial derivative of H we get,

$$\frac{d\xi_1}{dt} = 1 + \xi_1\{d_1 + (1-\eta_1 u_1(t))\beta y - (1-\eta_2 u_2(t))\gamma\} - \xi_2(1-\eta_1 u_1(t))\beta y - \xi_3 cyw$$
$$\frac{d\xi_2}{dt} = -1 + \xi_1(1-\eta_1 u_1(t))\beta x - \xi_2\{(1-\eta_1 u_1(t))\beta x - a - pz\} - \xi_3\{cxw - cq_1 w\} - \xi_4 cq_2 w$$
$$\frac{d\xi_3}{dt} = 1 - \xi_3\{cxy - cq_1 y - b + (1-\eta_3 u_2(t))\gamma_1\} - \xi_4 cq_2 y$$
$$\frac{d\xi_4}{dt} = \xi_2 py + \xi_4 h. \tag{24}$$

Hence the optimality of the system consists of the state system along with the adjoint system. Also it depends on the initial conditions and the transversality condition which satisfy $\xi_i(t_f) = 0$ and $x(0) = x_0, \ y(0) = y_0, \ w(0) = w_0, \ z(0) = z_0$.

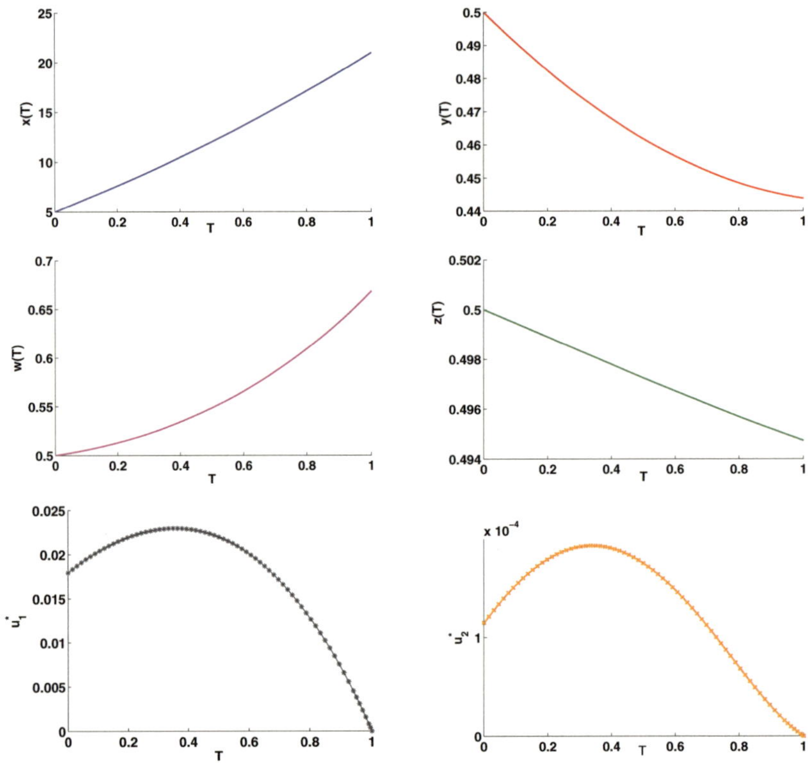

Fig. 9. This figure shows the system behavior for the Optimal treatment schedule of the control variable $u_1(t)$ and $u_2(t)$ for $R = 10$, $P = 50$, and $\eta_1 = 0.8$, $\eta_2 = 0.4$, $\eta_3 = 0.1$. All other parameter values are same as Table 1.

6. Conclusion

In this research article we have considered a mathematical model of immune system representing the response of a HIV infected individual in presence of HAART and IL-2. We have studied how the immune system recovers by applying IL-2 as an immune activator along with HAART. We have also observed the effect of delay in activation of uninfected $CD4^+T$ populations through IL-2 therapy. We have noticed the control therapy, which is more effective with respect to cost and also less side effect. Here analytical as well as numerical approaches have been observed. We have also noticed that, the rational behind concomitant administration of IL-2 with HAART is to augment host immune responses through prevention of destruction of the immunity system without stimulation of HIV replication. In the beginning of our research article, our mathematical model of HIV dynamics in presence of HAART and IL-2 suggest the existence of three equilibrium conditions : $E_1(x_1, 0, 0, 0)$, $E_2(x_2, y_2, 0, 0)$ and $E^*(x^*, y^*, w^*, z^*)$. Our analytical studies first indicates the infection free steady state or uninfected equilibrium, where $CD4^+T$ cells are healthy and no infected cell population exists and there is no HIV-specific CTL immune response. The second equilibrium condition is not a very desirable one since there is no immune response even in presence of HIV antigen. The third equilibrium state or infected steady state is said to be exist at certain limiting values of infected cell population in presence of HAART and IL-2. We also studied the stability of the system for different equilibrium points. Further a time delay has been introduced into the existing model to account for the activation of immune response through infected CD4$^+$T cells. In that study, we noticed that delay induced system has no useful delay effect which changes its stability. From optimal control studies, several interesting results have been obtained. As weight factors (R and P) increase from 0.1 to 10 and 0.5 to 50 respectively, there is a significant increase in the uninfected cell population with very little effect on the count of infected cells. The increase in the weight factors does not produce proportionate increase in the precursor CTL population and increase in effectiveness of HAART or IL-2 as denoted by η, is not manifested by remarkable change in precursor CTL number. The CTL effector population is found to decrease in all the cases. Thus, optimal control approach will help in designing an innovative cost-effective safe therapeutic regimen of HAART and IL-2 where the uninfected cell population will be enhanced with simultaneous decrease in the infected cell population. Moreover, successful immune reconstitution can also be achieved with increase in precursor CTL population. Mathematical modeling of viral dynamics thus enables maximization of therapeutic outcome even in case of multiple therapies with specific goal of reversal of immunity impairment.

From our above discussion of the results, it is clear that, though incorporation of time delay into the existing model (1) to account for time lag in activation of CTL_p did not exhibit any biologically significant interpretation, however, adoption of optimal control strategy in optimization of therapeutic regime of combination therapy of HAART and IL-2 was found to be really satisfactory in terms of enhancing the life expectancy of HIV-afflicted patients by improving the uninfected T cell count.

7. References

Wodarz, D.; Nowak, M.A. (1999). Specific therepy regimes could lead to long term immunological control to HIV, *Proc. Natl. Acad. Sci. USA*, Vol. 96, No. 25, pp. 14464-14469.

Srivastava, P.K.; Banerjee, M.; Chandra, P. (2010). A primary infection model for HIV and immune response with two discreat time delays, *Differ Equ Dyn Syst*, Springer.

Pontryagin, L.S.; Boltyanskii, V.G.; Gamkrelidze, R. V.; Mishchenko, E. F. (1986). Mathematical Theory of Optimal Processes, *Gordon and Breach Science Publishers*, Vol. 4.

Culshaw, R.V.; Ruan, S. (2000). A delay -differentianal equation model of HIV-1 infection of CD4$^+$T-cells, *Math. Biosci.*, Vol. 165, pp. 425-444.

Fleming, W.; Rishel, R. (1975). Deterministic and Stochastic optimal controls, *Springer-Verlag*, Chapter 3, pp. 545-562.

Swan, G. M. (1984). Application of Optimal Control Theory in Biomedicine, *CRC Press*.

Sereti, I.; Anthony, K.B.; Martinez-Wilson H.; Lempicki R. Adelsberger, J.; Metcalf, J.A.; Hallahan; C.W.; Follmann, D.; Davey, R.T.; Kovacs, J.A.; & Lane H.C. (2004). IL-2 induced CD4+ T-cell expansion in HIV-infected patients is associated with long-term decreases in T-cell proliferation, *Blood* , 104, pp. 775-780.

Smith, K.A. (2001). Low-dose daily interleukin-2 immunotherapy: accelerating immune restoration and expanding HIV-specific T-cell immunity without toxicity AIDS, *suppl 1*, vol. 15, pp. S28-S35.

Banerjee, S. (2008). Immunotherapywith Interleukin-2: A Study Based On Mathematical Modeling, *Int. J. Appl. Math. Comput. Sci.*, vol. 18, pp. 389-398.

Marchettia, G.; Meroni, L.; Molteni, C.; Bandera, A.; Franzetti, F.; Galli, M.; Moroni, M.; Clericib, M.; & Gori, A. (2004). Interleukin-2 immunotherapy exerts a differential effect on CD4 and CD8 T cell dynamics, *AIDS*, vol.18, pp. 211-216.

De, Paoli P. (2001). Immunological effects of Interleukin-2 therapy in human immune-deficiency virus-positive subjects Clin. Diagn. Lab., *Immunol.*, vol. 8, pp. 671-677.

Sereti, I.; Sklar, P.; Ramchandani, M.S.; Read, S.W.; Aggarwal, V.; Imamichi, H.; Natarajan, V.; Metcalf, J.A.; Davey, R.T.; Kovacs, J.A.; DerSimonian, R.; & Lane, H.C. (2007). CD4+ T Cell Responses to Interleukin-2 Administration in HIV-Infected Patients Are Directly Related to the Baseline Level of Immune Activation, *J. Infect. Dis.*, vol.196 , pp. 677-683.

De, Paoli P.; Bortolin, M. T; Zanussi, S.; Monzoni, A.; Pratesi, C; $ Giacc M. (2001). Changes in thymic function in HIV-positive patients treated with highly active antiretroviral therapy and interleukin-2, *Clin Exp Immunol*, vol. 125, pp.440-446.

Marchettia, G.; Franzetti, F.; & Gori, A. (2005). Partial immune reconstitution following highly active antiretroviral therapy: can adjuvant interleukin-2 fill the gap?, *J. Antimicrob. Chemother.*, vol. 55, pp. 401-409.

Paredes, R.; deQuiros, J.C.L.B.; Fernandez-Cruz, Z.; Clotet, $ Lane, H.C. (2002). Potential role of interleukin-2 in patients with HIV infection, *AIDS Rev.*, vol. 4, pp. 36-40.

Roy Priti Kumar; Chatterjee Amar Nath. (2011). Effect of HAART on CTL Mediated Immune Cells: An Optimal Control Theoretic Approach, *Electrical Engineering and Applied Computing, Springer*, Vol. 90, pp.595-607.

Roy Priti Kumar; Chatterjee, A. N. (2011). Delay Model of HIV with Cure Rate During Long Term Disease Progression, *Electrical Engineering and Applied Computing, Springer*, Vol. 90, pp. 699-713.

Roy Priti Kumar; Chatterjee, A. N. (2010). T-cell Proliferation in a Mathematical Model of CTL Activity Through HIV-1 Infection, *Lecture Notes in Engineering and Computer Science, WCE, UK*, Vol. 1, pp. 615-620.

Roy Priti Kumar; Chatterjee, A. N. (2010). Delay effect in a Mathematical model of HIV infected T-cell against killing by CTL, *Bull. Cal. Math. Soc.*, Vol. 102(6), pp. 513-524.

Perelson, A.S; Nelson, P.W. (1999). Mathematical Analysis of HIV-1 Dynamics in Vivo, *SIAM Review*, Vol. 41, pp. 3-41.

Wodarz, D.; May, R.M.; Nowak, M.A. (2000). The role of antigen independent persistance of memory cytotoxic T lymphocytes, *Int Immunol*, Vol. 12, pp.467.

Bonhoeffer, S.; Coffin, J.M.; Nowak, M.A. (1997). Human Immunodeficiency Virus Drug Therapy and Virus Load, *Journal of Virology*, Vol. 71, pp. 3275–3278.

Nowak, M.A.; Bangham, C.R.M. (1996). A delay -differentianal equation model of HIV-1 infection of $CD4^{+}$T-cells, *Science*, Vol. 272(5258), pp. 74-79.

Kirschner, D. (1996). Using mathematics to underdtand HIV immune dynamics, *Notice of the AMS*.

Gumel, A. B.; Zhang, X. W.; Shivkumar, P. N.; Garba, M. L.; Sahai, B. M. (2002). A new mathematical model for assessing therapeutic strategies for HIV infection, *J. Theo. Medicin*, Vol. 4(2), pp. 147-155.

Herz, A. V. M.; Bonhoeffer, S.; Anderson, R. M.; May, R. M.; Nowak, M. A. (1996). Viral dynamicsin vivo; limitations on estimates of intracellular delay and virus decay, *Proc. Natl. Acad. Sci. USA*, Vol. 93, pp. 7247-7251.

6

Oxidative Stress in Human Health and Disease

Isaac K. Quaye
University of Botswana School of Medicine,
Faculty of Medicine and Health Sciences, Gaborone,
Botswana

1. Introduction

Oxidative stress arises when the antioxidant capacity of cells to scavenge the excess production of reactive oxygen species(ROS) falls short. It may also be due to changes in the redox status of the cell. In health, pro-oxidants engage in useful signaling pathways that are important for growth and cellular health. Overstimulation of signaling pathways leads to sustained pro-oxidant production in the form of ROS that disrupt cellular structures and impair function leading to disease. Normally, antioxidants counteract the activity of pro-oxidants to retain cellular homeostasis and therefore a state of health.

In this review the cellular sources of reactive oxygen species (ROS) will be discussed in addition to its effect on macromolecular structures, cellular function and health. The ROS referred to in the text are:superoxide, hydrogen peroxide, hydroxyl radicals; reactive nitrogen species (RNS) nitric oxide and peroxynitrite.

The primary source of ROS is molecular oxygen (O_2). In aerobic cells during electron transport about 10% of reducing equivalents from NADH leaks to produce superoxide ($O_2^{-}\cdot$) and hydrogen peroxide (H_2O_2). These diffuse out of mitochondria and form the starting materials for subsequent generation of ROS through a serial one electron acceptor process. RNS (NO) also fuel ROS generation through a similar interaction with cytochrome *c* oxidase to give rise to $O_2^{-}\cdot/H_2O_2$ or react with $O_2^{-}\cdot$ to generate peroxynitrite (ONOO-).

The oxidative stress effect on health is discussed from the point of view of infectious/communicable diseases, non-infectious/non communicable diseases, genetic diseases and oxidant stress factors (mutation/hemolysis).

The respective infectious/communicable and non communicable diseases that are discussed are malaria, HIV/AIDS, and diabetes, obesity, sickle cell disease and ageing. Except for ageing, the biology of the diseases is briefly outlined and host immunological responses to the disease state that augments ROS generation and its effects are discussed.

The review ends with a brief on oxidative stress and ageing and a summary of how oxidative stress is at the core of the physiological processes that maintain a healthy body and longevity.

2. ROS activity in normal cell function

The designation 'reactive oxygen species' refers to the unpaired electrons on an oxygen atom, molecule or ion that confers reactivity to the species (1, 2). By this definition oxygen molecule is the weakest radical as the ground state has two unpaired electrons (1) although it is unreactive. Multicellular organisms maintain a network of signals to ensure growth, defense and repair. These signals begin outside of the cell, with ligand receptor interaction, followed by conformational changes in the receptor that enables it to be activated through phosphorylation by kinases and inhibition of phosphatases (3, 4). The signal is then carried by second messengers for transduction into the cell nucleus (5, 6). Transcription factors constitute the terminal signal receivers to initiate gene expression critical for normal cell function. ROS act as second messengers in signal transduction in normal housekeeping cell functions (7, 8). ROS signaling can also be through regulation of ion channels, in particular potassium and calcium ion channels to modulate nerve conduction and apoptosis (9).

In normal cell function ROS is generated constitutively by non-phagocytic cells and in response to injury, trauma or infection by phagocytic cells (10, 11). A common functional attribute of the two sources of ROS is that moderate amounts is largely associated with signaling activity while increasing amounts is important in cellular defense and or repair (12). Moderate amounts of ROS are generated through electron transport, vascular smooth muscle cell (VSMC) and endothelial cell (EC) activities (13). Other cellular sources of ROS that may be limited by the changes in cellular metabolic activity include lipoxygenases, cyclooxygenase, cytochrome P450 enzyme activities and lipid peroxidation (7).

2.1 ROS generation in non phagocytic conditions

Non phagocytic generation of superoxide occurs constitutively and intracellularly in fibrobrast , smooth muscle cells (14), renal mesanglial cells (15), hematopoietic stem cells, neurons, hepatocytes, vascular endothelium and for the cellular organelles mitochondria, peroxisomes and the cytochrome P450 system. When generated, ROS participate in the maintenance of baseline signal transduction needed for normal cell function in the absence of activation (16-18). The non phagocytic oxidases (NOX) are transmembrane proteins that transport electrons across cell membranes to reduce oxygen to superoxide. To date six human isoforms have been isolated (Nox 1, 3, 4, 5, and Duox 1 and 2) (19, 20). They utilize a system that is dependent on NADPH, although, NADH can also be used as substrate (21). As a result they are referred to as NAD(P)H oxidases (12, 22). A large component of the non-phagocytic ROS is from mitochondria during electron transport under normal physiological conditions (23). The primary ROS is superoxide generated from reduction of oxygen. It has a short half-life and so its availability is limited, making it a poor signaling molecule (24). In low pH environments as in phagosomes however, the reactivity of superoxide is enhanced by conversion to hydrogen peroxide (25). Unlike superoxide, hydrogen peroxide which is generated from superoxide dismutation (26), is stable and can selectively diffuse through membrane pores to stimulate distant targets, including downstream kinases (27, 28). It also activates the antioxidant function of p53 which potentiates the activity of glutathione peroxidase to convert it to water (29). A summary of ROS generation in the mitochondria in normal physiology and some effects attributed to ROS is presented in Figure 1.

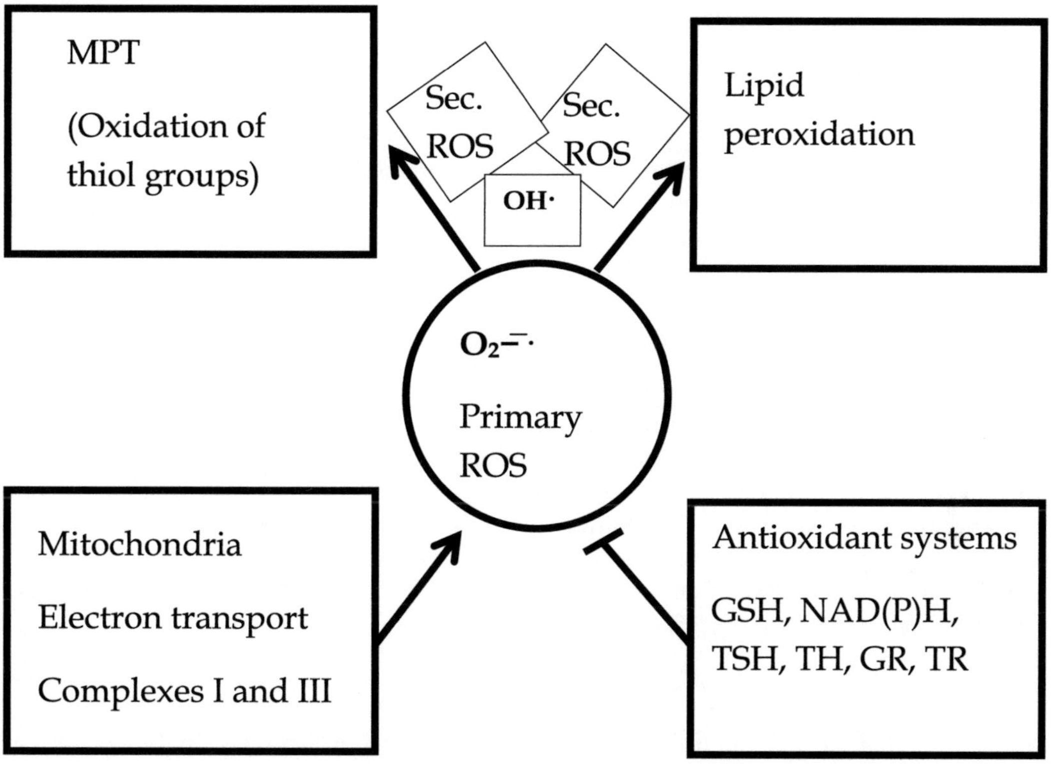

Fig. 1. Mitochondrial ROS generation sites by partial reduction of oxygen through a series of one electron acceptance and a role in oxidative stress effects.

2.2 ROS generation in the electron transport chain

At the end of the electron transport chain, molecular oxygen receives 4 electrons and is reduced to water providing energy for ATP synthesis. When oxygen is incompletely oxidized through the sequential acceptance of one electron, it gives rise to oxygen radicals that are more reactive than the molecule. These are in order of one electron acceptance, $O_2^{-}\cdot$, H_2O_2 and $OH^{\cdot}$ (30, 31). Acquisition of an electron by molecular oxygen generates $O_2^{-}\cdot$ as the primary ROS. The sites in the electron transport chain known to significantly contribute to ROS are complex I and III. Complex I ROS production is mediated by NADH coenzyme Q reductase while in complex III ROS production is through the binding of NO to ubiquinol cytochrome *c* oxidase to produce $O_2^{-}\cdot$ and H_2O_2 (31-33). Mitochondrial nitric oxide synthase produces NO, the primary RNS which reacts with $O_2^{-}\cdot$ to give peroxynitrite. Therefore NO production is central to the generation of $O_2^{-}\cdot$ and H_2O_2 in the electron transport chain (34, 35). Mitochondria also functions as an oxygen sensor under hypoxia to produce hydrogen peroxide which stabilizes hypoxia inducible factor (HIF) to modulate its effect on hypoxia (36-38). HIF is degraded by the hydroxylation of prolyl residues and requires iron as an obligatory cofactor, so when ROS oxidizes iron, it is unavailable for hydroxylation thereby retaining cellular response to hypoxia (38). In normal cellular metabolism, low to moderate ROS/RNS are generated as part of the signaling pathways, cellular response to growth and in innate and adaptive immune response against danger signals (39).

2.3 ROS generation in VSMC and EC

ROS generation in non-phagocytic cells other than mitochondria, is through the activity of non-phagocytic NAD(P)H oxidase (Nox) following ligand binding to the cognate receptor (cytokines, growth factor and G-protein coupled receptor agonists, e.g. angiotensin II) (40, 41). Of particular note is the binding of vascular endothelial growth factor (VEGF), platelet derived growth factor and epidermal growth factor (EGF) to their cognate receptors that lead to receptor dimerization, auto-phosphorylation and signaling to activate redox sensitive transcription factors (eg. NF-κB) responsible for the expression of target genes (40).

2.4 Functional significance of ROS/RNS generation

ROS generated by non-phagocytic cells channel signals to induce cell migration, proliferation and vessel wall formation (42). This activity is particularly important for angiogenesis and in ischemia/reperfusion response (27). In order to sustain signal transduction, ROS generated from ligand receptor interactions can oxidize cysteine residues in phosphatases to inhibit their function and sustain signal transduction to the nucleus (43, 44). Within the endothelial cell (EC), hydrogen peroxide or angiotensin II (Ang II) stimulation of ROS production activates eNOS to produce NO which facilitates cell migration and proliferation (2, 45, 46).

2.5 ROS and danger sensing

The cells of the innate immune system sense danger by recognizing highly conserved pathogen associated molecular patterns (PAMP) present on all the major pathogens; bacteria, parasites, viruses and yeast, or danger associated molecular patterns (DAMP) through germ line encoded pattern recognition receptors (PRR) (47-50). While PAMP enables ROS generation in response to an infection, DAMP enables cellular response to danger (damage, stress) in the absence of an infection (51-53). These molecules that signal cell damage or stress include ATP, nucleotides and uric acid (54). Through ligand receptor interactions and phagocytosis, ROS signaling molecules (hydrogen peroxide and superoxide) are generated intracellularly to promote signaling cascades on one hand and/or activate inflammasome (55). The inflammasome is a descriptive term for cytosolic pattern recognition receptors belonging to members of the caspase-1 activating platform, nucleotide oligomerization domain (NOD) like receptor family (NLR) or AIM2 DNA binding proteins (56, 57). The proteins activate the expression of pro-inflammatory cytokines (IL-1β and IL-18) necessary to amplify ROS generation against pathogen elimination or containment through pyroptosis (57, 58). ROS can be generated extracellularly when a ligand binds to a receptor. This source of phagocytic ROS is through NADPH oxidase, largely in neutrophils engaged in phagocytosis, when activated by PAMP. Activated neutrophils undergo a burst of ROS production to eliminate the offending organism (59).

3. ROS in oxidative stress

Oxidative stress arises when the activity of oxidant species (ROS) overwhelms the cells capacity to counteract with antioxidants (60-65). In oxidative stress, excess ROS ($O_2^{-}\cdot$, H_2O_2, $OH\cdot$) are involved in three main activities:

a. Causing damage to cellular macromolecules (DNA, proteins and membrane lipids) due to their chemical reactivity,
b. Causing changes in membrane potential, which in the inner mitochondrial membrane directly causes mitochondrial permeability transition (MTP) and
c. Acting as a sink for cellular antioxidants.

Whereas superoxide and hydrogen peroxide target Fe-S clusters and cysteine residues respectively, hydroxyl radical appears to be indiscriminate on targets, including oxidation of thiol groups in membrane proteins, making it the most damaging oxygen species (66-68).

a. ROS effect on macromolecules

DNA damage

The type of DNA damage attributed to ROS species may fall into several forms: single and double strand breaks; (69), sister chromatid exchange, DNA-DNA and DNA protein cross links and base modifications (71). Single strand breaks may be due to oxidation of phosphodiester bonds by direct abstraction of hydrogen by OH· from the deoxyribose-phosphodiester backbone giving rise to abnormal 3′ and 5′ ends which are not recognized by DNA polymerases (72). The bases may undergo hydroxylation or part of the ring may open up particularly for pyrimidine bases (73). Hydroxyl radicals also interact with DNA bases to form adducts. For instance reaction with guanine generates 8-oxo-7,8-dihydro-2′-deoxyguanosine (8-oxodG) adducts (74). Peroxynitrites generated from the reaction between NO and superoxide also react with guanine to form adducts (8-nitodG) (66, 71, 75, 76). The formation of DNA adducts can lead to loss of the bases giving rise to apurinic or apyrimidinic (AP) sites (77, 78). These adducts also contribute to accelerated telomere shortening, which regulates senescence. They can also lead to G→T transversion and microsatellite instability, a recipe for cell transformation (79). ROS attacks DNA to form hydroperoxides and peroxides (80-82). Lipid peroxidation by ROS is mediated through the Fenton reaction ($Fe^{2+} + H_2O_2 = Fe^{3+} + OH\cdot$) to produce lipid hydroperoxides (LOOH) and 4-hydroxynonenal (4-HNE) (1, 67, 83). These reactive metabolites impair membrane function and lead to changes in Ca^{2+} flux (84). They also serve as signaling molecules for activating or inhibiting apoptosis through the activity of serine/threonine kinase Akt in the PI3K/Akt pathway (85). Lipid peroxides are the major end products for stress induced oxidative damage that mediate apoptosis (86).

Protein damage

Oxidative ROS damage of proteins can lead to disruption of several vital cellular activities such as replication, transcription, and protein synthesis (78, 87, 88). The breakdown of amino acids occurs largely through the reactivity of hydroxyl radicals. Hydroxyl radical is generated by Fenton Chemistry through superoxide in the Haber-Weiss reaction ($O_2^{\cdot-} + H_2O_2 \rightarrow O_2 + \cdot OH + OH^-$) (88). It attacks amino acids abstracting hydrogen atom from the alpha carbon to generate the alkyl radical as the primary radical (89). This then undergoes a series of reactions to generate alkyl peroxide and alkoxyl radicals. These radicals not only disrupt the protein backbone but also engage in peptide bond cleavages to disrupt protein function (90). ROS can also oxidize almost all amino acid side chains, in particular sulphur containing amino acids, cysteine and methionine (1, 91). Other well-known targets are glutamyl and prolyl side chains to induce peptide bond cleavage. RNS also contribute to amino acid oxidation (nitration of tyrosine residues, nitrosation of cysteine sulfhydryl groups and oxidation of methionine) through the activity of peroxynitrite generated from a reaction between NO and superoxide (87). Oxidized amino acids have a higher tendency to cross link which affects folding and function. A major physiological impact of protein oxidation is accelerated ageing (92-94). This is attributed to increased degradation of oxidized proteins, limiting function (83, 87, 91, 95).

b. ROS and changes in mitochondrial membrane potential

Oxidation of mitochondrial membrane sulfhydryl groups is associated with membrane permeability transitional states (65). Mitochondrial membrane permeability transition (MPT) occurs when the inner membrane becomes non selectively permeable leading to accumulation of Ca^{2+}, loss of matrix components, impairment in mitochondrial function, excessive fluid accumulation and outer membrane burst (64, 96, 97). This leads to loss of cytochrome *c* and a drive towards apoptosis (96, 97). Currently, it has been shown that changes in mitochondrial redox status due to oxidation of NAD(P)H by ROS serves as the starting point for MPT (64, 98). NAD(P)H is critical for maintaining mitochondrial redox status through reduction of oxidized glutathione (GSSH) and thioredoxin (TSSH) necessary for reducing thiol groups in the inner membrane (27, 99, 100). Oxidized thiol groups in membrane proteins, cross link and aggregate to form the non selective permeability pores that disrupt mitochondrial function (101).

4. ROS in infectious diseases

4.1 Oxidative stress in malaria

Malaria is caused by parasites belonging to the genus *Plasmodium*. In humans four major species are responsible for the disease: *P. falciparum, P. vivax, P. ovale,* and *P. malariae* (102). Recently, *P. knowlesi* has been shown to be a major cause of malaria in parts of South East Asia (Borneo) (103, 104).The parasites are obligate and belong to the Phylum Apicomplexa (105). *P. falciparum* accounts for most severe malaria globally (106). The major vector for parasite transmission is the female anopheline mosquito (107). During a blood meal, sporozoites are inoculated under the skin and travel through the blood stream, liver sinusoids to settle in a hepatocyte after traversing several (108-111). This journey usually takes approximately 1 hour (112). Each sporozoite in a parasitophorous vacuole in the liver divides to generate between 10,000 to 30,000 merozoites (110). In *P. ovale, P. malariae,* and *P. vivax* some sporozoites turn to hypnozoites which can remain dormant for months or several years and then get reactivated (113, 114). Merozoite maturation occurs within two weeks in a process called tissue shizogony. The merozoites invade RBCs and develop into ring forms, trophozoites and blood schizonts which repeat the cycle of RBC invasion leading to significant hemolysis. The cycle repeats every 48 hours for *P. falciparum, P. ovale,* and *P vivax* called tertian malaria and every 72 hours for *P. malariae* called quartan malaria. Each RBC can harbor up to 20 trophozoites. Following a cycle of blood schizogony some merozoites develop into gametocytes which are the sexual forms. These are taken up in a next meal to undergo sexual reproduction and eventually generate sporozoites ready for inoculation(115) .

4.2 Generation of ROS in plasmodium infection

When Plasmodium species infects an individual, the clinical presentation may be described as uncomplicated (asymptomatic or mild) or complicated (severe). In uncomplicated malaria host exposure to the parasite is significant enough to generate protective immunity such that the parasite burden is limited (116). This is usually seen in endemic areas (116, 117). In contrast, in low endemicity and low parasite exposure, because of lack or low host immune response, infection can lead to severe disease. It has been shown that whether an infection is uncomplicated or severe, there is a higher generation of ROS that is host and parasite derived (118). Host derived ROS generation arises from interaction of parasite ligands with host receptors during sporozoite invasion leading to phagocytosis and activation of NADPH dependent oxidases for ROS release (119). In addition polymorphonuclear neutrophil attraction to the site of infection and activation is associated with significant release of ROS as a defense mechanism for parasite clearance (120-122). This mechanism also occurs during blood schizogony to inhibit merozoite invasion of RBCs. During the period of blood schizogony, significant quantities of heme are released into circulation that overwhelms the scavenging activity of hemopexin, so that free heme is available to induce further neutrophil migration and catalyze its activation (123). Free heme also binds to and oxidizes lipoproteins in membranes increasing RBC breakdown (124, 125). Malaria parasites release a large quantity of ROS in the infected RBC in the process of converting heme to hemozoin for heme detoxification (126). It has been shown that hemozoin (Pf, Hz) mediates peroxidation of unsaturated fatty acids and contributes to the production of 4-hydroxynonenal (HNE) which reacts with proteins to form adducts disrupting their function (127). The impact of disrupted protein function is down regulation of receptors required for gene expression and cell division. This is suggested to be a factor in decreased erythropoiesis and malaria induced anemia. An additional source of ROS recently identified is from infected rbc membrane microparticles which enable activation of macrophages and increase ROS generation.

4.3 Oxidative stress in HIV infection

The classical pathway of HIV infection is through binding of the envelope glycoprotein to CD4+ cells mediated by the coreceptors CXCR4 and CCR5 chemokine receptors (128) .HIV-1 isolates that replicate primarily in activated CD4 T-lymphocytes in vitro are said to be T-tropic whereas isolates replicating in primary macrophages are M-tropic (129). Dual tropism is shown by isolates with the ability to infect both cells efficiently. CXCR4 and CCR5 act as coreceptors for T-tropic and M-tropic isolates respectively (129-131). CCR5 target cells appear to be important in the early phase of transmission switching to CXCR4 as the disease progresses (129, 132). For the most part however both receptors are expressed on known target cells (CD4+ T cells, monocyte/macrophages, dendritic cells, Langerhans cells and rectal and vagina mucosa) (133). Recently it has been shown that HIV-1 can be transmitted into cells directly by a tunneling mechanism independent of receptor functions (134). HIV-1 has been divided into nine subtypes called clade A-D, F-H, J and K based on variation in the viral envelope. Clade B is predominant in Europe, the Americas and Australia, while the rest are found in Africa and Asia (135).

A common comorbidity in HIV infection is dementia, which is a combination of behavioral, cognitive, and motor dysfunction following HIV infection (134, 136). It is estimated that in adults below the age of 40, HIV accounts for the most cause of dementia (137, 138). Data accumulated to date shows that oxidative stress is an underlying cause of HIV associated dementia (HAD) (139). Brain polyunsaturated fatty acids readily undergo peroxidation by free radicals to generate the 4-HNE which breaks bonds in cysteine, histidine and lysine residues to disrupt protein function (140). 4-HNE also disrupts mitochondrial function to generate ROS aggravating oxidative stress in the process (141). Lipid peroxidation and protein oxidation also contribute to the generation of carbonyl groups, which characterize HIV dementia (142, 143). Some of the proteins that are affected due to lipid peroxidation include ATPases and glucose transporters. HIV regulatory protein Tat and structural protein gp120 are known to exert neurotoxicity by increasing ROS generation and lipid peroxidation (140). HIV gp41 is documented to induce iNOS expression and NO generation to react with superoxide forming peroxynitrite. Peroxynitrites cause nitration of tyrosine residues to disrupt protein function while its decomposition gives rise to hydroxyl radicals, a highly potent lipid peroxidizing agent (138). Over production of NO has been suggested to also increase HIV-1 replication. HIV-1 infection not only causes an increase in ROS generation but also leads to depletion of protective antioxidants in particular, glutathione (138, 144). Thus HIV disease is characterized by chronic oxidative stress which drives disease pathogenesis.

5. ROS in non communicable diseases

5.1 ROS in type 2 diabetes

Diabetes is a metabolic disease caused by derangement in carbohydrate and lipid metabolism due to defects in insulin secretion, action or both (145). Two major forms are defined, type 1 and 2. Type 1 is due to an absolute deficiency in insulin secretion attributed to autoimmune destruction of the β cells of the Islet and genetic factors (145, 146). Type 2 is a combination of insulin resistance and inadequate compensatory insulin secretory response. It is now confirmed that diabetes is an inflammatory disease with elevated plasma concentrations of IL-6, CRP, orosomucoid and sialic acid (146-148).

5.2 ROS in pancreatic β cell damage

In type 1 diabetes β cell damage partly initiates from cellular response to the danger signal, dsRNA which leads to overexpression of Toll like receptors (TLR3, 4). The TLR then activates redox sensitive transcriptions factors including NF-kB (149).The major source of ROS in pancreatic β cells is from mitochondria and activity of non phagocytic NADPH oxidase (98, 150, 151). When ROS generation is high, the β cell which is known to have lower levels of antioxidants (catalase, glutathione peroxidase and superoxide dismutase) compared to other cell types is damaged leading to decreased insulin secretion. It is also reported that autoimmune activities fuel an inflammatory phenotype to damage β cells. In insulin sensitive tissues glucose is transported intracellularly by specific membrane transporters (GLUT). Once inside the cell glucose is phosphorylated by glucokinase and goes through the glycolytic pathway (152, 153). Increased glycolytic activity feeds into higher ATP production, closure of K+ channels and increased intracellular Ca^{2+} which can stimulate ROS generation by mitochondria (153). The increased Ca^{2}+ flux can also promote NADPH oxidase activity to produce more ROS (154). As previously noted, low levels of ROS generated by glucose metabolism, is important for glucose stimulated insulin secretion while higher levels damage β cells of the Islets and induce insulin resistance through activation of redox sensitive intracellular signaling pathways (6). Changes in glucose and lipid metabolism contribute to ROS generation through the formation of diacylglycerol (DAG), advanced glycation end products (AGE), increased polyol formation and increased hexosamine pathway flux (155, 156). The polyol pathway involves the conversion of glucose to sorbitol when hyperglycemia persists. Metabolism of sorbitol generates fructose in a dehydrogenation reaction so that the NADH/NAD+ ratio increase favoring DAG synthesis. DAG potently stimulates protein kinase C, for activating non phagocytic NADPH oxidases (157). In addition increase in mitochondrial NADH/NAD ratio increases the proton gradient and probability of electron donation to molecular oxygen to generate superoxide (156). The β cell is insulin independent for glucose uptake so under elevated plasma glucose, the cells fail to down regulate glucose entry by insulin resistance. Free available reducing sugars (eg.glucose), can react with free amino groups to form a Schiffs base which rearranges into an Amadori glycation product (158-160). When accumulated in proteins, these AGEs modify protein function and or contribute to generation of ROS thereby damaging the cell (151). Another mechanism is the hexosamine pathway flux which functions under normal metabolism but is increased under hyperglycemia. In this process glucose metabolism in glycolysis is channeled into glucosamine phosphate from fructose 6-phosphate. The end product of the pathway is UDP-N-acetylglucosamine, which acts as a substrate for glycosylation of intracellular proteins, including transcription factors (161). Therefore, the expression of several genes including insulin is affected.

5.3 ROS and insulin resistance

In general insulin resistance leads to a sustained inflammatory state (162). Overt insulin resistance occurs from an initial impairment in insulin mediated glucose up take (IGT) (146, 163, 164). If this state is sustained, the impaired insulin response becomes blunted to constitute resistance (146, 164-166). In the end the blunted response leads to overt type 2 diabetes as glucose uptake is severely compromised leading to derangement in lipid metabolism (167, 168). Target tissues (muscle and adipose tissues) may fail to respond to insulin because of the diminished secretion or decreased sensitivity. Hyperglycemia, raised serum free fatty acids (FFA) and increased inflammatory phenotype indicated by high TNFα, CRP, IL-6 and IL-1β ((165, 167, 169) predominate in insulin resistance. High FFAs repress translocation of GLUT4 transporters to the plasma membrane and resistance to insulin mediated glucose uptake in muscle and adipose tissues, particularly (167). High FFA gives rise to elevated fatty acid metabolites; DAG, ceramides and fatty acyl CoA which activate protein kinase C resulting in activation of serine/threonine cascades (170). In skeletal muscle and adipose tissue the insulin receptor is phosphorylated at tyrosine sites upon binding by insulin (171, 172). The receptor in turn causes phosphorylation of substrates: insulin receptor substrate 1 and 2 (IRS1 and IRS2), which activates PI3-kinase, Akt/protein kinase B to recruit GLUT4 to the plasma membrane for glucose uptake ((167, 173). Elevated lipid metabolites scuttle this mechanism, and instead cause phosphorylation of serine sites on insulin receptor substrates, which inhibit their activation of phosphatidyl-inositol 3-kinase (PI3-kinase) and induce failure of transport of GLUT4 to the cell membrane (150, 171, 174). Also these metabolites decrease downstream signaling activities whereby insulin receptor substrates are activated for insulin secretion and response. ROS can also mediate these responses by inhibiting insulin receptor substrates 1 and 2 (IRS-1, and IRS-2) tyrosine auto-phosphorylation, while increasing phosphorylation of serine sites (173-175). Inhibition of tyrosine phosphorylation limits gene expression, cell growth and differentiation of the Islets.

5.4 ROS in obesity

Obesity is defined as a body mass index greater than or equal to 30 kg/m^2 (176). It is established to be a state of chronic low grade inflammatory disease (meta-inflammation) grouped together with insulin resistance, type 2 diabetes, cardiovascular disease and fatty liver disease as the metabolic syndrome (167). Excess calories stored in adipose tissue, causes it to expand, accompanied by infiltration of macrophages (176-179). The macrophages drive production of pro-inflammatory cytokines (TNFα, IL-6. iNOS, TGF-β, MCP-1) through toll like receptor 4 (TLR4) and so present the inflammatory phenotype (176, 180). In addition, increasing adiposity is associated with changes in the expression of adipokines (leptin, adiponectin, IL-6, resistin and TNF-α) which regulate energy intake and insulin sensitivity (176). With the exception of adiponectin, the expression of all the adipokines is increased with increasing fat mass (166, 178, 181). Adiponectin promotes insulin sensitivity by reducing fat and glucose storage. In Obese individuals, insulin resistance is characterized by upregulation of TNF-α by resident macrophages, a mechanism that is similar to that seen in type 2 diabetes (177). The location of the increased fat mass is known to affect the degree of inflammation. While visceral adipocity exacerbates, lower body fat mass has limited effect (177, 182). Enhanced DAG synthesis also affects downstream signaling pathways required to synthesize protein for Islet cell differentiation. As result islet cell differentiation is limited; this in turn affects insulin secretion and regulation of metabolic pathways (173).

5.5 ROS in sickle cell disease

Sickle cell disease arises from a mutation in the beta globin gene with substitution of glutamate for lysine at the 6th codon of β-globin to give hemoglobin S (HbS) variant (183-185). A homozygous HbSS is referred to as sickle cell anemia, while a heterozygous globin mutant with HbS constitutes sickle cell disease (186). The abnormal Hb has defining characteristics: it undergoes polymerization under low oxygen tension, precipitates when polymerized leading to generation of ROS which oxidizes the rbc membrane and makes it fragile and brittle (187). In sickle cell disease, the vascular endothelium becomes dysfunctional and shows increased inflammatory state, adhesiveness, and activation, concomitant with decreased NO bioavailability (188, 189). The disease makes subjects amenable to ischemic stroke, ischemia reperfusion injury, chronic renal disease, pulmonary hypertension, priapism, fetal wastage and growth retardation (190).

The propensity towards sickling is greatly enhanced if the transit time of rbc in the capillaries is increased. In the inflammatory state such delays become common place leading to severer hemolytic episodes and 'crisis'. Sickle cell anemia has high hemolytic episodes. The average life span of a normal rbc of 120 reduces to 14 days in sickle cell disease (190). The enhanced hemolysis contributes significantly to instigate a proinflammatory phenotype as free heme and hemoglobin are strong oxidants (191). Heme can donate electrons or Fe to membrane lipids through the fenton reaction to generate ROS that contributes to membrane damage and sustained hemolysis(188). Under sustained hemolytic conditions, the cellular mechanisms for scavenging hemoglobin and heme are overwhelmed (haptoglobin and hemopexin respectively) so that free heme and Hb are present intravascularly to initiate inflammation (192, 193). Extravascular hemolysis arising from ineffective scavenging of rbcs worn out or damaged, and ineffective erythropoiesis also contribute to heme and Hb leak into circulation. So in essence, sickle cell anemia is a typical systemic proinflammatory disease with sustained ROS production. Typical sources of ROS include activated NADPH oxidases from activated monocytes and endothelium, increased Xanthine oxidase expression and diminished NO availability (194, 195, 196). Activated endothelium increase expression of adhesion molecules for binding leukocytes and rbcs which contribute to hemostasis, rbc lysis and increased inflammatory phenotype (194).

5.6 ROS and endothelial dysfunction

The endothelium is the organ situated at the interface between the wall of the blood vessel and blood stream, functioning as a sensor for modulating vasomotor function, hemostasis and inflammation (197). Endothelial dysfunction refers to impairment of these functions associated with vascular remodeling and vascular growth, but more commonly to impairment of endothelium dependent vasodilation due to depletion of NO in the vessel wall (198). The factors released by the endothelium may lead to vasodilation or constriction. Some of these factors are NO, prostacycling, C-type natriuretic peptide, and endothelium derived hyper polarizing factors which act as vasodilators. ROS along with Ang II, endothelin 1 (ET-1) and thromboxane A_2, act as vasoconstrictors and up regulate adhesion molecules, intercellular adhesion molecule (ICAM-I), vascular cell adhesion molecule (VCAM-I) and E-selectin (197). The major sources of ROS in the endothelium are mitochondria, lipoxygenases, cyclooxygenases, cytoP450s, xanthine oxidases and NADPH oxidases (2, 14, 198, 199).

5.7 NO depletion and endothelium

In endothelial dysfunction NO synthesis is reduced. This affects vasodilation, inflammation and hemostasis. NO synthesis is by eNOS using L-arginine as substrate in the endothelium. Suggested mechanism for reduced NO synthesis is substrate unavailability, reduced eNOS synthase activity and quenching of NO when synthesized (200-204). ROS constitutes a major quencher of NO bioavailability. Reaction of NO with superoxide generates peroxynitrite which in turn reacts with proteins, lipids, and eNOS cofactor tetrahydrobiopterin (BH_4). By oxidizing BH_4 to generate BH_2, eNOS synthase activity is uncoupled, so that instead of producing NO, more ROS is generated from increased reductase activity of eNOS (199, 205). ROS up regulates the expression of adhesion molecules, ICAM-1, VCAM-1 and chemoattractant molecules (MCP-1) for neutrophil and macrophage attraction and activation (206, 207). eNOS synthase may also be competitively inhibited by asymmetric dimethylarginine (ADMA). It has been shown that increased ADMA concentration correlates with high blood pressure (BP) as renal plasma flow is impaired while flow resistance is increased leading to high BP (208, 209). As protein degradation increases in the cell, ADMA concentration also rises and is excreted in the kidneys or degraded to citrulline by the enzyme dimethylarginine dimethylaminohydrolase (DDAH) (208, 210, 211). As DDAH concentration increases in the cell, ADMA levels correspondingly decrease, associated with increased eNOS activation and reduced BP (211). Recently, the degree of endothelial dysfunction has been shown to inversely correlate with amount of endothelial progenitor cells in circulation. Endothelial progenitor cells have the capacity to develop into endothelial cells and are used to repair endothelial lesions (212, 213).

5.8 ROS in ageing

The free radical theory of ageing postulates that accumulated cellular damage by ROS over a period of time is associated with shortened life span (214). This includes effect on telomere shortening, dementia, accumulation of glycation end products and changes in signaling pathways that affect cellular function. A rise in the intracellular ROS generation as outlined previously damages cells, macromolecules and affects signaling pathways (1, 39, 214). These cumulatively drive cellular ageing.

6. Summary

Cumulative evidence shows that ROS is like a 'double edged sword' that on one side enables normal physiological cellular functions to be sustained and provides defense against invading organisms. However when in excess shown as oxidative stress, it plays a destructive role leading to cellular damage, senescence or death. These life attributes make ROS an essential investigative target in the biochemistry and physiology of health and pathological mechanisms of disease.

7. References

[1] Valko M, Leibfritz D, Moncol J, Cronin MT, Mazur M, Telser J. Free radicals and antioxidants in normal physiological functions and human disease. Int J Biochem Cell Biol 2007;39:44-84.

[2] Taniyama Y, Griendling KK. Reactive oxygen species in the vasculature: molecular and cellular mechanisms. Hypertension 2003;42:1075-81.

[3] Ha H, Lee HB. Reactive oxygen species amplify glucose signalling in renal cells cultured under high glucose and in diabetic kidney. Nephrology (Carlton) 2005;10 Suppl:S7-10.

[4] Lee SR, Kwon KS, Kim SR, Rhee SG. Reversible inactivation of protein-tyrosine phosphatase 1B in A431 cells stimulated with epidermal growth factor. J Biol Chem 1998;273:15366-72.

[5] Reth M. Hydrogen peroxide as second messenger in lymphocyte activation. Nat Immunol 2002;3:1129-34.

[6] Bogeski I, Kappl R, Kummerow C, Gulaboski R, Hoth M, Niemeyer BA. Redox regulation of calcium ion channels: Chemical and physiological aspects. Cell Calcium 2011.

[7] Reth M, Wienands J. Initiation and processing of signals from the B cell antigen receptor. Annu Rev Immunol 1997;15:453-79.

[8] Mahadev K, Wu X, Zilbering A, Zhu L, Lawrence JT, Goldstein BJ. Hydrogen peroxide generated during cellular insulin stimulation is integral to activation of the distal insulin signaling cascade in 3T3-L1 adipocytes. J Biol Chem 2001;276:48662-9.

[9] Reth M, Dick TP. Voltage control for B cell activation. Nat Immunol 2010;11:191-2.

[10] Lau AT, Wang Y, Chiu JF. Reactive oxygen species: current knowledge and applications in cancer research and therapeutic. J Cell Biochem 2008;104:657-67.

[11] Endemann DH, Schiffrin EL. Nitric oxide, oxidative excess, and vascular complications of diabetes mellitus. Curr Hypertens Rep 2004;6:85-9.

[12] Bedard K, Krause KH. The NOX family of ROS-generating NADPH oxidases: physiology and pathophysiology. Physiol Rev 2007;87:245-313.

[13] Spooner R, Yilmaz O. The role of reactive-oxygen-species in microbial persistence and inflammation. Int J Mol Sci 2011;12:334-52.
[14] Griendling KK, FitzGerald GA. Oxidative stress and cardiovascular injury: Part I: basic mechanisms and in vivo monitoring of ROS. Circulation 2003;108:1912-6.
[15] Shiose A, Kuroda J, Tsuruya K, Hirai M, Hirakata H, Naito S, Hattori M, Sakaki Y, Sumimoto H. A novel superoxide-producing NAD(P)H oxidase in kidney. J Biol Chem 2001;276:1417-23.
[16] Starkov AA. The role of mitochondria in reactive oxygen species metabolism and signaling. Ann N Y Acad Sci 2008;1147:37-52.
[17] Balaban RS, Nemoto S, Finkel T. Mitochondria, oxidants, and aging. Cell 2005;120:483-95.
[18] Nabeebaccus A, Zhang M, Shah AM. NADPH oxidases and cardiac remodelling. Heart Fail Rev 2011;16:5-12.
[19] Guichard C, Pedruzzi E, Fay M, Ben Mkaddem S, Coant N, Daniel F, Ogier-Denis E. The Nox/Duox family of ROS-generating NADPH oxidases. Med Sci (Paris) 2006;22:953-9.
[20] Cai H, Griendling KK, Harrison DG. The vascular NAD(P)H oxidases as therapeutic targets in cardiovascular diseases. Trends Pharmacol Sci 2003;24:471-8.
[21] Kim JA, Neupane GP, Lee ES, Jeong BS, Park BC, Thapa P. NADPH oxidase inhibitors: a patent review. Expert Opin Ther Pat 2011;21:1147-58.
[22] Krause KH, Bedard K. NOX enzymes in immuno-inflammatory pathologies. Semin Immunopathol 2008;30:193-4.
[23] Bedard K, Lardy B, Krause KH. NOX family NADPH oxidases: not just in mammals. Biochimie 2007;89:1107-12.
[24] Reeves EP, Nagl M, Godovac-Zimmermann J, Segal AW. Reassessment of the microbicidal activity of reactive oxygen species and hypochlorous acid with reference to the phagocytic vacuole of the neutrophil granulocyte. J Med Microbiol 2003;52:643-51.
[25] Klebanoff SJ. Myeloperoxidase: friend and foe. J Leukoc Biol 2005;77:598-625.
[26] Geiszt M, Witta J, Baffi J, Lekstrom K, Leto TL. Dual oxidases represent novel hydrogen peroxide sources supporting mucosal surface host defense. FASEB J 2003;17:1502-4.
[27] Hoek JB, Rydstrom J. Physiological roles of nicotinamide nucleotide transhydrogenase. Biochem J 1988;254:1-10.
[28] Li JM, Shah AM. Mechanism of endothelial cell NADPH oxidase activation by angiotensin II. Role of the p47phox subunit. J Biol Chem 2003;278:12094-100.
[29] Fujita T, Maruyama M, Araya J, Sassa K, Kawagishi Y, Hayashi R, Matsui S, Kashii T, Yamashita N, Sugiyama E, Kobayashi M. Hydrogen peroxide induces upregulation of Fas in human airway epithelial cells via the activation of PARP-p53 pathway. Am J Respir Cell Mol Biol 2002;27:542-52.
[30] Genova ML, Bianchi C, Lenaz G. Structural organization of the mitochondrial respiratory chain. Ital J Biochem 2003;52:58-61.
[31] Genova ML, Pich MM, Biondi A, Bernacchia A, Falasca A, Bovina C, Formiggini G, Parenti Castelli G, Lenaz G. Mitochondrial production of oxygen radical species and the role of Coenzyme Q as an antioxidant. Exp Biol Med (Maywood) 2003;228:506-13.

[32] Bianchi C, Fato R, Genova ML, Parenti Castelli G, Lenaz G. Structural and functional organization of Complex I in the mitochondrial respiratory chain. Biofactors 2003;18:3-9.

[33] Nohl H, Jordan W. The mitochondrial site of superoxide formation. Biochem Biophys Res Commun 1986;138:533-9.

[34] Packer MA, Porteous CM, Murphy MP. Superoxide production by mitochondria in the presence of nitric oxide forms peroxynitrite. Biochem Mol Biol Int 1996;40:527-34.

[35] Szabo C, Ischiropoulos H, Radi R. Peroxynitrite: biochemistry, pathophysiology and development of therapeutics. Nat Rev Drug Discov 2007;6:662-80.

[36] Muller FU, Neumann J, Schmitz W. Transcriptional regulation by cAMP in the heart. Mol Cell Biochem 2000;212:11-7.

[37] Acker T, Fandrey J, Acker H. The good, the bad and the ugly in oxygen-sensing: ROS, cytochromes and prolyl-hydroxylases. Cardiovasc Res 2006;71:195-207.

[38] Bruick RK, McKnight SL. A conserved family of prolyl-4-hydroxylases that modify HIF. Science 2001;294:1337-40.

[39] Martins Chaves M, Rocha-Vieira E, Pereira dos Reis A, de Lima e Silva R, Gerzstein NC, Nogueira-Machado JA. Increase of reactive oxygen (ROS) and nitrogen (RNS) species generated by phagocyting granulocytes related to age. Mech Ageing Dev 2000;119:1-8.

[40] Griendling KK, Sorescu D, Ushio-Fukai M. NAD(P)H oxidase: role in cardiovascular biology and disease. Circ Res 2000;86:494-501.

[41] Basset O, Deffert C, Foti M, Bedard K, Jaquet V, Ogier-Denis E, Krause KH. NADPH oxidase 1 deficiency alters caveolin phosphorylation and angiotensin II-receptor localization in vascular smooth muscle. Antioxid Redox Signal 2009;11:2371-84.

[42] Chen KC, Zhou Y, Zhang W, Lou MF. Control of PDGF-induced reactive oxygen species (ROS) generation and signal transduction in human lens epithelial cells. Mol Vis 2007;13:374-87.

[43] Hunter T. Tyrosine phosphorylation: thirty years and counting. Curr Opin Cell Biol 2009;21:140-6.

[44] Hunter T, Sun H. Crosstalk between the SUMO and ubiquitin pathways. Ernst Schering Found Symp Proc 2008;(1):1-16.

[45] Diep QN, El Mabrouk M, Cohn JS, Endemann D, Amiri F, Virdis A, Neves MF, Schiffrin EL. Structure, endothelial function, cell growth, and inflammation in blood vessels of angiotensin II-infused rats: role of peroxisome proliferator-activated receptor-gamma. Circulation 2002;105:2296-302.

[46] Diep QN, Amiri F, Touyz RM, Cohn JS, Endemann D, Neves MF, Schiffrin EL. PPARalpha activator effects on Ang II-induced vascular oxidative stress and inflammation. Hypertension 2002;40:866-71.

[47] Matzinger P. An innate sense of danger. Ann N Y Acad Sci 2002;961:341-2.

[48] Medzhitov R, Janeway C,Jr. The Toll receptor family and microbial recognition. Trends Microbiol 2000;8:452-6.

[49] Medzhitov R, Janeway C,Jr. Innate immune recognition: mechanisms and pathways. Immunol Rev 2000;173:89-97.

[50] Andrews T, Sullivan KE. Infections in patients with inherited defects in phagocytic function. Clin Microbiol Rev 2003;16:597-621.

[51] Medzhitov R, Janeway C,Jr. Innate immunity. N Engl J Med 2000;343:338-44.

[52] Medzhitov R, Janeway CA,Jr. How does the immune system distinguish self from nonself? Semin Immunol 2000;12:185,8; discussion 257-344.

[53] Janeway CA,Jr. The immune system evolved to discriminate infectious nonself from noninfectious self. Immunol Today 1992;13:11-6.

[54] Piccini A, Carta S, Tassi S, Lasiglie D, Fossati G, Rubartelli A. ATP is released by monocytes stimulated with pathogen-sensing receptor ligands and induces IL-1beta and IL-18 secretion in an autocrine way. Proc Natl Acad Sci U S A 2008;105:8067-72.

[55] Dunne A. Inflammasome activation: from inflammatory disease to infection. Biochem Soc Trans 2011;39:669-73.

[56] Martinon F, Mayor A, Tschopp J. The inflammasomes: guardians of the body. Annu Rev Immunol 2009;27:229-65.

[57] Martinon F, Tschopp J. NLRs join TLRs as innate sensors of pathogens. Trends Immunol 2005;26:447-54.

[58] Bergsbaken T, Fink SL, Cookson BT. Pyroptosis: host cell death and inflammation. Nat Rev Microbiol 2009;7:99-109.

[59] Faurschou M, Borregaard N. Neutrophil granules and secretory vesicles in inflammation. Microbes Infect 2003;5:1317-27.

[60] Vurusaner B, Poli G, Basaga H. Tumor suppressor genes and ROS: complex networks of interactions. Free Radic Biol Med 2011.

[61] Lushchak VJ. Budding Yeast Saccharomyces as a model to study modification of proteins in eukaryotes.Acta Biochimica Polonica 2006;53:679-684

[62] Mena S, Ortega A, Estrela JM. Oxidative stress in environmental-induced carcinogenesis. Mutat Res 2009;674:36-44.

[63] Berk BC. Novel approaches to treat oxidative stress and cardiovascular diseases. Trans Am Clin Climatol Assoc 2007;118:209-14.

[64] Kowaltowski AJ, Castilho RF, Vercesi AE. Mitochondrial permeability transition and oxidative stress. FEBS Lett 2001;495:12-5.

[65] Zoratti M, Szabo I. The mitochondrial permeability transition. Biochim Biophys Acta 1995;1241:139-76.

[66] Marnett LJ, Riggins JN, West JD. Endogenous generation of reactive oxidants and electrophiles and their reactions with DNA and protein. J Clin Invest 2003;111:583-93.

[67] Davies KJ. An overview of oxidative stress. IUBMB Life 2000;50:241-4.

[68] Cadenas E, Davies KJ. Mitochondrial free radical generation, oxidative stress, and aging. Free Radic Biol Med 2000;29:222-30.

[69] Davies KJ. Oxidative stress, antioxidant defenses, and damage removal, repair, and replacement systems. IUBMB Life 2000;50:279-89.

[70] Hazen SL, d'Avignon A, Anderson MM, Hsu FF, Heinecke JW. Human neutrophils employ the myeloperoxidase-hydrogen peroxide-chloride system to oxidize alpha-amino acids to a family of reactive aldehydes. Mechanistic studies identifying labile intermediates along the reaction pathway. J Biol Chem 1998;273:4997-5005.

[71] Marnett LJ, Plastaras JP. Endogenous DNA damage and mutation. Trends Genet 2001;17:214-21.

[72] Cadet J, Carvalho VM, Onuki J, Douki T, Medeiros MH, Di Mascio PD. Purine DNA adducts of 4,5-dioxovaleric acid and 2,4-decadienal. IARC Sci Publ 1999;(150):103-13.
[73] Uchida K. Cellular response to bioactive lipid peroxidation products. Free Radic Res 2000;33:731-7.
[74] Wagner JR, Hu CC, Ames BN. Endogenous oxidative damage of deoxycytidine in DNA. Proc Natl Acad Sci U S A 1992;89:3380-4.
[75] Burney S, Niles JC, Dedon PC, Tannenbaum SR. DNA damage in deoxynucleosides and oligonucleotides treated with peroxynitrite. Chem Res Toxicol 1999;12:513-20.
[76] Burney S, Caulfield JL, Niles JC, Wishnok JS, Tannenbaum SR. The chemistry of DNA damage from nitric oxide and peroxynitrite. Mutat Res 1999;424:37-49.
[77] Halliwell B, Zhao K, Whiteman M. Nitric oxide and peroxynitrite. The ugly, the uglier and the not so good: a personal view of recent controversies. Free Radic Res 1999;31:651-69.
[78] Halliwell B. Free radicals, proteins and DNA: oxidative damage versus redox regulation. Biochem Soc Trans 1996;24:1023-7.
[79] Di Micco R, Fumagalli M, Cicalese A, Piccinin S, Gasparini P, Luise C, Schurra C, Garre' M, Nuciforo PG, Bensimon A, Maestro R, Pelicci PG, d'Adda di Fagagna F. Oncogene-induced senescence is a DNA damage response triggered by DNA hyper-replication. Nature 2006;444:638-42.
[80] Bartkova J, Bakkenist CJ, Rajpert-De Meyts E, Skakkebaek NE, Sehested M, Lukas J, Kastan MB, Bartek J. ATM activation in normal human tissues and testicular cancer. Cell Cycle 2005;4:838-45.
[81] Swenberg JA, Ham A, Koc H, Morinello E, Ranasinghe A, Tretyakova N, Upton PB, Wu K. DNA adducts: effects of low exposure to ethylene oxide, vinyl chloride and butadiene. Mutat Res 2000;464:77-86.
[82] Swenberg JA, Christova-Gueorguieva NI, Upton PB, Ranasinghe A, Scheller N, Wu KY, Yen TY, Hayes R. 1,3-butadiene: cancer, mutations, and adducts. Part V: Hemoglobin adducts as biomarkers of 1,3-butadiene exposure and metabolism. Res Rep Health Eff Inst 2000;(92):191,210; discussion 211-9.
[83] Davies KJ, Pryor WA. The evolution of Free Radical Biology & Medicine: a 20-year history. Free Radic Biol Med 2005;39:1263-4.
[84] Van der Vliet A, Bast A. Effect of oxidative stress on receptors and signal transmission. Chem Biol Interact 1992;85:95-116.
[85] Sharma LK, Fang H, Liu J, Vartak R, Deng J, Bai Y. Mitochondrial respiratory complex I dysfunction promotes tumorigenesis through ROS alteration and AKT activation. Hum Mol Genet 2011.
[86] Jing Y, Liu LZ, Jiang Y, Zhu Y, Guo NL, Barnett J, Rojanasakul Y, Agani F, Jiang BH. Cadmium Increases HIF-1 and VEGF Expression through ROS, ERK and AKT Signaling Pathways and Induces Malignant Transformation of Human Bronchial Epithelial Cells. Toxicol Sci 2011.
[87] Stadtman ER. Protein oxidation and aging. Free Radic Res 2006;40:1250-8.
[88] Liochev SI, Fridovich I. The Haber-Weiss cycle -- 70 years later: an alternative view. Redox Rep 2002;7:55,7; author reply 59-60.

[89] Pastor N, Weinstein H, Jamison E, Brenowitz M. A detailed interpretation of OH radical footprints in a TBP-DNA complex reveals the role of dynamics in the mechanism of sequence-specific binding. J Mol Biol 2000;304:55-68.
[90] Roubal WT, Tappel AL. Damage to proteins, enzymes, and amino acids by peroxidizing lipids. Arch Biochem Biophys 1966;113:5-8.
[91] Stadtman ER. Cyclic oxidation and reduction of methionine residues of proteins in antioxidant defense and cellular regulation. Arch Biochem Biophys 2004;423:2-5.
[92] Dalle-Donne I, Scaloni A, Giustarini D, Cavarra E, Tell G, Lungarella G, Colombo R, Rossi R, Milzani A. Proteins as biomarkers of oxidative/nitrosative stress in diseases: the contribution of redox proteomics. Mass Spectrom Rev 2005;24:55-99.
[93] Fossel M. The long run. J Anti Aging Med 2003;6:1-2.
[94] Hayflick L. How and why we age. Exp Gerontol 1998;33:639-53.
[95] Jenner A, England TG, Aruoma OI, Halliwell B. Measurement of oxidative DNA damage by gas chromatography-mass spectrometry: ethanethiol prevents artifactual generation of oxidized DNA bases. Biochem J 1998;331 (Pt 2):365-9.
[96] Green DR, Reed JC. Mitochondria and apoptosis. Science 1998;281:1309-12.
[97] Kowaltowski AJ, Vercesi AE. Mitochondrial damage induced by conditions of oxidative stress. Free Radic Biol Med 1999;26:463-71.
[98] Green DR, Amarante-Mendes GP. The point of no return: mitochondria, caspases, and the commitment to cell death. Results Probl Cell Differ 1998;24:45-61.
[99] Kowaltowski AJ. Alternative mitochondrial functions in cell physiopathology: beyond ATP production. Braz J Med Biol Res 2000;33:241-50.
[100] Hoek JB, Harada N, Moehren G, Tomsho M, Stubbs CD. The role of calcium and phospholipase A2 in glucagon-induced enhancement of mitochondrial calcium retention. Adv Exp Med Biol 1988;232:25-36.
[101] Lenartowicz E, Bernardi P, Azzone GF. Phenylarsine oxide induces the cyclosporin A-sensitive membrane permeability transition in rat liver mitochondria. J Bioenerg Biomembr 1991;23:679-88.
[102] Kantele A, Jokiranta TS. Review of cases with the emerging fifth human malaria parasite, Plasmodium knowlesi. Clin Infect Dis 2011;52:1356-62.
[103] Figtree M, Lee R, Bain L, Kennedy T, Mackertich S, Urban M, Cheng Q, Hudson BJ. Plasmodium knowlesi in human, Indonesian Borneo. Emerg Infect Dis 2010;16:672-4.
[104] Cox-Singh J, Davis TM, Lee KS, Shamsul SS, Matusop A, Ratnam S, Rahman HA, Conway DJ, Singh B. Plasmodium knowlesi malaria in humans is widely distributed and potentially life threatening. Clin Infect Dis 2008;46:165-71.
[105] Ralph SA, van Dooren GG, Waller RF, Crawford MJ, Fraunholz MJ, Foth BJ, Tonkin CJ, Roos DS, McFadden GI. Tropical infectious diseases: metabolic maps and functions of the Plasmodium falciparum apicoplast. Nat Rev Microbiol 2004;2:203-16.
[106] Newbold C, Warn P, Black G, Berendt A, Craig A, Snow B, Msobo M, Peshu N, Marsh K. Receptor-specific adhesion and clinical disease in Plasmodium falciparum. Am J Trop Med Hyg 1997;57:389-98.
[107] Patz JA, Strzepek K, Lele S, Hedden M, Greene S, Noden B, Hay SI, Kalkstein L, Beier JC. Predicting key malaria transmission factors, biting and entomological inoculation rates, using modelled soil moisture in Kenya. Trop Med Int Health 1998;3:818-27.

[108] Amino R, Thiberge S, Blazquez S, Baldacci P, Renaud O, Shorte S, Menard R. Imaging malaria sporozoites in the dermis of the mammalian host. Nat Protoc 2007;2:1705-12.
[109] Kappe SH, Kaiser K, Matuschewski K. The Plasmodium sporozoite journey: a rite of passage. Trends Parasitol 2003;19:135-43.
[110] Vaughan AM, Aly AS, Kappe SH. Malaria parasite pre-erythrocytic stage infection: gliding and hiding. Cell Host Microbe 2008;4:209-18.
[111] Yamauchi LM, Coppi A, Snounou G, Sinnis P. Plasmodium sporozoites trickle out of the injection site. Cell Microbiol 2007;9:1215-22.
[112] Frevert U, Usynin I, Baer K, Klotz C. Nomadic or sessile: can Kupffer cells function as portals for malaria sporozoites to the liver? Cell Microbiol 2006;8:1537-46.
[113] Imwong M, Snounou G, Pukrittayakamee S, Tanomsing N, Kim JR, Nandy A, Guthmann JP, Nosten F, Carlton J, Looareesuwan S, Nair S, Sudimack D, Day NP, Anderson TJ, White NJ. Relapses of Plasmodium vivax infection usually result from activation of heterologous hypnozoites. J Infect Dis 2007;195:927-33.
[114] Mueller I, Galinski MR, Baird JK, Carlton JM, Kochar DK, Alonso PL, del Portillo HA. Key gaps in the knowledge of Plasmodium vivax, a neglected human malaria parasite. Lancet Infect Dis 2009;9:555-66.
[115] Garcia LS. Malaria. Clin Lab Med 2010;30:93-129.
[116] Malaguarnera L, Musumeci S. The immune response to Plasmodium falciparum malaria. Lancet Infect Dis 2002;2:472-8.
[117] Marsh K, Forster D, Waruiru C, Mwangi I, Winstanley M, Marsh V, Newton C, Winstanley P, Warn P, Peshu N. Indicators of life-threatening malaria in African children. N Engl J Med 1995;332:1399-404.
[118] Delmas-Beauvieux MC, Peuchant E, Dumon MF, Receveur MC, Le Bras M, Clerc M. Relationship between red blood cell antioxidant enzymatic system status and lipoperoxidation during the acute phase of malaria. Clin Biochem 1995;28:163-9.
[119] Schofield L, Tachado SD. Regulation of host cell function by glycosylphosphatidylinositols of the parasitic protozoa. Immunol Cell Biol 1996;74:555-63.
[120] Dondorp AM, Angus BJ, Chotivanich K, Silamut K, Ruangveerayuth R, Hardeman MR, Kager PA, Vreeken J, White NJ. Red blood cell deformability as a predictor of anemia in severe falciparum malaria. Am J Trop Med Hyg 1999;60:733-7.
[121] Djeu JY, Serbousek D, Blanchard DK. Release of tumor necrosis factor by human polymorphonuclear leukocytes. Blood 1990;76:1405-9.
[122] Djeu JY, Matsushima K, Oppenheim JJ, Shiotsuki K, Blanchard DK. Functional activation of human neutrophils by recombinant monocyte-derived neutrophil chemotactic factor/IL-8. J Immunol 1990;144:2205-10.
[123] Jakeman GN, Saul A, Hogarth WL, Collins WE. Anaemia of acute malaria infections in non-immune patients primarily results from destruction of uninfected erythrocytes. Parasitology 1999;119 (Pt 2):127-33.
[124] Mohan K, Ganguly NK, Dubey ML, Mahajan RC. Oxidative damage of erythrocytes infected with Plasmodium falciparum. An in vitro study. Ann Hematol 1992;65:131-4.

[125] Mohan K, Dubey ML, Ganguly NK, Mahajan RC. Plasmodium falciparum: role of activated blood monocytes in erythrocyte membrane damage and red cell loss during malaria. Exp Parasitol 1995;80:54-63.
[126] Omodeo-Sale F, Motti A, Dondorp A, White NJ, Taramelli D. Destabilisation and subsequent lysis of human erythrocytes induced by Plasmodium falciparum haem products. Eur J Haematol 2005;74:324-32.
[127] Foldes J, Matyi A, Matkovics B. The role of free radicals and antioxidative enzymes in erythrocytes and liver cells in the course of Plasmodium berghei and Plasmodium vinckei infection of mice. Acta Microbiol Immunol Hung 1994;41:153-61.
[128] Marx PA, Chen Z. The function of simian chemokine receptors in the replication of SIV. Semin Immunol 1998;10:215-23.
[129] Berger EA, Murphy PM, Farber JM. Chemokine receptors as HIV-1 coreceptors: roles in viral entry, tropism, and disease. Annu Rev Immunol 1999;17:657-700.
[130] Alkhatib G, Combadiere C, Broder CC, Feng Y, Kennedy PE, Murphy PM, Berger EA. CC CKR5: a RANTES, MIP-1alpha, MIP-1beta receptor as a fusion cofactor for macrophage-tropic HIV-1. Science 1996;272:1955-8.
[131] Dragic T, Litwin V, Allaway GP, Martin SR, Huang Y, Nagashima KA, Cayanan C, Maddon PJ, Koup RA, Moore JP, Paxton WA. HIV-1 entry into CD4+ cells is mediated by the chemokine receptor CC-CKR-5. Nature 1996;381:667-73.
[132] Alkhatib G, Broder CC, Berger EA. Cell type-specific fusion cofactors determine human immunodeficiency virus type 1 tropism for T-cell lines versus primary macrophages. J Virol 1996;70:5487-94.
[133] Rottman JB, Ganley KP, Williams K, Wu L, Mackay CR, Ringler DJ. Cellular localization of the chemokine receptor CCR5. Correlation to cellular targets of HIV-1 infection. Am J Pathol 1997;151:1341-51.
[134] Eugenin EA, Osiecki K, Lopez L, Goldstein H, Calderon TM, Berman JW. CCL2/monocyte chemoattractant protein-1 mediates enhanced transmigration of human immunodeficiency virus (HIV)-infected leukocytes across the blood-brain barrier: a potential mechanism of HIV-CNS invasion and NeuroAIDS. J Neurosci 2006;26:1098-106.
[135] Navia BA, Jordan BD, Price RW. The AIDS dementia complex: I. Clinical features. Ann Neurol 1986;19:517-24.
[136] King JE, Eugenin EA, Buckner CM, Berman JW. HIV tat and neurotoxicity. Microbes Infect 2006;8:1347-57.
[137] Gonzalez-Scarano F, Martin-Garcia J. The neuropathogenesis of AIDS. Nat Rev Immunol 2005;5:69-81.
[138] Steiner J, Haughey N, Li W, Venkatesan A, Anderson C, Reid R, Malpica T, Pocernich C, Butterfield DA, Nath A. Oxidative stress and therapeutic approaches in HIV dementia. Antioxid Redox Signal 2006;8:2089-100.
[139] Turchan J, Sacktor N, Wojna V, Conant K, Nath A. Neuroprotective therapy for HIV dementia. Curr HIV Res 2003;1:373-83.
[140] Haughey NJ, Cutler RG, Tamara A, McArthur JC, Vargas DL, Pardo CA, Turchan J, Nath A, Mattson MP. Perturbation of sphingolipid metabolism and ceramide production in HIV-dementia. Ann Neurol 2004;55:257-67.
[141] Esterbauer H, Schaur RJ, Zollner H. Chemistry and biochemistry of 4-hydroxynonenal, malonaldehyde and related aldehydes. Free Radic Biol Med 1991;11:81-128.

[142] Butterfield DA. beta-Amyloid-associated free radical oxidative stress and neurotoxicity: implications for Alzheimer's disease. Chem Res Toxicol 1997;10:495-506.

[143] Butterfield DA, Howard BJ, Yatin S, Allen KL, Carney JM. Free radical oxidation of brain proteins in accelerated senescence and its modulation by N-tert-butyl-alpha-phenylnitrone. Proc Natl Acad Sci U S A 1997;94:674-8.

[144] Gaskill PJ, Calderon TM, Luers AJ, Eugenin EA, Javitch JA, Berman JW. Human immunodeficiency virus (HIV) infection of human macrophages is increased by dopamine: a bridge between HIV-associated neurologic disorders and drug abuse. Am J Pathol 2009;175:1148-59.

[145] American Diabetes Association. Diagnosis and classification of diabetes mellitus. Diabetes Care 2011;34 Suppl 1:S62-9.

[146] Dabelea D, Pihoker C, Talton JW, D'Agostino RB,Jr, Fujimoto W, Klingensmith GJ, Lawrence JM, Linder B, Marcovina SM, Mayer-Davis EJ, Imperatore G, Dolan LM, SEARCH for Diabetes in Youth Study. Etiological approach to characterization of diabetes type: the SEARCH for Diabetes in Youth Study. Diabetes Care 2011;34:1628-33.

[147] Duncan BB, Schmidt MI, Pankow JS, Ballantyne CM, Couper D, Vigo A, Hoogeveen R, Folsom AR, Heiss G, Atherosclerosis Risk in Communities Study. Low-grade systemic inflammation and the development of type 2 diabetes: the atherosclerosis risk in communities study. Diabetes 2003;52:1799-805.

[148] Schmidt MI, Duncan BB. Diabesity: an inflammatory metabolic condition. Clin Chem Lab Med 2003;41:1120-30.

[149] Rasschaert J, Ladriere L, Urbain M, Dogusan Z, Katabua B, Sato S, Akira S, Gysemans C, Mathieu C, Eizirik DL. Toll-like receptor 3 and STAT-1 contribute to double-stranded RNA+ interferon-gamma-induced apoptosis in primary pancreatic beta-cells. J Biol Chem 2005;280:33984-91.

[150] Newsholme P, Haber EP, Hirabara SM, Rebelato EL, Procopio J, Morgan D, Oliveira-Emilio HC, Carpinelli AR, Curi R. Diabetes associated cell stress and dysfunction: role of mitochondrial and non-mitochondrial ROS production and activity. J Physiol 2007;583:9-24.

[151] Newsholme P, Keane D, Welters HJ, Morgan NG. Life and death decisions of the pancreatic beta-cell: the role of fatty acids. Clin Sci (Lond) 2007;112:27-42.

[152] Newsholme P, Bender K, Kiely A, Brennan L. Amino acid metabolism, insulin secretion and diabetes. Biochem Soc Trans 2007;35:1180-6.

[153] Bender K, Newsholme P, Brennan L, Maechler P. The importance of redox shuttles to pancreatic beta-cell energy metabolism and function. Biochem Soc Trans 2006;34:811-4.

[154] Kruman I, Guo Q, Mattson MP. Calcium and reactive oxygen species mediate staurosporine-induced mitochondrial dysfunction and apoptosis in PC12 cells. J Neurosci Res 1998;51:293-308.

[155] Bosch RR, Janssen SW, Span PN, Olthaar A, van Emst-de Vries SE, Willems PH, Martens JMG, Hermus AR, Sweep CC. Exploring levels of hexosamine biosynthesis pathway intermediates and protein kinase C isoforms in muscle and fat tissue of Zucker Diabetic Fatty rats. Endocrine 2003;20:247-52.

[156] Buse MG, Robinson KA, Gettys TW, McMahon EG, Gulve EA. Increased activity of the hexosamine synthesis pathway in muscles of insulin-resistant ob/ob mice. Am J Physiol 1997;272:E1080-8.
[157] Brownlee M. Biochemistry and molecular cell biology of diabetic complications. Nature 2001;414:813-20.
[158] Coughlan MT, Yap FY, Tong DC, Andrikopoulos S, Gasser A, Thallas-Bonke V, Webster DE, Miyazaki J, Kay TW, Slattery RM, Kaye DM, Drew BG, Kingwell BA, Fourlanos S, Groop PH, Harrison LC, Knip M, Forbes JM. Advanced Glycation End Products Are Direct Modulators of {beta}-Cell Function. Diabetes 2011;60:2523-32.
[159] Iborra RT, Machado-Lima A, Castilho G, Nunes VS, Abdalla DS, Nakandakare ER, Passarelli M. Advanced Glycation in macrophages induces intracellular accumulation of 7-ketocholesterol and total sterols by decreasing the expression of ABCA-1 and ABCG-1. Lipids Health Dis 2011;10:172.
[160] Madian AG, Myracle AD, Diaz-Maldonado N, Rochelle NS, Janle EM, Regnier FE. Determining the Effects of Antioxidants on Oxidative Stress Induced Carbonylation of Proteins. Anal Chem 2011.
[161] Gabriely I, Yang XM, Cases JA, Ma XH, Rossetti L, Barzilai N. Hyperglycemia induces PAI-1 gene expression in adipose tissue by activation of the hexosamine biosynthetic pathway. Atherosclerosis 2002;160:115-22.
[162] Dandona P, Aljada A, Mohanty P, Ghanim H, Hamouda W, Assian E, Ahmad S. Insulin inhibits intranuclear nuclear factor kappaB and stimulates IkappaB in mononuclear cells in obese subjects: evidence for an anti-inflammatory effect? J Clin Endocrinol Metab 2001;86:3257-65.
[163] Eizirik DL, Colli ML, Ortis F. The role of inflammation in insulitis and beta-cell loss in type 1 diabetes. Nat Rev Endocrinol 2009;5:219-26.
[164] Fernandez-Real JM, Pickup JC. Innate immunity, insulin resistance and type 2 diabetes. Trends Endocrinol Metab 2007.
[165] Feve B, Bastard JP, Vidal H. Relationship between obesity, inflammation and insulin resistance: new concepts. C R Biol 2006;329:587,97; discussion 653-5.
[166] Das UN. Obesity, metabolic syndrome X, and inflammation. Nutrition 2002;18:430-2.
[167] Steinberg GR. Inflammation in obesity is the common link between defects in fatty acid metabolism and insulin resistance. Cell Cycle 2007;6:888-94.
[168] Steinberg GR, Jorgensen SB. The AMP-activated protein kinase: role in regulation of skeletal muscle metabolism and insulin sensitivity. Mini Rev Med Chem 2007;7:519-26.
[169] Zulet MA, Puchau B, Navarro C, Marti A, Martinez JA. Inflammatory biomarkers: the link between obesity and associated pathologies. Nutr Hosp 2007;22:511-27.
[170] Saltiel AR, Kahn CR. Insulin signalling and the regulation of glucose and lipid metabolism. Nature 2001;414:799-806.
[171] Chiang SH, Baumann CA, Kanzaki M, Thurmond DC, Watson RT, Neudauer CL, Macara IG, Pessin JE, Saltiel AR. Insulin-stimulated GLUT4 translocation requires the CAP-dependent activation of TC10. Nature 2001;410:944-8.
[172] Saltiel AR. New perspectives into the molecular pathogenesis and treatment of type 2 diabetes. Cell 2001;104:517-29.

[173] Hotamisligil GS, Peraldi P, Budavari A, Ellis R, White MF, Spiegelman BM. IRS-1-mediated inhibition of insulin receptor tyrosine kinase activity in TNF-alpha- and obesity-induced insulin resistance. Science 1996;271:665-8.
[174] Paris M, Bernard-Kargar C, Vilar J, Kassis N, Ktorza A. Role of glucose in IRS signaling in rat pancreatic islets: specific effects and interplay with insulin. Exp Diabesity Res 2004;5:257-63.
[175] Hotamisligil GS, Budavari A, Murray D, Spiegelman BM. Reduced tyrosine kinase activity of the insulin receptor in obesity-diabetes. Central role of tumor necrosis factor-alpha. J Clin Invest 1994;94:1543-9.
[176] Nathan C. Epidemic inflammation: pondering obesity. Mol Med 2008;14:485-92.
[177] Bastard JP, Maachi M, Lagathu C, Kim MJ, Caron M, Vidal H, Capeau J, Feve B. Recent advances in the relationship between obesity, inflammation, and insulin resistance. Eur Cytokine Netw 2006;17:4-12.
[178] Drevon CA. Fatty acids and expression of adipokines. Biochim Biophys Acta 2005;1740:287-92.
[179] Trayhurn P, Wood IS. Signalling role of adipose tissue: adipokines and inflammation in obesity. Biochem Soc Trans 2005;33:1078-81.
[180] Onat A, Ayhan E, Hergenc G, Can G, Barlan MM. Smoking inhibits visceral fat accumulation in Turkish women Relation of visceral fat and body fat mass to atherogenic dyslipidemia, inflammatory markers, insulin resistance, and blood pressure. Metabolism 2009.
[181] Steinberg GR, Kemp BE. Adiponectin: starving for attention. Cell Metab 2007;6:3-4.
[182] Bastard JP, Maachi M, Van Nhieu JT, Jardel C, Bruckert E, Grimaldi A, Robert JJ, Capeau J, Hainque B. Adipose tissue IL-6 content correlates with resistance to insulin activation of glucose uptake both in vivo and in vitro. J Clin Endocrinol Metab 2002;87:2084-9.
[183] Kauf TL, Coates TD, Huazhi L, Mody-Patel N, Hartzema AG. The cost of health care for children and adults with sickle cell disease. Am J Hematol 2009.
[184] Adams-Graves P, Ostric EJ, Martin M, Richardson P, Lewis JB,Jr. Sickle cell hospital unit: a disease-specific model. J Healthc Manag 2008;53:305,15; discussion 316-7.
[185] Aliyu ZY, Kato GJ, Taylor J,4th, Babadoko A, Mamman AI, Gordeuk VR, Gladwin MT. Sickle cell disease and pulmonary hypertension in Africa: a global perspective and review of epidemiology, pathophysiology, and management. Am J Hematol 2008;83:63-70.
[186] Hebbel RP. Adhesion of sickle red cells to endothelium: myths and future directions. Transfus Clin Biol 2008;15:14-8.
[187] Eaton WA, Hofrichter J. Hemoglobin S gelation and sickle cell disease. Blood 1987;70:1245-66.
[188] Reiter CD, Wang X, Tanus-Santos JE, Hogg N, Cannon RO,3rd, Schechter AN, Gladwin MT. Cell-free hemoglobin limits nitric oxide bioavailability in sickle-cell disease. Nat Med 2002;8:1383-9.
[189] Gladwin MT, Schechter AN, Ognibene FP, Coles WA, Reiter CD, Schenke WH, Csako G, Waclawiw MA, Panza JA, Cannon RO,3rd. Divergent nitric oxide bioavailability in men and women with sickle cell disease. Circulation 2003;107:271-8.
[190] Hebbel RP. The systems biology-based argument for taking a bold step in chemoprophylaxis of sickle vasculopathy. Am J Hematol 2009;84:543-5.

[191] Wu CJ, Krishnamurti L, Kutok JL, Biernacki M, Rogers S, Zhang W, Antin JH, Ritz J. Evidence for ineffective erythropoiesis in severe sickle cell disease. Blood 2005;106:3639-45.

[192] Taylor JG 6, Nolan VG, Mendelsohn L, Kato GJ, Gladwin MT, Steinberg MH. Chronic hyper-hemolysis in sickle cell anemia: association of vascular complications and mortality with less frequent vasoocclusive pain. PLoS ONE 2008;3:e2095.

[193] Muller-Eberhard U, Javid J, Liem HH, Hanstein A, Hanna M. Plasma concentrations of hemopexin, haptoglobin and heme in patients with various hemolytic diseases. Blood 1968;32:811-5.

[194] Sultana C, Shen Y, Johnson C, Kalra VK. Cobalt chloride-induced signaling in endothelium leading to the augmented adherence of sickle red blood cells and transendothelial migration of monocyte-like HL-60 cells is blocked by PAF-receptor antagonist. J Cell Physiol 1999;179:67-78.

[195] Houston M, Estevez A, Chumley P, Aslan M, Marklund S, Parks DA, Freeman BA. Binding of xanthine oxidase to vascular endothelium. Kinetic characterization and oxidative impairment of nitric oxide-dependent signaling. J Biol Chem 1999;274:4985-94.

[196] Wood KC, Hsu LL, Gladwin MT. Sickle cell disease vasculopathy: a state of nitric oxide resistance. Free Radic Biol Med 2008;44:1506-28.

[197] Endemann DH, Schiffrin EL. Endothelial dysfunction. J Am Soc Nephrol 2004;15:1983-92.

[198] Cai H, Harrison DG. Endothelial dysfunction in cardiovascular diseases: the role of oxidant stress. Circ Res 2000;87:840-4.

[199] Griendling KK, FitzGerald GA. Oxidative stress and cardiovascular injury: Part II: animal and human studies. Circulation 2003;108:2034-40.

[200] Griendling KK, Sorescu D, Lassegue B, Ushio-Fukai M. Modulation of protein kinase activity and gene expression by reactive oxygen species and their role in vascular physiology and pathophysiology. Arterioscler Thromb Vasc Biol 2000;20:2175-83.

[201] Griendling KK, Ushio-Fukai M. Reactive oxygen species as mediators of angiotensin II signaling. Regul Pept 2000;91:21-7.

[202] Higashi Y, Noma K, Yoshizumi M, Kihara Y. Endothelial Function and Oxidative Stress in Cardiovascular Diseases. Circ J 2009.

[203] Higashi Y, Noma K, Yoshizumi M, Kihara Y. Endothelial Function and Oxidative Stress in Cardiovascular Diseases. Circ J 2009.

[204] Kato GJ, Hebbel RP, Steinberg MH, Gladwin MT. Vasculopathy in sickle cell disease: Biology, pathophysiology, genetics, translational medicine, and new research directions. Am J Hematol 2009;84:618-25.

[205] Wood KC, Hebbel RP, Lefer DJ, Granger DN. Critical role of endothelial cell-derived nitric oxide synthase in sickle cell disease-induced microvascular dysfunction. Free Radic Biol Med 2006;40:1443-53.

[206] De Caterina R, Libby P, Peng HB, Thannickal VJ, Rajavashisth TB, Gimbrone MA,Jr, Shin WS, Liao JK. Nitric oxide decreases cytokine-induced endothelial activation. Nitric oxide selectively reduces endothelial expression of adhesion molecules and proinflammatory cytokines. J Clin Invest 1995;96:60-8.

[207] Libby P. Inflammation in atherosclerosis. Nature 2002;420:868-74.

[208] Boger RH, Bode-Boger SM, Szuba A, Tsao PS, Chan JR, Tangphao O, Blaschke TF, Cooke JP. Asymmetric dimethylarginine (ADMA): a novel risk factor for endothelial dysfunction: its role in hypercholesterolemia. Circulation 1998;98:1842-7.

[209] Boger RH, Bode-Boger SM, Phivthong-ngam L, Brandes RP, Schwedhelm E, Mugge A, Bohme M, Tsikas D, Frolich JC. Dietary L-arginine and alpha-tocopherol reduce vascular oxidative stress and preserve endothelial function in hypercholesterolemic rabbits via different mechanisms. Atherosclerosis 1998;141:31-43.

[210] Achan V, Broadhead M, Malaki M, Whitley G, Leiper J, MacAllister R, Vallance P. Asymmetric dimethylarginine causes hypertension and cardiac dysfunction in humans and is actively metabolized by dimethylarginine dimethylaminohydrolase. Arterioscler Thromb Vasc Biol 2003;23:1455-9.

[211] Dayoub H, Achan V, Adimoolam S, Jacobi J, Stuehlinger MC, Wang BY, Tsao PS, Kimoto M, Vallance P, Patterson AJ, Cooke JP. Dimethylarginine dimethylaminohydrolase regulates nitric oxide synthesis: genetic and physiological evidence. Circulation 2003;108:3042-7.

[212] Hill JM, Zalos G, Halcox JP, Schenke WH, Waclawiw MA, Quyyumi AA, Finkel T. Circulating endothelial progenitor cells, vascular function, and cardiovascular risk. N Engl J Med 2003;348:593-600.

[213] Szmitko PE, Fedak PW, Weisel RD, Stewart DJ, Kutryk MJ, Verma S. Endothelial progenitor cells: new hope for a broken heart. Circulation 2003;107:3093-100.

[214] Finkel T, Holbrook NJ. Oxidants, oxidative stress and the biology of ageing. Nature 2000;408:239-47.

7

Worldwide Trends in Infectious Disease Research Revealed by a New Bibliometric Method

Hiromi Takahashi-Omoe[1] and Katsuhiko Omoe[2]
[1]*National Institute of Science and Technology Policy (NISTEP)*
[2]*Iwate University*
Japan

1. Introduction

Infectious diseases cause serious public health problems and their threat has been increasing. This is because these diseases are now spreading geographically much faster than at any time in history as a result of the highly mobile, interdependent, and interconnected society (World Health Organization [WHO], 2007). In addition, it is distressing that outbreaks of emerging infectious diseases such as severe acute respiratory syndrome, Nipah virus infection, and West Nile fever have been occurring at an unprecedented rate of one or more per year in animal and human populations since the 1970s (Brown, 2004; WHO, 2007). As a recent example, the 2009 H1N1 pandemic caused by a new subtype of influenza virus inflicted damage on people around the world. Because of these reasons, infectious disease research has been promoted primarily by developed countries to provide effective countermeasures against the diseases.

Infectious disease research has become more sophisticated and diversified. For example, the identification of natural reservoirs of emerging disease pathogens requires an interdisciplinary approach among microbiology, ecology, zoology, and other fields. The risk analysis of epidemic norovirus infection requires data regarding not only the virological properties of the virus but also wastewater management and hygienic conditions. In studies on influenza in Japan, a variety of basic and applied research approaches such as analysis of pathogenesis, vaccine development, clinical investigation of prepandemic vaccines, and surveys of the route of virus transmission via migratory birds have been conducted (Figure 1) (Takahashi-Omoe & Omoe, 2009). Toward building further strategies for infectious disease research at domestic and international levels, the real trends in such studies should be grasped systematically.

As a measure to grasp trends in various research fields including infectious disease research, quantitative surveys of research articles, as an application of bibliometrics, have been conducted using scientific literature databases such as the Web of Science® (Thomson Reuters), Scopus™ (Elsevier B.V.), and PubMed (National Library of Medicine). The results of surveys provide the information needed for decision makers, public policymakers, researchers, and business leaders (Statistics Canada, 1998).

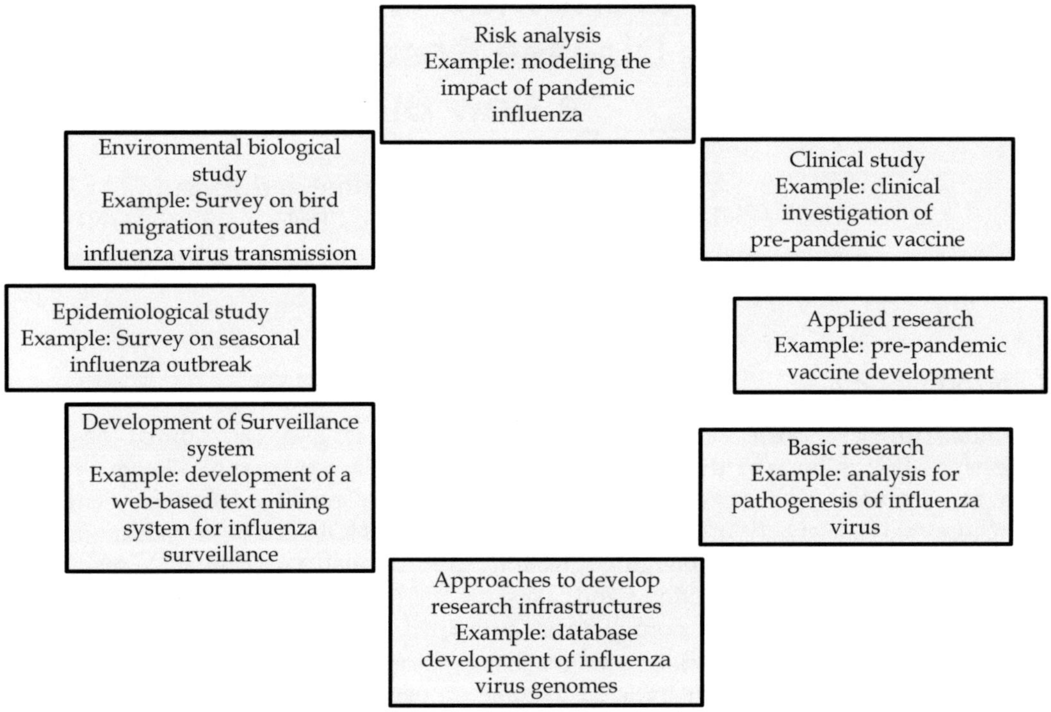

Fig. 1. An example of studies on influenza in Japan.

Regarding quantitative surveys in infectious disease research, in addition to specific diseases such as acquired immune deficiency syndrome (AIDS; caused by the human immunodeficiency virus [HIV]) (Patra & Chand, 2006; Uthman, 2008), tuberculosis (Ramos et al., 2008), and malaria (Garg et al., 2009), infectious diseases in general (Bliziotis et al., 2005; Ramos et al., 2004; Ramos et al., 2009) have been targeted. These studies demonstrated that the US, EU, and other specific world regions or nations showed a gradual increase in the publication of research articles, contributing to an increased grasp of general trends in infectious disease research in the world. However, the studies did not adequately demonstrate the real research trends in the non-English-speaking world because of limitations regarding journal selection for surveys of research articles. Previous studies were more likely to survey research articles in journals registered in the "Infectious Disease Category" of the Science Citation Index Expanded™ in the Web of Science® (the SCI Infectious Disease Category) (Thomson Reuters, 2011) and articles in international English-language journals, resulting in an underestimation of articles in non-English or regional journals that were published in the EU and Asia. Such limitations of bibliometric studies have been discussed in previous reports about the trends in infectious disease research

(Ramos et al., 2004), microbiology (Vergidis et al., 2005), and public health (Soteriades & Falagas, 2006). For example, Ramos et al. reported that European countries such as Germany, France, Italy and Spain had a long tradition of scientific publication in their own languages and might be penalized in comparative studies relying on the SCI (Ramos et al., 2004). Vergidis et al. also noted that journal selection based on the SCI particularly affected the survey results for Eastern Europe and Japan because scientists in these regions tended to publish their findings in regional journals more than scientists in others regions (Vergidis et al., 2005).

To improve on previous bibliometric analyses, we previously developed a method using 100 journals specializing in infectious disease research (infectious disease journals) (Takahashi-Omoe et al., 2009). These 100 journals, which were selected on the basis of keywords that exhaustively covered various infectious disease research fields, are published in various countries and written in various languages. Using these journals, we succeeded in surveying actual research trends in Asia between 1998 and 2006 without underestimating the number of articles in non-English and regional journals in comparison with surveys based on journals registered in the SCI Infectious Disease Category. This method using 100 journals has demonstrated the prospect for a more exhaustive survey of infectious disease research with less bias among nations and regions, although it is not perfect in comprehensiveness, similar to other bibliometric methods.

In this chapter, the features and usability of a new method using these 100 journals are being introduced, and the latest worldwide trends in infectious disease research is being presented as a practical application of the method.

2. Development of a survey method for infectious disease research

The 100 infectious disease journals used in this survey method were selected as described in section 2.1. The journals were assessed by their usability by comparison with journals registered in the SCI Infectious Disease Category as described in section 2.3.

2.1 Selection of 100 infectious disease journals

At the inception of selecting infectious disease journals, the Scopus™ database (as of 2011, the SciVerse Scopus, Elsevier B.V.; registered in January 2008) was used as a source. This is an abstract and citation database of the scientific literature that includes over 18,000 peer-reviewed journals.

On the basis of the Scopus™ database, infectious disease journals were screened using English keywords directly linked to disease control in detection, prevention, diagnosis, and medical care (A–E) (Figure 2). The keywords were chosen to select journals specifically focusing on infectious disease (A), general infectious diseases or infectious diseases belonging to specific categories (B), the field of clinical microbiology (C), the development of medicines (D), and overall technology development for disease control (E). In addition, related journals in the field of public health were selected on the basis of the author's experience (F).

In parallel, non-English journals were screened using Japanese, Chinese, French, German, Italian, Spanish, and Turkish keywords corresponding to the keywords in A–E. To screen

Korean journals, English keywords were used because almost all journal titles (89 of 91 journals) were registered in English or both English and Korean (in Roman letters) in the Scopus™ database. In the survey with English and non-English keywords, an approach based on both partial matching (for a search of journal titles that contain the keywords) and complete matching (for a search of titles that perfectly matches the keywords) was introduced to capture journal titles involving inflected forms of the keywords.

Through this screening, 264 candidates were selected, of which 240 were selected by English keywords and 24 by non-English words. The 264 journals were published in 30 countries and written in 12 languages: English, Japanese, Chinese, Korean, French, German, Italian, Spanish, Turkish, Polish, Russian, and Croatian. The list of journals can be found in our previous report (Takahashi- Omoe et al., 2009).

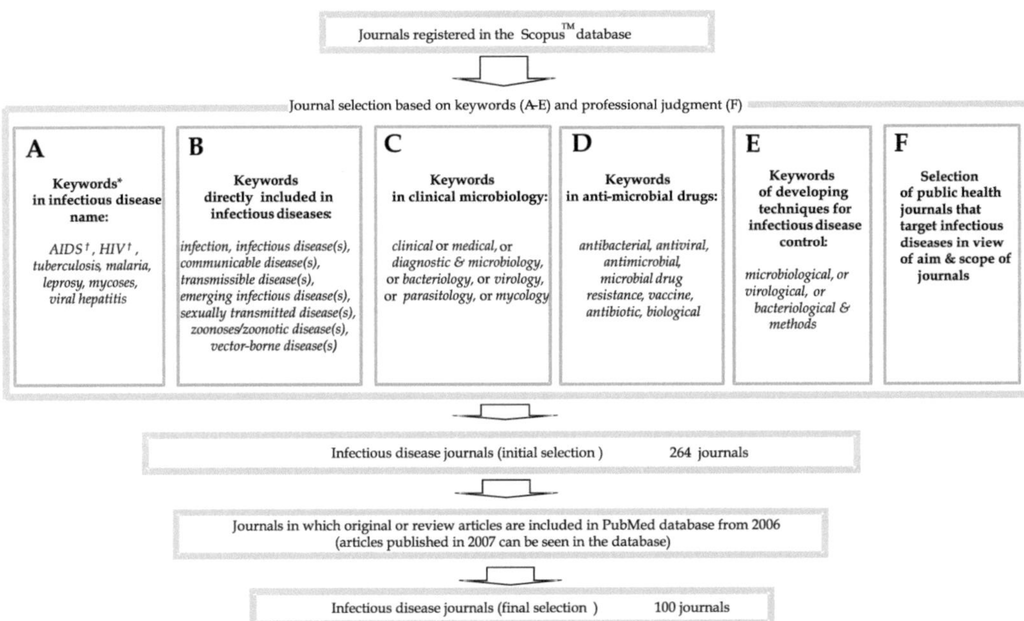

Fig. 2. Framework for selecting 100 infectious disease journals. *All keywords in A (excluding HIV); infection, infectious disease, communicable disease, sexually transmitted disease, and zoonosis in B; and antibacterial, antiviral, antimicrobial, vaccine, and antibiotic in D were translated into French, German, Italian, Spanish, Turkish, Chinese (in Roman letters), and Japanese (in Roman letters) to select journals written in non-English languages. †Journals regarding research on AIDS and HIV were selected according to the "Infectious Disease Category" of the Science Citation Index Expanded™ because several journals specializing in social-scientific and policy studies on patients could not be excluded by only the keywords "AIDS" and "HIV."

Subsequently, 100 of the 264 journals were selected on the basis of the usability of the PubMed database for indexing them. This was done to emphasize the further usability of the present survey method; the PubMed database is freely accessible and widely used, and the selected journals have continued in print through 2006 and beyond. The 100 journals listed in Table 1 were published in 18 countries and written in English and 7 non-English

AIDS	Diagnostic Microbiology and Infectious Disease	Journal of Acquired Immune Deficiency Syndromes (1999)	Malaria Journal
AIDS Patient Care and STDs	Emerging Infectious Diseases	The Japanese Journal of Antibiotics	Médecine et Maladies Infectieuses
The AIDS Reader	EnfermedadesInfecciosasy MicrobiologíaClínica	Japanese Journal of Infectious Diseases	Medical Microbiology and Immunology
AIDS Research and Human Retroviruses	Epidemiologyand Infection	Nihon Hansenby? Gakkai zasshi (Japanese Journal of Leprosy)	Medical Mycology
AIDS Reviews	European Journal of Clinical Microbiology & Infectious Diseases	Nihon Ishinkin Gakkai zasshi (Japanese Journal of Medical Mycology)	Microbes and Infection
American Journal of Infection Control	Expert Review of Vaccines	The Journal of Antibiotics	Microbial Drug Resistance
The American Journal of Tropical Medicine and Hygiene	FEMS Immunology and Medical Microbiology	The Journal of Antimicrobial Chemotherapy	Mycoses
Annals of Tropical Medicine and Parasitology	Genetic Vaccines and Therapy	Journal of Clinical Microbiology	The Pediatric Infectious Disease Journal
Antimicrobial Agents and Chemotherapy	HIV Clinical Trials	Journal of Clinical Virology	ProblemyTuberkuleza Boleznei Legkikh
Annals of Clinical Microbiology and Antimicrobials	HIV Medicine	Journal of Communicable Diseases	Reviews in Medical Virology
Antiviral Chemistry & Chemotherapy	Human Vaccines	The Journal of Hospital Infection	Scandinavian Journal of Infectious Diseases
Antiviral Research	Indian Journal of Leprosy	Journal of Immune Based Therapies and Vaccines	Sexually Transmitted Diseases
Antiviral Therapy	Indian Journal of Medical Microbiology	The Journal of Infection	Sexually Transmitted Infections
Biologicals	Infection	Journal of Infection and Chemotherapy	Surgical Infections
BMC Infectious Diseases	Infection and Immunity	The Journal of Infectious Diseases	The Brazilian Journal of Infectious Diseases
Canada communicable disease report	Infection Control and Hospital Epidemiology	Journal of Medical Microbiology	Transplant Infectious Disease
Clinical and Vaccine Immunology	Infectious Disease Clinics of North America	Journal of Medical Virology	Travel Medicine and Infectious Disease
Clinical Infectious Diseases	Infectious Diseases in Obstetrics and Gynecology	Journal of Microbiological Methods	Tropical Medicine & International Health
Clinical Microbiology and Infection	Infectious Disorders Drug Targets	Wei mian Yu gan ran za zhi (Journal of Microbiology, Immunology, and Infection)	Tuberculosis
Clinical Microbiology Reviews	International Journal of Antimicrobial Agents	Journal of Vector borne Diseases	Tuberkulozve Toraks
Communicable Diseases Intelligence	International Journal of Hygiene and Environmental Health	Journal of Viral Hepatitis	Vaccine
Comparative Immunology, Microbiology and Infectious Diseases	International Journal of Infectious Diseases	Journal of VirologicalMethods	Vector-borne and Zoonotic Diseases
Current HIV Research	International Journal of Medical Microbiology	Kansenshogakuzasshi (The Journal of the Japanese Association for Infectious Diseases)	Zhonghua jie he he hu xi za zhi (Chinese Journal of Tuberculosis and Respiratory Diseases)
Current Infectious Disease reports	International Journal of STD & AIDS	Kekkaku (Tuberculosis)	Zhonghua shi yan he lin chuang bing du xue za zhi (Chinese Journal of Experimental and Clinical Virology)
Current Opinion in Infectious Diseases	The International Journal of Tuberculosis and Lung Disease	The Lancet Infectious Diseases	
		Leprosy Review	

Table 1. List of the 100 infectious disease journals.

languages: Japanese, Chinese, French, German, Spanish, Turkish, and Russian. Forty-eight of the journals matched the journals in the SCI Infectious Disease Category. The remaining 52 journals were newly selected and included 15 Asian journals, comprising 3 journals written in Japanese, 2 in Chinese, 7 in English, and 3 in both English and Japanese or Chinese. The breakdown of the 100 journals corresponding to categories A to F is given in Figure 1: 21 were in A, 35 in B, 16 in C, 17 in D, 2 in E, and 3 in F (94 journals). Six of the journals belonged to 2 categories: 2 in A and B, 2 in B and C, 1 in B and D, and 1 in C and D.

2.2 Survey method using the 100 infectious disease journals

Using the 100 journals described in section 2.1 and the PubMed database, a method was developed to survey the actual number of research articles per infectious disease journal, publication year, and country where the first author of the article originated.

In this method, original articles and reviews were surveyed as research articles (hereafter, the term "research articles" includes both original articles and reviews); the former group was considered as an indicator of research activity, and the latter group was considered an appreciation of research results. As it was considered that highly valued scientists were given more opportunities to write reviews, meaning that their research results had attracted a good opinion and had relatively good qualities, reviews were also targeted in addition to original research articles. On the basis of the concept that the number of reviews might be indicative of research quality, the number of reviews was surveyed separately from the number of original articles.

The "Limits" function of the PubMed database was integrated into this survey method. The function contains tags for limiting the journal name (*[Jour]*), affiliation of author (*[ad]*), publication date (*[PPDAT]* for print date and *[EPDAT]* for electronic publication date), and publication type (*[pt]*). Concerning the publication date, the print date for journals that had both print and electronic versions was prioritized. Detailed information whether each infectious disease journal was surveyed on the basis of the print publication date or electronic publication date can be found in our previous report (Takahashi-Omoe et al., 2009).

For example, the following text to search for research articles published on "*AIDS*" during 2006 and first author of which lived in Japan was applied: *AIDS [Jour] AND journal article [pt] AND Japan [ad] AND 2006 [PPDAT]*.

2.3 Usability of the survey method

2.3.1 Method of usability analysis

To ascertain whether the 100 newly selected journals could survey a wide range of infectious disease research articles, the 100 journals and the journals of the SCI Infectious Disease Category were compared from the viewpoint of the difference in the proportion of Asian research articles relative to the world total. A usability analysis of the 100 journals intended for Asian articles was appropriate because research articles in non-English or regional journals published in the EU and Asia tend to be underestimated as described in the "Introduction."

The actual number of research articles in the 100 journals in 1998–2006 was surveyed using the PubMed database. The target Asian countries were Japan, China, India, Taiwan, Korea,

Singapore, Malaysia, Indonesia, Vietnam, Thailand, and the Philippines. The world total number of articles was also surveyed. Articles registered in the SCI category were surveyed in a manner similar to those in the 100 journals.

2.3.2 Results of the usability analysis

Concerning the proportion of Asian articles relative to the world total, it was revealed that a survey of the 100 journals revealed a consistently higher percentage than the SCI Infectious Disease Category in 1998–2006. The total number of Asian research articles accounted for 12% of the world total in the survey of the 100 journals (actual numbers of Asian and worldwide research articles were 14,156 and 118,158, respectively, as described in this paragraph) (Table 2) and 6.9% in the survey of SCI Infectious Disease Category (4,621 and 66,518, respectively) (Table 3). Each year during the study period, the proportion of original articles of Asian origin relative to the world total was approximately 8.6%–14.2% in the 100 journals and 4.7%–9.3% in the SCI category, and that of reviews of Asian origin was approximately 4.2%–6.9% in the 100 journals and 1.0%–3.9% in the SCI category (Table 2 and 3).

From these findings, it was demonstrated that a survey method using the 100 journals could identify more research articles and avoid underestimation of the numbers of articles in regional and non-English journals. Therefore, this method was considered beneficial to grasp the overall trends in infectious disease research in comparison with previous bibliometric studies based on journals registered in the SCI Infectious Disease Category.

Year/original articles or reviews	**1998/ OR**	**1998/ RV**	**1999/ OR**	**1999/ RV**	**2000/ OR**	**2000/ RV**	**2001/ OR**	**2001/ RV**	**2002/ OR**	**2002/ RV**
Total number of articles in Asian countries	830	48	1079	54	1330	60	1389	74	1516	66
Total number of articles in the world	9,661	1,013	10,430	1,237	10,764	1,442	10,919	1,484	11,032	1,405
Proportion of Asian articles relative to the world total (%)	8.6	4.7	10.3	4.4	12.4	4.2	12.7	5.0	13.7	4.7

Year/original articles or reviews	**2003/ OR**	**2003/ RV**	**2004/ OR**	**2004/ RV**	**2005/ OR**	**2005/ RV**	**2006/ OR**	**2006/ RV**	**1998-2006/ OR**	**1998-2006/ RV**	**1998-2006/ OR+RV**
Total number of articles in Asian countries	1605	107	1825	96	1847	99	2010	105	13452	705	14156
Total number of articles in the world	12,239	1,584	12,896	1,580	13,246	1,580	14,121	1,525	105,308	12,850	118,158
Proportion of Asian articles relative to the world total (%)	13.1	6.8	14.2	6.1	13.9	6.3	14.2	6.9	12.8	5.5	12.0

Table 2. Total number of articles in Asian countries and the world, and the proportion of Asian articles relative to the world total in 100 infectious disease journals in 1998–2006. OR is original articles, and RV is reviews.

Year/original articles or reviews	1998/ OR	1998/ RV	1999/ OR	1999/ RV	2000/ OR	2000/ RV	2001/ OR	2001/ RV	2002/ OR	2002/ RV
Total number of articles in Asian countries	259	7	365	14	438	20	450	25	472	28
Total number of articles in the world	5,489	697	5,847	805	6,256	919	6,262	976	6,243	864
Proportion of Asian articles relative to the world total (%)	4.7	1.0	6.2	1.7	7.0	2.2	7.2	2.6	7.6	3.2

Year/original articles or reviews	2003/ OR	2003/ RV	2004/ OR	2004/ RV	2005/ OR	2005/ RV	2006/ OR	2006/ RV	1998-2006/ OR	1998-2006/ RV	1998-2006/ OR+RV
Total number of articles in Asian countries	480	26	617	38	629	33	698	21	4,412	209	4,621
Total number of articles in the world	6,615	932	7,039	981	7,163	1,043	7,510	877	58,424	8,094	66,518
Proportion of Asian articles relative to the world total (%)	7.3	2.8	8.8	3.9	8.8	3.2	9.3	2.4	7.6	2.6	6.9

Table 3. Total number of articles in Asian countries and the world, and the proportion of Asian articles relative to the world total in the SCI Infectious Disease Category during 1998–2006. OR is original articles, and RV is reviews.

3. Worldwide trends in infectious disease research

As the method using 100 infectious disease journals was demonstrated to be beneficial as described in section 2.3.2, worldwide trends in infectious disease research were subsequently surveyed using the method.

3.1 Survey method

The number of research articles in the 100 infectious disease journals in 2001–2010 was surveyed on country-by-country and year-by-year bases and analyzed for relative comparisons among countries, yearly change, and the relationship between socioeconomic as well as science and technology factors.

Specifically, in a similar manner as described in section 2.2, the actual number of research articles was surveyed using the "Limits" function of the PubMed database. The targeted countries were the US, EU countries (the UK, France, Germany, Italy, Spain, and the Netherlands), and Asian countries (Japan, China, and India). These 6 EU and 3 Asian countries were selected on the basis of the higher production of infectious disease research articles in the areas, which has been previously reported (the EU and Asian top countries) (Ramos et al., 2009; Takahashi-Omoe et al., 2009). In addition, the US was reported to produce the most articles in the SCI Infectious Disease Category in 1995–2002 (Bliziotis et al., 2005). Therefore, a survey for these 10 countries was considered appropriate to grasp the worldwide trends in infectious disease research.

In the case of the UK, articles from England, Wales, Scotland, and Northern Ireland were grouped together, and the following limitation was set in the affiliation field of the PubMed database: UK[ad] OR United Kingdom[ad] OR Great Britain[ad] OR (England[ad] NOT New England[ad]) OR (Wales[ad] NOT New South Wales[ad]) OR Scotland [ad] OR (N Ireland[ad] OR Northern Ireland[ad]). For example, the following text was applied to search for research articles published on "*AIDS*" in 2010 and the first author of which lived in the UK: *AIDS [Jour] AND journal article [pt] AND (UK[ad] OR United Kingdom[ad] OR Great Britain[ad] OR (England[ad] NOT New England[ad]) OR (Wales[ad] NOT New South Wales[ad]) OR Scotland [ad] OR (N Ireland[ad] OR Northern Ireland[ad])) AND 2010 [PPDAT].*

As a further analysis of worldwide trends, the number of research articles registered in the 100 journals in 2001–2010 was weighted according to socioeconomic factors (the population and gross domestic product [GDP]) and science and technology factors (the number of researchers in research and development [R&D] and health expenditure per capita) of each country. Annual data for the population, GDP, number of researchers in R&D, and health expenditure of 10 countries were obtained from the World Bank. Detailed information about these socioeconomic and science and technology factors can be found in the World Bank database (The World Bank, 2011). Specifically, researchers in R&D are defined as professionals engaged in the conception or creation of new knowledge, products, processes, methods, or systems and in the management of the projects concerned, including postgraduate PhD students engaged in R&D. Health expenditure is derived from a sum of public and private health expenditures as a ratio of total population and covered the provision of health services (preventive and curative), family planning activities, nutrition activities, and emergency aid designated for health but did not include provision of water and sanitation.

Using the non-parametric correlation statistical test (Spearman's Rank Correlation test), the numbers of research articles were analyzed in relation to the socioeconomic and science and technology factors. Statistical analyses were performed using SPSS Statistics (version 17.0; SPSS Japan Inc., Tokyo, Japan).

3.2 Survey result

3.2.1 Leading countries in the number of research articles

The total number of infectious disease research articles throughout the world in the 100 infectious disease journals was 148,435 in 2001–2010 (Table 4). Among 10 countries, the US published the most infectious disease research articles (41,055 articles, 27.7% of the world total). This total far outpaced that of the second leading country, the UK (10,893 articles, 7.3%). France and Japan were the third and fourth most productive countries (7,711 [5.2%] and 7,582 articles [5.1%], respectively).

When original articles and reviews were viewed separately, the US remained the top country in terms of research article production, being responsible for 26.8% and 34.9% of original articles and reviews in the world, respectively (Table 5). The UK was a distant second, publishing 6.9% of original articles and 11.1% of reviews. Japan had a relatively higher percentage of original articles (5.4%) and was third in productivity, followed by France (5.2% of original articles). Interestingly, Spain and China produced an equal percentage of original articles (3.5%). Regarding reviews, it was remarkable that Asian countries had relatively lower percentages than the EU countries. In particular, the number of reviews originating from China totaled 118, which was 0.7% of the world total and the lowest proportion among the 10 countries.

At the domestic level, the proportion of reviews among the total number of articles was highest in the UK (16.4%), followed by the US (13.7%) and Germany (12.2%). Five EU countries had proportions exceeding 10%, whereas all 3 Asian countries had proportions less than 10%, including Japan (6.6%).

Countries	Original articles	Reviews	Original articles & reviews
World	132,282	16,153	148,435
US	35,425	5,630	41,055
UK	9,106	1,787	10,893
France	6,884	827	7,711
Germany	5,457	756	6,213
Italy	4,129	484	4,613
Spain	4,587	464	5,051
The Netherland	3,172	353	3,525
Japan	7,081	501	7,582
China	4,618	118	4,736
India	3,337	187	3,524

Table 4. Total number of research articles originating from the US, EU, and Asian countries in 100 infectious disease journals in 2001–2010. The numeric data show the number of original articles and reviews.

	Relative to the domestic total number		Relative to the total number of OR, RV, or OR+RV of the world		
	OR /OR+RV	RV /OR+RV	OR/OR	RV/RV	OR+RV /OR+RV
US	86.3	13.7	26.8	34.9	27.7
UK	83.6	16.4	6.9	11.1	7.3
France	89.3	10.7	5.2	5.1	5.2
Germany	87.8	12.2	4.1	4.7	4.2
Italy	89.5	10.5	3.1	3.0	3.1
Spain	90.8	9.2	3.5	2.9	3.4
The Netherlands	90.0	10.0	2.4	2.2	2.4
Japan	93.4	6.6	5.4	3.1	5.1
China	97.5	2.5	3.5	0.7	3.2
India	94.7	5.3	2.5	1.2	2.4

Table 5. Relative comparison of the number of articles originating from the US, EU, and Asian countries in 100 infectious disease journals in 2001–2010. The numeric data indicate percentages. OR: original articles, RV: reviews.

3.2.2 Yearly change in the number of research articles

As shown in Figure 3, the number of original articles across the world increased from 2001 to 2010. By contrast, the numbers from the US and the UK did not remarkably change, regardless of their high numbers. The increase in the total number of original articles across the world resulted from the increase in articles from China as shown in Fig. 4, or perhaps other countries that were not surveyed in this study.

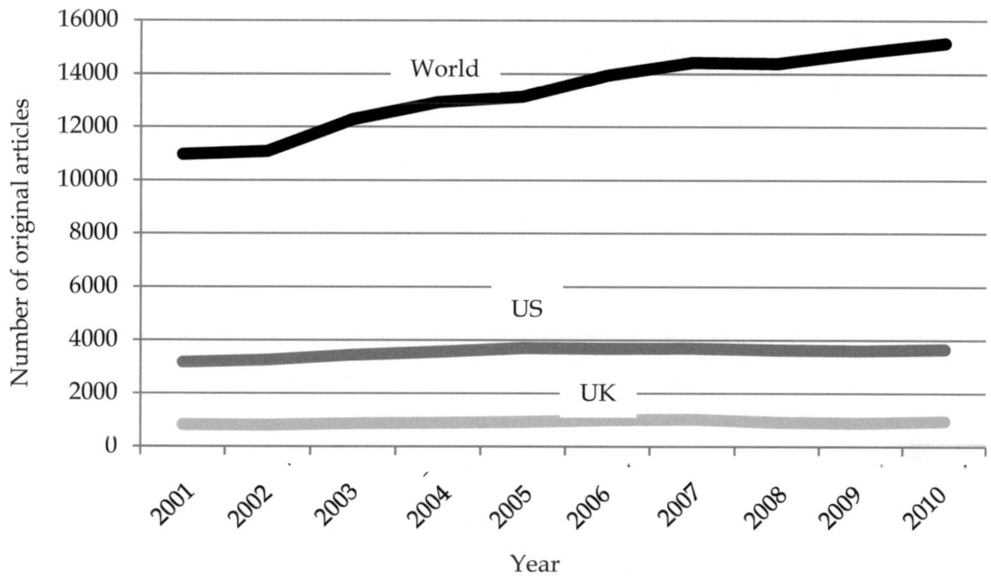

Fig. 3. Number of original articles in 100 infectious disease journals originating from the world, US, and UK in 2001–2010.

As noted previously, the number of original articles originating from China remarkably increased during this same period (Figure 4). The number in 2010 was more than 3-fold higher than that in 2001, including remarkable growth in the number of articles over the last 5–6 years. The concrete number of original articles from China exceeded that from Germany in 2008 (616 vs. 539 articles), Japan in 2009 (733 vs. 711 articles), and France in 2010 (809 vs. 764 articles).

Concerning the number of reviews, no noticeable increase was revealed in the world or the US and UK totals during the study period (Figure 5). The number from France showed a 2-fold increase in 2002–2006, but a slight decline since 2007. By contrast, the numbers from China and India remarkably increased from 2001 to 2010 (approximately 8.3-fold and 5.7-fold), but their numbers were lower than other countries (Figure 6). In addition, the number from Italy relatively increased among 10 countries (approximately 2.3-fold).

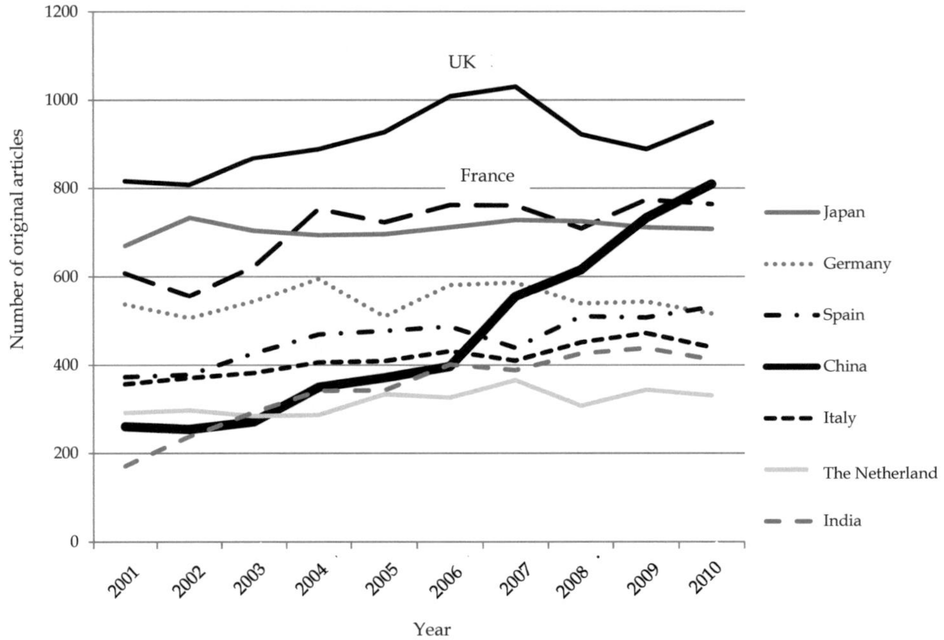

Fig. 4. Number of original articles in 100 infectious disease journals originating from the EU and Asian countries in 2001-2010.

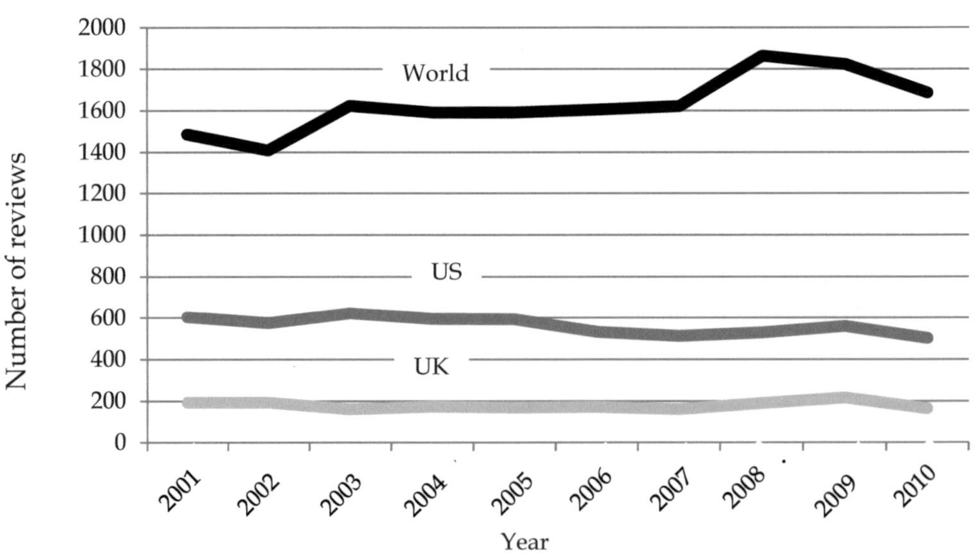

Fig. 5. Number of reviews in 100 infectious disease journals originating from the world, US, and UK in 2001-2010.

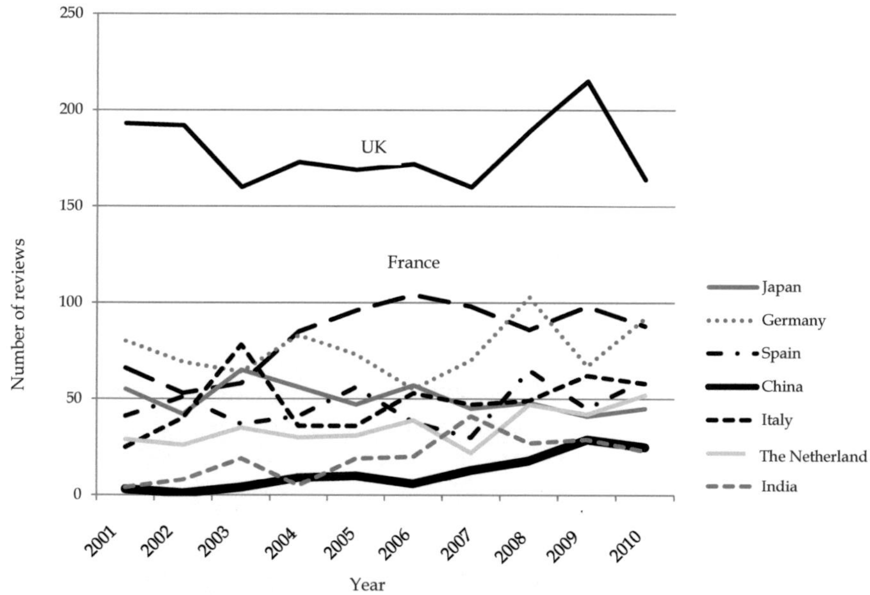

Fig. 6. Number of reviews in 100 infectious disease journals originating from the EU and Asian countries in 2001–2010.

3.2.3 Research productivity from the socioeconomic viewpoint

As a further analysis of publications of infectious disease research, the number of research articles was compared among 10 countries in terms of socioeconomic factors, the population, and GDP of each country.

Regarding the population, the ratio of the number of original articles to the population of individual countries exhibited a median value of 9 publications/1 million population/year (range, 0.3–19.3) in 2001–2009. Using population-adjusted ratios, the Netherlands (median value of 19.3) and the UK (14.9) were the most productive countries (Figure 7). The ratio of the number of reviews exhibited a median value of 0.9 publications/1 million population/year (range, 0–2.8). Using population-adjusted ratios, the UK ranked first (2.8), followed by the Netherlands (2.0) and the US (1.9). No statistically significant correlation were found between the average population and the number of original articles (Spearman's correlation coefficient = 0.213, p = 0.554) or reviews (Spearman's correlation coefficient = −0.097, p = 0.789) in the 10 countries in 2001–2009.

Regarding the ratio of the number of original articles to the GDP, the median value was 3.2 publications/10 billion GDP/year (range, 1.5–4.8) in 2001–2009. According to GDP-adjusted ratios for original articles, the Netherlands (4.8), India (4.2), and the UK (4.1) were highly productive (Figure 8). The ratio of the number of reviews exhibited a median value of 0.4 publications/10 billion GDP/year (range, 0–0.8) in 2001–2009. According to GDP-adjusted ratios for reviews, the UK (0.8) and the Netherlands (0.5) were most productive. A statistical correlation was found between the average GDP and the number of original articles (Spearman's correlation coefficient = 0.778, p = 0.008), but no statistically significant correlation between the average GDP and the number of reviews was observed (Spearman's correlation coefficient = 0.576, p = 0.082) in the 10 countries.

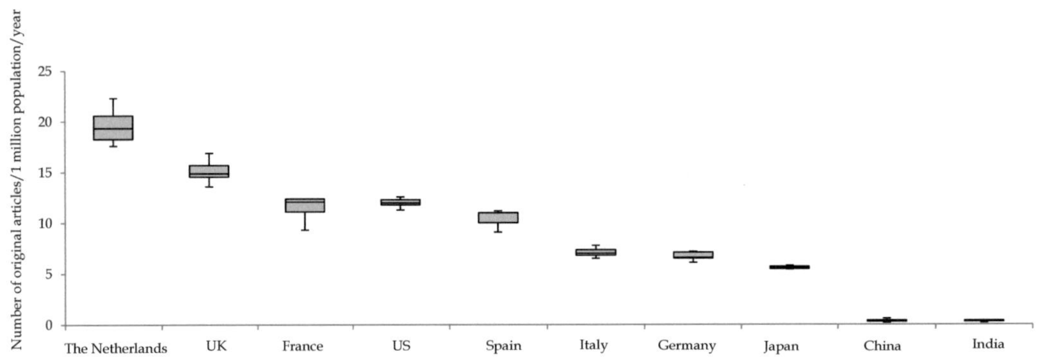

Fig. 7. Publication of original articles in 100 infectious disease journals by population in 2001–2009. Upper horizontal lines, dots, and lower horizontal lines in the boxes represent the first, second (median), and third quartiles, respectively. Whiskers represent the extension of values up and down.

In summary, we demonstrated that the Netherlands and the UK were most productive among the 10 countries when adjusting the production of original articles and reviews according to socioeconomic factors such as the population and GDP of each country.

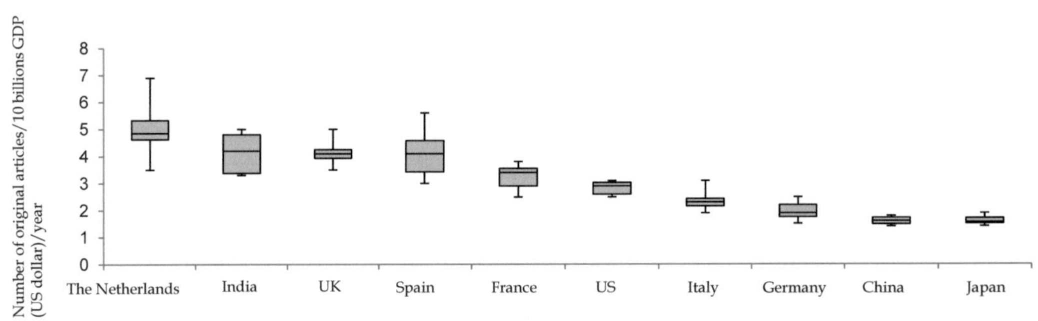

Fig. 8. Publication of original articles in 100 infectious disease journals by GDP in 2001–2009. Upper horizontal lines, dots, and lower horizontal lines in the boxes represent the first, second (median), and third quartiles, respectively. Whiskers represent extension of values up and down.

3.2.4 Research productivity from the science and technology viewpoint

In addition to socioeconomic factors, science and technology factors, represented by the number of researchers in R&D and health expenditure per capita, were applied to analyze the research productivity of each country.

The ratio of the number of original articles to the number of researchers in R&D exhibited a median value of 0.3 publications/number of researchers per 100 thousand people/year (range, 25.1–1.2) in 2001–2007. Using the number of researchers-adjusted ratios, India (median value of 25.1) was the most productive country (Figure 9). The ratio of the number of reviews exhibited a median value of 0.3 publications/number of researchers per 100 thousand people/year (range, 0.1–1.4) in 2001–2007. When adjusting the production of reviews according to the number of researchers, India ranked first (1.4), followed by the US (1.3). There were statistically significant correlations between the average number of researchers and original articles (Spearman's correlation coefficient = 0.802, p = 0.005) and reviews (Spearman's correlation coefficient = 0.806, p = 0.005) in the 10 countries in 2001–2007.

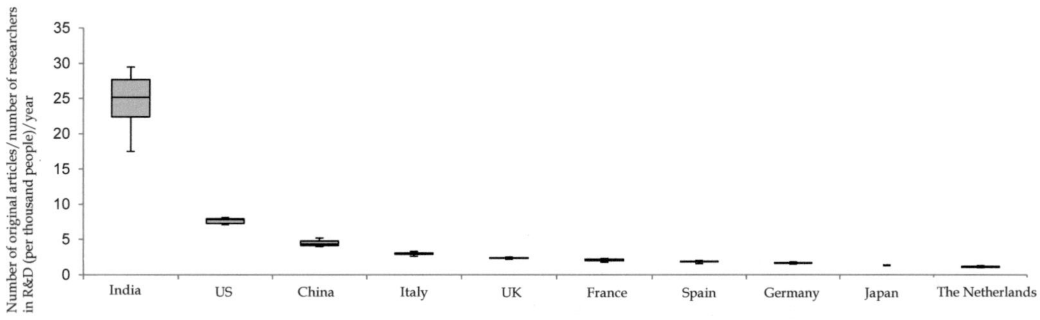

Fig. 9. Publication of original articles in 100 infectious disease journals according to the number of researchers in R&D in 2001–2007. Upper horizontal lines, dots, and lower horizontal lines in the boxes represent the first, second (median), and third quartiles, respectively. Whiskers represent the extension of values up and down. The survey period was 2001–2007 because data for the 10 countries were not fully gained from the World Bank data source in 2008–2009.

Concerning the ratio of the number of original articles to the health expenditure per capita, the median value was 2.3 publications/10 dollars health expenditure per capita/year (range, 0.8–113.2). For health expenditure-adjusted ratios, India (113.2) and China (45.5) were highly productive (Figure 10).

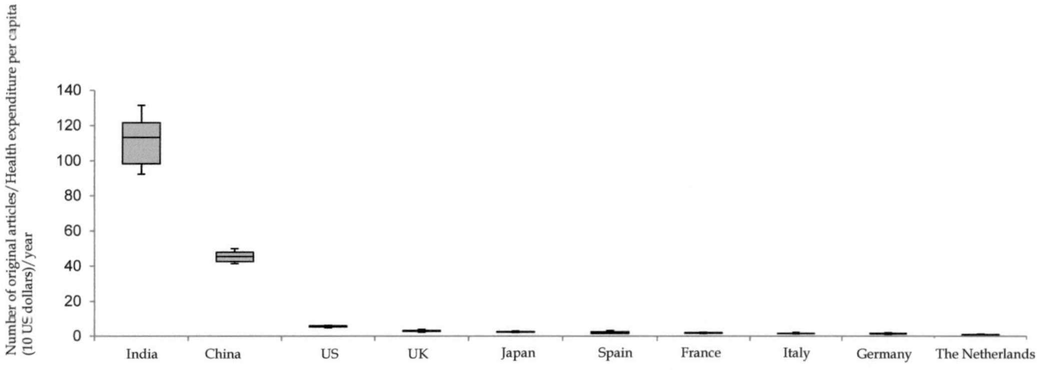

Fig. 10. Publication of original articles in 100 infectious disease journals according to health expenditure per capita in 2001–2009. Upper horizontal lines, dots, and lower horizontal lines in the boxes represent the first, second (median), and third quartiles, respectively. Whiskers represent the extension of values up and down.

The ratio of the number of reviews exhibited a median value of 0.2 publications/10 dollars health expenditure per capita/year (range, 0.1–6.3). When adjusting the production of reviews according to the health expenditure per capita, India (6.3) and China (1.2) were the most productive countries. There was no statistical correlation between the average of the health expenditure per capita and the number of original articles (Spearman's correlation coefficient = 0.407, $p = 0.243$), but a statistical correlation between the average of the health expenditure per capita and the number of reviews was observed (Spearman's correlation coefficient = 0.697, $p = 0.025$) for the 10 countries.

Generally, India was the most productive according to science and technology factors such as the number of researchers and health expenditure of each country. The US and China were ranked in the top three for both researcher- and health expenditure-adjusted ratios.

3.3 General overview of worldwide trends in infectious disease research

Through a bibliometric analysis using the 100 infectious disease journals described previously, 5 features were highlighted as the worldwide research trends in 2001–2010.

3.3.1 Vigorous infectious disease research around the world

We demonstrated that increasing numbers of infectious disease research articles were published around the world. This result was similar to previous bibliometric data reported by Bliziotis et al., although their study targeted journals registered in the SCI Infectious Disease Category and published in 1995–2002 (Bliziotis et al., 2005). It can be said that infectious disease research has been evidently vigorous without the influence of survey methods.

3.3.2 US as the leading country in infectious disease research

Our survey demonstrated that the US was the leading country in infectious disease research, as the US produced the highest percentage of total research articles (27.7% of the world total). The UK ranked second (7.3% of the world), but its output was dwarfed by that of the US. Ramos et al. also reported these 2 countries as the leading countries (Ramos et al., 2009) based on their study on journals registered in the SCI Infectious Disease Category covering the period of 2002–2007 (Bliziotis et al., 2005). These results from surveys based on 100 infectious journals and journals in the SCI Infectious Disease Category demonstrated that the US and the UK had an undisputed lead in infectious disease research productivity.

3.3.3 The Netherlands, India, and China as productive countries in the field of infectious disease research according to socioeconomic and science and technology factors

The US and the UK dominated the field of infectious disease research according to the global share of research articles, but the Netherlands, India, and China were considered productive countries when adjusting the production of original articles for socioeconomic factors and science and technology factors.

3.3.4 Developing infectious disease research in China

According to our findings, the productivity of infectious disease research in terms of a noticeable increase in the number of produced original articles was observed for China.

Significantly, China overtook France and Japan regarding the number of original articles in 2010 and 2009, respectively. However, China had the lowest proportion of reviews among the 10 countries. This trend might indicate that infectious disease research in China was developing and that it has not come to be well recognized.

3.3.5 More appreciated outputs of infectious disease research from the US and the top EU countries

Through this method, it became clear that the US and the top EU countries produced relatively higher proportions of reviews than the top Asian countries. Even Japan, which produced the most research articles in Asia, produced fewer reviews than the UK, France, and Germany. It could be speculated that the research output from the US and the top EU countries was more appreciated than those from top Asian countries.

4. Conclusion

This chapter presented the recent worldwide trends in infectious disease research as a practical application of a method using 100 infectious disease journals. The trends in 2001–2010 included vigorous research, with the US and the UK being the most active countries. Given the research productivity based on socioeconomic and science and technology factors, the Netherlands, India, and China had relatively high productivity. The developing research in China and more appreciated research outputs from the top EU countries were also significant. Based on these survey results, further content analysis of infectious disease research articles may be necessary to build future research strategies for effective disease control.

5. Acknowledgment

The study introduced in this chapter was supported by Japan Grants-in Aid for Scientific Research (KAKENHI) (research project number 23580435).

6. References

Bliziotis, I.A.; Paraschakis, K.; Vergidis, P.I.; Karavasiou, A.I. & Falagas, M.E. (2005).
Worldwide trends in quantity and quality of published articles in the field of infectious diseases. *BMC Infectious Diseases*, Vol.5, No.16, ISSN 1471-2334

Brown, C. (2004). Emerging zoonoses and pathogens of public health significance–an overview. *Revue scientifique et technique (International Office of Epizootics)*, Vol.23, No.2, pp. 435-42, ISSN 0253-1933

Elsevier B.V. (2011). SciVerse Scopus, Available from http://www.info.sciverse.com/scopus/about

Garg, K.C.; Kumar, S.; Madhavi, Y. & Bahl, M. (2009). Bibliometrics of global malaria vaccine research. *Health Information and Libraries Journal* Vol.26, pp.22-31, ISSN 1471-1834

Patra, S.K. & Chand, P. (2007). HIV/AIDS research in India: A bibliometric study. *Library & Information Science Research* Vol.29, pp.124-134, ISSN 0740-8188

Ramos, J.M.; Gutiérrez, F.; Masía, M. & Martín-Hidalgo, A. (2004). Publication of European union research on infectious diseases (1991-2001): A bibliometric evaluation.

European Journal of Clinical Microbiology & Infectious Diseases, Vol.23, pp.180-184, ISSN 0934-9723

Ramos, J.M.; Masía, M.; Padilla, S. & Gutiérrez, F. (2009). A bibliometric overview of infectious diseases research in European countries (2002-2007). *European Journal of Clinical Microbiology & Infectious Diseases*, Vol.28, pp.713-716, ISSN 0934-9723

Ramos, J.M.; Padilla, S.; Masía, M. & Gutiérrez, F. (2008). A bibliometric analysis of tuberculosis research indexed in PubMed, 1997-2006. *International Journal of Tuberculosis and Lung Disease*, Vol.12, pp.1461-1468, ISSN 1027-3719

Soteriades, E.S. & Falagas M.E. (2006). A bibliometric analysis in the fields of preventive medicine, occupational and environmental medicine, epidemiology, and public health. *BMC Public Health*, Vol.6, No.301, ISSN 1471-2458

Statistics Canada (1998). *Bibliometric analysis of scientific and technological research: A user's guide to the methodology*, Canada, Available from http://www.statcan.gc.ca/pub/88f0006x/88f0006x1998008-eng.pdf

Takahashi-Omoe, H. & Omoe, K. (2009). Regulatory and scientific framework for zoonosis control in Japan–contributing to International Health Regulations (2005). *Revue scientifique et technique (International Office of Epizootics)*,Vol.28, pp.957-973, ISSN 0253-1933

Takahashi-Omoe, H.; Omoe, K. & Okabe, N. (2009). New journal selection for quantitative survey of infectious disease research: application for Asian trend analysis. *BMC Medical Research Methodology*, Vol.9, No.67, ISSN 1471-2288

Thomson Reuters (2011). Science Sitation Index Expanded, Available from http://science.thomsonreuters.com/cgi-bin/jrnlst/jloptions.cgi?PC=D

Uthman, O.A. (2008). HIV/AIDS in Nigeria: a bibliometric analysis. *BMC Infectious Diseases*, Vol. 8, No.19, ISSN 1471-2334

Vergidis, P.I.; Karavasiou, A.I.; Paraschakis, K.; Bliziotis, I.A.; Falagas M.E. (2005). Bibliometric analysis of global trends for research productivity in microbiology. *European Journal of Clinical Microbiology & Infectious Diseases*, Vol. 24, pp.342-345, ISSN 0934-9723

World Bank. (2011). Data, Inficators, Available from http://data.worldbank.org/indicator

World Health Organization. (2007). *The World Health Report 2007, A Safer Future: Global Public Health Security in the 21st Century*, Geneva, Switzerland, Available from http://www.who.int/whr/2007/whr07_en.pdf

Part 2

Immuno-Kinetics and Vaccination

8

Chemokine Responses to Hepatitis C Virus and Their Impact in Mediating the Treatment Responses of Antiviral Treatment

Jon Florholmen and Rasmus Goll
Research group of Gastroenterology and Nutrition,
Institute of Clinical Medicine, University of Tromsø, Tromsø
Department of Medical Gastroenterology,
University Hospital North Norway, Tromsø,
Norway

1. Introduction

The hepatitis C virus (HCV) is a global health challenge with strong regional implications (Shepard et al, 2005). Currently, about 170 million people throughout the world are chronically HCV infected and it is the most important cause of liver disease worldwide. During the last 30 years the mode of transmission in industrial countries has changed from infection by medical use of contaminated blood products to infection by shared utensils by drug abusers. The incidence of HCV infection in Europe increased during the 1990`s (Rantala & van de Laar, 2008). It is unknown if this trend of increased incidence in Europe and worldwide has persisted after 2000.

Following acute HCV infection approximately 80 % of adults and between 50 to 60% of children develop chronic disease (Vogt et al, 1999). The reasons for the ineffective clearance of HCV virus is unknown, but most likely there are viral escape factors and host factors such as inappropriate immune based viral clearance. Progression of chronic HCV infection occurs in a proportion of infected subjects in a sequence via liver fibrosis to liver cirrhosis and finally death due either to liver failure or to hepatocellular carcinoma (HCC). The rate of progression is affected by various factors such as age at infection, gender, alcohol consumption, and co-infection particularly with human immunodeficiency virus (HIV), but also with hepatitis B virus (HBV) (Poynard et al, 2001). When compensated cirrhosis is established, the probability of decompensation is estimated to be 15-17 % within 2-3 years. The burden of expenses to health services due to HCV related disease has been predicted to be considerable in the future. In 2004, 23 % of all liver transplantations in Europe were related to HCV infection. Most likely the incidence of decompensated cirrhosis and HCC will increase substantially in the next few decades, due to the steady increase of HCV positive persons-at-risk (Lehman & Wilson, 2009).

Chronic HCV infection is treated with a combination of pegylated interferon (peg-IFN)-α, and the synthetic nucleoside analogue ribavirin. By this combination sustained virological response (SVR) is achieved in between 40 % and 50 % for genotype 1 and as high as approximately 85 % for genotypes 2 and 3. Due to the limited success rate of this combined therapy approach, triple therapy options have been suggested. Thus, both protease inhibitors and polymerase inhibitors has been tested as addition to PEG-interferon and ribavirin. These drugs are not approved by the authorities as standard treatment since they are still under investigation. Depending of the efficacy of triple therapy, the future need for liver transplantation may be reduced, with a considerable impact on health expenditures.

Both viral and host factors are determinants for the spontaneous elimination or persistence of HCV. The high risk for chronic infection is most likely caused by a lack of a strong and specific immune response to viral antigens. On the other hand, an overly powerful immune response may lead to acute liver failure as seen in rare cases of hepatitis A and hepatitis B. The frequent mutations of HCV are challenging to the host immune response and results in a high risk for viral escape. In the recent years HCV research has been focused on the innate and adaptive response to the virus. Special attention has been put into the role of chemokines and their receptors which are responsible for recruitment of leukocytes from blood stream to the affected tissue. It has been proposed that this is one of the most critical immunological steps for an effective clearance of the virus. We have recently reported that in the antiviral treatment, SVR is dependent on a rapid (24 hours) chemokine response (Florholmen et al, 2011). This has initiated the present review of the immunological mechanisms against the HCV with a special emphasis on the chemokine response.

2. Aims

The first part of the chapter we will review the chemokine concept and its role in the HCV pathogenesis, their role in the innate and adaptive response to HCV leading to liver inflammation and liver fibrosis. The second part will concentrate on the chemokine response during antiviral treatment using interferon, ribavirin and the new nucleoside analogues.

3. Hepatitis C virus

HCV is a positive single stranded RNA virus with regions coding for structural peptides (an envelope, 9000 bases) and regions coding for non-structural (NS) peptides (1 – 5) (Myrmel et al, 2009). Eleven genotypes have so far been described and 6 are commonly diagnosed. The Genotypes 1, 4 and 6 respond to antiviral therapy (interferon (IFN) + ribavirin) with an SVR of 50 % and 85 %, respectively. The virus has a high production of estimated 1012 virions per day, with an average half-life of 2.7 h and a turn-over rate close to 99 %. The calculated annual mutation rate is in the order of 1.5–2.0 x10^3 nucleotide substitutions per site. Furthermore, the virus has no proofreading mechanisms. The naturally occurring mutations may thereby enhance resistance both to endogenous immune responses and to anti-HCV therapy. Mutations conferring resistance of hepatitis C virus to the new treatment agents, the NS3 protease inhibitors, have been described (Halfon & Locarnini, 2011). The various genotypes have not been associated to specific pathobiology. As described above, however, the pattern of genotype related resistance to therapy has been extensively documented. The molecular mechanisms of this resistance have been described to some extent. Of great interest is the interferon sensitivity-determining region (ISDR) in the non-structural NSR5 part of the virus genome. Amino acid substitutions in ISDR have been related to increased SVR of anti-HCV treatment (for review, see (Chayama & Hayes, 2011)).

4. Antiviral immune response

The immunological response to viral infection is a complex interplay between host tissue cells, the innate and adaptive immune responses. A series of mediators, systemic and paracrine, as well as cell-cell interaction will in most cases result in clearance of infection. Some viruses have developed strategies of immune evasion and can therefore establish chronic infections. In case of HCV infection, the resulting chronic inflammatory response is actually harmful to the host by driving development of fibrosis, cirrhosis, and liver failure or HCC.

Viral pathogens can enter the host in several ways, the mucosal membranes being the most frequently used. A few viruses mainly spread via direct inoculation in the bloodstream, HCV being a classic example. Each type of virus has its preferred host cell type based on specific homing mechanisms. The HCV tropism for hepatocytes and internalization process is partly characterised and involve cluster of differentiation (CD) 81 and Claudin-1 (Thorley et al, 2010).

Viral pathogens do not have metabolism and rely on modifying the host cell production apparatus to its own benefit. A range of defensive mechanisms has been developed in response to this strategy. The end result from these mechanisms is mostly death by lysis or apoptosis of the infected cell, while at the same time restricting spread of the infectious agent to neighbouring cells in the infected site. A short overview of the general immune response to viral infection with special emphasis on mechanisms related to the anti-HCV response will be given in the following.

Leukocyte trafficking is a very important feature of the immune system allowing for the immune cells to patrol the entire host organism and thereby detect any intruding microorganism, bacteria or virus. The ability to generate a rapid local response when an intruder has been detected is based on homing mechanisms which mainly are triggered by early response cytokines and chemokines. As it turns out in the case of HCV infection, chemokines may also be central in generating an effective immune response following pharmacological intervention, as a swift chemokine response early in the course of treatment can predict a sustained virological response.

4.1 Innate receptor systems

The innate immune defence consists of several specialized cell types like dendritic cells (DC's) granulocytes, natural killer (NK) cells and macrophages. A common trait for these cell types is the pattern recognition receptors (PRR's) consisting of both intracellular and transmembrane subtypes. The nucleotide oligomerization domain (NOD) receptors are intracellular and the toll like receptors (TLR's) are transmembrane receptors primarily directed towards the extracellular compartment. These innate receptors detect common motifs from pathogenic microorganisms including both bacteria and viruses. Upon triggering the receptor an intracellular pathway common to most of the TLR's involve myeloid differentiation primary response gene 88 (MyD88) and interleukin-1 receptor-associated kinase (IRAK) kinases leading to activation of NF-κ-B and transcription of pro-inflammatory cytokines.

The professional antigen presenting cell i.e. dendritic cell carry an array of pattern recognition receptors and these cells are crucial for the initiation of an adaptive response. All cell lines of the adaptive system must be stimulated by DC's in order to raise a response. The DC determines the profile of the adaptive system depending on its cytokine secretion pattern.

Most viruses have specific binding strategies for entry into host cells. This leads to a tropism of the virus rendering specific target cells its point of attack depending on the homing mechanism. Subsequently the virus particle is disassembled. At this point intracellular receptors may detect the pathogen and trigger production of early viral response cytokines – mainly type I interferons like IFN-α and -β. A possible trigger of IFN production can be double stranded RNA which has been found to stimulate type I interferons in vitro. Intracellular TLR3 is likely triggered by viral dsRNA.

4.1.1 Interferons

The family of interferons consists of three subgroups of mediators with high sequence homology. The first interferons were described by their physiological effects i.e. their ability to *interfere* with viral replication in cell cultures. The type I interferons is a group of five members: IFN -α, -β, -ω, -κ, and limitin. IFN-α and IFN-β can be secreted by practically all infected cells types following viral infection and the production of these cytokines is therefore not restricted to immune competent cells.

Type I IFN has a common receptor IFN-αβ-R which signals via the JAK-STAT pathway (JAK is short for Janus Kinase, and STAT is short for Signal Transducer and Activator of Transcription) towards the *Interferon stimulated response element* ISRE in the cell nucleus and induce transcription of several interferon inducible genes which in turn increase degradation of viral RNA and inhibit translation processes. The secreted interferon acts on both the secreting cell (autocrine stimulation) and neighbouring cells (paracrine stimulation) thus inhibiting local spread of the viral infection. Furthermore, interferons up-regulate major histocompatibility complex I (MHC-I) and thereby enhance the display of viral antigens to the adaptive effector cells (see below). Interferons also activate NK cells and thereby facilitate killing of infected cells. Thus, the entry of a virus in a cell induce production of interferons which in turn help protect neighbouring cells from infection but also facilitate killing of the infected cell by NK cells and/or antigen specific cytotoxic T cells.

4.1.2 Natural killer cells

NK cells are part of the innate immune response, and have an important role in combating viral infections in the early phase until the specific adaptive cytotoxic response is raised. The NK cell is believed to distinguish infected from normal cells via an intricate process involving both stimulatory and inhibitory signalling. A set of immunoglobulin-like receptors (*K*iller cell *I*mmunoglobulin-like *R*eceptors: KIR's) and C-type lectins are involved in activation of the NK cell. A strong inhibitory signal is presentation of MHC-I on the cell surface which may be recognized by KIR's or CD94:NKG2. As part of the microbial survival strategy many viral infections inhibit MHC-I display in order to restrain presentation of antigens to the adaptive response. This strategy removes the inhibitory signal to NK cells and the infected cells display only activation signals to the NK cells and will be eliminated. Some viruses induce conformational change of MHC-I with the same result. Thus, the NK cell may be able to detect the infected cell even if it evades the adaptive response by cytotoxic CD8+ T cells (see below).

If stimulated by IFN-α or IFN-β the NK cell increase cytotoxic activity by a factor 20-100. The activated NK cell also secretes mediators important to direct the early response patterns in the tissue. The effector action of NK cells is completed by close binding to the infected cell and may use different pathways including lysis of the cell membrane by perforins or triggering of apoptosis by interaction between Fas (CD95) and FasL (CD95L). The role of NK cells in HCV infection has been reviewed recently (Cheent & Khakoo, 2011).

4.1.3 Adaptive immune response

The adaptive immune response is antigen specific and can identify foreign antigens with great sensitivity and specificity. It consists of both humoral and cellular parts, of which especially the former can enhance the function of the innate response. Opsonising antibodies can boost the performance of innate phagocytes like neutrophil granulocytes and macrophages, and also enhance the function of an NK cell mediated cytotoxic response. The specific adaptive responses are modulated in phases: in the early response phase, activated cells undergo clonal expansion. This is followed by an effector phase where the strike against the microorganism is delivered. Finally the response is attenuated after elimination of the infectious agent - this phase is controlled by regulatory T cells (see below). In the process of down regulating the adaptive response, a small population of memory cells will remain dormant. These memory cells will be able to launch a swift and efficient adaptive response if the host should encounter the same agent at a later time.

A common feature of the adaptive immune system is that the cells are unable to generate a response without help of the innate system or other parts of the adaptive response. The T cell receptor only recognizes its epitope in the context of an MHC molecule in combination with co-stimulatory factors. Each of the adaptive cell populations are restricted by specific mechanisms. T helper (Th) cells must be stimulated by their antigen presented on MHC-II by antigen presenting cells (APC's). Cytotoxic T cells must be triggered by their epitope presented on MHC-I by the target cell. B cells bind their antigen on the B-cell receptor and internalize it for degradation and presentation on the surface by MHC-II. This allows for co-stimulation by contact with, and cytokine secretion from, Th cells with the same specificity. In this way, the B cell can also present antigens for stimulation of Th cells. The local cytokine milieu at the time of stimulation determines which effector profile the stimulated Th cell will have: IFN-γ and interleukin (IL)-12A: Th1; IL-4: Th2; transforming growth factor-β: Th3; IL-6 and TGF-β: Th17; IL-10: T regulatory-1 (Tr1).

In a viral infection, the adaptive immune response is triggered by presented antigens towards a classic Th1 profile enhancing a cytotoxic effector response. The cytotoxic CD8+ T cell is antigen specific in contrast to the NK cell, and stimulation of this cell line is primarily by Th1 cytokines like IFN-gamma and IL12A. The specificity rely on the T cell receptor recognition of the antigen as presented in the groove of a MHC-I molecule on the surface of the cell in question. Also, the cytotoxic T cell and the innate NK cell tend to mirror the Th profile in the immune response at hand, so these effector cells secrete cytokines and tend to enhance the milieu given by Th cells.

The humoral part of the adaptive response also enhances the phagocyte and cytotoxic responses by a mechanism called opsonisation. Innate immune cells like neutrophil granulocytes, macrophages and NK cells carry receptors for the stem of the antibody (the FC part). Antibodies bind their target in the binding sites, and can crosslink the target to FC receptors on the innate cell. This way a viral particle on the surface of cells can be "visualized" to innate cells. Antibodies in blood, mucosal membranes, and the extracellular space also neutralise viral particles by binding.

4.1.4 Regulatory T cells

The regulatory T cells include distinct subpopulations of which some are non-specific ($CD25^{high}$ natural T_{reg}) and others are antigen specific (Tr1 and Th3). A common trait for regulatory T cells is the expression of forkhead family transcription factor FOXP3. The natural T_{reg}'s are generated in the thymus and characterised by a high expression of CD25 (IL-2 receptor). Natural T_{reg}'s seem to act primarily by direct cell contact similar to the actions of NK cells. In contrast, the antigen specific regulatory T cells act by secretion of cytokines like IL-10 and TGF-beta. The regulatory cytokines and direct cell contact actions keep an important brake on the immune system in general, as an uncontrolled pro-inflammatory response can lead to serious pathology and even organ destruction. Thus, the function of regulatory T cells is to balance the response of pro-inflammatory immune cells in order to keep homeostasis and avoid excessive tissue damage as well as resolving inflammation when the infection has been eliminated. The balance between pro- and anti-inflammatory stimuli is delicate. The perfect immune response is swift, efficient, and causes a minimum of damage to host cells. Of course this is a compromise and the balance may tip in either direction. In HCV infection, an overly powerful response would lead to acute liver failure and death; it has been suggested that the development of cirrhosis in longstanding HCV infection is a result of an overly aggressive chronic inflammation (Larrubia et al, 2008).

4.2 Homing and chemotaxis

All of the cell types described above must be recruited to the site of infection in order to perform their part of the anti-microbial response. Though the adaptive humoral response and antibody production in most cases takes place in the regional lymph nodes, the B cells and Th cells must still be recruited and activated. The recruitment of leukocytes to the site of infection is an intricate process controlled by homing mechanisms. Some central mechanisms of leukocyte homing will be presented in the following.

Chemotaxis is a basic behaviour seen in bacteria, primitive organisms, and several cell types in the immune system. The definition of chemotaxis is that the cell in question moves towards a higher concentration of a given chemotactic compound. As the name implies, chemokines are chemotactic compounds and a cell releasing chemokines will attract the attention of nearby immune cells.

4.2.1 Chemokines

The chemokines are a family of highly homologous small proteins with a common *Greek key* structure. These mediators have a key role in the earliest phases of infection. They can be released by many cell types in response to infectious agents and to physical damage. Chemokines can recruit cells of both innate and adaptive lines to the site of infection.

The chemokines can be divided into two main subgroups: the CC group (at least 27 members named CCL1-28) with 2 adjacent cystein residues close to the amino-terminal, and the CXC group (at least 17 members named CXCL1-17) in which the two cystein residues are spaced by a single amino-acid. This structural difference is important because each subgroup has its own set of receptors. Some receptor cross-reaction within subgroup occurs, and each chemokine may react with more than one of the receptors of the group. In addition to these main groups a few chemokines of C and CX3C group with their own receptor types have been described.

4.2.2 Chemokine receptors

The chemokine receptors have a common structure with a 7-transmembrane helix coupled to G-protein intracellular signalling. The subfamilies each have a set of chemokine receptors expressed on target cells. So far, ten CC receptors (CCR1-10) and seven CXC receptors (CXCR1-7) have been described. The system of chemokines and their receptors is quite complex and so far only partly described. However, at least theoretically, different chemokine secretion profiles combined with the receptor profiles of the target cells allow for close regulation of the homing process according to the infectious agent.

4.2.3 Chemokine effects

The chemokines trigger conformational change in the adhesion molecules (leukocyte integrins) on cell surface of leucocytes, thereby enabling a stable binding of the leukocyte to intercellular adhesion molecules (ICAM's) on the vessel wall. When the leukocyte is bound to the vessel wall it is able to squeeze between endothelial cells and enter the tissue. The cells first recruited are neutrophils, then later comes monocytes and immature dendritic cells. The chemokine activation also includes arming of the cells as effectors.

4.2.4 Homing

Upon chemokine activation endothelial cells present selectins and ICAM's on the luminal surface. Leukocytes tend to roll along the endothelial surface due to weak binding between endothelial selectin and leukocyte sialyl-Lewis^x (s-Le^x) blood group antigen. If the leukocyte integrin profile matches the ICAM a strong binding is established. This binding is enhanced further by conformational changes in the leukocyte integrin triggered by chemokine stimulation. When the cell is tightly bound, extravasation by diapedesis can be initiated. After extravasation, further movement along a chemotactic gradient to the site of infection follows.

The endothelial cells will be further activated by early response cytokines like tumor necrosis factor (TNF)-α. The chemokine activation of the neutrophil granulocyte will also stimulate the oxidative burst, which is a characteristic of the effector profile in this cell type.

4.2.5 Chemokines in the adaptive immune response

Certain chemokine receptors are expressed in certain immune profile cells. Thus a Th1 chemokine receptor set can be defined: CCR5 and CXCR3; while CCR3, CCR4 and CCR8 are linked to Th2 responses (Larrubia et al, 2008). Therefore, in a viral infection a certain subset of chemokines are especially interesting, as the Th1 response is considered the adequate and efficient response type. Ligands for the CXCR3 (Interferon gamma induced protein 10 (IP-10), Monokine induced by gamma interferon (Mig), Interferon-inducible T-cell alpha chemoattractant (I-TAC)) and CCR5 (Regulated on Activation, Normal T Expressed and Secreted (RANTES), macrophage inflammatory protein (MIP)-1-alpha, and MIP-1-beta) are theoretically crucial for the initiation of response and resolution of infection. Indeed, a frame shift mutation on the CCR5 receptor increases susceptibility to HCV infection (Woitas et al,

2002). In effect, both theoretical and experimental data support the crucial role of the chemokine response for mounting an efficient resolution of the viral infection.

4.3 Special immunobiological features of the liver

The liver is an immunotolerant organ with constitutive high expression of IL-10 and TGF-β (Crispe et al, 2006; Manigold & Racanelli, 2007). The sinusoids are inhabited by a special type of 'pit cells'; large granular lymphocytes of the NK cell trait. Data from mouse studies indicate that the NK cells of the liver tend to secrete more regulatory cytokines and less pro-inflammatory cytokines than their peripheral counterparts (Cheent & Khakoo, 2011; Lassen et al, 2010). When the HCV virus enters this environment, a proper immune response must be launched, and to this end a massive recruitment of different types of immune cells is needed. Cells of the innate immune system such as dendritic cells and NK cells are important for the initial response and stimulation of a proper adaptive Th1 response including antigen specific T helper cells, cytotoxic T cells and B cells as well as inducible regulatory T cells. All of these cell types must be recruited from the circulation and to this end an array of chemotactic signals are activated.

Chemokines have local effects on endothelium activating processes for trans-endothelial migration, and the leucocytes also have chemokine receptors activating leukocytes rolling and binding of selectins to integrin receptors. Thus chemokines have an important role in infection response allowing extravasation of leucocytes to the site of infection. As the liver has some inherent immunetolerance as mentioned above, this recruitment of external cells is especially important. Furthermore, considering the treatment of HCV with peg-IFN-α and Ribavirin the therapy may be efficient by altering the profile and composition of inflammatory cells in the liver. In this respect, the leukocyte recruitment seems have a key role in resolution of the infection.

4.3.1 Immune response to HCV infection

HCV has parenchymal liver cells as primary target utilizing CD81, claudin-1, and possibly the LDL receptor. After binding of to a target cell, the viral particle is internalized and disassembled in the cytoplasm. HCV virus has developed strategies to evade some of the basic antiviral mechanisms described above. The early IFN-β response can be blunted by cleaving adaptor proteins necessary for activating IFN transcription, and can also inhibit the JAK-STAT pathway thus inhibiting the intracellular effector events after stimulation by IFN-α.

Relatively recently a new series of λ-interferons have been described. These include the highly homologous IL-28A (IFN-λ-2), IL-28B (IFN-λ-3) and IL-29 (IFN-λ-1). Especially IL-28B has turned out to be interesting in regard to HCV infection. It seems that a firm IL-28B response is necessary for viral clearing, and that CC genotype in the rs12979860 single nucleotide polymorphism (SNP) (The Duke) in the promoter of the IL-28B gene is associated with a higher rate of spontaneous resolution of infection and also can predict response to treatment with peg-IFN-α (Langhans et al, 2011).

4.3.2 Chemokines in the context of HCV infection

Considering the immunotolerant milieu of the liver, an efficient immune response against a pathogen like HCV must be based on a considerable influx of fresh immune cells. In this respect, the chemokine response is crucial and may be one of the main factors that determine if the infection becomes chronic or is spontaneously resolved. One of the effects of peg-IFN-α therapy is to increase the pro-inflammatory response including the chemokine response allowing for fresh Th1 cells, B cells, NK cells, and dendritic cells to engage the virus. As such, the chemokine response can be seen as a common marker for a step-up in the immune response in initiation of treatment. Whether observed chemokine responses are directly triggered by the peg-IFN-α or result from a general increase in immunologic activity in the liver remains to be determined. However, as a biological marker of sustained virological response, the early rise in chemokine activity is interesting.

5. Treatment of hepatitis C

As described in the Introduction, peg-IFN-α in combination with the nucleoside analogue ribavirin is the standard treatment of HCV infection. Upcoming new drugs are albumin-INF-α, and nucleoside analogues or protease inhibitors, and nucleoside analogue/non-nucleoside analogue polymerase inhibitors. In general, these agents act via inhibitory mechanisms on the HCV gene to reduce the viral replication. These new anti HCV drugs exert their effects directly on the virus replication: protein kinase inhibitors on NS3A/B and polymerase inhibitors on NS5A/B (for review, see (Vezali et al, 2011)).

5.1 IFN-α

The mechanisms of action of peg-IFN-α are through indirect activating of the immune system and a direct antiviral mechanism at the interferon-sensitive sites of the HCV inhibiting the transcription. These mechanisms of action are rather complex and beyond the scope of this presentation. Briefly, peg-INF-α triggers a cascade of intracellular events including activations of IFN-inducible genes and increased synthesis of IFN-induced proteins (Katze et al, 2002). These proteins such as RNA-dependent protein kinase inhibit intracellular virus replication by a RNA-degrading mechanism. Peg-IFN-α also inhibits the viral replication indirectly via an immune response and most likely via activation of immune cells. These are complex mechanisms such as increased MHC-I expression and activation of immune cells with cytokine secretion. Finally, peg-IFN-α also induces an immuno-modulation in the favour of a Th1 response and an inhibition of a Th2 response (see fig 1, for review, see (Vezali et al, 2011)).

5.2 Ribavirin

The exact mode of action of ribavirin is unknown. As ribavirin alone does not inhibit the virus replication, a synergistic action together with IFN-α has been proposed. The proposed mechanisms of actions of ribavirin are: 1. an indirect host change of Th profile from a Th2 to a Th1 profile. 2. A direct inhibitory effect on the NS5B encoded RNA dependent RNA polymerase (for review, see (Lau et al, 2002)) (figure 1)

6. Chemokines in antiviral therapy

As described above, the chemokines play a pivotal role in the chemotactic immune response to HCV by acting via their specific receptors on immune active cells. The role of chemokines in the antiviral treatment is so far only incompletely understood. Of special interest for the

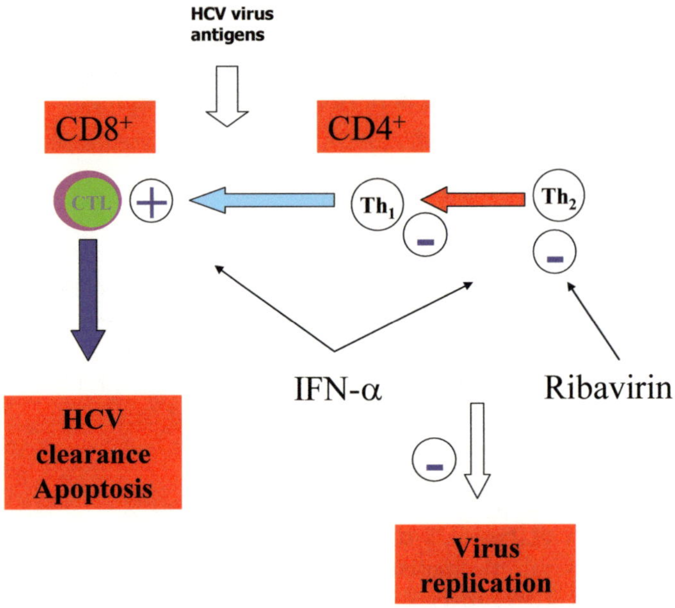

Fig. 1. Targets for antiviral therapy.

hepatic immunity is the CC chemokines macrophage inflammatory protein (MIP) -α (CCL3), MIP-1β (CCL4) and Regulated on Activation, Normal T Expressed and Secreted (RANTES) (CCL5). These chemokines are expressed by the portal vessel endothelium and recruit macrophages and lymphocytes into the liver (Ahlenstiel et al, 2004; Kusano et al, 2000). In the following we present the role of chemokines at baseline and as an early predictor of antiviral responses and clearance of the virus.

6.1 Chemokines at baseline

In one small sample sized study baseline levels before anti-HCV treatment serum levels of MIP-1β could predict a significant effect on SVR, but not eotaxin, MIP-1α, RANTES (CCL5) and IL-8 (Yoneda et al, 2011). Serum levels of MIP-3α (Yamauchi et al, 2002) have also been associated with a positive prognostic response. Moreover, increase of CXCR3 expressing CD8+ cells during treatment has been associated with achievement of viral control (Larrubia et al, 2007). Of interest was that a substitution in the ISDR was associated with response to treatment. In contrast, another study showed that baseline IL-8 level was inversely related to the response to therapy i.e. the higher IL-8 levels, the lower chance of SVR (Akbar et al, 2011). In a broad screening study of baseline CCL and CXCL chemokines, only CXCL10 was significantly associated to lack of SVR (Moura et al, 2011). In another study high CXCL10 gene expression during treatment (Sixtos-Alonso et al, 2011) and plasma level (Moura et al, 2011) were negative predictors of SVR. Finally, in two other studies baseline levels of IP10 were associated with a negative prognostic response to treatment with peg-IFN-α and ribavirin (Butera et al, 2005; Lagging et al, 2006). Interestingly, as the CCL 3-5 are produced in the portal vascular endothelium while IP-10 is produced mainly in sinusoidal endothelium and hepatocytes surrounding lobular inflammation (Zeremski et al, 2007).

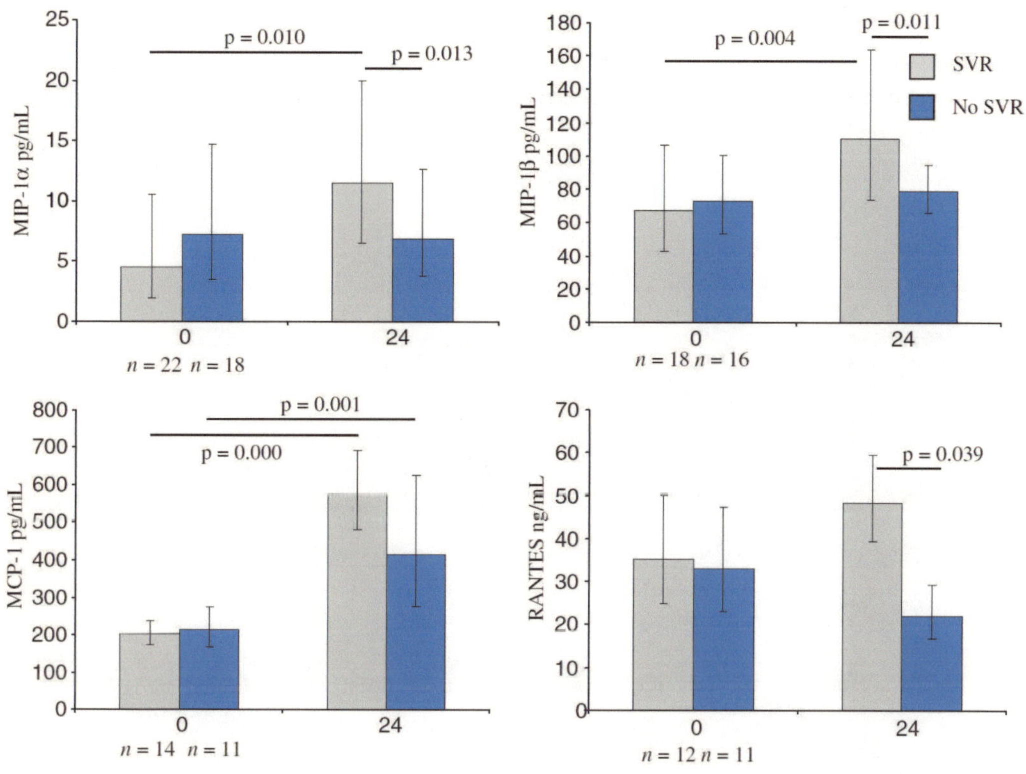

Fig. 2 Early serum chemokine responses to the treatment of chronic HCV infection. (Florholmen et al, 2011)

It is hard to interpret these apparent contradictional results of how chemokine levels can predict the response to treatment. It is of interest to note that the chemokines predicting an effective viral clearance are the CC-chemokines expressed by the portal vessel endothelium. The other chemokines predicting a lack of effect of antiviral treatment are recruited from other sources. These chemokines reflect an apparent state of viral resistance, but further studies are needed to reveal the mechanisms of action.

6.2 Early chemokine response

It is expected that an initial strong immune response is critical for a successful viral clearance in the anti HCV treatment. As far we know only one study have investigated early (24 hrs) chemokine responses during anti-HCV treatment. An early response of MIP-1α, MIP-1β, and RANTES may predict a sustained virological treatment response. MCP-1 was significantly increased but could not discriminate between SVRs and non-SVRs (Fig. 2) (Florholmen et al, 2011). However, the receiver-operator characteristic (ROC) analyses for MIP-1α, MIP-1β shows that alone, these chemokines are not suitable for clinical decisions like termination of therapy due to probable non-response (Fig. 3). Therefore, this study indicates that an early response of chemokines can be critical for an effective virus clearance during the anti-HCV treatment.

The chemokine studies mentioned above have to be interpreted with some caution both due to small sample sizes and that none of them were designed for prognostics and stratified for confounding factors.

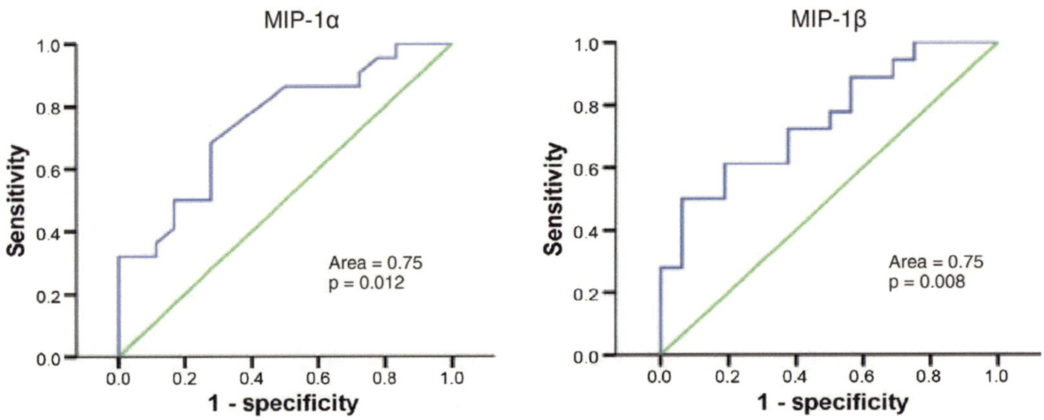

Fig. 3. ROC analysis of early chemokine response as predictor of sustained virological response (Florholmen et al, 2011).

7. New antiviral agents

The new antiviral agents based on inhibition of proteases and polymerases exert their effects on the various NS regions of the HCV genome described above. Ribavirin also has effects on an indirect mechanism of host T-cell mediation with a change from a Th2 to a Th1 profile. So far there is no evidence that the new antiviral drugs have direct suppressive effects on the HCV. Experiences from treatment of HIV show that there is a need of combination of two or more therapeutical molecules to prevent development of resistant HCV strains. So far there is an increase of SVR from 40-50 % to 75 % going from duo-therapy to triple-therapy of patients with HCV genotype 1. It would be of great interest to know if the new triple-therapy is dependent on an additional chemokine-based viral clearance for an effective treatment response. Therefore, we are waiting for further studies.

8. Concluding remarks

Chemokines seem to play a pivotal role in the immune response to HCV both to induce a spontaneous clearance during an active infection but also during the immunotherapy with peg-IFN-α and ribavirin. The mechanisms of action of chemokines are complex and still far from being fully understood. The understanding of both the successful treatment and the apparent resistance mechanisms with a virus escape from the chemokines and other immune factors is still incomplete. Most of the CC chemokines seem to play an important role in the anti virus attack. However, for other chemokines including some CXC-chemokines, increased secretions represent an apparent state of antiviral resistance to therapy. This paradox is so far poorly understood, but different compartments of chemokine production for the CC and the CXC chemokines may be a clue. It seems that the CC chemokines located in the portal vein may play a pivotal role for en effective clearance of the HCV, and the early chemokine response during antiviral treatment may be used as prognostic biomarkers. However, most of all there is a need of future studies relating viral kinetics to the chemokine responses in vivo, experimental in vitro models may contribute to a more comprehensible understanding of the role of chemokines in HCV infection.

9. References

Ahlenstiel,G.; Woitas,R.P.; Rockstroh,J., & Spengler,U. (2004). CC-chemokine receptor 5 (CCR5) in hepatitis C--at the crossroads of the antiviral immune response?, *The Journal of Antimicrobial Chemotherapy*, Vol. 53, No.6, pp. 895-898, ISSN 0305-7453.

Akbar,H.; Idrees,M.; Butt,S.; Awan,Z.; Sabar,M.F.; Rehaman,I.u.; Hussain,A., & Saleem,S. (2011). High baseline interleukine-8 level is an independent risk factor for the achievement of sustained virological response in chronic HCV patients, *Infection, Genetics and Evolution: Journal of Molecular Epidemiology and Evolutionary Genetics in Infectious Diseases*, Vol. 11, No.6, pp. 1301-1305, ISSN 1567-7257.

Butera,D.; Marukian,S.; Iwamaye,A.E.; Hembrador,E.; Chambers,T.J.; Di Bisceglie,A.M.; Charles,E.D.; Talal,A.H.; Jacobson,I.M.; Rice,C.M., & Dustin,L.B. (2005). Plasma chemokine levels correlate with the outcome of antiviral therapy in patients with hepatitis C, *Blood*, Vol. 106, No.4, pp. 1175-1182, ISSN 0006-4971.

Chayama,K. & Hayes,C.N. (2011). Hepatitis C virus: How genetic variability affects pathobiology of disease, *Journal of Gastroenterology and Hepatology*, Vol. 26 Suppl 1, pp. 83-95, ISSN 1440-1746.

Cheent,K. & Khakoo,S.I. (2011). Natural killer cells and hepatitis C: action and reaction, *Gut*, Vol. 60, No.2, pp. 268-278, ISSN 1468-3288.

Crispe,I.N.; Giannandrea,M.; Klein,I.; John,B.; Sampson,B., & Wuensch,S. (2006). Cellular and molecular mechanisms of liver tolerance, *Immunological Reviews*, Vol. 213, pp. 101-118, ISSN 0105-2896.

Florholmen,J.; Kristiansen,M.G.; Steigen,S.E.; Sørbye,S.W.; Paulssen,E.J.; Kvamme,J.M.; Konopski,Z.; Gutteberg,T., & Goll,R. (2011). A rapid chemokine response of macrophage inflammatory protein (MIP)-1-alpha, MIP-1-beta and the regulated on activation, normal T expressed and secreted chemokine is associated with a sustained virological response in the treatment of chronic hepatitis C, *Clinical Microbiology and Infection: The Official Publication of the European Society of Clinical Microbiology and Infectious Diseases*, Vol. 17, No.2, pp. 204-209, ISSN 1469-0691.

Halfon,P. & Locarnini,S. (2011). Hepatitis C virus resistance to protease inhibitors, *Journal of Hepatology*, Vol. 55, No.1, pp. 192-206, ISSN 0168-8278.

Katze,M.G.; He,Y., & Gale,M., Jr. (2002). Viruses and interferon: a fight for supremacy, *Nature Reviews.Immunology*, Vol. 2, No.9, pp. 675-687, ISSN 1474-1733.

Kusano,F.; Tanaka,Y.; Marumo,F., & Sato,C. (2000). Expression of C-C chemokines is associated with portal and periportal inflammation in the liver of patients with chronic hepatitis C, *Laboratory Investigation; a Journal of Technical Methods and Pathology*, Vol. 80, No.3, pp. 415-422, ISSN 0023-6837.

Lagging,M.; Romero,A.I.; Westin,J.; Norkrans,G.; Dhillon,A.P.; Pawlotsky,J.M.; Zeuzem,S.; von Wagner,M.; Negro,F.; Schalm,S.W.; Haagmans,B.L.; Ferrari,C.; Missale,G.; Neumann,A.U.; Verheij-Hart,E., & Hellstrand,K. (2006). IP-10 predicts viral response and therapeutic outcome in difficult-to-treat patients with HCV genotype 1 infection, *Hepatology (Baltimore, Md.)*, Vol. 44, No.6, pp. 1617-1625, ISSN 0270-9139.

Langhans,B.; Kupfer,B.; Braunschweiger,I.; Arndt,S.; Schulte,W.; Nischalke,H.D.; Nattermann,J.; Oldenburg,J.; Sauerbruch,T., & Spengler,U. (2011). Interferon-lambda serum levels in hepatitis C, *Journal of Hepatology*, Vol. 54, No.5, pp. 859-865, ISSN 0168-8278.

Larrubia,J.R.; Benito-Martinez,S.; Calvino,M.; Sanz-de-Villalobos,E., & Parra-Cid,T. (2008). Role of chemokines and their receptors in viral persistence and liver damage during chronic hepatitis C virus infection, *World Journal of Gastroenterology: WJG*, Vol. 14, No.47, pp. 7149-7159, ISSN 1007-9327.

Larrubia,J.R.; Calvino,M.; Benito,S.; Sanz-de-Villalobos,E.; Perna,C.; Perez-Hornedo,J.; Gonzalez-Mateos,F.; Garcia-Garzon,S.; Bienvenido,A., & Parra,T. (2007). The role of CCR5/CXCR3 expressing CD8+ cells in liver damage and viral control during persistent hepatitis C virus infection, *Journal of Hepatology*, Vol. 47, No.5, pp. 632-641, ISSN 0168-8278.

Lassen,M.G.; Lukens,J.R.; Dolina,J.S.; Brown,M.G., & Hahn,Y.S. (2010). Intrahepatic IL-10 maintains NKG2A+Ly49- liver NK cells in a functionally hyporesponsive state, *Journal of Immunology (Baltimore, Md.: 1950)*, Vol. 184, No.5, pp. 2693-2701, ISSN 1550-6606.

Lau,J.Y.N.; Tam,R.C.; Liang,T.J., & Hong,Z. (2002). Mechanism of action of ribavirin in the combination treatment of chronic HCV infection, *Hepatology (Baltimore, Md.)*, Vol. 35, No.5, pp. 1002-1009, ISSN 0270-9139.

Lehman,E.M. & Wilson,M.L. (2009). Epidemic hepatitis C virus infection in Egypt: estimates of past incidence and future morbidity and mortality, *Journal of Viral Hepatitis,* Vol. 16, No.9, pp. 650-658, ISSN 1365-2893.

Manigold,T. & Racanelli,V. (2007). T-cell regulation by CD4 regulatory T cells during hepatitis B and C virus infections: facts and controversies, *The Lancet Infectious Diseases,* Vol. 7, No.12, pp. 804-813, ISSN 1473-3099.

Moura,A.S.; Carmo,R.A.; Teixeira,A.L.; Teixeira,M.M., & Rocha,M.O.d.C. (2011). Soluble inflammatory markers as predictors of virological response in patients with chronic hepatitis C virus infection treated with interferon-alpha plus ribavirin, *Memórias Do Instituto Oswaldo Cruz,* Vol. 106, No.1, pp. 38-43, ISSN 1678-8060.

Myrmel,H.; Ulvestad,E., & Asjø,B. (2009). The hepatitis C virus enigma, *APMIS: Acta Pathologica, Microbiologica, Et Immunologica Scandinavica,* Vol. 117, No.5-6, pp. 427-439, ISSN 1600-0463.

Poynard,T.; Ratziu,V.; Charlotte,F.; Goodman,Z.; McHutchison,J., & Albrecht,J. (2001). Rates and risk factors of liver fibrosis progression in patients with chronic hepatitis c, *Journal of Hepatology,* Vol. 34, No.5, pp. 730-739, ISSN 0168-8278.

Rantala,M. & van de Laar,M.J.W. (2008). Surveillance and epidemiology of hepatitis B and C in Europe - a review, *Euro Surveillance: Bulletin Européen Sur Les Maladies Transmissibles = European Communicable Disease Bulletin,* Vol. 13, No.21, 1560-7917.

Shepard,C.W.; Finelli,L., & Alter,M.J. (2005). Global epidemiology of hepatitis C virus infection, *The Lancet Infectious Diseases,* Vol. 5, No.9, pp. 558-567, ISSN 1473-3099.

Sixtos-Alonso,M.S.; Sanchez-Munoz,F.; Sanchez-Avila,J.F.; Martinez,R.A.; Dominguez Lopez,A.; Vargas Vorackova,F., & Uribe,M. (2011). IFN-stimulated gene expression is a useful potential molecular marker of response to antiviral treatment with Peg-IFN-alpha 2b and ribavirin in patients with hepatitis C virus genotype 1, *Archives of Medical Research,* Vol. 42, No.1, pp. 28-33, ISSN 1873-5487.

Thorley,J.A.; McKeating,J.A., & Rappoport,J.Z. (2010). Mechanisms of viral entry: sneaking in the front door, *Protoplasma,* Vol. 244, No.1-4, pp. 15-24, ISSN 1615-6102.

Vezali,E.; Aghemo,A., & Colombo,M. (2011). Interferon in the treatment of chronic hepatitis C: a drug caught between past and future, *Expert Opinion on Biological Therapy,* Vol. 11, No.3, pp. 301-313, ISSN 1744-7682.

Vogt,M.; Lang,T.; Frösner,G.; Klingler,C.; Sendl,A.F.; Zeller,A.; Wiebecke,B.; Langer,B.; Meisner,H., & Hess,J. (1999). Prevalence and clinical outcome of hepatitis C infection in children who underwent cardiac surgery before the implementation of blood-donor screening, *The New England Journal of Medicine,* Vol. 341, No.12, pp. 866-870, ISSN 0028-4793.

Woitas,R.P.; Ahlenstiel,G.; Iwan,A.; Rockstroh,J.K.; Brackmann,H.H.; Kupfer,B.; Matz,B.; Offergeld,R.; Sauerbruch,T., & Spengler,U. (2002). Frequency of the HIV-protective CC chemokine receptor 5-Delta32/Delta32 genotype is increased in hepatitis C, *Gastroenterology,* Vol. 122, No.7, pp. 1721-1728, ISSN 0016-5085.

Yamauchi,K.; Akbar,S.M.F.; Horiike,N.; Michitaka,K., & Onji,M. (2002). Increased serum levels of macrophage inflammatory protein-3alpha in chronic viral hepatitis:

prognostic importance of macrophage inflammatory protein-3alpha during interferon therapy in chronic hepatitis C, *Journal of Viral Hepatitis*, Vol. 9, No.3, pp. 213-220, ISSN 1352-0504.

Yoneda,S.; Umemura,T.; Joshita,S.; Ichijo,T.; Matsumoto,A.; Yoshizawa,K.; Katsuyama,Y.; Ota,M., & Tanaka,E. (2011). Serum chemokine levels are associated with the outcome of pegylated interferon and ribavirin therapy in patients with chronic hepatitis C, *Hepatology Research: The Official Journal of the Japan Society of Hepatology*, Vol. 41, No.6, pp. 587-593, ISSN 1386-6346.

Zeremski,M.; Petrovic,L.M., & Talal,A.H. (2007). The role of chemokines as inflammatory mediators in chronic hepatitis C virus infection, *J Viral Hepat.*, Vol. 14, No.10, pp. 675-687, ISSN

9

Immunological Pathogenesis of Septic Reactions and Elimination of Triggers and Mediators of Inflammation

Irina Shubina, Natalia Anisimova, Elena Gromova,
Irina Chikileva and Mikhail Kiselevsky
NN Blokhin Russian Cancer Research Center
Russia

1. Introduction

Modern intensive therapy is armed with very sophisticated methods, however sepsis is still one of the most challenging issues of medicine. Death rate in patients caused by sepsis remains high and reaches about 30-80% (Yegenaga I. et al., 2004). This problem is especially important in oncology, as every sixth septic patient has a diagnosis of cancer; and the death risk of such patients is 30% higher (Angus D.C. et al., 2001).

The established bacteriologic paradigm of sepsis implies an infectious component for its development. The priority in the pathogenesis of this disease has been assigned to microorganisms, and therefore sepsis is regarded primarily as an infective disease. However, over the last decades there have appeared tendencies for an essential revision in the understanding of mechanisms of sepsis development; inflammatory reactions of the organism are now regarded as important as infection. In particular, according to a current definition, approved by American College of Chest Physicians/Society of Critical Care Medicine (ACCP/SCCM) Consensus Conference, "sepsis is a systemic inflammatory response syndrome developing in response to an invasion of different pathogenic microorganisms, which is diagnosed if an infective agent and two or more signs of the systemic inflammatory response are present" (USA, Chicago, 1991).

Systemic inflammatory response syndrome (SIRS) includes the whole set of the clinical manifestations of systemic inflammatory response (SIR), which is a generalized form of inflammatory reaction and is formed as a result of an excessive immune cell activation that produce different types of mediators (cytokines, leukotrienes, thromboxanes, etc.). SIRS is a necessary component of sepsis, however, it is not the same, as SIRS may be induced by different non-infective causes such as trauma, pancreatitis, etc. Thus, signs of systemic infection are necessary to prove diagnosed sepsis. Besides, it should be taken into account that bacteremia is not pathognomonic to sepsis. The rate of diagnosed bacteremia even in the most serious cases does not exceed 45% if accurate techniques of blood sampling and modern microbiologic methods are applied. Detection of microorganisms in the patient's peripheral blood with no clinical and laboratory test conclusion of SIRS may be considered as transitory bacteremia that is not necessarily caused by septic process. Some authors recommend differentiating localized focus of infection from true sepsis even if it is associated with the symptoms of systemic inflammatory reaction. In about half of cases (30-60%) when clinical symptoms of sepsis were evident, it was impossible to isolate live microorganisms from the blood or find the focus of infection.

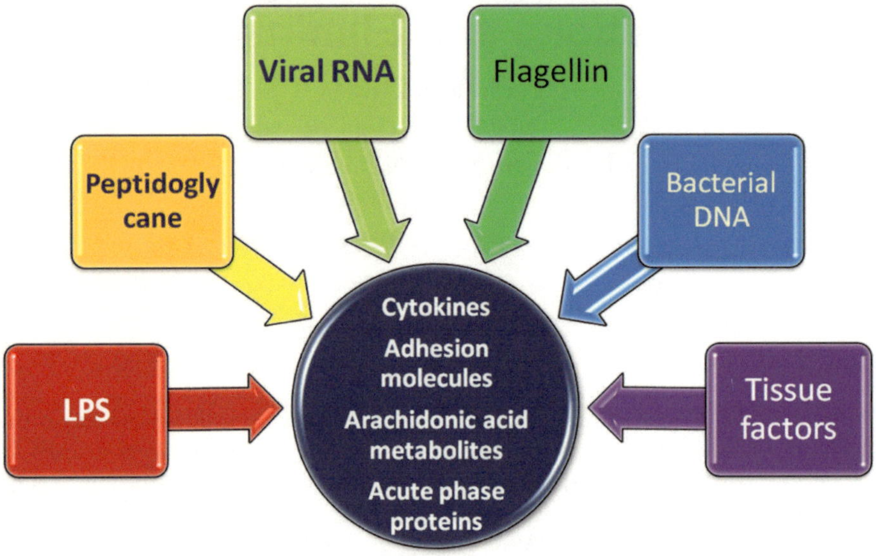

Fig. 1. Triggering factors and mediators of sepsis.

The disease status that demonstrates the whole set of septic symptoms but lack of infection is regarded like pseudosepsis or sepsis-like syndrome. Trigger factors initiating systemic inflammatory response might be derivatives of microorganisms (exo- or endotoxins) rather than microorganisms themselves, or even factors of non-infective origin including endogeneous factors (such as tissue factors, elastin, thrombin, etc.), which appear primarily during organ or tissue damage (Fig. 1) as a result of traumas, burns, etc.

Clinical symptoms of sepsis as well as organ or multi-organ dysfunction syndrome (MODS) may develop in response to endo- and exotoxins of microorganisms in the absence of bacteremia (septicemia) or localized focus of infection. The macroorganism reaction to bacterial products displays totally the whole symptom complex that is characteristic for bacterial sepsis. LPS poisoning does not only induce clinical presentations of sepsis and septic (endotoxic shock), but leads to pathomorphologic changes characteristic for septic conditions (Angus D.C. et al., 2001).

Present understanding of sepsis states that it is a systemic inflammatory response of the macroorganism, which develops as a result of interaction of the immune system with bacteria or their toxins and is mediated by the over-expression of a complex of humoral factors: cytokines and other substances (platelet activation factor, metabolites of arachidonic acid, endotelin-1, and complement components). Local tissue damage during SIRS arises from the release of active oxygen forms, proteases and escalation of cytokine synthesis. Such vision of sepsis pathogenesis suggests that new diagnostic and prognostic markers of this condition should be identified in patient's immunologic parameters. Following this concept, new therapeutic strategies of inactivation or elimination of SIR triggers and mediators are being developed.

2. Bacterial toxins: triggers of inflammation

Infective agents have various factors of virulence which can affect protective reactions of the body. In septic and inflammatory conditions cascade of events initiated by microbes and their products may develop out of control. Immune effectors recognize pathogens, firstly, by innate immunity receptors detecting different pathogen-associated molecular patterns that include various components of microbial cell wall (such as, LPS -lipopolysaccharide, peptidoglycan, lipoteichoic acid, mannan, flagellin, bacterial DNA, viral double-helical RNA, glucan and intracellular components, etc.)

Bacterial toxins, primarily LPS of gram-negative bacteria, have significant impact on activating mechanisms of inflammation and may induce or potentiate systemic inflammatory response in the absence of microbial cells. In particular, it was shown that in humans LPS in the minimal dose (4 ng/kg) initiates release of inflammatory mediators, alterations of hemostasis and fall of the blood pressure resulting from the decrease of the cardiac output and vascular resistance. Sepsis-like conditions were described in volunteers after injections of high endotoxin doses as well as in patients receiving therapies based on LPS-immunomodulators (Laurenzi L. et al., 2004, Zucker T. et al., 2004). Sepsis-like syndrome is observed in patients after cardiac surgery, closed injury, and in patients resuscitated after cardiac arrest.

One of the major mechanisms of infection is penetration of normal microflora and substances including endotoxins into blood circulation from the natural organism biocoenoses, mainly from the bowels (Annane D. et al., 2005). Translocation of bacteria and their toxins into the bloodstream might be caused by changes in the mucous intestine tunic (Moore F.A. , 1999). Nevertheless, impairment of the intestine permeability most often has a secondary origin and results from the SIR to trauma, surgical stress, burn, high-dose antibiotic therapy and other damaging factors (Deitch E.A.&Bridges R.M. , 1987, Balzan S.et al., 2007). In cancer patients, risk of bacterial toxin translocation increases due to disorders of the intestine mucous barrier function caused by the major disease and especially, by anti-tumor aggressive therapy. An additional unfavorable factor is older age of patients because of the age-related changes in the intestines permeability. These patients, despite of the widely accepted view about immunity involution and down-regulation of immune reactions in the elderly, demonstrate an enhanced response to bacterial toxins. For example, patients over 65 have a more significant drop of the blood pressure after injections of minimal LPS doses (2 ng/kg) compared with younger individuals. The phenomenon is apparently linked to the systemic chronic inflammatory reaction of the elderly, associated with a higher initial level of pro-inflammatory factors.

When LPS enters blood circulation, it partly links to the LPS-binding protein (LBP) and the newly formed complex interacts with CD14-positive cells, such as macrophages. LPB potentiates LPS transport to receptors of macrophages (CD14) and stimulates functional activity of these innate immunity effectors (Takeshita S. et al., 2002). The endotoxin-shipping function in the blood also refers to the soluble circulating macrophage CD14-receptors. A number of studies showed an increase in these markers in patients with sepsis, including cancer patients (Myc A. et al., 1997, Nijhuis C. S. et al., 2003).

Our data show that LPS serum concentration increases in patients with sepsis aggravated by organ failure or MODS. Particularly, in contrast to healthy volunteers, whose blood almost lacks LPS, patients with kidney or hepatic failure with no symptoms of SIRS showed moderate increase of LPS serum concentrations (0,1-0,2 IU/ml), while patients with sepsis and septic shock had markedly increased blood serum concentrations of this bacterial toxin - median parameter in the group was 0,55 IU/ml, sometimes reaching 6,25 IU/ml (Fig. 2).

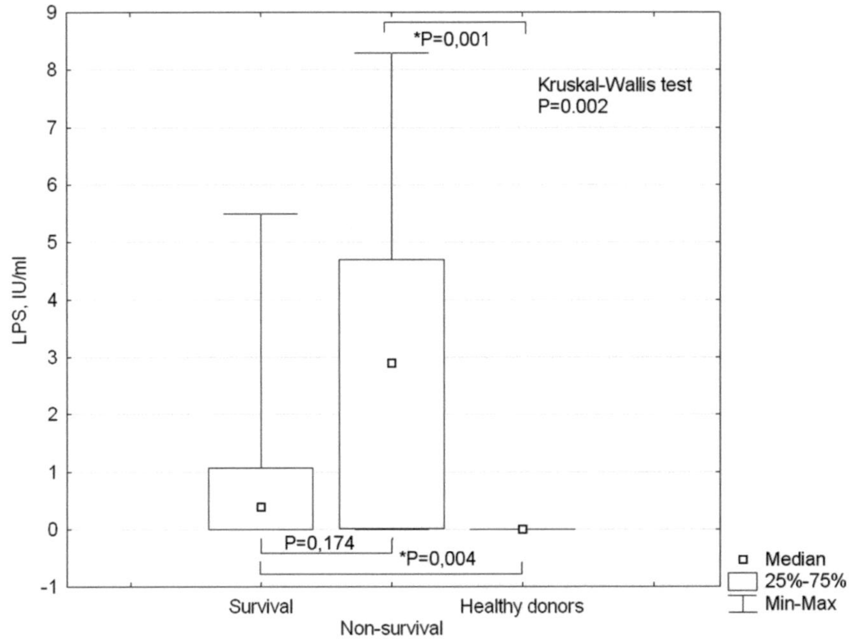

Fig. 2. Comparative analysis of LPS serum level in groups of survival and died patients with sepsis and in healthy volunteers.

A high LPS concentration in peripheral blood is generally associated with a drop of LPB level. In patients with sepsis the ratio of blood serum concentrations LPS/LPB is on average ten-fold higher than in healthy individuals. Therefore, dynamic growth of LPS concentration and decrease of LPB level in sepsis may be considered as negative prognostic factors.

3. Cytokines

Over the last years, a lot of data have been accumulated that discuss the role of endogenic bioregulators of different origin (cytokines, kinins, phospholipids, arachidonic acid metabolites, etc.) in development of structural and functional alterations leading to systemic inflammatory reactions and sepsis. Immune mediators - cytokines have an absolutely important role in inflammation pathogenesis. Their high biologic activity and a small difference between effective and toxic concentrations make them key factors both in natural physiologic processes and pathologic conditions. As it was mentioned earlier, a triggering mechanism of SIRS, besides bacteria and/or their toxins, might be a trauma, including surgical intervention. With no microbial components it may also initiate an inflammatory cascade, leading to cellular damage and organ dysfunctions. Different endogenous factors, so-called alarmins, which are activated by tissue damage (for example, necrotic cells, RNA, urine acid crystals, etc.), may bind leucocyte receptors and induce systemic inflammatory response or "sepsis with no infective agent". A term "alarmin" was suggested by J. Oppenheim for endogenous stress molecules that provide signals about tissue and cell damage (Oppenheim J.J.& Yang D., 2005).

Thus, excessive concentrations of these endogenous modulators provoke development of pathophysiologic abnormalities leading to organ failure or MODS. However, despite numerous studies looking at prognostic or diagnostic significance of cytokine concentrations in the serum of patients with purulent and septic complications, there is still disagreement on the topic. Serum cytokine low levels are registered in the peripheral blood of many patients regardless clinical symptoms of sepsis or septic shock. At the same time, some authors report data of increased concentrations of several cytokines such as interleukin(IL)-8, tumor necrosis factor (TNF)α, IL-6 in the peripheral blood of patients with sepsis (Calandra T.et al., 1990, Anderson R.&Schmidt R., 2010, Gaïni S. et al., 2006).

Risk of SIRS development is extremely high in cancer patients, as the necessary extensive surgery stimulates release of pro-inflammatory cytokines that may promote development of systemic inflammatory response (Hildebrand F. et al., 2005, Lenz A. et al., 2007). Some authors suggested diagnostic and prognostic significance of TNFα serum level (Calandra T., 1990). The results showed both increased as well as similar to the control group concentrations of TNFα in serum of patients with severe sepsis. An unfavorable course of the septic process was observed in the cases of low basic TNFα level or its negative dynamics (TNFα level dropped from 30,4 ± 2,7 pg/ml to 15,8 ± 6,3 pg/ml). Originally high TNFα in the blood of septic patients (1020,7 ± 30,1 pg/ml) was considered as a "cytokine cascade out of control". They also presented data demonstrating that intensive therapy in the group of patients with originally high TNFα concentration leaded to its significant decrease (from 680,4 ± 32,7 pg/ml to 450 ± 16,7 pg/ml), which was associated with favorable prognosis. TNFα level varied in a wide range from 50 to 3500 pg/ml in patients with septic shock. Median TNFα level was 180 pg/ml in the group of survived patients; and 330 pg/ml in the group of the deceased. On the basis of these data, contradictory conclusions were made about prognostic significance of pro-inflammatory cytokine serum levels in general and TNFα, in particular. However, many researchers agree that both high and low TNFα serum levels in critical conditions may be regarded as a poor prognostic parameter (Martin C.et al., 1994, Quinn J.V.&Slotman G.J., 1999).

According to our data, only the concentration of IL-6 was significantly increased in the peripheral blood of cancer patients with sepsis (Table 1). The highest mediator levels were observed in patients with septic shock. A probable cause of the pro-inflammatory cytokine increase in the patients' blood could be its overproduction by the resident macrophages, in particular, by the hepatic Kupffer cells. Besides TNFα, IL-6 is one of the probable markers of severity of an infective or non-infective stress. It induces production of a wide range of proteins of the acute phase that regulate inflammation process. In septic shock, the cytokine may directly affect organs and tissues; in particular, it may suppress myocardium. Various studies investigated the role of this cytokine in pathogenesis of septic shock, MODS and other systemic processes and its prognostic significance; however, their conclusions are somewhat contradictory (Anderson R.&Schmidt R., 2010, Pinsky M.R., 2004).

Groups	IL-6	IL-8	IL-10	INFγ	TNFα	TNF β	IL-1β	IL-4	IL-17
Cancer patients with sepsis	203* 61÷494	17 6÷130	48 31÷163	0 0÷16	4 0÷30	4 4÷26	1 0÷28	6 3÷13	31 0÷73
healthy volunteers	0 0÷1	3 0÷11	80 0÷108	2 0÷16	0 0÷0	0 0÷9	0 0÷0	10 2÷12	9 6÷19

* – significant difference compared to the control group of healthy volunteers ($P<0.01$)

Table 1. Cytokine profile of cancer patients with sepsis compared to healthy volunteers (median, 25th ÷75th quartiles), pg/ml.

On the whole, the above data suggest that determination of free cytokine serum concentrations in the peripheral blood of patients with septic complications presents little information, except for IL-6, which is statistically significantly increased in patients with sepsis, and, especially, with septic shock. Therefore IL-6 is the only serum cytokine, which concentration might be recommended as a marker for sepsis. A possible reason of low importance of the cytokine profile determination in sepsis may be due to the fact that commercially available kits are designed to evaluate concentrations of free (soluble) cytokines only. It is a serious obstacle for the estimation of the total cytokine concentrations secreted into the blood circulation. Even if free cytokines are not detected in the blood, their receptor-bound complexes may be circulating. As a result, "hidden cytokinemia" - high cytokine concentrations non-detectable by conventional methods - may take place.

Therefore, low levels of serum cytokines do not necessarily reflect the true mediator concentrations in blood serum and may result not only from insufficient activity of immune effectors of cancer patients, but also from specific binding with increased concentrations of cytokine soluble receptors. A number of studies reported on the statistically significant increase of concentrations of soluble cytokine receptors: TNF receptors (sTNF-R I and sTNF-R II) (Zhang B.et al., 1998), IL-1 – sIL-1 RII (Müller B., 2002) and decrease of soluble IL-6 receptor (sIL-6 R) (Frieling J.T.M.et al., 1995, Zeni F. et al., 1995) in patients with sepsis. However, other researchers presented different results (Barber M.D.et al, 1999).

The data of our studies showed that only sTNF-RI (p55) serum level was significantly more enhanced in cancer patients with sepsis compared with control group of healthy volunteers. However, the comparative analysis of cytokine and their soluble receptor concentrations in the blood of survived and deceased patients with sepsis showed that simultaneous increase of IL-6, IL-8, IL-10, sTNF-RI, sIL-1RII and sIL-6R was associated with poor prognosis. Probably, the mentioned facts result from the so-called "cytokine storm" and reflect the extreme imbalance of the immune system in sepsis leading to the fatal outcome. This suggestion is supported by the increased level of both pro-inflammatory cytokines (IL-6, IL-8) and anti-inflammatory IL-10 in the patients died from sepsis

Comparative studies of immunocompetent cell potential for cytokine secreting presented more precise data. The level of spontaneous production of these endogenous bioregulators characterizes the original physiologic activity of the blood cells. The intensity of the stimulated cytokine production helps to determine the potential reactivity in response to a possible infection.

The obtained data from our studies showed that blood cells of septic cancer patients with spontaneous overproduction of certain cytokines (IL-6, IL-8) are mostly non-responsive to any stimulation. The observation suggests that immune effectors in this group of patients are over-stimulated.

The inflammatory reaction in response to trauma or infection is induced mainly by innate immunity and develops rapidly at the early stage. Endogenous inflammation mediators synthesized by immune cells in response to microbial components or tissue factors are released within few minutes and may peak within 1-3 hours in peripheral blood. These factors play a major role in the formation of the protective response to infection (they enhance bactericidal activity of phagocytes, promote recruitment of leukocytes to the infection site, stimulate hemopoiesis, and cause fever). However, inflammatory over-reaction leads to an excessive release of inflammatory mediators both of peptide (cytokines) and lipid nature (metabolites of membrane lipids –leukotrienes, thromboxanes, platelet activation factor). These substances, besides protective functions, are highly toxic and may cause hemodynamic imbalance, metabolic and pathologic alterations that are characteristic for sepsis and septic shock. Activation of anti-inflammatory factors, as well as of inhibitors of inflammatory mediators (prostaglandin E2, IL-1Ra, IL-10 and TGF-β), takes place during SIRS and is considered as compensatory anti-inflammatory syndrome, a protective response limiting tissue damage by endogenous pro-inflammatory factors. On the other hand, prevalence of anti-inflammatory mediators may lead to immune suppression and anergy of immune cells (Keel M.&Trentz O., 2005). Evidently, both hyper- and hypo-inflammatory phases may follow each other or develop independently from each other, according to the original reactivity of the organism. Both conditions of hyper- and hyporeactivity are equally dangerous and may cause fatal outcome.

4. Functional activity of leukocytes

So far a lot of data have been collected to characterize immune status of cancer patients with suppurative septic complications (Martin C., 1994, Quinn J.V.&Slotman G.J., 1999, Anderson R.&Schmidt R., 2010, Pinsky M.R. et al., 2004, Zhang B. et al, 1998, Frieling J.T.M.et al., 1995). Although most of the studies look at parameters of humoral immunity, particularly, at assessment of cytokine profile, a higher interest has been seen in studying functions of immune competent cells over the last years. Special attention is aimed at effectors of innate immunity (natural killers, granulocytes and monocytes), which play a key role in pathogenesis of sepsis (Zeerleder S., 2005). A number of authors show an increasing suppression of cellular immunity with septic background that reveals as decreased function of immune competent cells due to high rate of immunosuppressive agents (IL-10) and decrease of regulatory peptides (IL-12). On the other hand, there are data that prove enhanced production of pro-inflammatory cytokines (IL-8, TNFα, IL-6, IL-1β) in cancer patients, which level is many times higher than that in healthy individuals (Rigato O.et al., 1996, Kumar A.T. et al., 2009). The logic consequence of this phenomenon may be higher cellular functioning, mostly - innate immunity effector cells function. In the environment of bacteriemia and bacterial toxicity these cells are responsible for natural resistance to infectious agents. However their super activation triggers cascade hyperproduction of inflammatory mediators which initiate SIRS (Angus D.C. et al., 2001, Hildebrand F. et al., 2005).

The results of our studies showed that cancer patients with sepsis have a significant increase of natural killer (NK) cells activity as compared with cancer patients having no sepsis or healthy volunteers. These data comply with results of other authors who demonstrated an enhanced function of NK in patients with sepsis (Giamarellos-Bourboulis E.J.et al., 2006, Yoneda O. et al., 2000). The observed phenomenon seemed to be associated with the enhanced rate of IL-12 in blood serum of patients with severe sepsis or septic shock due to the fact that IL-12 stimulates NK and T-killer cells cytotoxicity as a result of secreting molecules involved in cytolytic reactions (gransymes A and B) (Zeerleder S., et al. 2005).

Neutrophils are the first line of protection against acute infections and play an important role in pathogenesis of sepsis (Segal A.W. , 2005). On the one hand they are major players in eliminating infectious microorganisms, on the other hand - an excessive release of oxidants and proteases by neutrophils leads to damaging organs and tissues. Neutrophils are involved both in inflammatory processes and natural immunity effects migrating to the site of infection or inflammation to eliminate infectious agents. Besides that they produce signals about invasion of a foreign agent to alert effectors of innate immunity. These signals induce activation of other cells, such as, monocytes/ macrophages as well as epithelial and mast cells and trombocytes. On activation neutrophils generate various chemotaxic factors attracting macrophages. Because of their common origin neutrophils and macrophages have common functions (phagocytosis, similar behavioral kinetics in infectious and inflammatory process, anti-microbial and immunomodulating functions). Activated neutrophils releasing chemokines stimulate and recruit to the inflammation site monocytes and macrophages and may effect on macrophage differentiation into pro- or anti-inflammatory subtype (type I or type II macrophages). In addition to release of pro-inflammatory cytokines neutrophils also secrete reactive oxygen radicals that induce acute tissue destruction, such as lung destruction in acute reactive distress syndrome (ARDS) or pneumonia (Kumar V. et al., 2010). Besides phagocytosis and secretion of anti-bacterial molecules neutrophils form so-called extra-cellular traps. Extra-cellular traps are formed from the decondensated chromatin and the contents of some granule, as well as from the cytoplasmic proteins and can interact both with gram-negative and gram-positive bacteria leading to destruction of virulent factors and killing bacteria. However the excessive reaction of innate immunity following bacterial infection may lead to immune suppression in the end. Part of this condition is impairment of neutrophil phagocytic activity, which is the major component determining the status of anti-infectious defense (Kumar V. et al., 2010, Giamarellos-Bourboulis E.J. et al., 2010, Volk H.D. et al., 1999).

Patients with sepsis and the background of neutrophil sequestration can often develop complications in tissues, such as ARDS, and excessive activation of neutrophils is associated with lung destruction (Kumar V. et al., 2010, Giamarellos-Bourboulis E.J. et al., 2010).

There is a number of data that demonstrate long-term cellular over-production of pro-inflammatory cytokines (IL-8, TNFα, IL-6, IL-1β) in cancer patients with sepsis, which can effect neutrophil functions (Martin C. et al., 1994, Zhang B. et al., 1998, Frieling J.T.M. et al., 1995, Barber M.D. et al., 1999, Rigato O. et al., 1996, Segal A.W., 2005). The results revealed that in most cases the phagocytotic activity of neutrophils of cancer patients with sepsis (phagocytic index and phagocytic number) were higher than those of healthy volunteers (in 2,6 and 6,3 times, respectively) (Fig. 3a,b, Fig.4 a,b). This phenomenon may be the results of increased production of pro-inflammatory cytokines, in particular IL-8: key cytokine involved in recruitment of neutrophiles into the inflammation site and stimulating their function (Hammond M.E. et al., 1995).

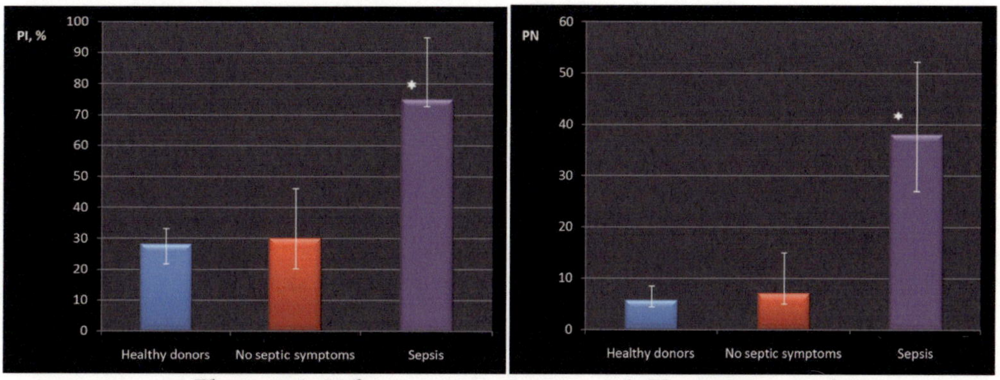

a Phagocytic index b Phagocytic number

*– values that have reliable difference from those of healthy volunteers (p<0,05).

Fig. 3. Parameters of phagocytosis rate of blood granulocytes in cancer patients with sepsis and patients with no septic symptoms in comparison with healthy volunteers (median, 25%÷75%).

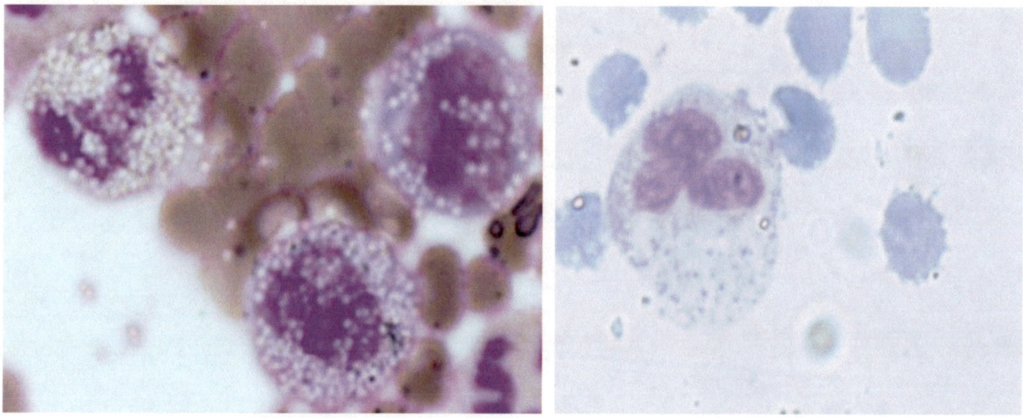

a b

Fig. 4. Microphotos of neutrophils in peripheral blood of healthy volunteers (a) and cancer patient with sepsis (b) after incubation with latex particles (t=40 min).

Patients with sepsis have a significant increase in activation of oxygen dependent mechanisms of phagocytes as compared to those of patients with no complications or healthy volunteers (5-fold and 15-fold, respectively) that points to a high rate of activation of intracellular bactericidal systems when there is septic process (Fig. 5).

Hydrogen peroxide combined with myeloperoxidase (enzyme of primary neutrophil granules) and halogen ions forms an effective bactericidal system that kills bacteria by halogenation of the cellular wall (Zychlinsky A. et al., 2003). But phagocytes release these endogenous active substances into the inter-cellular medium so that they also destroy self-tissues and thus they become involved in developing organ dysfunction or MODS (Thomas S. et al., 2004).

Previous studies suggest that the basis for MODS in critical conditions is the impairment of vessel endothelium, which was the result of active function of immune competent cells induced by microbial products. Therefore super-activation of effectors of innate immunity (neutrophils, natural killers) may be considered as an important link in pathogenesis of organ or multi-organ dysfunction syndrome.

Excessive reaction of innate immune system after contact with bacterial infection can lead to immune suppression. A part of this condition is the disorder in phagocytic function of neutrophils, which to a high extent determines anti-infectious defense (Volk H.D. et al., 1999, Alves-Filho J.C. et al., 2010, Giamarellos-Bourboulis EJ et al., 2010).

One of the results of the developing immune suppression in patients with sepsis can be decreased number of lymphocytes that is associated with their sequestration in the inflammation site or their apoptotic death as a result of the excessive production of pro-apoptotic factors. Clinical studies showed marked T-cell lymphopenia with its maximum within a few days. Absolute and relative number of CD4+ and CD8+ T-lymphocytes reduces. At the same time percentage of B-lymphocytes in the peripheral blood goes up (Murphy R.&DeCoursey T. E., 2006, Holub M. et al., 2000). Essential alterations were observed in NK examination (Emoto M. et al., 2002, Kerr A.R., et al., 2005).

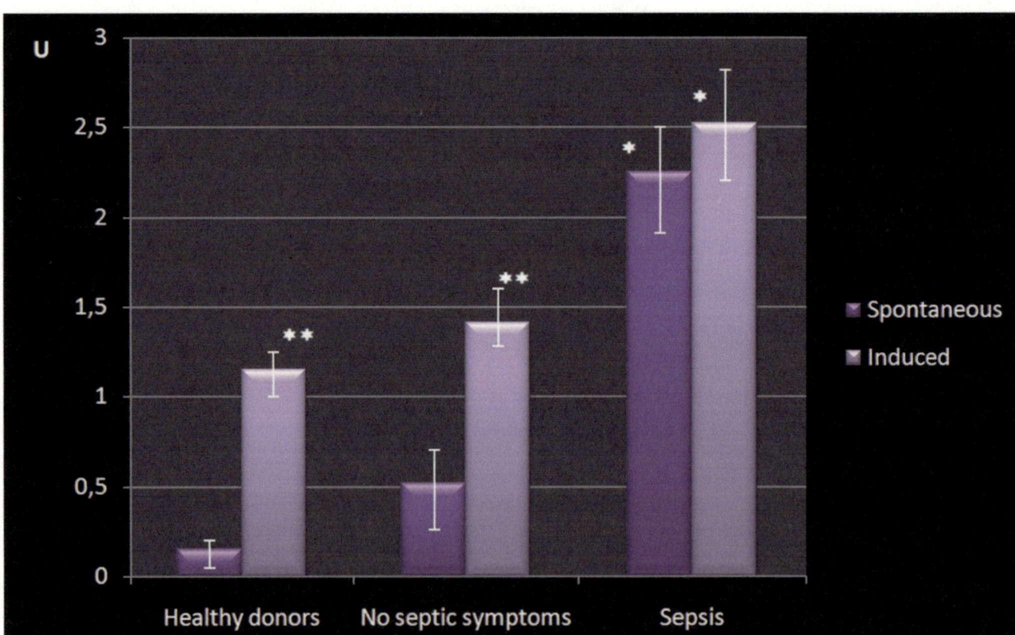

*– values that have reliable difference from control (p<0,05);

**– results of the induced NB-test reliably different from the results of spontaneous NB-test (p<0,05).

Fig. 5. Rate of metabolic activity of neutrophils in peripheral blood of cancer patients in comparison with those of healthy volunteers in spontaneous and induced NB-test (nitrone blue test) (median, 25%÷75%).

Peripheral blood NK number enhances at the early stage of sepsis in patients with sepsis (Giamarellos-Bourboulis E.J. et al., 2006), while in patients with septic shock their relative number decreases (Holub M. et al., 2000).

5. Apoptosis of the immune cells after trauma

Apoptosis of various immune cells is an important part of immune suppression development in response to an emergency situation (trauma, burns, infection). Suppression of active immunity due to the death of monocytes, macrophages and lymphocytes can enhance risk of opportunistic infections. Moreover, a higher rate of apoptosis in lymphoid tissues and parenchyma organs may lead to disorders in cellular homeostasis and the following inadequate response of the organism as a whole including development of MODS.

Clinical and experimental studies of trauma and burns showed that enhanced production of endogenous mediators of inflammation (heat shock proteins, free oxygen radicals, NO, TNF, IL-1 and IL-6) could activate signaling pathways of apoptosis in different immune cells. Increased expression of apoptotic markers on T-cells (Fas и FasL) was observed in patients who underwent surgery that makes reason for lymphopenia leading to a higher risk of post-surgical infections. However, some authors reported about decrease of apoptotic marker on leukocytes in sepsis and SIRS (Härter L. et al., 2003, Sayeed M.M., 2004, Papathanassoglou E.D.E. et al., 2005, Jimenez M.F., et al. 1997, Lee WL & Downey GP. , 2001). The expression level of this marker on neutrophils correlates with the severity of the inflammation (Fialkow L. et al., 2006). Apparently, alterations in apoptosis regulation as the process responsible for the elimination of fading cells play an essential role in pathogenesis of sepsis and multi-organ dysfunction syndrome (Pierozan P. et al.,2006, Mahidhara R. et al, 2000).

6. Platelets in sepsis

Platelets may be considered as a linking chain between innate immunity and homeostasis. Activated platelets can form clusters in blood circulation system that leads to thromboses and their sequestration in microcirculation often leads to dessiminated inter-vessel blood coagulation.

Systemic capillary thrombosis in situation of inter-vessel blood coagulation is one of the reasons for multi-organ dysfunction. Moreover, extended and long-term activation of the coagulation system results in exhausted factors of coagulation and platelet function, which causes increased bleeding.

7. Immunoglobulins

Imbalance of humoral immunity that develops in sepsis presents quantitative and qualitative changes in serum immunoglobulins. A lot of authors report about reduction of immunoglobulins A, G, M and their subtype levels in SIRS (Kyles B.D.M.& Baltimore J., 2005, Tabata N. et al., 1995). The results of a prospective study (Dietz S. et al., 2010) of 543 patients with sepsis demonstrated that half of them had physiological normal IgG level in peripheral blood (6,1-11,9 g/dL). However intra-venous infusion of immunoglobulins in patients with systemic inflammatory processes is widely used (Berlot G. et al, 2007, Jenson H.B., 1998, Pildal J.& Gotzsche P.C., 2008). On the other hand, some authors state that there was no reliable increase of survival in patients with sepsis after treatment with exogenous immunoglobulins (Alejandria M.M. et al., 2002, Werdan K., 1999).

8. Immunological imbalance in patients with sepsis

At present there is a standpoint of the massive inflammatory reaction as a result of systemic release of cytokines that is the basic cause for MODS (Goris J.A. et al., 1985). A MODS is the result of endothelial cell damage, impairment of vessel penetrative capacity, micro circular disorders with developing cellular hypoxia and finally, cell apoptosis with the release of immune or necrotic proteins. Kidneys and gastro-intestinal tract are highly sensitive to micro-circular disorders, which lead to necrosis of renal tubules that enhances concentration of serum creatinine, develops oliguria or anuria and necrosis of intestine fringes. Excessive inflammatory reaction may change to areactivity that leads to immune suppression (and even to immunological paralysis) and joining secondary infection. Pathological morphological analysis often cannot detect correspondence between histological results and the grade of organ dysfunction registered in patients who died from sepsis. The number of dead tissue cells of heart, kidneys, liver and lungs can be insignificant to reflect the marked organ dysfunctions. Apparently, most symptoms of organ dysfunctions in patients with sepsis can be due to "cell hibernation" or "cell stunning" in the way it happens in myocardial ischemia (Sawyer DB & Loscalzo J., 1985). Reactions that are observed in septic conditions can be also seen in other pathological processes that are not directly linked to effects of microbes or their products, such as trauma, shock, advanced surgical interventions. Therefore the correct definition of sepsis is crucial because different approach to understanding sepsis leads to different treatment strategy (primarily, anti-bacterial) and directly effects the outcome. Biological response to microbial components at the beginning of SIRS and sepsis is considered to be immunological reaction of the body in order to reduce the number of pathogens. However unrestricted and excessive production of pro- and anti-inflammatory mediators plays the major role in pathogenesis of sepsis and MODS. Therefore treatment of sepsis should involve control of mediators of inflammatory cascade. Microbial components (such as endotoxin, etc.) and other mediators of inflammation (cytokines, chemokines, leukotriens, thromboxanes, platelet activating factor) that induce systemic inflammatory syndrome should be eliminated at the early stage of sepsis. Some authors proposed restriction of excessive activation of immune system of patients with sepsis by inhibiting various elements of inflammatory cascade. Monoclonal antibodies against LPS and TNF and other biological regulatory factors were offered to achieve the desired effect. However randomized clinical studies did not show clinical effectiveness of such agents (Vincent J.-L.&Abraham E., 2006). Another promising approach is the use of selective haemosorption with LPS-absorbers that allow elimination of a large part of bacterial toxins and inflammatory mediators from patient's peripheral blood.

9. Haemosorption with LPS-adsorber for elimination of triggers and mediators of inflammation in patients with sepsis and SIRS

Endotoxin (lipopolysaccharide, LPS) is well known as the main biological substance causing Gram-negative septic shock. The lack of clinical success in anti-endotoxin therapies with antibodies determined the development of extracorporeal methods aimed at reducing the circulating endotoxin level by adsorption. Theoretically such procedures could prevent progression of the systemic inflammatory reaction due to the elimination of inflammation trigger factors and mediators (cytokines, bacterial exo- and endotoxins) from the patient's body. The necessity of eliminating a wide spectrum of substances characterized by different physical and chemical features from blood stipulates the application of non-selective and non-specific methods such as haemosorption. In current clinical practice some devices for haemosorption are used as specific (LPS) adsorbers. Launched in 2006 the Alteco® LPS Adsorber (Alteco Medical AB, Sweden; class IIa medical device) is based on a tailor-made synthetic peptide which is non-toxic and adsorbs endotoxin selectively in a recommended single 2-h treatment with a blood flow of 100–200 ml/min and activated clotting time of ≥180 s (information provided by the manufacturer).

Data available confirmed an effective reduction in the LPS level in the patients' blood after this procedure (Yaroustovsky M, 2009, Andersen T.H., 2009). In particular, Kulabukhov VV et al. demonstrated almost total elimination of LPS from the patient's blood (from 1.44 EU/ml before treatment to 0.03 EU/ml post treatment) (Kulabukhov VV., 2008). This effect was accompanied by a reduction in procalcitonin and inflammatory cytokines levels. Also, an obvious improvement was observed in the patient's haemodynamics.

The same results were shown in the work of T. Ala-Kokko et al.(T. Ala-Kokko, 2009). The mean total duration of vasopressor infusion was 46 h shorter in the treatment group compared with the control group (95% CI, 104–12 h, $p = 0.165$), with an average vasopressor requirement period of 17.4 ± 6.8 h (95% CI, 5.8–23.8 h) following the start of adsorption treatment. The level of LPS decreased in all cases except in one study patient and all were without vasopressors at 24 h. The decrease in the Sequential Organ Failure Assessment (SOFA) score was 3.4 ± 1.7 from baseline to 24 h after the treatment. The average period of hospital stay was 3.4 days shorter in the treatment group (95% CI, 21.7–14.8 days, $p = 0.881$).

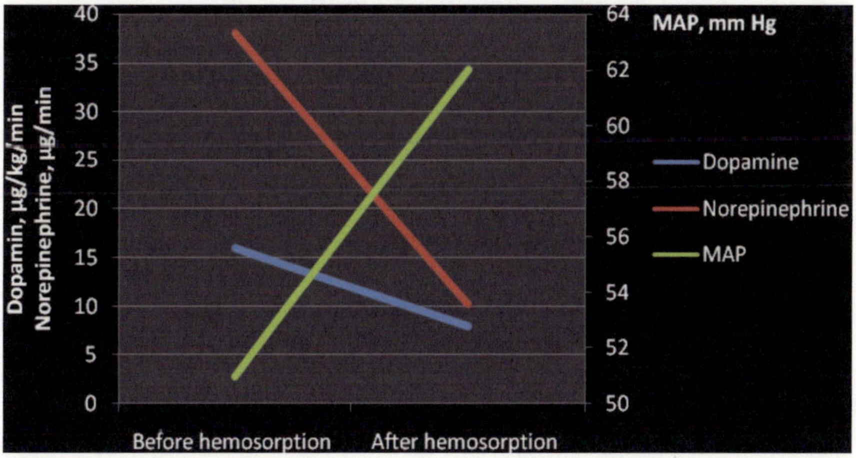

Fig. 6. Inverse correlation of MAP dynamics and vasopressor requirement before and after haemosorption by Alteco.

We studied LPS adsorbers for treating 7 patients with sepsis or septic shock. During the course of extracorporeal detoxification a number of clinical parameters were estimated.

These were temperature, mean arterial pressure (MAP), central venous pressure (CVP), the percentage of available haemoglobin saturated with oxygen (SaO_2), the fraction of inspired oxygen (FiO_2), the partial pressure of oxygen in arterial blood (PaO_2), PaO_2/FIO_2 ratio (an index to characterize the acute respiratory distress syndrome), severe hypoxaemia (insufficient oxygen content in blood), the biochemical parameters of blood (lactate, procalcitonin (PCT)), and concentrations of LPS and cytokines in blood. The requirement for vasopressors (Dopamine, Norepinephrine) was also evaluated.

Data shown in Table 2 and Figure 6 unambiguously demonstrated a pronounced tendency towards the oxygen saturation of haemoglobin (SaO_2) and normalization of the oxygen index (decreasing FiO2 on 22%). This was associated with a rise in MAP and a decrease in CVP. Normalization of cardio-vascular system function led to a reduction in the requirement for vasopressors.

Parameters	Before hemosorption	After hemosorption	p
CVP, mm Hg	16±5.0	12±4.1	>0.05
SaO_2 ,%	87±6.1	94±5.9	>0.05
FiO_2 ,%	77±32.3	55±15.4	<0.05*
PaO_2/FiO_2	160±70.9	200±54.1	<0.05*
PCT ng/ml	22±14.3	12±6.0	>0.05
Lactate, mmol/l	4.3±1.3	4.5±3.2	>0.05

* Significant difference

Table 2. Clinical parameters before/after haemosorption by Alteco.

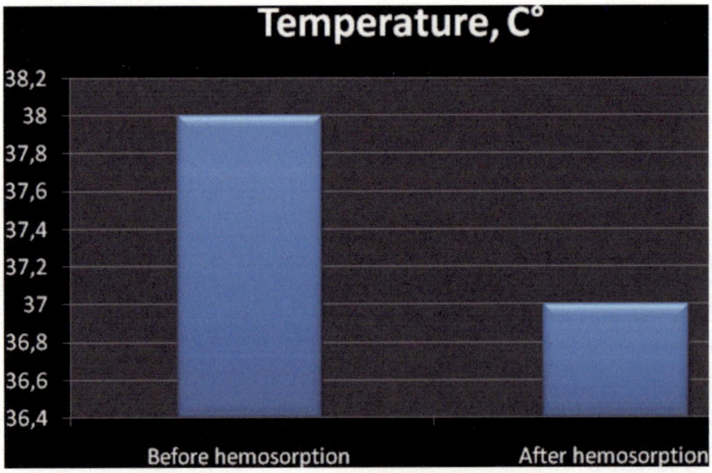

Fig. 7. The body temperature values for patients before and after haemosorption by Alteco.

The significant increase in the respiratory index (PaO2/FiO2) after haemosorption evidenced the improvement of oxygen diffusion through the alveoli-capillary membrane.

As a result, normalization of integral indices, such as body temperature and blood PCT level, was observed (Fig.7).

The level of LPS, the key trigger signal for system inflammatory reaction, decreased by a factor of 2 to 3 versus control after haemosorption (Fig.8).

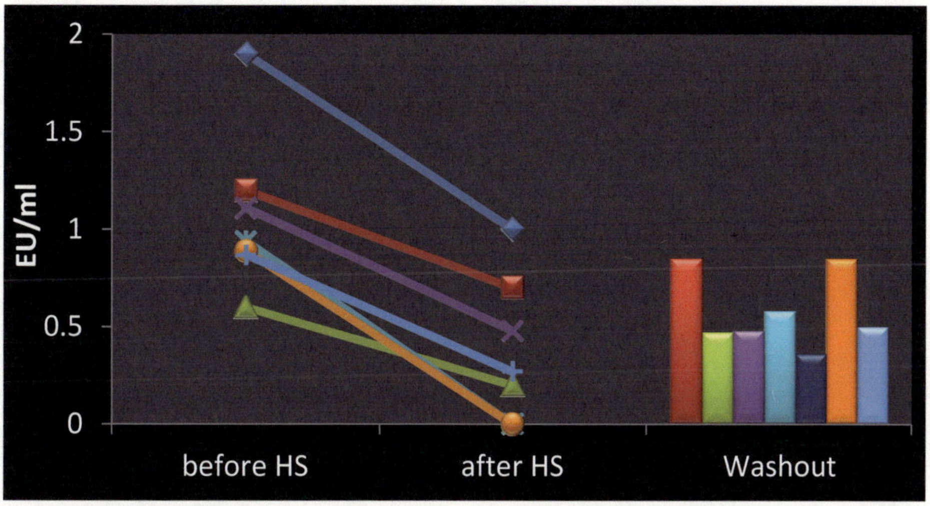

Fig. 8. LPS level in the blood of patients with sepsis before and after haemosorption by Alteco.

As hypercytokinaemia determines the development of SIRS, it seems to be possible that reducing cytokine levels (IL-8, IL-1β, IL-6, IL-10 etc) in blood may block the generalization of this pathological process or interrupt the cascade of cytokine storm. We studied the influence of haemosorption on the cytokine content in blood (Fig. 9).

Equal portions of sorbent were suspended in equal volumes of physiological solution (0.9% NaCl) and put onto the shaker during temperature control. High levels of some cytokines (IL-6, IL-8, IL-12, INFγ and TNF) were indicated in the supernatant (Fig.9).

We also investigated washouts from a sorbent after the termination of the haemosorption procedure. There were no well-developed specific conditions for the extraction and quantitative estimation of the characteristics of the sorbent.

This approach was especially informative in cases in which the level of analyte was higher in the blood after haemosorption than before the treatment (see examples in Fig. 9). Moreover, an increase in the concentration of some soluble cytokine receptors (sIL-1 II R, sIL-6 R) was observed in patient blood after haemosorption (Fig. 10).

We assumed that this phenomenon was determined by the release of cytokines from their complexes with receptors or proteins during the course of haemosorption.

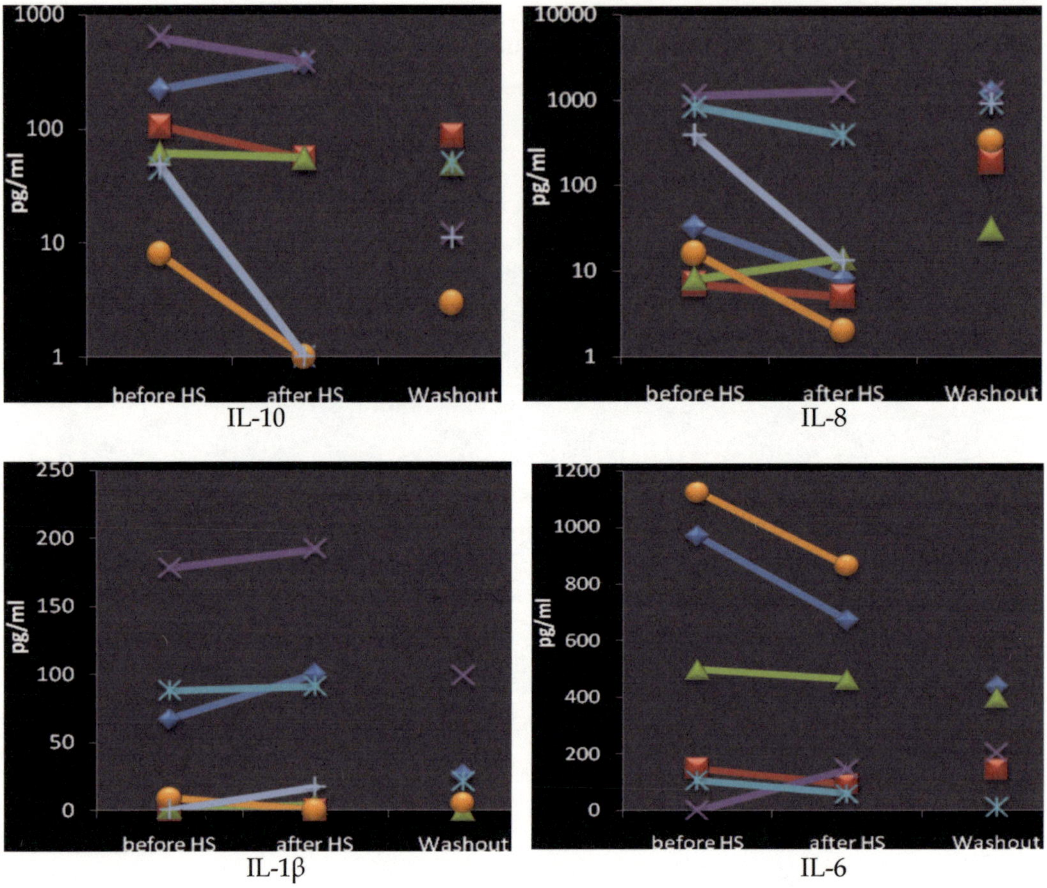

Fig. 9. The levels of cytokines in the blood of patients with sepsis before and after haemosorption by Alteco.

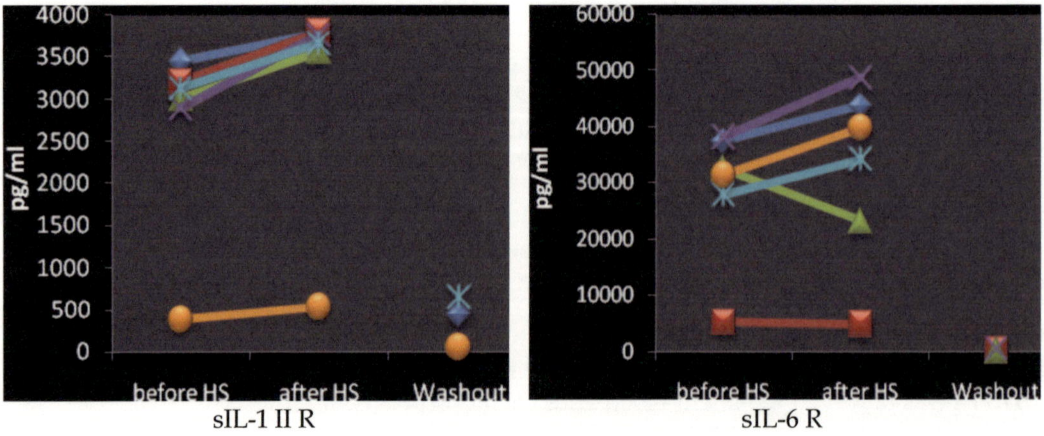

Fig. 10. Serum levels of soluble receptors in the blood of patients with sepsis before and after haemosorption by Alteco.

Our results indicated that low levels of serum cytokines revealed by ELISA did not reflect the real content of these mediators of inflammation in the blood of patients with septic complications. Perhaps a high secretion of cytokines was accompanied by an increase in the expression of congruent receptors, which bound a significant quantity of free cytokines in ligand-receptor complexes capable of dissociation. We showed that extracorporeal detoxification using the Alteco device allowed the elimination not only of free cytokines, but also the majority of bound endogenous bioregulators from cytokine/receptor complexes. Removal of the trigger factor (LPS) along with a wide range of pro- and anti-inflammatory cytokines, and possibly with other inflammation mediators (leukotrienes, thromboxanes, C-reactive protein) led to the interruption of the systemic inflammatory reaction, which was regarded as positive clinical effect of haemosorption for extracorporeal detoxification. Correlation analysis demonstrated a close connection between the concentrations in blood of LPS and TNFα ($p = 0.050$), LPS and IL-8 ($p = 0.050$). During the study, a 28-day survival of 9 critical patients was 96%, only 1 patient died after the procedure.

Taking into account a high correlation of normalized clinical parameters and the dynamics of LPS level and the serum profile of cytokines, the testing parameters (serum levels of IL-6,TNFα, IL-8) could be considered additional indicators of patient's status during the course of treatment, including methods of extracorporeal detoxification.

We assumed that changes in serum concentrations of cytokines after haemosorption might influence the functional activity of immune cells. Neutrophils and natural killers (NK) play a crucial role in pathogenesis of organ and multi-organ failures in case of sepsis. Our results demonstrated a pronounced tendency towards normalization of the functional activity of these innate immunity effectors after haemosorption by Alteco. Thus, phagocytic number (PN) and phagocytic index (PI) decreased after haemosorption in 1.3 – 2.1 times and 2.1 – 2.6 times, respectively. A reduction in spontaneous neutrophil activity was also observed. This parameter indicates the intensity of oxygen-dependent phagocytosis associated with the release of free radicals destroying the adjacent cells including endothelium. Moreover, the decrease was observed in the super-aggressive non-specific reaction of NK: index of cytotoxic activity (ICA) reduced after haemosorption from 75-90% to 54-58% (normal for healthy volunteers). This effect of normalizing functional activity of neutrophils and NK is likely connected with the elimination of LPS molecules and cytokines from peripheral blood.

Stimulation of immune cells for a long period could lead to exhaustion of their killing activity, resulting in the circulation of leukocytes that are unable to provide defence functions, such as termination of phagocytosis and killing transformed cells. These "ballast" cells do not express apoptosis receptor CD95 on their surface membrane, and consequently they cannot be eliminated from system circulation.

It was shown previously that prolongation of life of leukocytes could produce tissue and organ damage in case of SIRS and sepsis. A change in apoptosis regulation may influence pathogenesis of sepsis and multi-organ failure. We demonstrated the increase in CD45+CD95+ cell number (from 21-24% to 38-40%) after haemosorption. After the treatment, the number of CD45+CD66b+CD95+ neutrophils was higher by 32-42%, which correlated with an increase in the number of phagocytes able to terminate oxygen-dependent phagocytosis. Correlation analysis revealed a strong connection between these parameters ($p=0.0086$).

Therefore, reduction of the functional activity of leukocytes (PN, PI, ICA) to the level of that of healthy individuals and simultaneous increase in CD95+ leukocyte level could be considered a favourable prognostic factor.

The obtained results demonstrated that the LPS adsorber could effectively eliminate a wide range of the factors from peripheral blood (such as LPS, cytokines, etc.), which mediate all the stages of systemic inflammatory reaction in the body. Significant improvement of the performance status of patients with sepsis was observed after extracorporeal detoxification with LPS adsorber. This was the normalization of cardio-respiratory functions and reduction in hyperthermia and vasopressor requirement, normalization of MAP and concentration of gases in peripheral blood.

10. Conclusion

The discussed data and information show that cancer patients with sepsis have an enhanced serum level of LPS as compared to healthy volunteers. There is a close link between a decreased serum level of LPB along with the 10-fold reduction of LPB/LPS ratio and poor prognosis in cancer patients with sepsis. A characteristic cytokine profile of septic condition demonstrated that IL-6, IL-18 and soluble receptor sTNF RI concentrations significantly exceeded those of healthy volunteers and therefore high serum concentrations of IL-6, IL-8, IL-10, sTNF RI, sIL-1 RII, and sIL-6 R could be suggested as markers of sepsis for cancer patients.

In conclusion, triggers and mediators of inflammation secreted by immune cells play a crucial role in pathogenesis of SIRS and sepsis. Management of the inflammatory cascade should be considered an essential part of the complex approach to the treatment of systemic suppurative septic complications.

11. References

Alejandria M.M., Lansang M.A., Dans L.F., Mantaring J.B.V. Intravenous immunoglobulin for treating sepsis and septic shock. Cochrane Database Syst Rev. 2002;CD001090.

Alves-Filho J.C., Spiller F., Cunha F.Q. Neutrophil paralysis in sepsis. Shock. 2010;34 (Suppl 1):15-21.

Andersen T.H., Jensen T.H., Andersen L.W. Adjunctive therapy of severe sepsis and septic shock in adults Current Anaesthesia & Critical Care Volume 20, Issues 5-6, 2009, P. 254-258

Anderson R., Schmidt R. Clinical biomarkers in sepsis. Front Biosci (Elite Ed). 2010 1;2:504-520.

Anderson R., Schmidt R. Clinical biomarkers in sepsis. Front Biosci (Elite Ed). 2010 1;2:504-20.

Angus D.C., Linde-Zwirble W.T., Lidicker J., Clermont G., Carcillo J., Pinsky M.R. Epidemiology of severe sepsis in the United States: analysis of incidence, outcome, and associated costs of care. Crit Care Med. 2001; 29: 1303–1310.

Annane D, Bellissant E, Cavaillon J-M. Septic shock. Lancet. 2005; 365: 63-78.

Balzan S., Quadros C. D. A., Cleva R.D., Zilberstein B., Cecconello I. Bacterial translocation: Overview of mechanisms and clinical impact Issue J Gastroenterol Hepatol. 2007; 22(4): 464–471.

Barber M.D., Fearon K.C., Ross J.A. Relationship of serum levels of interleukin-6, soluble interleukin-6 receptor and tumour necrosis factor receptors to the acute-phase protein response in advanced pancreatic cancer. Clin Sci (Lond). 1999 ;96(1):83-87.

Barber M.D., Fearon K.C., Ross J.A. Relationship of serum levels of interleukin-6, soluble interleukin-6 receptor and tumour necrosis factor receptors to the acute-phase protein response in advanced pancreatic cancer. Clin Sci (Lond). 1999 ;96(1):83-87.

Berlot G., Bacer B., Piva M., Lucangelo U., Viviani M. Immunoglobulins in sepsis Adv In Sepsis. 2007; 6 (2): 41-46.

Calandra T., Baumgartner J.D., Grau G.E., Wu M.M., Lambert P.H., Schellekens J., Verhoef J., Glauser M.P. Prognostic values of tumor necrosis factor/cachectin, interleukin-1, interferon-alpha, and interferon-gamma in the serum of patients with septic shock. J Infect Dis. 1990;161(5):982-987.

Deitch EA, Bridges RM. Effect of stress and trauma on bacterial translocation from the gut. J Surg Res 1987; 42 (5): 536–42

Dietz S., Lautenschlaeger C., Mueller-Werdan U., Werdan K. Low levels of immunoglobulin G in patients with sepsis or septic shock: a signum mali ominis? Crit Care. 2010; 14(Suppl 1): P26.

Emoto M., Miyamoto M., Yoshizawa I., Emoto Y., Schaibe U.E., Kita E., Kaufmann S.H.E. Critical role of NK cells rather than $V\alpha14$+NKT cells in lipopolysaccharide-induces lethal shock in mice. J Immunol. 2002; 169:1426-1432.

Fialkow L., Filho L.F., Bozzetti M.C., Milani A.R., Filho E.M.R., Ladniuk R.M., Pierozan P., de Moura R.M.,Prolla J.C., Vachon E., Downey G.P. Neutrophil apoptosis: a marker of disease severity in sepsis and sepsis-induced acute respiratory distress syndrome Crit Care. 2006; 10(6): R155.

Frieling J.T.M., Van Deuren M., Wijdenes J. Circulating interleukin-6 receptor in patients with sepsis syndrome. J Infect Dis 1995; 171:469-472.

Frieling J.T.M., Van Deuren M., Wijdenes J. Circulating interleukin-6 receptor in patients with sepsis syndrome. J Infect Dis 1995; 171:469-472.

Gaïni S., Koldkjaer O.G., Pedersen C., Pedersen S.S. Procalcitonin, lipopolysaccharide-binding protein, interleukin-6 and C-reactive protein in community-acquired infections and sepsis: a prospective study. Crit Care. 2006;10(2):R53.

Giamarellos-Bourboulis E.J. What is the pathophysiology of the septic host upon admission? Int J Antimicrob. Agents. 2010;36 (2):S2-54.

Giamarellos-Bourboulis E.J., Tsaganos T., Spyridaki E., Mouktaroudi M., Plachouras D., Vaki I., Karagianni V., Antonopoulou A., Veloni V., Giamarellou H. Early changes of CD4-positive lymphocytes and NK cells in patients with severe Gram-negative sepsis. Crit Care. 2006; 10: R166.

Giamarellos-Bourboulis EJ What is the pathophysiology of the septic host upon admission? Int J Antimicrob Agents. 2010 Dec;36 Suppl 2:S2-54;

Goris J.A., te Boekhorst T.P.A., Nuytinck J.K.S. Multiple organ failure: generalized autodestructive inflammation? Arch. Surg. 1985; 120:1109-1115.

Hammond M.E., Lapointe G.R., Feucht P.H., Hilt S., Gallegos C.A., Gordon C.A., Giedlin M.A., Mullenbach G., Tekamp-Olson P. IL-8 induces neutrophil chemotaxis predominantly via type I IL-8 receptors. J Immunol. 1995;155(3):1428-1433.

Härter L., Mica L., Stocker R., Trentz O., Keel M. Mcl-1 correlates with reduced apoptosis in neutrophils from patients with sepsis. J Am Coll Surg. 2003;197:964–973.

Hildebrand F., Pape H.C., Krettek C. The importance of cytokines in the posttraumatic inflammatory reaction Unfallchirurg. 2005;108(10):793-794, 796-803.

Holub M., Kluèkova Z., Beneda B., Hobstová J., Hužička I., Pražák J., Lobovská A. Changes in lymphocyte subpopulations and CD3+/DR+ expression in sepsis. Clin Microbiol Infect. 2000; 6: 657-660.

Jenson H.B., Pollock B.H. The role of intravenous immunoglobulin for the prevention and treatment of neonatal sepsis. Semin Perinatol. 1998;22:50-63.

Jimenez M.F., Watson W.G., Parodo J., Evans D., Foster D., Steinberg M., Rotstein O.D., Marshall J.C. Dysregulated expression of neutrophil apoptosis in the systemic inflammatory response syndrome. Arch Surg. 1997;132:1263–1270.

Keel M., Trentz O. Pathophysiology of polytrauma, Injury. 2005;36: 691–709.

Kerr A.R., Kirkham L.A.S., Kadioglu A., Andrew P.W., Garside P., Thompson H., Mitchell T.J. Identification of a detrimental role for NK cells in pneumococcal pneumonia and sepsis in immunocompromised hosts. Microbes Infect. 2005; 7:845-852.

Kulabukhov VV. Use of an endotoxin adsorber in the treatment of severe abdominal sepsis. Acta Anaesthesiol Scand. 2008 Aug;52(7):1024-5.

Kumar A.T., Sudhir U., Punith K., Kumar R., Ravi Kumar V.N., Rao M.Y. Cytokine profile in elderly patients with sepsis. Indian J Crit Care Med 2009;13:74-78.

Kumar V., Sharma A. Neutrophils: Cinderella of innate immune system. Int Immunopharmacol. 2010; 10: 1325-1334.

Kyles B.D.M., Baltimore J. Adjunctive use of plasmapheresis and intravenous immunoglobulin therapy in sepsis: a case report american journal of critical care. 2005; 14 (2): 109-112.

Laurenzi L., Natoli S., Di Filippo F., Calamaro A. Systemic and haemodynamic toxicity after isolated limb perfusion (ILP) with TNF-alpha. J Exp Clin Cancer Res. 2004;23(2): 225-231.

Lee WL, Downey GP. Neutrophil activation and acute lung injury. Curr Opin Crit Care. 2001;7:1–7

Lenz A., Franklin G.A., Cheadle W.G. Systemic inflammation after trauma Injury. 2007 Dec;38(12): 1336-1345.

Mahidhara R., Billiar T.R. Apoptosis in sepsis. Crit Care Med. 2000;28:N105–N113.

Martin C., Saux P., Mege J.L., Perrin G., Papazian L., Gouin F. Prognostic values of serum cytokines in septic shock. Intensive Care Med. 1994;20(4):272-977.

Martin C., Saux P., Mege J.L., Perrin G., Papazian L., Gouin F. Prognostic values of serum cytokines in septic shock. Intensive Care Med. 1994;20(4):272-977.

Moore F.A. The role of the gastrointestinal tract in postinjury multiple organ failure// Am. J. Surg. 1999; 178: 449–453.

Müller B., Peri G., Doni A., Perruchoud A.P., Landmann R., Pasqualini F., Mantovan A. High circulating levels of the IL-1 type II decoy receptor in critically ill patients with sepsis: association of high decoy receptor levels with glucocorticoid administration. J Leukocyte Biol. 2002;72:643-649

Murphy R., DeCoursey T. E. Charge compensation during the phagocyte respiratory burst. Bioenergetics. 2006; 1757(8): 996-1011.

Myc A., Buck J., Gonin J., Reynolds B., Hammerling U., Emanuel. The level of lipopolysaccharide-binding protein is significantly increased in plasma in patients with the systemic inflammatory response syndrome. Clin Diagn Lab Immunol. 1997; 4:113–116.

Nijhuis C. S., Vellenga E., Daenen S.J., Graaf W.T., Gietema J.A., Groen H. J., Kamps W.A., Bont E. Lipopolysaccharide-binding protein: a possible diagnostic marker for Gram-negative bacteremia in neutropenic cancer patients Intensive Care Medicine 2003; 29, 12: 2157-2161.

Oppenheim J.J., Yang D. Alarmins: chemotactic activators of immune responses. Curr Opin Immunol. 2005; 17: 359-365.

Papathanassoglou E.D.E., Moynihan J.A., McDermott M.P., Ackerman M.H. Expression of Fas (CD95) and Fas ligand on peripheral blood mononuclear cells in critical illness and association with multiorgan dysfunction severity and survival. Crit Care Med. 2001;29:709–718.

Pildal J., Gotzsche P.C. Polyclonal immunoglobulin for treatment of bacterial sepsis: a systematic review. Clin Infect Dis. 2004;39:38-46.

Pinsky M.R. Pathophysiology of sepsis and multiple organ failure:pro- versus anti-inflammatory aspects. Contrib. Nephrol. 2004; 144: 31-43.

Quinn J.V., Slotman G.J. Platelet-activating factor and arachidonic acid metabolites mediate tumor necrosis factor and eicosanoid kinetics and cardiopulmonary dysfunction during bacteremic shock. Crit Care Med. 1999;27(11):2485-2494.

Rigato O., Ujvari S., Castelo A., Salomão R. Tumor necrosis factor alpha (TNF-α) and sepsis: Evidence for a role in host defense. Infection. 1996; 24: 314–318.

Rigato O., Ujvari S., Castelo A., Salomão R. Tumor necrosis factor alpha (TNF-α) and sepsis: Evidence for a role in host defense. Infection. 1996; 24: 314–318.

Sawyer DB, Loscalzo J. Myocardial hibernation: restorative or preterminal sleep? Circulation. 2002; 105(13): 1517-1519.

Sayeed M.M. Delay of neutrophil apoptosis can exacerbate inflammation in sepsis patients: cellular mechanisms. Crit Care Med. 2004;32:1604–1606.

Segal A.W. How neutrophils kill microbe. Ann Rev Immunol 2005;23:197–223.

Segal A.W. How neutrophils kill microbe. Ann Rev Immunol 2005;23:197–223.

T. Ala-Kokko, J. Koskenkari and J. Laurila, Lipopolysaccharide adsorber in abdominal septic shock, Crit Care 13 (Suppl. 1) (2009), p. 280.

Tabata N., Azuma E., Masuda S.-I., Ido M., Sakurai M. Transient low level of IgG3 induced by sepsis Pediatrics International. 1995; 37(2): 201–202.

Takeshita S., Tsujimoto H., Kawase H., Kawamura Y., Sekine I. Increased Levels of lipopolysaccharide binding protein in plasma in children with kawasaki disease Clin Diagn Lab Immunol. 2002; 9(1): 205–206.

Thomas S., Balasubramanian K. A. Role of intestine in postsurgical complications: involvement of free radicals. Free Rad Biol Med. 2004; 36 (6): 745-756.

Vincent J.-L., Abraham E. The last 100 years of sepsis Am J Resp Crit Care Med. 2006; 173: 256-263.

Volk H.D., Reinke P., Döcke W.D. Immunological monitoring of the inflammatory process: Which variables? When to assess. Eur J Surg Suppl. 1999; 584:70-72.

Werdan K. Immunoglobulins in Sepsis: Therapeutic Use of Immunoglobulins. Sepsis. 1999; 3, 3:239-245.

Yaroustovsky M, Abramyan M, Popok Z, Nazarova E, Stupchenko O, Popov D, Plushch M, Samsonova N. Preliminary report regarding the use of selective in complex cardiac surgery patients with extensive sepsis and prolonged intensive care stay. Blood Purif. 2009;28(3):227-33.

Yegenaga I., Hoste E., Van Biesen W., Vanholder R., Benoit D., Kantarci G., Dhondt A., Colardyn F., Lameire N.: Clinical characteristics of patients developing ARF due to sepsis/systemic inflammatory response syndrome: Results of a prospective study. Am J Kidney Dis. 2004; 43 :817 –824.

Yoneda O., Imai T., Goda S., Inoue H., Yamauchi A., Okazaki T., Imai H., Yoshie O., Bloom E.T., Domae N., Umehara H. Fractalkine-mediated endothelial cell injury by NK Cells. J Immunol. 2000; 164: 4055-4062.

Zeerleder S., Hack C.E., Caliezi C., van Mierlo G., Eerenberg-Belmer A., Wolbink A., Wuillenmin W.A. Activated cytotoxic T cells and NK cells in severe sepsis and septic shock and their role in multiple organ dysfunctio. Clin Immunol. 2005;116(2): 158-165.

Zeni F., Tardy B., Vindimian M., Pain P., Gery P., Bertrand J.C. Soluble interleukin-6 receptor in patients with severe sepsis. J Infect Dis. 1995;172(2):607–608.

Zhang B., Huang Y.H., Chen Y., Yang Y., Hao Z.L., Xie S.L. Plasma tumor necrosis factor-α, its soluble receptors and interleukin-1β levels in critically burned patients. Burns. 1998;24(7):599-603.

Zhang B., Huang Y.H., Chen Y., Yang Y., Hao Z.L., Xie S.L. Plasma tumor necrosis factor-α, its soluble receptors and interleukin-1β levels in critically burned patients. Burns. 1998;24(7):599-603.

Zucker T., Kriger G. Sepsis-like syndrome caused by the Russian medication pyrogenal (Salmonella typhi endotoxin). J Exp Clin Cancer Res. 2004; Isr Med Assoc J. 2003; 5(10):750-751.

Zychlinsky A., Weinrauch Y., Weiss J. Introduction: Forum in immunology on neutrophils. Microbes and Infection. 2003; 5(14): 1289-1291.

10

Studies on the Association of Meningitis and Mumps Virus Vaccination

Alejandra Lara-Sampablo[1,2], Nora Rosas-Murrieta[2], Irma Herrera-Camacho[2], Verónica Vallejo-Ruiz[1], Gerardo Santos-López[1] and Julio Reyes-Leyva[1]*

[1]*Laboratorio de Biología Molecular y Virología, Centro de Investigación Biomédica de Oriente, Instituto Mexicano del Seguro Social, Metepec, Puebla;*

[2]*Centro de Química, Instituto de Ciencias, Benemérita Universidad Autónoma de Puebla, Puebla, México*

1. Introduction

Mumps is an acute viral infection caused by a member of the *Rubulavirus* genus in the *Paramyxoviridae* family. Although it is mostly a childhood disease, with peak incidence occurring among those aged 5–9 years, mumps virus (MuV) may also affect teenagers. MuV is known to affect the salivary glands causing parotid swelling; however, it can also produce an acute systemic infection involving glandular, lymphoid and nervous tissues, leading to some important complications such as pancreatitis, oophoritis orchitis, mastitis, nephritis and thyroiditis. The main central nervous system (CNS) complication of mumps virus infection is aseptic meningitis (in up to 15% of cases); it is also associated rarely with encephalitis, hydrocephalus and sensorineural deafness (affecting approximately 5/100 000 mumps patients) (Carbone & Rubin, 2007; Hviid et al., 2008; Plotkin & Rubin, 2007; World Health Organization [WHO], 2007).

Massive vaccination programs have decreased the incidence of MuV infection worldwide, before the introduction of live attenuated mumps virus vaccines, mumps was the main cause of virus-induced disease in the CNS of children; indeed, the annual incidence of mumps in the absence of immunization was in the range of 100–1000 cases/100 000 people. Although vaccination programs have decreased the incidence of mumps virus infection, outbreaks have not been completely eliminated (WHO, 2007). The main problems associated with MuV vaccination are lack of protection due to vaccine failure and presentation of secondary adverse complications due to the use of relatively virulent vaccine strains; indeed, L-Zagreb, Leningrad-3 and Urabe AM9 strains have been associated with post-vaccinal aseptic meningitis (Brown et al., 1991; Dourado et al., 2000; Galazka et al., 1999; Goh, 1999). The unacceptably high rate of vaccine associated meningitis and parotitis cases has resulted in vaccine withdrawal and public resistance to mumps vaccination (Schmitt et al., 1993). In consequence, mumps epidemics have re-emerged, and the incidence is rising in several countries (Choi, 2010; Dayan et al., 2008).

2. Wild-type mumps virus natural infection and CNS involvement

2.1 Mumps virus

Mumps virus (MuV) is a member of the *Rubulavirus* genus of the *Paramyxoviridae* family. Mumps virions are pleomorphic particles ranging from 100 to 600 nm in size, consisting of a helical ribonucleocapsid surrounded by a host cell-derived lipid envelope. Full-length genome is a non-segmented, single-stranded RNA of negative polarity that consists of 15,384 nucleotides containing 7 genes that code for the nucleoprotein (NP), phosphoprotein (P), matrix (M), fusion (F), small hydrophobic (SH), hemagglutinin-neuraminidase (HN), and large (L) proteins. The genomic organization of the virus from 3′ to 5′ ends is NP-P-M-F-SH-HN-L (Lamb & Parks, 2007; Pringle, 1997).

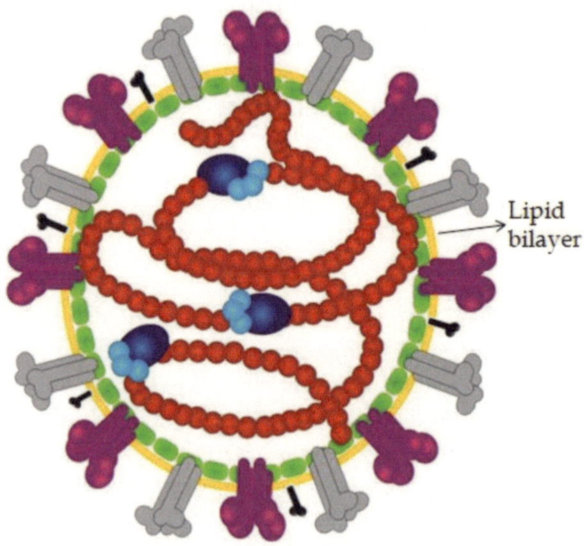

Viral protein	Biological activity	Viral protein	Biological activity
Nucleoprotein (NP)	Protects genomic RNA from cellular proteases; determines helical structure of capsid	Small hydrophobic (SH)	Unknown function. This protein has been involved in evasion of the host anti-viral response
Phosphoprotein (P)	Forms part of the transcriptase complex.	Fusion (F)	Virus-to-cell and cell-to-cell fusion
Large (L)	Forms part of the transcriptase complex	Hemagglutinin-Neuraminidase (HN)	Viral attachment and entry. Prevention of self-agglutination
Matrix (M)	Virion assembly		

Fig. 1. Schematic diagram of mumps virus (not drawn to scale). On the surface of the viral membrane 3 glycoproteins are anchored: HN, F and SH. The M protein is located inside of the viral envelope. In the center of the virion is the ribonucleoprotein complex formed by the nucleocapside (NP:RNA) and viral RNA polymerase (P:L). Information based on the references: Carbone & Rubin, 2007; Santos-López et al., 2004.

A schematic diagram of the virion and functions of viral proteins are shown in figure 1. On the surface of viral particles and infected cells are projected two glycoproteins, F and HN, which are transmembrane glycoproteins of types I and II, respectively. HN glycoprotein is responsible for mumps virus attachment; it binds to sialic acid-containing cell receptors. Its neuraminidase (sialidase) activity releases the sialic acid residues from viral progeny to prevent self-aggregation during budding; HN glycoprotein also activates the F glycoprotein, which promotes the fusion between viral and cell membranes (Carbone & Rubin, 2007; Lamb & Parks, 2007).

SH is an integral membrane protein without well-known properties; despite this, SH protein has been reported to block the TNFα mediated apoptotic signaling pathway; therefore it has been involved in evasion of the host anti-viral response (Wilson et al., 2006), so it has been proposed as a virulence factor, however, this issue is still controversial (T. Malik et al., 2011; Woznik et al., 2010). Likewise, the sequence of the mumps virus SH gene varies greatly from strain to strain and has therefore been used in molecular epidemiological studies to group mumps virus strains (Orvell et al., 1997).

Inside the envelope lies a helical nucleocapsid core containing the RNA genome and the NP, P, and L proteins, which are involved in virus replication. NP protein is an RNA-binding protein that coats and protects full-length viral (-) sense genomic and (+) sense antigenomic RNAs to form the helical nucleocapsid template (Carbone & Rubin, 2007; Lamb & Parks, 2007). Each NP protein interact with 6 nucleotides of the viral genome, therefore a full-length genome polyhexameric may be required for efficient viral replication (process known as, Rule of Six) (Kolakofsky et al., 1998, 2005; Vulliemoz & Roux, 2001). P and L proteins form an enzymatic complex with RNA-dependent RNA polymerase activity; where L protein has the catalytic domain for RNA polymerization, whereas P protein functions as a cofactor for L protein and is able to bind the ribonucleoprotein complex (RNA-NP) (Kingston et al., 2004; Lamb & Parks, 2007).

M protein resides between the envelope and the nucleocapside core; this is the most abundant protein in the virion, and it serves to physically link the ribonucleocapsid with the host cell membrane to promote the viral assembly process (Carbone & Rubin, 2007; Lamb & Parks, 2007).

Two nonstructural proteins, V and I, are encoded by the P gene and are synthesized as a result of co-transcriptional editing of messenger RNA (mRNA) (Carbone & Rubin, 2007; Paterson & Lamb, 1990). In this process the viral polymerase moves repeatedly (process known as, stuttering) in a region known as "editing site" of the P gene, which is rich in citidine nucleotides (3'CCCCCC 5') inserting some non-template guanidine (G) nucleotides in the nascent transcript (Hausmann et al., 1999; Paterson & Lamb, 1990; Vidal et al., 1990). This editing mechanism involves the production of mRNAs whose ORFs are altered by insertion of G residues (Figure 2); so, the translation of full-transcript (unedited) encodes a V protein, which plays a role in circumventing the interferon (IFN) mediated antiviral responses by blocking IFN signaling and limiting IFN production (Didcock et al., 1999a, 1999b; Fujii et al., 1999; Rodriguez et al., 2003; N. H. Rosas-Murrieta et al., 2010); while, mRNAs generated by inserting 2 and 4 G residues encode a P and I proteins respectively. The generated proteins have the same N-terminus, but differ in their C-terminus (Lamb & Parks, 2007).

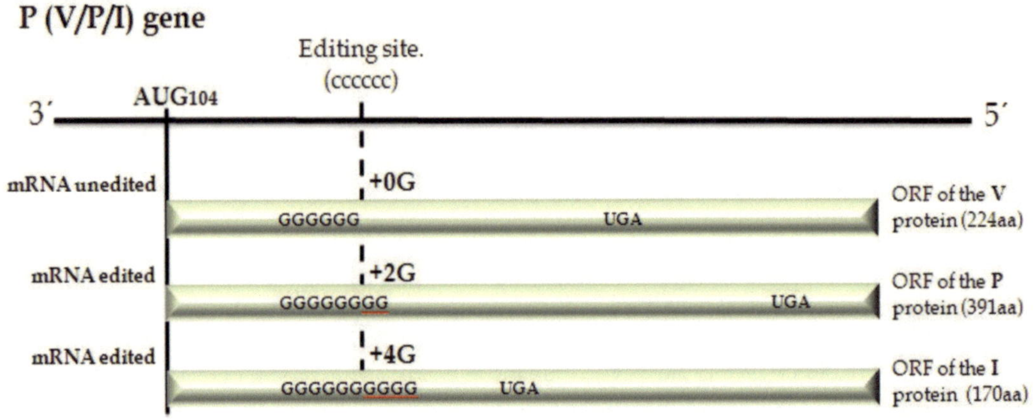

Fig. 2. Schematic representation of mumps virus P gene and mRNA editing mechanism (not drawn to scale). By a stuttering mechanism in the editing site of P gene, the viral polymerase introduces non-template G residues in the nascent transcript, which generates mRNAs with different ORFs, so, the translation of full-transcript (unedited) encodes a V protein, while mRNAs generated by inserting 2 and 4 G residues encode P and I proteins respectively. AUG and UGA sequence indicate the start and stop codons, respectively. Information based on the references: Hausmann et al., 1999; Lamb & Parks, 2007; Paterson & Lamb, 1990; Vidal et al., 1990.

2.2 Viral pathogenesis and invasion central nervous system

Natural infection with mumps virus is restricted to humans and is transmitted via the respiratory mucosa by direct contact, droplet spread or contaminated fomites. The incubation period is about 15 to 24 days (average 19 days). Infected patients become most contagious 1 to 2 days before onset of clinical symptoms and continue for several days afterwards (Hviid et al., 2008). Mumps virus initially infects the upper-respiratory-tract mucosa where it undergo a first replication cycle and then the progeny viruses spread to local lymph nodes where they undergo a second replication followed by a systemic spread with involvement of glandular, nervous and other target organs (figure 3) (Carbone & Rubin, 2007; Enders, 1996; Plotkin & Rubin, 2007).

The main clinical manifestation of mumps is parotid swelling. However, parotitis is not a primary or necessary step of mumps virus infection. Mumps virus can also infect urinary tract, genital organs, pancreas, kidney and central nervous system (CNS). It is not yet well-known how mumps virus spreads to the CNS, however, studies in newborn hamster model suggest that virus spreads by passage of infected mononuclear cells across the epithelium to epithelial cells of the choroid plexus (Fleischer & Kreth, 1982; Wolinsky et al., 1976). Alternatively, direct spread of virus is possible. At this site virus is replicated and released persistently from ependymal and choroidal cells, followed by deeper spread into the brain parenchyma causing encephalitis and several neurological complications. There are few data on the histopathology of the brain in mumps encephalitis (since death is rare). The data show the characteristic picture of a parainfectious process, characterized by perivenous demyelinisation and perivascular infiltration with mononuclear cells (Hviid et al., 2008).

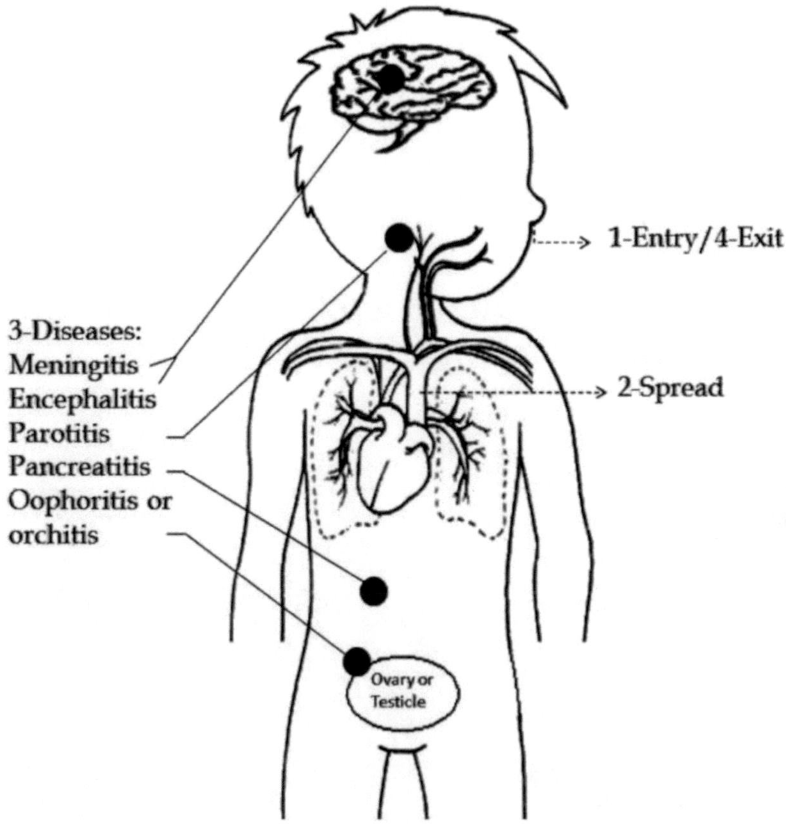

Fig. 3. Pathogenesis of mumps virus infection. Mumps virus is acquired trough the upper-respiratory-tract mucosa (1); where it undergo a first replication, after that new viruses spread (2) to local lymph nodes followed by a systemic spread with involvement of glandular and nervous tissues causing various diseases (3); finally virus is transmitted to another person through droplets or fomites (4). Based on the reference, Enders, 1996.

2.3 Aseptic meningitis and other neurological complications of mumps

Infection of the CNS is the most common extra-salivary gland manifestation of mumps virus infection, being aseptic meningitis the most frequent complication. Although the disease is usually mild should not be underestimated, mumps meningitis affects to 10%-15% of individuals infected by MuV, which is characterized by the sudden onset of fever with signs and symptoms of meningeal involvement as evidenced by changes in cerebrospinal fluid properties, including pleocytosis in absence of bacteria (Bonnet et al., 2006; Plotkin & Rubin, 2007).

Another less frequent but more serious complication of mumps virus infection is encephalitis (0.02-0.3% cases), which can lead to permanent neurologic damage including paralysis, seizures, hydrocephalus and even cause death. Likewise mumps virus infection is a major cause of sensorineural deafness in childhood and affects five per 100,000 patients (Bonnet et al., 2006; Hviid et al., 2008; Plotkin & Rubin, 2007; WHO, 2007).

3. Mumps vaccination

Safe and efficacious vaccines against mumps - based on live, attenuated viral strains - have been available since the 1960s. In most regions of the world the annual incidence of mumps in absence of vaccination ranges from 100 to 1000 per 100 000 of the general population (WHO, 2007). In 2010, the World Health Organization indicated that 61% of countries (figure 4) have incorporated mumps vaccination into their national immunization programs, in most cases using combined measles–mumps–rubella (MMR) vaccine (WHO, 2010).

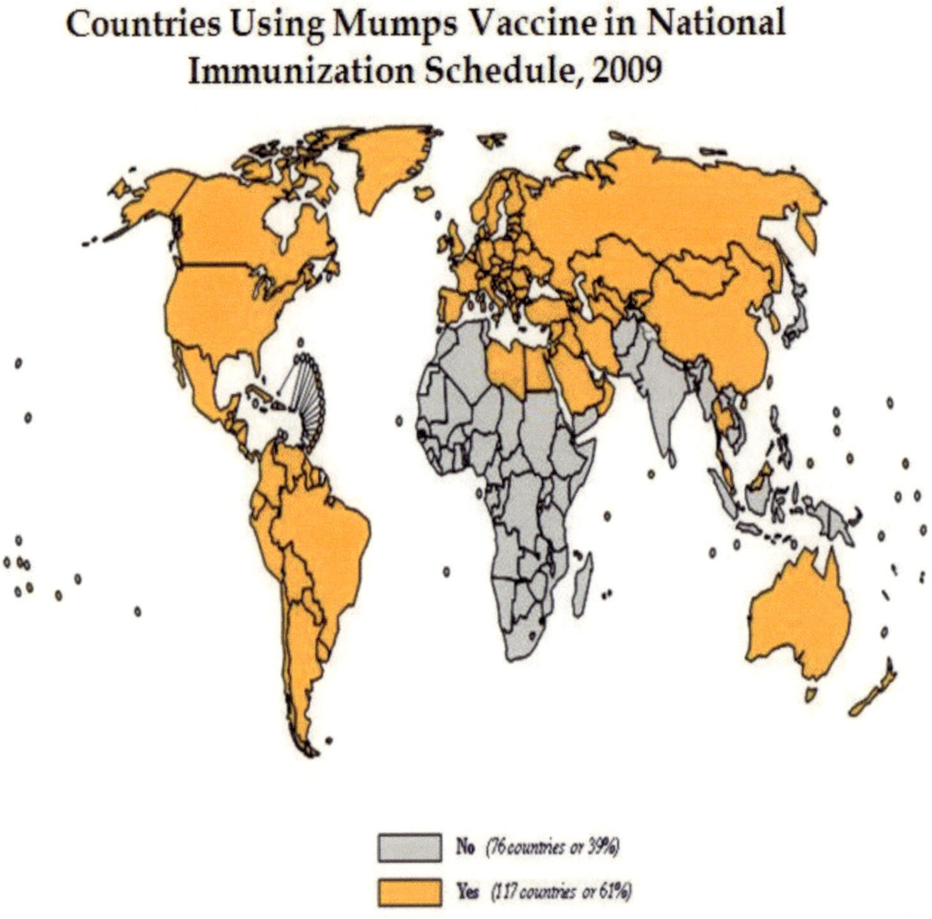

Fig. 4. Countries that have incorporated mumps vaccination in their national immunization programs. Yellow and gray indicate the countries immunized (61%) and unimmunized (39%) respectively. Source: WHO/IVB database, 193 WHO Member States, Data as of July 2010. Date of slide: 19 August 2010.

3.1 Effects of vaccination on epidemic mumps

Use of mumps vaccine (usually administered in measles-mumps-rubella or measles-mumps-rubella-varicella vaccines) is the best way to prevent mumps. Mumps immunization has been effective at controlling epidemic mumps infection and complications associated with it has been drastically reduced,. This is the reason why the WHO defined viral mumps as a disease preventable by vaccination (vaccine-preventable) (WHO, 2007). In countries where there is no vaccination against mumps, its incidence remains high, with epidemic peaks every 2–5 years and those aged 5–9 years consistently being the most affected. In the pre-vaccine era, mumps was a common infectious disease with a high annual incidence, usually >100 per 100 000 population (Dayan et al., 2008; Galazka et al., 1999). It was a very common disease in U.S. children, with as many as 300,000 cases reported every year. After the introduction of mumps virus vaccine in United States in 1967, cases dropped by 98%, from 152,209 cases in 1968 to 2982 cases in 1985. Since 1989, the incidence of mumps has declined, with 266 reported cases in 2001. This decrease is probably due to the fact that children have received a second dose of mumps vaccine (part of the two-dose schedule for measles, mumps, rubella or MMR). Studies have shown that the effectiveness of mumps vaccine ranges from 73% to 91% after 1 dose vaccines and from 79% to 95% after 2 doses. However, we can not let our guard down against viral mumps (Centers for Disease Control and Prevention [CDC], 2010a).

Despite mumps epidemics have decreased from the incorporation of mumps vaccine, in the late 1980s, mumps outbreaks have occurred in both unvaccinated and vaccinated adolescents and young adults. From October 1988 to April 1989 a mumps epidemic was reported in Douglas County, Kansas; of the 269 cases, 208 (77.3%) occurred among primary and secondary school students, of whom 203 (97.6%) had documentation of mumps vaccination. These data suggested that both mumps vaccine failure and the lack of vaccination have contributed to the relative resurgence of mumps. Therefore a change in immunization policy was recommended to two-dose schedule of measles-mumps-rubella vaccine, which should help reduce the occurrence of mumps outbreaks in highly vaccinated populations (Hersh et al., 1991). The widespread use of a second dose of mumps vaccine among U.S. schoolchildren beginning in 1990 was followed by low reports of mumps cases; which was established at 2010 elimination goal, however, various mumps outbreaks have been reported in several countries at different years (Brockhoff et al., 2010; CDC, 2010b; Cheek et al., 1995; Dayan et al., 2008; Dayan & Rubin, 2008; Park et al., 2007; Vandermeulen et al., 2009; Vandermeulen et al., 2004). These reports have suggested that secondary vaccine failure played an important role in mumps outbreaks, thus a more effective mumps vaccine or changes in vaccine policies may be considered to prevent future outbreaks.

3.2 Vaccine strains: preparation, attenuation, induced immune

Mumps vaccines are available in the form of live attenuated virus and may be given alone or in combination with measles and rubella vaccines, according to recommendations from the World Health Organization (WHO, 2007). Mumps viruses are attenuated by adaption in embryonated chicken eggs, chicken or quail embryo fibroblasts or human diploid cells. Through these processes virus mutants are selected because of their increased ability to replicate under new culture conditions but with a reduced capacity to produce disease but stimulating immunity in the natural host (Brown & Wright, 1998; Plotkin & Rubin, 2007).

There are more than 10 strains of mumps virus used as vaccines (Table 1), which induce different levels of seroconversion (80-99%) and protective efficacy (70-95%). Nowadays, the most often used vaccine strains are Jeryl Lynn, RIT 4385, Urabe-AM9, L-Zagreb and Leningrad-3 (Bonnet et al., 2006). The first live attenuated mumps virus vaccine, Jeryl Lynn

B (introduced in the U.S.A in 1967), represents an ideal vaccine because it induces neutralizing antibodies in 95%-98% of vaccinees and few side effects have been associated with its application (Carbone & Rubin, 2007). The Jeryl Lynn strain was attenuated by passage in embryonated hen's eggs and chicken embryo cell culture (Plotkin & Rubin, 2007). The RIT 4385 mumps vaccine was derived from a Jeryl Lynn clone (JL-1) by passage through chicken embryo fibroblast cultures. Comparative studies of the RIT 4385 and Jeryl–Lynn vaccines showed similar seroconversion rates (96-98% for RIT 4385 and 97% for Jeryl Lynn) although the geometric mean titre was significantly higher among recipients of the Jeryl–Lynn vaccine (Crovari et al., 2000; Kanra et al., 2000; Lim et al., 2007). The Urabe Am9 strain was developed by the Biken Institute in Japan from an isolate obtained from the saliva of a mumps patient. Urabe Am9 strain preparations are produced either in the amnion of embryonated hen's eggs or in chicken embryo cell cultures. Seroconversion rates in children aged 12–20 months range from 92–100%. The Rubini mumps vaccine virus was derived from a mumps isolate obtained from the urine of a child in Switzerland in 1974. Comparative efficacy of Rubini, Jeryl-Lynn and Urabe strain mumps vaccine were 80.7, 54.4 and -55.3%, respectively. Thus, Rubini vaccine was discontinued due to poor efficacy (Goh, 1999; Ong et al., 2005). The Leningrad-3 strain was developed in the 1950s in guinea pig kidney cell cultures, with further passages in Japanese quail embryo cultures. The Leningrad-3 vaccine strain has achieved seroconversion rates of 89–98% in children aged 1–7 years and protective efficacy ranged from 92% to 99%. The Leningrad-3 mumps virus was further attenuated in Croatia by adaptation and passages on chicken embryo fibroblast cell cultures. The new mumps strain, designated L-Zagreb, is used in Croatia and India (Bonnet et al., 2006; Plotkin & Rubin, 2007; WHO, 2007).

Vaccine strain	Cell substrate	Sero-conversión	Protective efficacy	Manufacturer	Main area of distribution
Jeryl-Lynn	CWE	80-100%	72.8- 91%	Merck	Worldwide
RIT 4385	CWE	96-98.1%		GlaxoSmithKline	Worldwide
Leningrad- 3	QEF	89-90%	92-99%	Bacterial Medicine Institute, Moscow	Russia
Leningrad-Zagreb	CEF	89-98%	92-99%	Institute of Immunology of Zagreb	Yugoslavia
Urabe AM9	EHE CEF	92-100%	54.4%- 93%	Sanofi Pasteur Biken	Worldwide Japan
Rubini	HDCS	N I	0-33%	Swiss Serum Institute	Discontinued
Hoshino	CEF	N I	N I	Kitasato Institute	Japan
Torii	CEF	N I	N I	Takeda Chemicals	Japan
Miyahara	CEF	N I	N I	Chem-Sero Therapeutic Research Institute	Japan
NL M-46	CEF	N I	N I	Chiba	Japan
S-12	HDCS	N I	N I	Razi State Serum and Vaccine Institute	Iran

NI, No Information; CEF, chicken embryo fibroblasts; HEF, human embryo fibroblasts; QEF, quail embryo fibroblasts; EHE, embryonated hen's eggs; HDCS, human diploid cells.
Information based on the following references: Bonnet et al., 2006; Dayan & Rubin, 2008; Dourado et al., 2000; Galazka et al., 1999; Lim et al., 2007; Peltola et al., 2007; Plotkin & Rubin, 2007; WHO, 2007.

Table 1. Live attenuated mumps vaccine stains.

4. Adverse reactions

In general, adverse reactions to mumps vaccination are rare and mild. Apart from slight soreness and swelling at the injection site, local reactions, low-grade fewer, parotitis, and rashes are the most common adverse events. Occasionally, orchitis and sensorineural deafness have been observed after mumps virus vaccination (WHO, 2007).

In a comparative study of the Jeryl Lynn, Urabe, and Leningrad-Zagreb strains in MMR combination vaccines, the frequency of parotitis in vaccinated children was 0-5%, 1-3%, and 3-1%, respectively, compared with 0-2% in unvaccinated controls (Hviid et al., 2008).

A recent study reported adverse reactions following immunization with MMR vaccine that contain the live attenuated mumps virus Hoshino strain; Parotitis was the most frequent event occurring in 1.8% of recipients, followed by fever and convulsions (0.03%), convulsions (0,16%), encephalopathy (0,004%), and anaphylactic reactions (0,004%) in children vaccinated at 12 months and at 4 to 6 years of age (Esteghamati et al., 2011).

4.1 Post vaccine meningitis

One of the most frequent side effects associated with mumps virus vaccine is aseptic meningitis which is also the most frequent complication of naturally acquired mumps infection (Table 2). In November 2006, the Global Advisory Committee on Vaccine Safety (GACVS) reviewed adverse events following mumps vaccination with special reference to the risk of vaccine associated aseptic meningitis (WHO, 2007). Cases of aseptic meningitis and estimates of incidence rates have been reported following the use of the Urabe Am9, Leningrad–Zagreb, Hoshino, Torii and Miyahara strains from various surveillance systems and epidemiological studies. The reported rate of aseptic meningitis that occurs after vaccination ranges widely, from approximately 1 in 1.8 million doses for the Jeryl Lynn strain to as high as 1 in 1000 for the Leningrad-3 strain (Bonnet et al., 2006). However, due to the variability of the methods used in the different studies, no clear conclusion can be drawn on the differences in risk for this complication among these strains.

Urabe AM9 strain was introduced in Canada and UK in 1986 as part of the MMR vaccine. In September 1992, the Urabe AM9-strain was withdrawn from the market worldwide following data indicating a higher rate of vaccination-related cases of meningitis (Schmitt et al., 1993). Despite this, Urabe AM9 strain continued in use several years later in some developing countries including but not limited to Mexico and Brasil (Dourado et al., 2000; Santos-López et al., 2006).

The first reports suggesting a relationship between MMR vaccine (which contained mumps virus strain Urabe AM9, measles virus strain Schwarz and rubella virus strain RA 27/3) and aseptic meningitis showed an estimated incidence of 1/62,000 administered doses (Furesz & Contreras, 1990). Reports of meningitis in patients immunized with Urabe AM9 strain range from 1/233,000 to 16.6/10,000 administered doses (Kimura et al., 1996; Schmitt et al., 1993). An outbreak of aseptic meningitis following the mass immunization campaign with an Urabe-containing vaccine was reported, with an estimated risk of aseptic meningitis 1 per 14,000 doses. This study confirms a link between measles-mumps-rubella vaccination and aseptic meningitis (Dourado et al., 2000). Likewise, no serious adverse effects have been

Vaccine strain	Genetic heterogeneity	Cases of aseptic meningitis/dose administered	Estimated cases of meningitis/100,000 dose	Reference
Jeryl-Lynn	Composed of two distinct viral strains: JL1 and JL2 (Amexis et al., 2002)	0.1/100,000 to 2/500,000	0,1 to 0,4	Bonnet et al., 2006; Makela et al., 2002
Urabe AM9	Composed of quasispecies mix, (Sauder et al., 2006)	1/233,000 to 16.6/10,000	0,4 to 166	Dourado et al., 2000; Furesz & Contreras, 1990; Kimura et al., 1996; Miller et al., 2007; Rebiere & Galy-Eyraud, 1995; Schmitt et al., 1993; Sugiura & Yamada, 1991
Leningrad-3	Composed more than one viral variant (Boriskin et al., 1992)	2/10,000 to 1/1000	20 to 100	Cizman et al., 1989; Plotkin & Rubin, 2007; WHO, 2007
Leningrad-Zagreb	Composed of two major variants: A and B. (Kosutic-Gulija et al., 2008)	1/19,247 to 1/ 3,390	5,1 to 29,5	Arruda & Kondageski, 2001; da Cunha et al., 2002; da Silveira et al., 2002; Phadke et al., 2004
RIT 4385	One strain, clone JL1 (Tillieux et al., 2009)	1/525,312	0,19	Bonnet et al., 2006; Schlipkoter et al., 2002

Table 2. Genetic heterogeneity and Incidence of postvaccine aseptic meningitis.

related to vaccination with RIT 4385 mumps virus strain (Lim et al., 2007). Little epidemiological information is available for other vaccines. Leningrad-Zagreb strain-containing vaccines have been associated with a high rate of aseptic meningitis (da Cunha et al., 2002; da Silveira et al., 2002); however, other reports indicate no evidence to link Leningrad-Zagreb strain with aseptic meningitis (Kulkarni et al., 2005; Sharma et al., 2010). Although high rates of aseptic meningitis ((1/1000 vaccine recipients) have been reported for vaccines containing Leningrad-3 mumps virus strain the evidence confirming causal association is limited (Cizman et al., 1989).

5. Virulence and attenuation of mumps virus strains

Problems with attenuated virus vaccines generally reflect under- or over-attenuation or lack of efficacy respectively. Different studies have attempted to establish molecular markers allow discrimination between an attenuated strain and a virulent strain, nevertheless, the genetic basis for attenuation are still not completed known for any of the mumps vaccines. Likewise the lack the laboratory studies that assure the absence of residual neurotoxicity in mumps vaccine has been a serious problem, as demonstrated by the occurrence of aseptic meningitis in recipients of certain vaccine strains. Thus, some vaccines found to be neuroattenuated in monkeys were later found to be neurovirulent in humans when administered in large numbers (Rubin & Afzal, 2011).

5.1 Genetic characterization of post vaccination virus isolates (Helvetica, 9pt, bold)

The first reports suggesting a relationship between Urabe AM9 strain with the occurrence of aseptic meningitis, suffer however of a lack of molecular markers to discriminate between vaccine- (attenuated) and wild-type strains of the virus, making it difficult to differentiate whether the patient had an infection caused by vaccine or wild type virus. Several laboratories were able to differentiate Urabe AM9 strain from wild-type isolates of mumps virus by RT-PCR and partial sequence analysis of the P, SH, F and HN genes, confirming that mumps virus isolates from post-vaccination meningitis correspond to Urabe AM9 strain, establishing a causal association of virus strain with post-vaccination meningitis (Brown et al., 1991; Forsey et al., 1990; Yamada et al., 1990).

Analysis of cDNA sequences of several isolates from vaccine-associated meningitis and parotitis cases demonstrated that Urabe AM9 strain consisted of a mixture of virus variants that could be distinguished based on the sequence of the hemagglutinin-neuraminidase gene (HN) at nt 1,081 (nt 7,616 of the genome). Viruses containing an A residue at nt 1081 and encoding a lysine at amino acid position 335 were isolated from cases of post-vaccination parotitis or meningitis whereas viruses containing a G residue at nt 1081 that codes for a glutamic acid (aa 335) were not associated with post-vaccination disease, suggesting A_{1081} (K^{335}) was a marker of neurovirulence and G_{1081} (E^{335}) was a marker of attenuation (Brown et al., 1996). The identification of an A residue at position 1081 in the HN gene sequenced from samples of either patients with post-vaccination meningitis (Afzal et al., 1998; Wright et al., 2000) and patients infected with the wild-type strain (Cusi et al., 1998), supported the previous hypothesis.

However, this hypothesis was questioned by other researchers, reporting that some UrabeAM9 vaccine lots encoding K^{355} did not lead to adverse events in vaccinees (Amexis et al., 2001; Mori et al., 1997). Moreover, K^{335} was also found in the HN glycoprotein of the Jeryl Lynn vaccine strain, a widely used vaccine not associated with aseptic meningitis (Mori et al., 1997). Nonetheless, Jeryl Lynn strain differs from Urabe AM9 at more than 900 nucleotides, so its safety is likely determined by a number of other genetic changes.

By comparison of the HN gene sequences of several Urabe AM9 vaccine derived isolates, Afzal et al., showed that those sequences differed at several other sites (M89V; N464K; N498D), complicating the interpretation of the initial findings (Afzal et al., 1998). Moreover, heterogeneity at position 464 in the HN glycoprotein (Asn464/Lys) was also reported from sequence analysis of Urabe AM9 vaccine virus and post-vaccination meningitis isolates (Afzal et al., 1998; Amexis et al., 2001; Wright et al., 2000). Further, it was shown that Urabe-AM9 strain is constituted by several virus quasispecies that differ in distinct sites all along their genome, with several amino acids changes in the NP, P, L (involved in replication/transcription), F and HN proteins (involved in the recognition, fusion and release of virus in infected cells), as well as in the intergenic region NP-P (Shah et al., 2009). Sauder et al., showed that genetic heterogeneity at the specific genome sites have a profound effect on the neurovirulent phenotype of Urabe-AM9 strain (Sauder et al., 2006), suggesting there is not a unique genetic marker responsible for virus attenuation, rather the combination of mutations may be necessary for an adequate viral attenuation (Amexis et al., 2001; Sauder et al., 2006; Shah et al., 2009).

Different vaccine strains exhibit high degree of nucleotide heterogeneity (table 2) across their entire genome making it impossible to determine which genetic change is associated with neurovirulence or neuroattenuation. At respect, the Jeryl Lynn strain contains a mixture of two substrains (JL1 and JL2) that presented 414 nucleotide differences (2.69%), leading to 87 amino acid substitutions (1.67%). Subsequent passage of Jeryl Lynn strain in Vero or CEF cell cultures resulted in rapid selection of the major component JL1, while growth in embryonated chicken eggs (ECE) favored accumulation of the minor component JL2 (Afzal et al., 1993; Amexis et al., 2002; Chambers et al., 2009). Meanwhile, Leningrad-3 strain was characterized as heterogenic on the basis of plaque morphology and with several ambiguities in P and F genes (Boriskin et al., 1992). L-Zagreb vaccine strain was developed by further subcultivation of Leningrad-3 mumps vaccine strain in primary culture of chicken embryo fibroblast (CEF) and its heterogeneity was identified throughout the entire genome (Kosutic-Gulija et al., 2008).

5.2 Structural, functional and antigenic analysis of mumps virus proteins

Mumps vaccine strains, including L-Zagreb, Leningrad-3 and Urabe AM9, have been associated with a high incidence of post-vaccination aseptic meningitis. Although several researchers have focused to study the genetic basis of mumps virus strains virulence/attenuation, there is not genetic marker that help to discriminate between a virulent strain and an attenuated strain. Previous analyses confirmed that Jeryl Lynn, Urabe-AM9, Leningrad-3 and L-Zagreb mumps virus strains are genetically heterogeneous, where each nucleotide changes may contribute to neurovirulence-neuroattenuation of the vaccine. Therefore, caution should be exercised when evaluating genetic markers because more than one nucleotide can influence the attenuation or virulence of a vaccine (Sauder et al., 2006). By other side, functional analysis of point mutations gives relevant information about the properties of a virus variant. A point mutation from guanine (G) to adenine (A) at nucleotide position 1081 in the hemagglutinin-neuraminidase (HN) gene has been associated with neurovirulence of Urabe AM9 mumps virus vaccine. This mutation corresponds to a glutamic acid (E) to lysine (K) change at position 335 in the HN glycoprotein. We have experimentally demonstrated that two variants of Urabe AM9 strain (HN-A_{1081} and HN-G_{1081}) differ in their replication efficiency in cell culture, where HN-A_{1081} variant was efficiently replicated in both human neuroblastoma cells (SHSY5Y) and newborn rat brain (10^5 and 10^4 PFU respectively), whereas HN-G_{1081} variant was replicated at low titers (10^2 PFU in both cases) (Santos-Lopez et al., 2006). These findings can be explained in part by differences in cell receptor binding affinity of each variant, where HN-A_{1081} variant showed highest affinity towards α2-6 linked sialic acids that are highly expressed in human nerve cells, whereas HN-G_{1081} viral variant showed higher affinity towards α2-3 linked sialic acids that are less expressed in nerve cells, however this latter variant also recognized α2-6 linked sialic acid but with lesser affinity than HNA_{1081} virus (Reyes-Leyva et al., 2007). Controversially, two mumps virus that differ at position 335 (K/E) of HN protein exhibited similar growth kinetics in neuronal (SHSY5Y) and non neuronal cell lines (Vero cells) and similar neurotoxicity when tested in rats models. This suggests that amino acid 335 is not a crucial determinant of Urabe neurovirulence, nevertheless this point mutation can not be excluded as contributing to vaccine virulence (Sauder et al., 2009).

Likewise, we have performed a structure-function analysis of that amino acid substitution, suggesting that the E/K interchange does not affect the structure of the sialic acid binding motif; however, the electrostatic surface differs drastically due to an exposed short alpha helix. Consequently, this mutation may affect the accessibility of HN to substrates and membrane receptors of the host cells (Santos-Lopez et al., 2009). These results suggest that the change K335E affects the biological activity of HN glycoprotein, conferring neurotropism for HN-A_{1081} viral variant as previously proposed (Brown et al., 1996; Wright et al., 2000). Amino acid 335 is located at an important domain of HN glycoprotein that involves the recognition of an antigenic site, thus all virus variants that possess a Glu at position 335 were completely neutralized, while those containing Lys escaped neutralization (Afzal et al., 1998).

Using a rat based model of mumps neurovirulence, Shah et al. demonstrated that viral variants with a Glu at position 335 of HN glycoprotein is significantly attenuated (hydrocephalus 1.37% ± 0.50) compared to a virus isolated from a patient with post-vaccination meningitis (hydrocephalus 4.70%±0.77) and compared with wild type (hydrocephalus 11.47%±1.16) which have Lys at this position (Shah et al., 2009).

The importance of amino acid 464 in the HN glycoprotein was demonstrated by mumps virus reverse genetic, which showed that N464S substitution is involved in virus replication in nerve cells (SH-SY5Y) (Ninomiya et al., 2009). Crystal structure studies of the HN glycoprotein of a closely related paramyxovirus Newcatle disease virus, indicates that amino acid position 466 may be at or near the active site of the HN protein (Crennell et al., 2000), thus the substitution around this site (464) might affect enzymatic activity of HN protein and might change the cell specificity of mumps virus. Amino acids 464-466 form a potential N-liked glycosylation site given that substitutions at this site were predicted to result in loss of N-linked glycosylation, and affect virus tropism and virulence (Rubin et al., 2003). Similarly, Malik et al., demonstrated that Ser-466Asp substitution in the HN protein resulted in decreased receptor binding and neuraminidase activity, Ala91Thr change in the fusion protein resulted in decreased fusion activity, and that Ile736Val substitution in the polymerase resulted in increased replication and transcriptional activity (Malik et al., 2007; Malik et al., 2009).

A study based on the extent of hydrocephalus induced in the rat brain after intracerebral vaccine inoculation showed that expression of the F gene of the neurovirulent Kilman strain alone was sufficient to induce significant levels of hydrocephalus, this experiment confirms the importance of surface glycoproteins in neuropathogenesis (Lemon et al., 2007). Moreover, recent studies done in the rat model demonstrated the ability of nucleoprotein/matrix protein of the Jeryl Lynn vaccine strain to significantly neuroattenuate wild-type 88-1961 strain, which is highly neurovirulent (Sauder et al., 2011)

6. Innate immune response against mumps virus infection

Innate immune response acts as a first line of defense during viral infections, through immunoregulatory mechanisms that increase own innate immune response and stimulate an adaptive immune response. After viral infection, intracellular signaling events are activated and innate cytokine expression are induced as interleukins (IL), tumor necrosis factor (TNF) and interferon (IFN) (Biron & Sen, 2007; Pestka, 2007).

Type-I IFNs (IFN-α/β) are a superfamily of cytokines that were discovered as a result of their induction by and action against virus infections. The interaction between Toll-like receptors (TLR) and pathogen-associated molecular patterns (as genomic RNA and viral proteins), triggers the activation cell signaling pathways that promote activation of some transcription factors such as IRF3 and NFκB, which are necessary to induce expression of IFN-β. Analogously, RNA helicase molecules (RIG-I and mda-5) trigger TLR-independent pathways that respond to viral nucleic acids (such as dsRNA) generated in the cytoplasm by viral replication, causing activation of IRF3 and NFκB, wich also promote the synthesis of IFN-β (Conzelmann, 2005; Honda et al., 2005; Randall & Goodbourn, 2008; Xagorari & Chlichlia, 2008).

The biological activities of IFNs are initiated by the recognition of IFN-α/β receptor (composed of the products of the IFNAR1 and IFNAR2 genes) on the cell surface, which results in the activation of a signaling pathway known as Jak/STAT pathways. This starts by activation of tysosine kinases Tyk2 and Jak1 located in the cytoplasmic tail of IFNAR1 and IFNAR2 subunits respectively (de Weerd et al., 2007; Randall & Goodbourn, 2008). Activation of the signal transduction occurs when Tyk2 phosphorylates Tyr^{466} residue on IFNAR1, creating a docking site for STAT2, which is then phosphorylates on Tyr^{690}. Phosphorylated STAT2 protein associates with STAT1, inducing its phosphorylation on Tyr^{701} by JAK1. Phosporylated Stat2 and Stat1 proteins form a stable heterodimer that creates a nuclear localization signal (NLS) that permits the transport of these dimers into the nucleus until their dephosphorylation (Randall & Goodbourn, 2008; Schindler et al., 2007). In addition, IFNAR2 subunit is acetylated at Lys399 and promotes the acetylation of IRF9, which is essential to DNA binding (Tang et al., 2007). Association of STAT1-STAT2 heterodimer with IRF9 constitutes ISGF3 (IFN-stimulated gene factor 3) a heterotrimeric transcription factor that binds to the IFN-stimulated response element (ISRE), present in the promoters of several IFN-stimulated genes (ISG). The final step of this signaling pathway is the induction of gene transcription whose expression establishes the antiviral state (Biron & Sen, 2007; Randall & Goodbourn, 2008; Schindler et al., 2007; Sen, 2001).

Numerous ISG products have been described such as Caspases, which are involved in cell death; Protein kinase R (PKR) that inhibits both cellular and viral translation, through phosphorylation of NF-κB and eIF2α factor; 2´5´-oligoadenylate synthetase (OAS) that binds to and activates the RNase L, which promotes the degradation cellular and viral RNAs; Mx protein that binds nucleocapsid-like structures, thereby restricting virus replication and assembly (Honda et al., 2005; Randall & Goodbourn, 2008).

6.1 Mumps virus and evasion of innate immune response

Several viruses have evolved strategies to circumvent the antiviral state stimulated by IFN through the expression of proteins that antagonize components of the Jak-Stat signaling pathway, such as the V protein of paramyxoviruses (Gotoh et al., 2002; Randall & Goodbourn, 2008). As mentioned, mumps virus P gene codes for three polypeptides: V, I and P. Their mRNAs are translated by use of overlapping reading frames (ORFs) via cotranscriptional insertion of nontemplated guanidine nucleotides (mRNA edition) (Lamb & Parks, 2007; Paterson & Lamb, 1990). Mumps virus V protein is a nonstructural protein that counteracts the IFN-induced antiviral response by different mechanisms. In some paramyxoviruses V protein interacts with and inhibits the activity of mda-5 (Andrejeva et al., 2004), but not RIG-I (Komatsu et al., 2007); in other viruses V inhibits interferon-mediated antiviral response through degradation of STAT proteins and thus promotes viral replication (Gotoh et al., 2002; Horvath, 2004; Randall & Goodbourn, 2008).

We have shown that two variants of Urabe AM9 vaccine strain (HN-A$_{1081}$ and HN-G$_{1081}$) that were initially characterized by their difference in the HN gene nt 1081, also differ in their replication efficiency in nerve cells, where HN-A$_{1081}$ variant preferentially infects nerve cells, whereas HN-G$_{1081}$ variant has limited replication in this cells (Santos-Lopez et al., 2006); These results were associated with differences in the virus binding affinity towards cell receptors and enzymatic activity (Reyes-Leyva et al., 2007). Further experiments showed that differences in sensitivity to IFN determined the replication rate of Urabe AM9 mumps virus variants in nerve cells, where HN-G$_{1081}$ variant was more sensitive to interferon (from 102.5 to 101.3 TCID50) than HN-A$_{1081}$ variant (from 103.5 to 102.6 TCID50). Moreover HN-A$_{1081}$ virus reduced the transcription of cellular IFN responsive genes such as STAT1, STA2, p48 and MxA in both unprimed and IFN-primed cells, whereas HN-G$_{1081}$ virus just reduced MxA transcription. Sensitivity to IFN was associated with insertion of a non-coded glycine at position 156 in the V protein (V$_{Gly}$) of HN-G$_{1081}$ virus variant, whereas resistance to IFN was associated with preservation of wild-type phenotype in the V protein (V$_{WT}$) of HN-A$_{1081}$ virus variant (Rosas-Murrieta et al., 2007). Functional analysis of Gly 156 insertion suggested that V$_{WT}$ protein may be more efficient than V$_{Gly}$ protein to inactivate both the IFN signaling pathway and antiviral response due to differences in their finest molecular interaction with STAT proteins (Rosas-Murrieta et al., 2010).

On the other hand the activation of the JAK-STAT pathway by IFN simultaneously activates other processes regulated by IFN such as apoptosis. We studied the relationship between V protein variants of Urabe AM9 vaccine strain and IFN-α induced apoptosis. Our results indicated that V proteins decrease the levels of caspases and DNA fragmentation, suggesting that V$_{WT}$ protein is a better modulator of apoptosis than Vgly in the vaccine strain (Rosas-Murrieta et al., 2011).

7. Conclusions

Several strains of mumps virus used as attenuated vaccines have been associated with post-vaccination meningitis. Experimental data indicates that neurovirulence is a complex issue that involves multiple components either viral or cellular. Further studies are in progress to recognize the role of these in viral attenuation and virulence.

8. References

Afzal, M.A.; Pickford, A.R.; Forsey, T.; Heath, A.B. & Minor, P.D. (1993). The Jeryl Lynn vaccine strain of mumps virus is a mixture of two distinct isolates. *J Gen Virol*, Vol.74 (Pt 5), pp.917-920, ISSN 0022-1317

Afzal, M.A.; Yates, P.J. & Minor, P.D. (1998). Nucleotide sequence at position 1081 of the hemagglutinin-neuraminidase gene in the mumps Urabe vaccine strain. *J Infect Dis*, Vol.177, No.1, pp.265-266, ISSN 0022-1899

Amexis, G.; Fineschi, N. & Chumakov, K. (2001). Correlation of genetic variability with safety of mumps vaccine Urabe AM9 strain. *Virology*, Vol.287, No.1, pp.234-241, ISSN 0042-6822

Amexis, G.; Rubin, S.; Chizhikov, V.; Pelloquin, F.; Carbone, K. & Chumakov, K. (2002). Sequence diversity of Jeryl Lynn strain of mumps virus: quantitative mutant analysis for vaccine quality control. *Virology*, Vol.300, No.2, pp.171-179, ISSN 0042-6822

Andrejeva, J.; Childs, K.S.; Young, D.F.; Carlos, T.S.; Stock, N.; Goodbourn, S. & Randall, R.E. (2004). The V proteins of paramyxoviruses bind the IFN-inducible RNA helicase, mda-5, and inhibit its activation of the IFN-beta promoter. *Proc Natl Acad Sci U S A*, Vol.101, No.49, pp.17264-17269, ISSN 0027-8424

Arruda, W.O. & Kondageski, C. (2001). Aseptic meningitis in a large MMR vaccine campaign (590,609 people) in Curitiba, Parana, Brazil, 1998. *Rev Inst Med Trop Sao Paulo*, Vol.43, No.5, pp.301-302, ISSN 0036-4665

Biron, C.A. & Sen, G. (2007). Innate responses to viral infections, In: *Fields Virology*, D.M. Knipe & P.M. Howley (Eds.), pp. 250-277, Lippincott Williams & Wilkins, ISBN 0781760607.

Bonnet, M.C.; Dutta, A.; Weinberger, C. & Plotkin, S.A. (2006). Mumps vaccine virus strains and aseptic meningitis. *Vaccine*, Vol.24, No.49-50, pp.7037-7045, ISSN 0264-410X

Boriskin, Y.S.; Yamada, A.; Kaptsova, T.I.; Skvortsova, O.I.; Sinitsyna, O.A.; Takeuchi, K.; Tanabayashi, K. & Sugiura, A. (1992). Genetic evidence for variant selection in the course of dilute passaging of mumps vaccine virus. *Res Virol*, Vol.143, No.4, pp.279-283, ISSN 0923-2516

Brockhoff, H.J.; Mollema, L.; Sonder, G.J.; Postema, C.A.; van Binnendijk, R.S.; Kohl, R.H.; de Melker, H.E. & Hahne, S.J. (2010). Mumps outbreak in a highly vaccinated student population, The Netherlands, 2004. *Vaccine*, Vol.28, No.17, pp.2932-2936, ISSM 1873-2518

Brown, E.G.; Dimock, K. & Wright, K.E. (1996). The Urabe AM9 mumps vaccine is a mixture of viruses differing at amino acid 335 of the hemagglutinin-neuraminidase gene with one form associated with disease. *J Infect Dis*, Vol.174, No.3, pp.619-622, ISSN 0022-1899

Brown, E.G.; Furesz, J.; Dimock, K.; Yarosh, W. & Contreras, G. (1991). Nucleotide sequence analysis of Urabe mumps vaccine strain that caused meningitis in vaccine recipients. *Vaccine*, Vol.9, No.11, pp.840-842, ISSN 0264-410X

Brown, E.G. & Wright, K.E. (1998). Genetic studies on a mumps vaccine strain associated with meningitis. *Rev Med Virol*, Vol.8, No.3, pp.129-142, ISSN 1099-1654

Carbone, K.M. & Rubin, S. (2007). Mumps virus, In: *Fields Virology*, D.M. Knipe & P.M. Howley (Eds.), pp. 1528-1551, Lippincott Williams & Wilkins, ISBN 0781760607.

CDC. Basics and Common Questions: What Would Happen If We Stopped Vaccinations?, Available from: http://www.cdc.gov/vaccines/vac-gen/whatifstop.htm#mumps

CDC (October 2010). Mumps outbreaks, In: *Mumps*, Available from: http://www.cdc.gov/mumps/outbreaks.html

Cizman, M.; Mozetic, M.; Radescek-Rakar, R.; Pleterski-Rigler, D. & Susec-Michieli, M. (1989). Aseptic meningitis after vaccination against measles and mumps. *Pediatr Infect Dis J*, Vol.8, No.5, pp.302-308, ISSN 0891-3668

Conzelmann, K.K. (2005). Transcriptional activation of alpha/beta interferon genes: interference by nonsegmented negative-strand RNA viruses. *J Virol*, Vol.79, No.9, pp.5241-5248, ISSN 0022-538X

Crennell, S.; Takimoto, T.; Portner, A. & Taylor, G. (2000). Crystal structure of the multifunctional paramyxovirus hemagglutinin-neuraminidase. *Nat Struct Biol*, Vol.7, No.11, pp.1068-1074, ISSN 1072-8368

Crovari, P.; Gabutti, G.; Giammanco, G.; Dentico, P.; Moiraghi, A.R.; Ponzio, F. & Soncini, R. (2000). Reactogenicity and immunogenicity of a new combined measles-mumps-rubella vaccine: results of a multicentre trial. The Cooperative Group for the Study of MMR vaccines. *Vaccine*, Vol.18, No.25, pp.2796-2803, ISSN 0264-410X

Cusi, M.G.; Santini, L.; Bianchi, S.; Valassina, M. & Valensin, P.E. (1998). Nucleotide sequence at position 1081 of the hemagglutinin-neuraminidasegene in wild-type strains of mumps virus is the most relevant marker of virulence. *J Clin Microbiol*, Vol.36, No.12, pp.3743-3744, ISSN 0095-1137

Chambers, P.; Rima, B.K. & Duprex, W.P. (2009). Molecular differences between two Jeryl Lynn mumps virus vaccine component strains, JL5 and JL2. *J Gen Virol*, Vol.90, No.Pt 12, pp.2973-2981, ISSN 1465-2099

Cheek, J.E.; Baron, R.; Atlas, H.; Wilson, D.L. & Crider, R.D., Jr. (1995). Mumps outbreak in a highly vaccinated school population. Evidence for large-scale vaccination failure. *Arch Pediatr Adolesc Med*, Vol.149, No.7, pp.774-778, ISSN 1072-4710

Choi, K.M. (2010). Reemergence of mumps. *Korean J Pediatr*, Vol.53, No.5, pp.623-628, ISSN 2092-7258.

da Cunha, S.S.; Rodrigues, L.C.; Barreto, M.L. & Dourado, I. (2002). Outbreak of aseptic meningitis and mumps after mass vaccination with MMR vaccine using the Leningrad-Zagreb mumps strain. *Vaccine*, Vol.20, No.7-8, pp.1106-1112, ISSN 0264-410X.

da Silveira, C.M.; Kmetzsch, C.I.; Mohrdieck, R.; Sperb, A.F. & Prevots, D.R. (2002). The risk of aseptic meningitis associated with the Leningrad-Zagreb mumps vaccine strain following mass vaccination with measles-mumps-rubella vaccine, Rio Grande do Sul, Brazil, 1997. *Int J Epidemiol*, Vol.31, No.5, pp.978-982, ISSN 0300-5771.

Dayan, G.H.; Quinlisk, M.P.; Parker, A.A.; Barskey, A.E.; Harris, M.L.; Schwartz, J.M.; Hunt, K.; Finley, C.G.; Leschinsky, D.P.; O'Keefe, A.L.; Clayton, J.; Kightlinger, L.K.; Dietle, E.G.; Berg, J.; Kenyon, C.L.; Goldstein, S.T.; Stokley, S.K.; Redd, S.B.; Rota, P.A.; Rota, J.; Bi, D.; Roush, S.W.; Bridges, C.B.; Santibanez, T.A.; Parashar, U.; Bellini, W.J. & Seward, J.F. (2008). Recent resurgence of mumps in the United States. *N Engl J Med*, Vol.358, No.15, pp.1580-1589, ISSN 1533-4406.

Dayan, G.H. & Rubin, S. (2008). Mumps outbreaks in vaccinated populations: are available mumps vaccines effective enough to prevent outbreaks? *Clin Infect Dis*, Vol.47, No.11, pp.1458-1467, ISSN 1537-6591

de Weerd, N.A.; Samarajiwa, S.A. & Hertzog, P.J. (2007). Type I interferon receptors: biochemistry and biological functions. *J Biol Chem*, Vol.282, No.28, pp.20053-20057, ISSN 0021-9258

Didcock, L.; Young, D.F.; Goodbourn, S. & Randall, R.E. (1999a). Sendai virus and simian virus 5 block activation of interferon-responsive genes: importance for virus pathogenesis. *J Virol*, Vol.73, No.4, pp.3125-3133, ISSN 0022-538X

Didcock, L.; Young, D.F.; Goodbourn, S. & Randall, R.E. (1999b). The V protein of simian virus 5 inhibits interferon signalling by targeting STAT1 for proteasome-mediated degradation. *J Virol*, Vol.73, No.12, pp.9928-9933, ISSN 0022-538X.

Dourado, I.; Cunha, S.; Teixeira, M.G.; Farrington, C.P.; Melo, A.; Lucena, R. & Barreto, M.L. (2000). Outbreak of aseptic meningitis associated with mass vaccination with a urabe-containing measles-mumps-rubella vaccine: implications for immunization programs. *Am J Epidemiol*, Vol.151, No.5, pp.524-530, ISSN 0002-9262

Enders, G. (1996). Paramyxoviruses, In: *Medical Microbiolog*, S. Baron (Ed), The University of Texas Medical Branch at Galveston, ISBN-10: 0-9631172-1-1, Galveston, Texas.

Esteghamati, A.; Keshtkar, A.; Heshmat, R.; Gouya, M.M.; Salar Amoli, M.; Armin, S. & Mahoney, F. (2011). Adverse reactions following immunization with MMR vaccine in children at selected provinces of Iran. *Arch Iran Med*, Vol.14, No.2, pp.91-95, ISSN 1029-2977.

Fleischer, B. & Kreth, H.W. (1982). Mumps virus replication in human lymphoid cell lines and in peripheral blood lymphocytes: preference for T cells. *Infect Immun*, Vol.35, No.1, pp.25-31, ISSN 0019-9567

Forsey, T.; Mawn, J.A.; Yates, P.J.; Bentley, M.L. & Minor, P.D. (1990). Differentiation of vaccine and wild mumps viruses using the polymerase chain reaction and dideoxynucleotide sequencing. *J Gen Virol*, Vol.71 (Pt 4), pp.987-990, ISSN 0022-1317.

Fujii, N.; Yokosawa, N. & Shirakawa, S. (1999). Suppression of interferon response gene expression in cells persistently infected with mumps virus, and restoration from its suppression by treatment with ribavirin. *Virus Res*, Vol.65, No.2, pp.175-185, ISSN 0168-1702

Furesz, J. & Contreras, G. (1990). Vaccine-related mumps meningitis--Canada. *Can Dis Wkly Rep*, Vol.16, No.50, pp.253-254, ISSN 0382-232X

Galazka, A.M.; Robertson, S.E. & Kraigher, A. (1999). Mumps and mumps vaccine: a global review. *Bull World Health Organ*, Vol.77, No.1, pp.3-14, ISSN 0042-9686.

Goh, K.T. (1999). Resurgence of mumps in Singapore caused by the Rubini mumps virus vaccine strain. *Lancet*, Vol.354, No.9187, pp.1355-1356, ISSN 0140-6736

Gotoh, B.; Komatsu, T.; Takeuchi, K. & Yokoo, J. (2002). Paramyxovirus strategies for evading the interferon response. *Rev Med Virol*, Vol.12, No.6, pp.337-357, ISSN 1052-9276

Hausmann, S.; Garcin, D.; Delenda, C. & Kolakofsky, D. (1999). The versatility of paramyxovirus RNA polymerase stuttering. *J Virol*, Vol.73, No.7, pp.5568-5576, ISSN 0022-538X

Hersh, B.S.; Fine, P.E.; Kent, W.K.; Cochi, S.L.; Kahn, L.H.; Zell, E.R.; Hays, P.L. & Wood, C.L. (1991). Mumps outbreak in a highly vaccinated population. *J Pediatr*, Vol.119, No.2, pp.187-193, ISSN 0022-3476

Honda, K.; Yanai, H.; Takaoka, A. & Taniguchi, T. (2005). Regulation of the type I IFN induction: a current view. *Int Immunol*, Vol.17, No.11, pp.1367-1378, ISSN 0953-8178

Horvath, C.M. (2004). Weapons of STAT destruction. Interferon evasion by paramyxovirus V protein. *Eur J Biochem*, Vol.271, No.23-24, pp.4621-4628, ISSN 0014-2956

Hviid, A.; Rubin, S. & Muhlemann, K. (2008). Mumps. *Lancet*, Vol.371, No.9616, pp.932-944, ISSN 1474-547X

Kanra, G.; Ceyhan, M. & Ozmert, E. (2000). Reactogenicity and immunogenicity of a new measles-mumps-rubella vaccine containing RIT 4385 mumps virus strain in healthy Turkish children. *Turk J Pediatr*, Vol.42, No.4, pp.275-277, ISSN 0041-4301.

Kimura, M.; Kuno-Sakai, H.; Yamazaki, S.; Yamada, A.; Hishiyama, M.; Kamiya, H.; Ueda, K.; Murase, T.; Hirayama, M.; Oya, A.; Nozaki, S. & Murata, R. (1996). Adverse events associated with MMR vaccines in Japan. *Acta Paediatr Jpn*, Vol.38, No.3, pp.205-211, ISSN 0374-5600.

Kingston, R.L.; Hamel, D.J.; Gay, L.S.; Dahlquist, F.W. & Matthews, B.W. (2004). Structural basis for the attachment of a paramyxoviral polymerase to its template. *Proc Natl Acad Sci U S A*, Vol.101, No.22, pp.8301-8306, ISSN 0027-8424.

Kolakofsky, D.; Pelet, T.; Garcin, D.; Hausmann, S.; Curran, J. & Roux, L. (1998). Paramyxovirus RNA synthesis and the requirement for hexamer genome length: the rule of six revisited. *J Virol*, Vol.72, No.2, pp.891-899, ISSN 0022-538X

Kolakofsky, D.; Roux, L.; Garcin, D. & Ruigrok, R.W. (2005). Paramyxovirus mRNA editing, the "rule of six" and error catastrophe: a hypothesis. *J Gen Virol*, Vol.86, No.Pt 7, pp.1869-1877, ISSN 0022-1317

Komatsu, T.; Takeuchi, K. & Gotoh, B. (2007). Bovine parainfluenza virus type 3 accessory proteins that suppress beta interferon production. *Microbes Infect*, Vol.9, No.8, pp.954-962, ISSN 1286-4579

Kosutic-Gulija, T.; Forcic, D.; Santak, M.; Ramljak, A.; Mateljak-Lukacevic, S. & Mazuran, R. (2008). Genetic heterogeneity of L-Zagreb mumps virus vaccine strain. *Virol J*, Vol.5, pp.79, ISSN 1743-422X

Kulkarni, P.S.; Phadke, M.A.; Jadhav, S.S. & Kapre, S.V. (2005). No definitive evidence for L-Zagreb mumps strain associated aseptic meningitis: a review with special reference to the da Cunha study. *Vaccine*, Vol.23, No.46-47, pp.5286-5288, ISSN 0264-410X

Lamb, R.A. & Parks, G.D. (2007). Paramyxoviridae: The viruses and their replication, In: *Fields Virology*, D.M. Knipe & P.M. Howley (Eds.), pp. 1450- 1497, Lippincott Williams & Wilkins, ISBN 0781760607.

Lemon, K.; Rima, B.K.; McQuaid, S.; Allen, I.V. & Duprex, W.P. (2007). The F gene of rodent brain-adapted mumps virus is a major determinant of neurovirulence. *J Virol*, Vol.81, No.15, pp.8293-8302, ISSN 0022-538X

Lim, F.S.; Han, H.H. & Bock, H.L. (2007). Safety, reactogenicity and immunogenicity of the live attenuated combined measles, mumps and rubella vaccine containing the RIT 4385 mumps strain in healthy Singaporean children. *Ann Acad Med Singapore*, Vol.36, No.12, pp.969-973, ISSN 0304-4602

Makela, A.; Nuorti, J.P. & Peltola, H. (2002). Neurologic disorders after measles-mumps-rubella vaccination. *Pediatrics*, Vol.110, No.5, pp.957-963, ISSN 1098-4275

Malik, T.; Shegogue, C.W.; Werner, K.; Ngo, L.; Sauder, C.; Zhang, C.; Duprex, W.P. & Rubin, S. (2011). Discrimination of mumps virus small hydrophobic gene deletion effects from gene translation effects on virus virulence. *J Virol*, Vol.85, No.12, pp.6082-6085, ISSN 1098-5514.

Malik, T.; Wolbert, C.; Mauldin, J.; Sauder, C.; Carbone, K.M. & Rubin, S.A. (2007). Functional consequences of attenuating mutations in the haemagglutinin neuraminidase, fusion and polymerase proteins of a wild-type mumps virus strain. *J Gen Virol*, Vol.88, No.Pt 9, pp.2533-2541, ISSN 0022-1317

Malik, T.H.; Wolbert, C.; Nerret, L.; Sauder, C. & Rubin, S. (2009). Single amino acid changes in the mumps virus haemagglutinin-neuraminidase and polymerase proteins are associated with neuroattenuation. *J Gen Virol*, Vol.90, No.Pt 7, pp.1741-1747, ISSN 0022-1317

Miller, E.; Andrews, N.; Stowe, J.; Grant, A.; Waight, P. & Taylor, B. (2007). Risks of convulsion and aseptic meningitis following measles-mumps-rubella vaccination in the United Kingdom. *Am J Epidemiol*, Vol.165, No.6, pp.704-709, ISSN 0002-9262.

Mori, C.; Tooriyama, T.; Imagawa, T. & Yamanishi, K. (1997). Nucleotide sequence at position 1081 of the hemagglutinin-neuraminidase gene in the mumps virus Urabe vaccine strain. *J Infect Dis*, Vol.175, No.6, pp.1548-1549, ISSN 0022-1899.

Ninomiya, K.; Kanayama, T.; Fujieda, N.; Nakayama, T.; Komase, K.; Nagata, K. & Takeuchi, K. (2009). Amino acid substitution at position 464 in the haemagglutinin-neuraminidase protein of a mumps virus Urabe strain enhanced the virus growth in neuroblastoma SH-SY5Y cells. *Vaccine*, Vol.27, No.44, pp.6160-6165, ISSN 1873-2518

Ong, G.; Goh, K.T.; Ma, S. & Chew, S.K. (2005). Comparative efficacy of Rubini, Jeryl-Lynn and Urabe mumps vaccine in an Asian population. *J Infect*, Vol.51, No.4, pp.294-298, ISSN 1532-2742

Orvell, C.; Kalantari, M. & Johansson, B. (1997). Characterization of five conserved genotypes of the mumps virus small hydrophobic (SH) protein gene. *J Gen Virol*, Vol.78 (Pt 1), pp.91-95, ISSN 0022-1317

Park, D.W.; Nam, M.H.; Kim, J.Y.; Kim, H.J.; Sohn, J.W.; Cho, Y.; Song, K.J. & Kim, M.J. (2007). Mumps outbreak in a highly vaccinated school population: assessment of secondary vaccine failure using IgG avidity measurements. *Vaccine*, Vol.25, No.24, pp.4665-4670, ISSN 0264-410X

Paterson, R.G. & Lamb, R.A. (1990). RNA editing by G-nucleotide insertion in mumps virus P-gene mRNA transcripts. *J Virol*, Vol.64, No.9, pp.4137-4145, ISSN 0022-538X

Peltola, H.; Kulkarni, P.S.; Kapre, S.V.; Paunio, M.; Jadhav, S.S. & Dhere, R.M. (2007). Mumps outbreaks in Canada and the United States: time for new thinking on mumps vaccines. *Clin Infect Dis*, Vol.45, No.4, pp.459-466, ISSN 1537-6591

Pestka, S. (2007). The interferons: 50 years after their discovery, there is much more to learn. *J Biol Chem*, Vol.282, No.28, pp.20047-20051, ISSN 0021-9258

Phadke, M.A.; Patki, P.S.; Kulkarni, P.S.; Jadhav, S.S. & Kapre, S.V. (2004). Pharmacovigilance on MMR vaccine containing L-Zagreb mumps strain. *Vaccine*, Vol.22, No.31-32, pp.4135-4136, ISSN 0264-410X.

Plotkin, S.A. & Rubin, S.A. (December 2007). Mumps vaccine In: *Vaccines*, Available from <http://www.thelancetglobalhealthnetwork.com/wp-content/uploads/2008/03/plotkins_ch020-x3611.PDF>

Pringle, C.R. (1997). The order Mononegavirales--current status. *Arch Virol*, Vol.142, No.11, pp.2321-2326, ISSN 0304-8608

Randall, R.E. & Goodbourn, S. (2008). Interferons and viruses: an interplay between induction, signalling, antiviral responses and virus countermeasures. *J Gen Virol*, Vol.89, No.Pt 1, pp.1-47, ISSN 0022-1317

Rebiere, I. & Galy-Eyraud, C. (1995). Estimation of the risk of aseptic meningitis associated with mumps vaccination, France, 1991-1993. *Int J Epidemiol*, Vol.24, No.6, pp.1223-1227, ISSN 0300-5771.

Reyes-Leyva, J.; Banos, R.; Borraz-Arguello, M.; Santos-Lopez, G.; Rosas, N.; Alvarado, G.; Herrera, I.; Vallejo, V. & Tapia-Ramirez, J. (2007). Amino acid change 335 E to K affects the sialic-acid-binding and neuraminidase activities of Urabe AM9 mumps virus hemagglutinin-neuraminidase glycoprotein. *Microbes Infect*, Vol.9, No.2, pp.234-240, ISSN 1286-4579

Rodriguez, J.J.; Wang, L.F. & Horvath, C.M. (2003). Hendra virus V protein inhibits interferon signaling by preventing STAT1 and STAT2 nuclear accumulation. *J Virol*, Vol.77, No.21, pp.11842-11845, ISSN 0022-538X

Rosas-Murrieta, N.; Herrera-Camacho, I.; Vallejo-Ruiz, V.; Millan-Perez-Pena, L.; Cruz, C.; Tapia-Ramirez, J.; Santos-Lopez, G. & Reyes-Leyva, J. (2007). Differential sensitivity to interferon influences the replication and transcription of Urabe AM9 mumps virus variants in nerve cells. *Microbes Infect*, Vol.9, No.7, pp.864-872, ISSN 1286-4579.

Rosas-Murrieta, N.H.; Herrera-Camacho, I.; Palma-Ocampo, H.; Santos-Lopez, G. & Reyes-Leyva, J. (2010). Interaction of mumps virus V protein variants with STAT1-STAT2 heterodimer: experimental and theoretical studies. *Virol J*, Vol.7, pp.263, ISSN 1743-422X.

Rosas-Murrieta, N.H.; Santos-Lopez, G.; Reyes-Leyva, J.; Jurado, F.S. & Herrera-Camacho, I. (2011). Modulation of apoptosis by V protein mumps virus. *Virol J*, Vol.8, pp.224, ISSN 1743-422X

Rubin, S.A. & Afzal, M.A. (2011). Neurovirulence safety testing of mumps vaccines--historical perspective and current status. *Vaccine*, Vol.29, No.16, pp.2850-2855, ISSN 1873-2518

Rubin, S.A.; Amexis, G.; Pletnikov, M.; Li, Z.; Vanderzanden, J.; Mauldin, J.; Sauder, C.; Malik, T.; Chumakov, K. & Carbone, K.M. (2003). Changes in mumps virus gene sequence associated with variability in neurovirulent phenotype. *J Virol*, Vol.77, No.21, pp.11616-11624, ISSN 0022-538X

Santos-Lopez, G.; Cruz, C.; Pazos, N.; Vallejo, V.; Reyes-Leyva, J. & Tapia-Ramirez, J. (2006). Two clones obtained from Urabe AM9 mumps virus vaccine differ in their replicative efficiency in neuroblastoma cells. *Microbes Infect*, Vol.8, No.2, pp.332-339, ISSN 1286-4579

Santos-López, G.; Hernández, J.; Borraz-Argüello, M.T.; Ramírez -Mendoza, H.; Vallejo, V. & Reyes-Leyva, J. (2004). Estructura, función e implicaciones patológicas de las proteínas del Rubulavirus porcino. *Arch. med. vet. [online]*, Vol.36, No.2, pp.119-136, ISSN 0301-732X.

Santos-Lopez, G.; Scior, T.; Borraz-Arguello Mdel, T.; Vallejo-Ruiz, V.; Herrera-Camacho, I.; Tapia-Ramirez, J. & Reyes-Leyva, J. (2009). Structure-function analysis of two variants of mumps virus hemagglutinin-neuraminidase protein. *Braz J Infect Dis*, Vol.13, No.1, pp.24-34, ISSN 1678-4391

Sauder, C.J.; Vandenburgh, K.M.; Iskow, R.C.; Malik, T.; Carbone, K.M. & Rubin, S.A. (2006). Changes in mumps virus neurovirulence phenotype associated with quasispecies heterogeneity. *Virology*, Vol.350, No.1, pp.48-57, ISSN 0042-6822

Sauder, C.J.; Zhang, C.X.; Link, M.A.; Duprex, W.P.; Carbone, K.M. & Rubin, S.A. (2009). Presence of lysine at aa 335 of the hemagglutinin-neuraminidase protein of mumps virus vaccine strain Urabe AM9 is not a requirement for neurovirulence. *Vaccine*, Vol.27, No.42, pp.5822-5829, ISSN 1873-2518.

Sauder, C.J.; Zhang, C.X.; Ngo, L.; Werner, K.; Lemon, K.; Duprex, W.P.; Malik, T.; Carbone, K. & Rubin, S.A. (2011). Gene-specific contributions to mumps virus neurovirulence and neuroattenuation. *J Virol*, Vol.85, No.14, pp.7059-7069, ISSN 1098-5514.

Schindler, C.; Levy, D.E. & Decker, T. (2007). JAK-STAT signaling: from interferons to cytokines. *J Biol Chem*, Vol.282, No.28, pp.20059-20063, ISSN 0021-9258

Schlipkoter, U.; Muhlberger, N.; von Kries, R. & Weil, J. (2002). Surveillance of measles-mumps-rubella vaccine-associated aseptic meningitis in Germany. *Infection*, Vol.30, No.6, pp.351-355, ISSN 0300-8126.

Schmitt, H.J.; Just, M. & Neiss, A. (1993). Withdrawal of a mumps vaccine: reasons and impacts. *Eur J Pediatr*, Vol.152, No.5, pp.387-388, ISSN 0340-6199

Sen, G.C. (2001). Viruses and interferons. *Annu Rev Microbiol*, Vol.55, pp.255-281, ISSN 0066-4227

Shah, D.; Vidal, S.; Link, M.A.; Rubin, S.A. & Wright, K.E. (2009). Identification of genetic mutations associated with attenuation and changes in tropism of Urabe mumps virus. *J Med Virol*, Vol.81, No.1, pp.130-138, ISSN 1096-9071.

Sharma, H.J.; Oun, S.A.; Bakr, S.S.; Kapre, S.V.; Jadhav, S.S.; Dhere, R.M. & Bhardwaj, S. (2010). No demonstrable association between the Leningrad-Zagreb mumps vaccine strain and aseptic meningitis in a large clinical trial in Egypt. *Clin Microbiol Infect*, Vol.16, No.4, pp.347-352, ISSN 1469-0691.

Sugiura, A. & Yamada, A. (1991). Aseptic meningitis as a complication of mumps vaccination. *Pediatr Infect Dis J*, Vol.10, No.3, pp.209-213, ISSN 0891-3668

Tang, X.; Gao, J.S.; Guan, Y.J.; McLane, K.E.; Yuan, Z.L.; Ramratnam, B. & Chin, Y.E. (2007). Acetylation-dependent signal transduction for type I interferon receptor. *Cell*, Vol.131, No.1, pp.93-105, ISSN 0092-8674

Tillieux, S.L.; Halsey, W.S.; Sathe, G.M. & Vassilev, V. (2009). Comparative analysis of the complete nucleotide sequences of measles, mumps, and rubella strain genomes contained in Priorix-Tetra and ProQuad live attenuated combined vaccines. *Vaccine*, Vol.27, No.16, pp.2265-2273, ISSN 0264-410X

Vandermeulen, C.; Leroux-Roels, G. & Hoppenbrouwers, K. (2009). Mumps outbreaks in highly vaccinated populations: What makes good even better? *Hum Vaccin*, Vol.5, No.7, pp.494-496, ISSN 1554-8619

Vandermeulen, C.; Roelants, M.; Vermoere, M.; Roseeuw, K.; Goubau, P. & Hoppenbrouwers, K. (2004). Outbreak of mumps in a vaccinated child population: a question of vaccine failure? *Vaccine*, Vol.22, No.21-22, pp.2713-2716, ISSN 0264-410X

Vidal, S.; Curran, J. & Kolakofsky, D. (1990). A stuttering model for paramyxovirus P mRNA editing. *EMBO J*, Vol.9, No.6, pp.2017-2022, ISSN 0261-4189

Vulliemoz, D. & Roux, L. (2001). "Rule of six": how does the Sendai virus RNA polymerase keep count? *J Virol*, Vol.75, No.10, pp.4506-4518, ISSN 0022-538X

WHO (February 2007). Mumps virus vaccines, In: *Weekly Epidemiological Record (WER)* Available from: http://www.who.int/wer/2007/wer8207/en/index.html

WHO (December 2010). Mumps, In: *Immunization surveillance, assessment and monitoring*, Available from:
http://www.who.int/immunization_monitoring/diseases/mumps/en/index.html

Wilson, R.L.; Fuentes, S.M.; Wang, P.; Taddeo, E.C.; Klatt, A.; Henderson, A.J. & He, B. (2006). Function of small hydrophobic proteins of paramyxovirus. *J Virol*, Vol.80, No.4, pp.1700-1709, ISSN 0022-538X.

Wolinsky, J.S.; Klassen, T. & Baringer, J.R. (1976). Persistence of neuroadapted mumps virus in brains of newborn hamsters after intraperitoneal inoculation. *J Infect Dis*, Vol.133, No.3, pp.260-267, ISSN 0022-1899.

Woznik, M.; Rodner, C.; Lemon, K.; Rima, B.; Mankertz, A. & Finsterbusch, T. (2010). Mumps virus small hydrophobic protein targets ataxin-1 ubiquitin-like interacting protein (ubiquilin 4). *J Gen Virol*, Vol.91, No.Pt 11, pp.2773-2781, ISSN 1465-2099.

Wright, K.E.; Dimock, K. & Brown, E.G. (2000). Biological characteristics of genetic variants of Urabe AM9 mumps vaccine virus. *Virus Res*, Vol.67, No.1, pp.49-57, ISSN 0168-1702

Xagorari, A. & Chlichlia, K. (2008). Toll-like receptors and viruses: induction of innate antiviral immune responses. *Open Microbiol J*, Vol.2, pp.49-59, ISSN 1874-2858.

Yamada, A.; Takeuchi, K.; Tanabayashi, K.; Hishiyama, M.; Takahashi, Y. & Sugiura, A. (1990). Differentiation of the mumps vaccine strains from the wild viruses by the nucleotide sequences of the P gene. *Vaccine*, Vol.8, No.6, pp.553-557, ISSN 0264-410X.

11

Synthetic Peptide Vaccines

Alexandr A. Moisa and Ekaterina F. Kolesanova
Institute of Biomedical Chemistry, Russian Academy of Medical Sciences
Moscow,
Russia

1. Introduction

Vaccination was discovered more than 200 years ago and quickly distributed around the whole Europe despite of the fact that mechanisms of protective effects of vaccines remained unclear for a long time. New vaccines appeared only at the end of XIX century and mainly during the last century after detailed studies of infectious processes, microorganisms inducing these infections, and mechanisms of immune defense. During this period many effective vaccines were developed; they controlled and even totally eliminated some dangerous infectious diseases (Makela, 2000). Now about 40 human diseases are controlled by vaccination (Uchaikin & Shamsheva, 2001). However, for some infections vaccine prophylaxis and vaccine therapy have not been developed yet. These include AIDS and hepatitis C (Barrett & Stanberry, 2009). Situation with these infections is complicated by lack of effective therapeutics, causing full elimination of the human immunodeficiency virus causing AIDS and therapeutics, which would be effective in all patients infected with hepatitis C virus (HCV) (Barrett & Stanberry, 2009). It results in the high chronization degree of these infections (almost 100% in the case of HIV infection and 70—80% in the case of HCV), which basically become lethal ones (Barrett & Stanberry, 2009). Numerous efforts to develop vaccines against these diseases still remain unsuccessful; however, problems associated with the development of such vaccines stimulated large-scale studies of the interaction of infectious agents with the immune system, mechanisms of the immune response, structural basis of immunogenicity and antigenicity, methodology and technology for the development of new generation vaccines.

Traditional vaccines are subdivided into alive (attenuated microorganisms or viral cultures), dead, or corpuscular (inactivated infectious agents) and subunit, or chemical vaccines (individual immunogenic components of infective agents) (Uchaikin & Shamsheva, 2001). The latter vaccines are free from side effects that appear after inoculation of the whole pathogenic agents. Traditional technology has been employed for the development of effective vaccines against many infections (Uchaikin & Shamsheva, 2001); however, now this technology tends to be avoided in many cases because the preparation and use of such vaccines is associated with some problems (Liljeqvist & Stahl, 1999), including:

- expensive cultivation of pathogenic bacteria, viruses or protozoa for industrial production of vaccines or immunogenic components;
- risk of infectious agent leaks;

- side effects during administration; first of all, increased reactogenicity, which cannot be excluded even in the case of subunit vaccines;
- expensive purification and detoxification of vaccine products;
- high genetic variability of an infectious agent; this complicates the detection of chemical components, which can induce an immune response against all its strains;
- significant structural changes of an infectious agent during its life cycle in the host organism that lead to the changes of its antigenic properties.

Solution of these problems requires elaboration of novel approaches to vaccine development based on knowledge of an antigenic structure of a pathogen, immune response of the host organism to the pathogen or its components, and mechanisms responsible for the modification of strength and direction of this response. Such combined approach that includes the arsenal of methods of bioinformatics, molecular biology, organic chemistry, experimental and clinical immunology is known as "reverse vaccinology". It is aimed at the identification, study of antigenic and immunogenic properties, construction and production of highly purified preparations of novel recombinant and synthetic immunogens and their use for the development of new generation vaccines (Rappuoli, 2001). Synthetic peptide vaccines considered in this review belong to vaccines developed by this approach. Here we do not discuss problems of the development of anticancer vaccines, because of special approaches required for that. One can address available papers, including reviews (Palena et al, 2006, Machiels et al, 2002, Garg et al., 2010) that describe this question.

2. What are peptide vaccines and what are their advantages?

Synthetic peptide vaccines represent fragments of protein antigen sequences, which are synthesized from amino acids and assembled into a single molecule or a supramolecular complex or just mechanically mixed; they are recognized by the immune system and induce the immune response (Sesardic, 1993). This immune response may involve either cytotoxic T-cells or B-cells (i.e. directed to elaboration of specific antibodies) or combine both possible pathways (Bijker et al., 2007). Fragments of protein molecules exhibiting B- and/or T-epitope activity are the main components of peptide vaccines, which determine the direction and specificity of the immune response. Such vaccines may also contain some individual compounds or supramolecular complexes (e.g. micelles, liposomes, polymer particles, etc.), which can nonspecifically or specifically activate certain stages of the immune response to peptides and therefore potentiate this response (Vogel & Alving, 2002). Increase in chemical stability of peptides is achieved by their attachment to carriers, which simultaneously act as activators of the immune response (Aguilar & Rodriguez, 2007).

Peptide vaccines are characterized by the following advantages over traditional vaccines based on dead pathogens, and also subunit and recombinant vaccines (Ben-Yedidia & Arnon, 1997; van der Burg et al., 2006):

- Relatively inexpensive and safe production technologies.
- Ability to induce the immune response to those structural elements of a protein antigen, which exhibit weak immunogenicity within the whole antigen molecule.
- High standardization.
- Lack of components possessing high reactogenicity (lipopolysaccharides, toxins).

- Possibility of removal of antigen fragments exhibiting allergenicity and cross-reactivity to own molecules of the vaccinated organism.
- Possibility of conjugation of various peptides from different antigens to the same carrier.

3. Steps for the synthetic peptide vaccine development

The development of a candidate synthetic peptide vaccine includes the following steps (Rappuoli, 2001, Sobolev et al., 2005):

1. Selection of immunoactive peptide fragments of protein antigen(s) of an infectious agent and construction of a peptide antigen (or several antigens).
2. Chemical synthesis of peptide antigens and their conjugation (if necessary) to a carrier.
3. Immunogenicity testing of resultant constructs on laboratory animals, determination of specificity of antibodies (elaborated to these constructs) and their protective properties.
4. Preclinical trials of selected antigens.
5. The development of the candidate vaccine and laboratory technology for its production and elaboration of samples for testing.
6. Preclinical and clinical trials of the candidate vaccine samples.

Steps 4—6 are usually determined by sanitary rules and methodical instructions approved by the corresponding governmental control services (in Russian Federation: State Sanitary and Epidemiologic Inspection (Sanitary Rules, 1995, 1998; Methodical Recommendations, 1998); in the USA: Food and Drug Administration (FDA)). Steps 1—3 are discussed in this review.

3.1 Selection of antigenic determinants for immunogenic constructs

First of all, one should take into account the type of the immune response directed to the pathogen neutralization and providing vaccine therapy and/or vaccine prophylaxis: cytotoxic response realized by specific cytotoxic T-lymphocytes, or specific humoral response, which involves the conversion of B-lymphocytes activated by a particular antigen into plasma cells that generate specific neutralizing antibodies (Sobolev et al., 2005). General features of mechanisms responsible for the formation of the specific immune response to various foreign antigens are comprehensively considered in textbooks (Male et al., 2006, Abbas & Lichtman, 2011). Taking into account these common mechanisms, vaccines directed to the generation of cytotoxic immune response should contain cytotoxic T-epitopes as obligatory components, which are often supplemented by class 1 T-helper epitopes (van der Burg et al., 2006). Vaccines that induce antibody formation should contain B-epitopes and T-helper epitopes as obligatory components (van der Burg et al., 2006). It is essential that the B-epitope components of such vaccines should originate from antigens from virulent strains and the generated antibodies should suppress virulence (Sesardic, 1993).

If antigens and virulence factors of an infectious agent remain unknown, it is possible to predict them by means of the "reverse vaccinology", which employs computer analysis of biopolymer structures (first of all their nucleotide and amino acid sequences of genome and proteome, respectively). The technology of this process has been highlighted in the reviews (Rappuoli, 2001, Sobolev et al., 2005, Barocchi et al., 2007). In order to prove the antigenicity and virulence of predicted protein molecules they are expressed and tested for the interaction with antibodies obtained from patients with corresponding infections and for their ability to cause pathological reactions in animals (Rappuoli, 2001). Now, high-throughput screening methods for antigen detection in microorganism proteomes have appeared. These include SERPA technology (SERological Proteome Analysis) and antigenome analysis (Klade, 2002; Ling et al., 2004; Tedeschi et al., 2009,Vytvytska et al., 2002, Målen et al., 2008; Glowalla et al., 2009; Meinke et al., 2005; Felgner et al., 2009; Fritzer et al., 2010). The first method consists in the separation of protein components of the cultivated infectious agent by two-dimensional electrophoresis followed by subsequent visualization of antigenically active proteins by immunoblotting with antibodies from sera of patients with corresponding diseases (Målen et al., 2008; Glowalla et al., 2009; Meinke et al., 2005; Felgner et al., 2009; Fritzer et al., 2010). The second approach includes preparation (by means of heterologous expression) of a library of proteins and their fragments encoded by the library of genome fragments of the infectious agent followed by subsequent testing of expressed proteins for antigenicity (evaluated by interaction with antibodies from sera of infected patients) and then for immunogenicity in experiments by immunizing laboratory animals (Felgner et al., 2009; Fritzer et al., 2010; Meinke et al., 2005). Antigenomic analysis excludes the cultivation of a pathogenic organism of interest; it is applicable in the case of microorganisms with small and completely sequenced genomes. To the contrary, SERPA technology is suitable for the determination and characterization of primary structures of the most diagnostically and therapeutically important antigens of infectious agents with incompletely sequenced genomes.

The next task consists in the identification of peptides corresponding to B- and T-epitopes. If tertiary structure of the peptide antigen and/or its sites involved in the binding with antibodies neutralizing its virulent properties are known, the task implies the selection and design of a peptide (or peptides) that is the best model of the already known B-epitope (Rodriguez et al., 2007, Haro et al., 2003). However, tertiary structures of antigens may be unknown; and also, this approach detects only B-epitopes, but not T-epitopes, recognized as linear peptides. Frequently, most probable B- and T-epitope selection is performed via the antigen amino acid sequence analysis with the help of bioinformatics approaches. The principal technology of this process has been well described in many reviews (Sobolev et al., 2005, Sobolev et al., 2003, He et al., 2010). It should be noted that computer-based epitope prediction capabilities are constantly extended: appearance of new information on mapped B- and T-epitopes results in the more exact specification of corresponding patterns and, consequently, in increased effectiveness of corresponding program products. New, more convenient interfaces are developed for servers containing epitope databases and prediction tools; the development of integrated servers allows to search for possible B- and T-epitopes and combine them into putative immunogenic constructions at one place (Sieker et al., 2009; Wiwanitkit, 2009; MacNamara et al., 2009; Lin et al., 2008; Perry et al., 2008; Roggen, 2006; Tian et al., 2009; Schuler et al., 2007).

However, accuracy of prediction of B- and T-helper epitopes from antigen amino acid sequences remains rather low, and many researchers prefer experimental identification of these epitopes (especially taking into account existing methods of high-throughput screening). Peptide scanning by means of partially overlapping fragments of protein antigen amino acid sequences obtained by multiple parallel synthesis allows to map both linear B-epitopes and also helper and cytotoxic T-epitopes (Castric & Cassels, 1997; Tribbick, 2002). B-epitopes are detected by testing peptides for their interaction with antisera obtained against the whole protein antigen and also sera of infected patients (there are many examples of such studies, for example, antigenic mapping of HCV envelope proteins (Kuzmina et al., 2009; Olenina et al., 2002)). Besides chemical synthesis, fragments of antigen amino acid sequences for B-epitope mapping are also obtained by genetic engineering approach: by means of construction of expression libraries of fragments as chimeras with easily expressed and purified proteins (Bongartz et al., 2009). Peptides of various lengths (from 6 to 20 and even more residues) are used for antigen scanning for B-epitopes; however, it should be noted that peptides longer than 10 residues may contain more than one linear B-epitope (Olenina et al., 2002). Besides the determination of linear B-epitopes attempts are undertaken to map and model conformational epitopes by synthetic and also phage display combinatorial peptide libraries that cover a large number of amino acid sequences from 6 to 15 residues (Pereboeva et al., 2000). In addition, B-epitopes may be determined by means of mass-spectrometry analysis of antigen-antibody complexes via the determination of an antigen site protected against proteolysis or modification by an antibody paratope (Castric & Cassels, 1997; Lu et al., 2009). Fragments of antigen molecules exhibiting T-epitope activity are detected by their ability to induce proliferation of T-lymphocytes in culture (Ahmed & Maeurer, 2009). Cytotoxic T-epitopes have a limited length (8—11 residues) and must have free N-terminal amino and C-terminal carboxyl groups; it is determined by the structure of the MHC I binding pocket. In the case of helper T-epitope determination, longer peptides, often with amidated C-terminal carboxyl groups, are used (Tribbick, 2002). The type of helper epitope activity (Th1 or Th2) is determined by ELISPOT technology. This technology allows large-scale screening of peptides, putative T-helper epitopes, via the determination of the cytokine profile (gamma-interferon, interleukins 2, 4, 10, etc) secreted by T-lymphocytes stimulated by corresponding peptides (Kalyuzhny, 2005; Wulf et al., 2009). Peptide vaccines usually contain such T-helper epitope, which exhibits affinity towards several most widespread (in a given population) Human Leukocyte Antigen (HLA) alleles (so-called universal, or promiscuous T-epitope), or an antigen fragment containing several overlapping T-epitopes of different specificity towards HLA (Sobolev et al., 2005, Panina-Bordignon et al., 1989; Jackson et al., 2002). Several cytotoxic T-epitopes with different specificity towards HLA are included into candidate peptide vaccines for induction of cytotoxic response (Bermúdes et al., 2007; Lauer et al., 2004).

3.2 Construction of peptide immunogen

Formation of a single immunogenic construction from predicted or experimentally determined B- and T-epitopes provides optimal recognition of all the components of this construction by the immune system. For example, the integration of a linear B-epitope and a helper T-epitope in a single molecule results in their penetration into the same B-lymphocyte, which will be converted into a plasma cell producing antibodies of a desired specificity (Moss et al., 2007). B- and T-epitopes may be located far away from each other in a parent protein antigen molecule; moreover, they may originate even from different proteins of the infectious agent and even from different microorganisms. For example, the universal human T-helper epitope of tetanus toxin, QYIKANSKFIGITE, is frequently used in immunogenic constructions in combinations with various peptide B-epitopes for high population coverage of a candidate vaccine (Panina-Bordignon et al., 1989). Combination of a fragment, which is supposed to induce a specific antibody, but is characterized by weak (if any) immunogenicity within the whole protein antigen, with the universal T-helper epitope allows the induction of such specific humoral response in the vaccinated organism that could not be achieved by the immunization with the whole antigen. It is one of advantages of peptide vaccines. Insertion of a short flexible linker between B- and T-epitopes provides a free rotation of the B- and T-helper parts versus each other and therefore promotes independent recognition by corresponding receptors of immunocompetent cells (Moss et al., 2007). In some cases overlapping B- and T-helper epitopes are used as they are located in the protein antigen molecule (e.g. synthetic peptide immunogens from protein VP1 of foot-and-mouth disease virus (Kupriianova et al., 2000)).

Synthetic immunogenic constructs can be represented by both linear oligopeptides and more complex structures such as branched dendrimers (so-called lysine "trees") (Tam, 1988; Van Regenmortel & Muller, 1999), cyclic or linear unbranched oligomers conjugated (via their side chain functional groups) with either individual B- and T-epitopes or such constructs as T-epitope—linker—B-epitope/B-epitope—linker-T-epitope (Jackson et al., 2002). Complex structures are less sensitive to proteolysis and therefore they have higher stability during administration to the body and form higher local concentrations of the immunogen (Sobolev et al., 2005). However, such structures are more difficult to obtain; in addition, their complex surface structure can interfere with the recognition of individual linear B-epitopes included into these constructs (Van Regenmortel & Muller, 1999). Optimal co-location of B- and T-epitopes is selected experimentally by comparing the immugenicity of constructs with different structures (Van Regenmortel & Muller, 1999). A general principle of the effective immune response to B-epitope consists in its close proximity to T-helper epitope(s). Binding of the B-epitope to a B-lymphocyte receptor seems to protect the neighboring T-helper epitope against endosomal cleavage (Moss et al., 2007).

Synthetic peptide vaccines based on cytotoxic and Th1-epitopes represent mechanical mixtures of peptides corresponding to various T-epitopes from one or several antigens of an infectious agent (Jackson et al., 2002). The design of monomolecular constructs is not required because in contrast to the B-T-epitope construction these T-epitopes can independently bind to various cells of the immune system.

The monomolecular immunogenic constructions can also include components with adjuvant functions (see below).

3.3 Immunogen synthesis

Peptide components for synthetic vaccines are obtained by means of solid phase peptide synthesis and peptide synthesis in solution (Sobolev et al., 2005, Sieker et al., 2009; Jackson et al., 2002, Tam, 1988; Van Regenmortel & Muller, 1999). In the case of constructs that include B- and T-helper epitopes representing rather long peptides (exceeding 20 residues) an automated solid phase synthesis or a combination of solid phase synthesis of separate immunogen fragments followed by their condensation into a single peptide in solution are preferable (Lloyd-Williams et al., 1997; Bruckdorfer et al., 2004; Mitsuaki et al., 1987; Rinnova et al., 1999). Solid phase peptide synthesis developed by Merrifield in the beginning of 1960th, now represents rather routine procedure due to numerous studies and automation of this process (Lloyd-Williams et al., 1997). The major advantage of solid phase synthesis over synthesis in solution consists in that there is no need in the purification of a resultant product after each round of peptide chain elongation. The product remains covalently bound to a polymer support up to the end of synthetic procedure, and unreacted components, activators and improper products are washed away by a solvent flow. It significantly accelerates the solid phase protein synthesis compared to the synthesis in solution (Bruckdorfer et al., 2004). Use of microwave irradiation significantly accelerates the solid phase synthesis process and increases its efficiency: synthesis of peptides of 40 residues long takes less than one day and results in good yields. It is especially useful for the synthesis of peptides, which tend to aggregate on the support (Sabatino & Papini, 2008). Of course, synthesis of each peptide requires experimental selection of the most effective protocol and initial amino acid derivatives, which allow to obtain the final product with a maximal yield (Lloyd-Williams et al., 1997). Now the most popular peptide synthesis employs amino acid derivatives protected at alpha-amino group with 9-fluorenyl(methoxycarbonyl) (FMOC). In contrast to synthesis using *tert*-butyl(oxycarbonyl)(BOC)-amino acid derivatives it does not require the use of such strong acid as HF to cleave the synthesized peptide from the support at the end of the process. FMOC-amino acids are preferably used in large-scale peptide synthesis that may yield tens and even hundred kilograms of peptides (Bruckdorfer et al., 2004). Since it is difficult to obtain long peptides (exceeding 30 residues) with good yield and separate them from contaminants differing by 1—2 residues, such peptides are synthesized as 2—3 fragments with protected side chain functional groups and then these fragments are linked together (in solution) into a single molecule (Mitsuaki et al., 1987; Rinnova et al., 1999). The same approach is used for conjugation of B-T-epitope constructions or individual epitopes with lysine dendrimers, cyclic or linear oligomer matrix structures. Methods of chemoselective cross-links used for conjugation of peptides with oligomer carriers are discussed elsewhere (Jackson et al., 2002). Non-disturbance of epitope structures during cross-linking is achieved via the introduction of additional modifiable groups or amino acid residues into synthesized peptides. Most frequently, conjugation is performed by thioalkylation (in this case cysteine residue is included into one component of the construct, whereas monochloroacetyl or maleimide group is included into another component), hydrazone or oxime formation (serine residue is included into one component, in which the CH_2OH group is oxidized to CHO by periodic acid, while monohydrazide of succinic or benzoic acid or aminooxyacetic acid residue is included into another component), and formation of thiazolidine or oxazolidine cycle (in this case the CH_2OH group of serine residue included into one component is oxidized to CHO and additional serine or cysteine residue is included into another component). In addition, some companies (e.g. Novabiochem and Bachem, both from Switzerland) produce supports for solid phase peptide synthesis with preformed lysine dendrimers, on which peptide synthesis can be performed.

3.4 Adjuvants for peptide vaccines

Formation of strong and long-term specific immune response to antigens is an important task for creation of any vaccine. It is achieved by an additional nonspecific stimulation of the immune system cells, specific targeted antigen delivery to the immunocompetent cells and their constant activation by the antigen due to its depositing and protection against protease cleavage. These functions are attributed to adjuvants (from Latin *adjuvans, adjuvantis*: aiding, helping), which are included into vaccine preparations (Aguilar & Rodriguez, 2007). In vaccines prepared from attenuated and killed infectious agents structural elements of the microorganisms such as cell walls, membranes and their components (polysaccharides, lipopolysaccharides, phospholipids, etc.) play the adjuvant role (Uchaikin & Shamsheva, 2001, Aguilar & Rodriguez, 2007). Subunit vaccines contain added adjuvants, which promote the depositing of antigens (via their adsorption) and nonspecific stimulation of the immune response (lymphocyte and macrophage attraction to the injection site due to the inflammatory reaction development); usually aluminium salts or hydroxide are used for this purpose (Aguilar & Rodriguez, 2007; Uchaikin & Shamsheva, 2001). Adjuvant selection becomes especially important during development of synthetic peptide vaccines, because peptides are usually well soluble in aqueous media, readily subjected to proteolysis and are not deposited at the administration site. Peptide constructs are targeted to the activation of immune response of a narrow specificity, and they do not provide attraction and activation of cells participating in the nonspecific immune response, which potentiate and direct the specific response. Aluminum hydroxide and salts poorly adsorb peptides, weakly activate immunocompetent cells and do not potentiate the immune response to peptide antigens (Jackson et al., 2002). Search for new adjuvants for peptide vaccines against human infectious diseases includes adjuvants approved to animal use and also immunomodulators (Aguilar & Rodriguez, 2007, Jackson et al., 2002).

Oil-based adjuvants, for example, Freund's complete adjuvant (which contains a suspension of killed *Mycobacterium tuberculosis* cells or their lipopolysaccharides in a mineral oil with lanolin) are used in laboratory studies of immunogenicity on animals for a long time. However, Freund's adjuvant is rather toxic, exhibits high reactogenicity and can induce formation of necrotic ulcers at the injection site (Allison & Byars, 1991). Now less toxic and reactogenic oil-based adjuvants (Montanide series) have been developed; they are used in some peptide vaccines that are under clinical trials (Ahmed & Maeurer, 2009; Roestenberg et al., 2008).

Saponins (e.g., QuilA, an extract from *Quillaja saponaria*, in which 23 different saponins have been identified), plant glycosides with surfactant properties, which form micelles in solution, are also used as adjuvants. QuilA is too toxic for use in humans, but its fraction QS-21, which is less toxic and induces an effective T-cell response against antigens, is considered as a prospective adjuvant for peptide vaccines (Allison & Byars, 1991; Kensil, 1996; Takahashi et al., 1990). Saponins are used as adjuvants in the immunostimulating complexes (abbreviated as ISCOMs), which represent mixed micelles of saponin and cholesterol of 40 nm in diameter where hydrophobic and amphipathic antigens are inserted. ISCOMs represent a convenient system for antigen delivery to antigen presenting cells; these particles can penetrate into such antigen-presenting cells as dendritic cells and macrophages, and hence increase the efficiency of antigen presentation (Allison & Byars, 1991; Singh et al., 2006).

Improvement in peptide antigen transport to antigen presenting cells also occurs using the polycations poly-L-lysine, poly-L-arginine and chitosan as adjuvants (Schlaphoff et al., 2007; Svirshchevskaya et al., 2009). Effectiveness of the polymeric polycation polyoxidonium (which has been shown to nonspecifically activate cell immune response (Khaitov & Pinegin, 2005)) as the adjuvant for synthetic peptide vaccines is still questionable (Olenina et al., 2003).

Currently adjuvants synthesized on the basis of pathogen-associated unique highly conserved molecular structures are widely used; they do not have analogues in macroorganisms and trigger nonspecific immune response via pattern-recognizing receptors (e.g. Toll like receptors) [Düesberg et al., 2002; Chua et al., 2007; Jackson et al., 2004]. Dipalmitoyl glyceryl-S-cysteine (Pam_2Cys) (Düesberg et al., 2002; Chua et al., 2007; Jackson et al., 2004; Deliyannis et al., 2006), a synthetic analogue of the lipid fragment of macrophage activating lipopeptide-2 isolated from *Mycoplasma fermentans* membranes (Zeng et al., 2002) is one of such structures. Pam_2Cys has been used in some candidate synthetic peptide vaccines against hepatitis C virus; these vaccines consist of cytotoxic HLA-A2-specific T-epitope of the HCV NS5B protein or of highly immunogenic hypervariable region 1 of HCV E2 envelope protein and a foreign CD4+ T-helper epitope (Engler et al., 2004; Torresi et al., 2007; Chua et al., 2008). Synthetic peptide constructs also contain the other lipid group, Pam_3Cys, which represents an N-terminal fragment of *E. coli* lipoprotein (Zeng et al., 2000; Müller et al., 2002). The immunogenic constructs based on the peptide covalently linked to Pam_3Cys induce an effective immune response after both parenteral and intranasal administration; the raised protective antibodies belong to immunoglobulin A type (Müller et al., 2002), which are important components of the mucosal immune response.

Frequently, peptide constructs containing fatty acid residues and also hydrophobic peptides are included into liposomes. Liposome-associated antigens are protected against proteolysis, they arrive directly to the antigen-presenting cells and this potentiates the immune response (Engler et al., 2004; Kaplun et al., 1999; Scheerlinck & Greenwood, 2006, 2008). Besides antigens, liposomes also contain proteins promoting liposome fusion with cell membranes, such as influenza virus hemagglutinin; such particles are known as virosomes (Kaplun et al., 1999; Scheerlinck & Greenwood, 2008). Virosomes use routes that are natural for viral particles and the antigen fragment is exposed on the surface of the antigen-presenting cells in the complex with MHC II (i.e. in the form recognized by T-helpers). Antigen incorporation into nanoparticles of 20—40 nm in size (virosomes, liposomes, ISCOMs) improves its presentation because such particles are readily absorbed by antigen-presenting dendritic cells (Jackson et al., 2004; Scheerlinck & Greenwood, 2006, 2008).

Besides liposomes and ISCOMs antigens may be also incorporated into biodegradable polymeric microspheres for storage and protection against proteolysis. Such microcapsules (size less than 10 (mu)m) that consist of polylactide, polyglycolide or their copolymer may be used for peroral antigen administration because they are insoluble in gastric juice and may provide gradual antigen release (Eldridge et al., 1991; Cox et al., 2006; Scheerlinck & Greenwood, 2006).

3.5 Evaluation of efficiency and protectivity of the immune response to synthetic peptide immunogens

Studies of peptide constructs begin with the determination of their immunogenicity (i.e. their ability to induce the immune response programmed during the design of these constructs) (Sobolev et al., 2005, Sobolev et al., 2003, Jackson et al., 2002). If a peptide immunogen includes B- and T-helper epitopes, it should induce production of antibodies against its B-epitope and also against the protein, which "borrowed" the fragment corresponding to this B-epitope; usually such experiments are performed on laboratory animals. The higher the proportion of animals developed such immune response (among total number of immunized animals) the more universal T-helper epitope included into the construct is. Immunogenicity of a mixture of peptides corresponding to cytotoxic T-epitopes is initially elucidated by appearance of cytotoxic T-lymphopcytes of a certain specificity in immunized animals (Kalyuzhny, 2005; Wulf et al., 2009). Subsequently, effectiveness of the cytotoxic immune response is evaluated in a mixed cell culture by the degree of infected cell killing by cytotoxic T-lymphocytes obtained from immunized animals or cell cultures stimulated by the investigated peptide immunogens (Lauer et al., 2004; Schlaphoff et al., 2007; Takahashi et al., 1990). Protectivity of the specific humoral response induced by peptide immunogen administration is determined by the neutralizing effect of antibodies on the penetration of an infectious agent to the target cell or by inactivation of a toxin produced by the infectious agent (Sobolev et al., 2005, Sobolev et al., 2003; Law et al., 2008). If animals are also susceptible to this disease an investigation of the protective effect of the immunization by the peptide antigen is performed on animals. Strains of small rodents are the most convenient animal models from the viewpoint of maintenance. However, there are situations when no laboratory animal is susceptible to a certain disease. In such cases severe combined immunodeficiency (SCID) mice with xenotransplanted human cells or tissues are used: in the case of malaria these are SCID mice with transplanted human erythrocytes (Badell et al., 2000), in the case of hepatitis C these are SCID mice with transplanted human hepatic tissue (Guévin et al., 2009; Zhu et al., 2006). Alternatively, researchers limit their experiments by testing protectivity of the immune response in cell cultures. For example, testing of virus neutralizing activity of antibodies produced in response to hepatitis C virus (HCV) antigens is performed in experiments by blockade of the entry of the virus or virus-like particles carrying HCV envelope proteins on their surfaces into primary hepatocytes or into hepatoma cell culture (Law et al., 2008).

It should be noted that not only the strength of the protective immune response but also its duration after the last immunogen administration is crucial. If an infectious agent exhibits high genetic variability, it is important to elucidate whether the immune response to a particular peptide immunogen is strain or isolate-specific. Only after this step of studies the synthetic peptide immunogenic construction may be submitted to preclinical and clinical trials (Rappuoli, 2001, Sobolev et al., 2005, Sobolev et al., 2003).

4. Examples of synthetic vaccines reaching stages of clinical trials

4.1 Peptide vaccines against malaria

Development of peptide vaccines against malaria started in 1970th and in spite of first unsuccessful attempts it is still considered as a perspective direction (Epstein et al., 2007). Malaria is caused by *Plasmodium* parasites, which undergo several developmental stages in the human body and each stage of its development is characterized by different protein and therefore antigenic structures. Forty perspective protective *Plasmodium* antigens have been identified and they are used for the development of various types of anti-malaria vaccines targeted to various stages of the parasite life cycle. Interest in the development of peptide vaccines is determined by genetic and therefore antigenic differences in local populations of *Plasmodium;* this does not allow to form the isolate-nonspecific protective immune response during administration of the whole infectious agent or its protein antigens than belong to one of many strains (Takala & Plowe, 2009). In addition, it is easier to develop a multiantigenic vaccine based on synthetic peptides, which would induce formation of the immune response against various stages of the parasite development (with minimal reactogenicity).

In 1980, clinical trials of the first synthetic anti-malaria vaccine Spf66 against *Pl. falciparum* in the asexual stage of development started (Urdaneta et al., 1998). This vaccine consisted of three fragments of three various surface antigens of the merozoite with the repeated PNAN fragment of sporozoite CS protein between them. However, efficiency of Spf66 in clinical trials significantly varied in dependence of geographical regions and subsequent trials were interrupted (Graves & Gelband, 2007).

Now three candidate vaccines against malaria are under various phases of clinical trials. Two of them contain long (> 70 amino acid residues) synthetic peptide immunogens inducing antibody production to two surface *Plasmodium* proteins at the shizont stage: merozoite surface protein 3 (MSP3) and glutamate rich protein (GLURP). These immunogens are MSP-3-LSP (Long synthetic protein) that represents the MSP-3 fragment including the residues 186-276 [Bouharoun-Tayoun, 1995] and GLURP-LPS that represents the GLURP fragment including the residues 85-213 (Dodoo et al., 2000; Theisen et al., 2000, 2001). These peptide immunogens were highly conservative for all plasmodium isolates; they induced formation of cytophilic antibodies of IgG1 and IgG3 subclasses; via opsonizing shizonts they attracted monocytes that caused shizont lysis (Theisen et al., 2001; Soe et al., 2004). Phase I clinical trials (Druilhe et al., 2005; Sirima et al., 2009) demonstrated formation of long (at least 1 year) immune response to these vaccines. At the moment Phase IIb clinical trial of the MSP3-LSP vaccine continues (http://www.amanet-trust.org/ext/reports /newsletters/issue23June08.pdf).

Preparations of the virosomal peptide vaccines PEV302 and PEV301 jointly developed by Swiss Tropical Institute and Pevion Biotech Ltd on the basis of fragments of the sporozoite CS protein and apical membrane antigen 1 (AMA-1) are under Phase I clinical trials (AMANET). PEV302 is a 39-mer cyclic peptide containing five highly conservative NPNA repeats of the CS protein; the peptide is conjugated with phosphatidylethanolamine and included into a phosphorlipid particle together with influenza virus hemagglutinin (Okitsu et al., 2007). PEV301 is a similar virosomal preparation that contains another (49-mer) peptide including rather conservative loop I of AMA-1 domain III, also conjugated with phosphatidylethanolamine. It was demonstrated that both peptide containing virosomal preparations induced production of antibodies inhibiting sporozoite invasion of liver cells and erythrocytes (Okitsu et al., 2007; Thompson et al., 2008).

4.2 Synthetic peptide vaccines against HCV

Hepatitis C virus (HCV) exhibits extremely high genetic variability and therefore employment of the traditional approach for vaccine development based on attenuated or inactivated virus strain is ineffective in the case of HCV (Barrett & Stanberry, 2009). This determines the need of nontraditional approaches for the development of anti-HCV vaccines, particularly, synthetic vaccines. HCV envelope proteins are characterized by high variability of their amino acid sequences and the presence of a large number of glycosyl residues similar to those present in host glycoproteins; this complicates the development of effective isolate-nonspecific neutralizing antibody production. At the same time the importance of the cytotoxic immune response in HCV eliminations in patients with spontaneous reconvalescence has been demonstrated (Freeman et al., 2003; Tester et al., 2005). It determined the interest in the development of therapeutic peptide vaccines stimulating the cytotoxic response to the virus. These candidate peptide anti-

HCV vaccines represent either a mixture of several peptides or a single multiepitope polypeptide.

4.2.1 Synthetic peptide vaccines based on CTL epitopes

IC41 is a therapeutic candidate vaccine developed by Intercell AG (Austria); it contains 5 synthetic peptides (2 fragments of the core protein, residues 23—44 and 132—140; 2 fragments of the nonstructural protein NS3, residues 1073—1081 and 1248-1261; one fragment of the NS4 protein, residues 1764—1786; all fragments are taken from HCV genotype I and numeration of amino acid residues is shown by the sequence of HCV polyprotein) and poly-L-arginine as the adjuvant stimulating penetration of the peptide antigens into cells. these peptides contain 3 T-helper epitopes (core protein, residues 23—44; NS3, residues 1248—1261; NS4, residues 1767—1786) and five HLA-A2-specific cytotoxic T-epitopes (core protein, residues 35-44 and 132—140; NS3 1073—1081; NS4, residues 1764—1772) (Schlaphoff et al., 2007). The fragments 23—44, 132—140, 1248—1261, 1764—1772 are conservative in various HCV genotypes (the identify of their sequences in the subtypes 1a, 1b, and 2 is not less than 87%) (Lauer et al., 2004). The NS3 fragment 1073—1081 differs in various HCV genotypes (the identity did not exceed 15%); however, vaccine developers used this peptide as one of effective T-epitopes typical for the HCV genotype 1a frequently detected in Europe (Firbas et al., 2006). Phase I clinical trials have shown that the IC41 vaccine induces formation of HCV-specific CD8+ T-lymphocytes in healthy patients and is well-tolerated in patients (Klade et al., 2008). In Phase II clinical trials HLA-A2 positive patients with chronic hepatitis C received 6 doses of the vaccine with a 4-week interval between doses; although the content of circulating HCV RNA was not decreased, the increase in HCV specific CD8+ specific lymphocytes was observed in 25% of patients (Lauer et al., 2004). In the other study 66% of patients with chronic hepatitis C (genotype 1) resistant to the standard therapy demonstrated a small but statistically significant decrease in HCV RNA observed 6 months after vaccination with IC41 (Klade et al., 2008).

Another CTL T-epitope-based vaccine was developed in Japan. It included a HLA-A2-restricted HCV core protein-derived 35-44 fragment as CTL T-epitope injected in an emulsion with incomplete Freund's adjuvant during Phase I clinical trial. About 25% patients (non-responders for the previous interferon plus ribavirin treatment) positively responded to vaccinations: alanine aminotransferase activity was lowered, and some patients showed the decline of viral load. However, all patients received more than 10 vaccinations, and some received even more than 50 injections of the peptide formulation (Yutani et al., 2009).

4.2.2 Virosome-based peptide vaccine

This vaccine developed by Pevion Biotech Ltd is under Phase I clinical trials. The virosome envelope consists of phospholipids with included influenza virus hemagglutinin and neuraminidase. The virosome contains a synthetic fragment of HCV core protein of 132 residues in length, which induced formation of virus specific cytotoxic T-cells producing [gamma]-interferon in HLA-A2.1 transgenic mice (Amacker et al., 2005).

4.3 Synthetic peptide vaccine against human papillloma virus, strain 16

This vaccine has been developed in the Center for Genetic Engineering and Biotechnology, Havana, Cuba, and undergoes Phase II clinical trial now. It consists of HLA-A2-restricted human papilloma virus strain 16 (HPV16) E7 T-epitope incorporated into very small size proteoliposomes. Four vaccinations with this vaccine resulted in the clearance from HPV16 in 3 out of 7 immunized patients and in complete or at least partial regression of cervical lesions caused by HPV infection (Solares et al., 2011).

4.4 Synthetic vaccine against foot-and-mouth disease

Although inactivated vaccine against foot-and-mouth disease (FMD) may effectively protect animals it has some serious drawbacks such as: a) slow formation of the immune response and existing risk of viral infection of vaccinated animals before the development of the adaptive immune response; b) appearance of virus carriers even after successful vaccination; c) difficulties with discrimination of vaccinated animals from convalescence and infected animals (Barrett & Stanberry, 2009).

During many years researchers try to develop alternative vaccines against FMD virus. Synthetic peptide vaccines based on the VP1 peptide fragments 135—160 and 200-213 containing virus neutralizing B-epitopes (Strohmaier et al., 1982) and the fragments of the same protein 20—41 and 170—189 containing T-helper epitopes (Collen et al., 1991; Volpina et al., 1993) are considered as possible variants. A synthetic vaccine based on the VP1 protein fragment 135—159 (FMD virus, strain 22) has been developed in M. M. Shemyakin and Yu. A. Ovchinnikov Institute of Biooeganic Chemistry (Russian Academy of Sciences); this vaccine provided antiviral protection within one year after a single immunization (Volpina et al., 1993, 1999). It is the only synthetic peptide vaccine approved in Russia for the use in veterinary (Volpina et al., 1999).

4.5 Dendrimeric peptide vaccine against swine fever virus

Three dendrimeric peptide constructs were prepared from three different fragments of the classical swine fever virus (CSFV) envelope protein E2 (as B-epitopes) and T helper epitope from the NS3 protein of the same virus (Tarradas et al., 2011). Each dendrimer contained four copies of one of the putative B-epitopes linked to the T-epitope. Intramuscular injections with these dendrimers significally reduced the pig lethality after the challenge with the lethal dose of CSFV though no netralizing antibodies were detected in animal blood.

5. Examples of peptide immunogens under current successful development

5.1 Peptide immunogens for universal anti-flu vaccines

Current influenza vaccines protect mostly against homologous virus strains. However, while facing the danger of new pandemics expected from the transmittance of mutated bird and swine flu viruses to humans, the development of a broadly protective anti-flu vaccine is of great importance. Several groups succeeded in preparing conserved synthetic peptide immunogens derived from hemagglutinin and matrix M2 protein of the influenza virus. These fragments were shown to be conserved in various virus strains. Corresponding synthetic peptides conjugated with carrier protein keyhole limpet hemocyanin were able to elicit broadly specific immune response in mice and protect them from the influenza infection caused by different virus strains (Stanekova et al., 2011; Wang et al., 2010).

5.2 Peptide immunogens for anti-HCV vaccines under development

Antibodies protective against HCV infection should attack HCV envelope proteins, since these proteins are responsible for targeting the virus into the host cells, where its replication occurs (Gal-Tanamy et al., 2009; Voisset & Dubuisson, 2004). However, HCV envelope proteins demonstrate the highest sequence variability, with regard to HCV genetic variants, among all viral proteins (Sobolev et al., 2000). Though the immunization with the full-size HCV envelope proteins can elicit virus-neutralizing antibodies, these antibodies are specific to certain HCV genetic variants, relative to the one, from which the envelope proteins used for immunization, are taken (Elmowalid et al., 2007; Alvarez-Lajonchere et al., 2009). Several highly conserved sites were determined in HCV envelope proteins E1 and E2 (Sobolev et al, 2000); however, most these sites did not elicit specific antibodies because of insufficient T-lymphocyte help resulting from the absence of T-helper epitopes in the vicinity. Conjugation of putative B-epitopes, derived from HCV envelope proteins, to promiscuous T-helper epitopes from other sources (Torresi et al., 2007) or to the carrier protein, keyhole limpet hemocyanin (El Awady et al., 2010; El Abd et al., 2011), resulted in the formation of immunogens capable of producing antibodies specific for the whole HCV envelope proteins and viral particles. However, the use of foreign T-epitopes and carrier proteins leads to the formation of T helper memory cells that are non-specific for HCV and hence, will not be activated upon HCV infection.

We performed a search for putative T-helper epitope motifs in HCV envelope proteins with the help of SYFPEITHI Database and detected several conserved fragments that contain a number of such motifs of different specificity with regard to HLA allele products. Hence these fragments can be considered as broadly specific T helper epitopes. Several artificial peptide constructs were made on the basis of one such E2 protein fragment (CR2; fragment designation here and in the table 1 in accordance with Sobolev et al., 2000) and three fragments from the same protein, shown to be responsible for the interaction of HCV with heparan-sulphates (Olenina et al., 2005). These artificial constructs were synthesized and tested for their immunogenicity on rats (table 1). The constructs were shown to be highly immunogenic in the absence of any carrier besides Freund's adjuvant and able to elicit antibodies that interacted with full-size envelope proteins. The mixture of all six constructs showed the comparable immunogenicity and enhanced ability in eliciting anti-E2 antibodies. Five out of six constructs as well as the mixture of constructs elicited antibodies capable of binding HCV from patient plasma(fig. 1) (Kolesanova et al., 2011).

5.3 Other important examples of peptide immunogens

An interesting example of the peptide immunogen has been developed for the candidate anti-anthrax vaccine. The current vaccines for anthrax though being efficient, require extensive immunization protocols, and one of the reasons for it is the absence of antibodies against the linear determinant in domain 2 of *Bacillus anthracis* protective antigen. Two multiple antigenic peptides composed of the fragment 304-319 (loop-neutralizing determinant) of *B. anthracis* protective antigen and a promiscuous T-helper epiope from *Pl.*

Peptide	Antibody titer*		
	Against peptide	Against E2 protein	Against E1E2 heterodimer
CR2-linker-CR3	1:32000	1:50-1:100 (3)	1:50-1:100 (3)
CR3-linker-CR2	1:8100	1:50-1:100 (3)	1:50-1:100 (3)
PRR1-linker-CR2	1:900	1:50 (1)	1:50 (1)
CR2-linker-PRR1	1:9200	1:50(2)	1:50(2)
CHR-linker-CR2	1:5600	1:50 (2)	1:50 (2)
CR2-linker CHR	1:2700	1:50 (1)	1:50 (1)
Mixture of 6	1:2000-1:24000 depending on peptide	1:150 (3)	1:100 (3)

* Numbers in brackets show the number of animal antisera samples containing corresponding antibodies. Number of rats in experimental groups – 5; the group immunized with mixture of the constructs consisted of 4 species.

Table 1. Artificial peptide constructs made from E2 HCV protein fragments and their immunogenicity testing results.

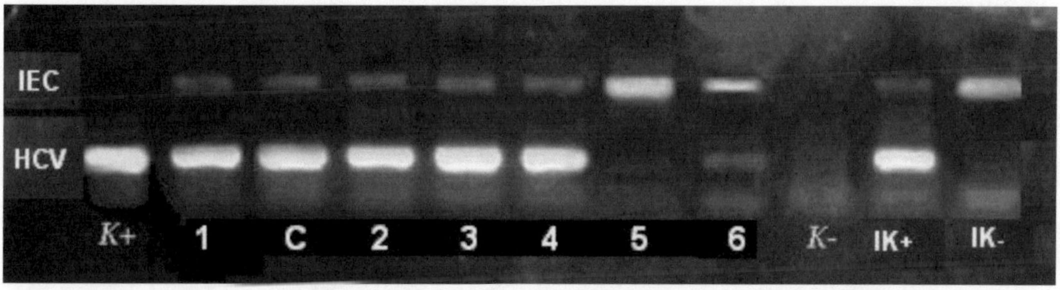

Fig. 1. HCV binding to antibodies elicited by artificial peptide constructs made from envelope protein E2 conserved fragments – PCR detection. Numbers in the line below designate the number of the construct used for the immunization (see table 1), C – mixture of all 6 constructs. K+ and K- - positive and negative control probes; IK+ and IK- - positive and negative internal controls; IEC – internal experiment control PCR product; HCV – HCV-derived PCR product.

falciparum were prepared with the B-T or T-B order of epitope determinants. Rabbits immunized with both constructs were efficiently protected from the lethal infection caused by aerosolized spores of B. anthracis. (Oscherwitz et al., 2010).

Peptide immunogens are also of interest as immunogens for anti-allergic vaccines. Since the aim of these vaccine preparation is to elicit antibodies that bind and clear off allergens from blood for preventing an allergic reaction, full-size allergen molecules can hardly be applied as immunogens. Allergen-derived epitope structures devoid of determinants responsible for causing allergic reactions are used instead. The development of the peptide immunotherapy peptide-based vaccine for cat allergy can be considered as one of such examples (Worm et al., 2011). Several peptides derived form the cat allergen Fel d1 that were identified as T-helper lymphocyte-stimulating molecules and synthesized, were safe and well tolerated in human volunteers. This vaccine was efficient in very small doses (3 nmols) and did not cause any allergic reactions that are caused by the full-size allergen molecule. Hence these peptide immunogens and the methodological basis for their development can be further used for the preparation of anti-allergic vaccines of other kinds.

6. Conclusions

Now there is a good background for the selection of immunogens targeted to those immune processes, which should be triggered by future vaccines. However, at the moment all known synthetic peptide vaccines against agents causing infectious diseases in man are at various stages of clinical trials (http://clinicaltrials.gov/ct2/results?term=vaccine). This situation is associated with the following circumstances: difficulties in reproduction of native conformation of protein antigenic sites, some B-cell epitopes recognized by neutralizing antibodies are discontinuous rather than linear ones; peptides are easily subjected to proteolysis. Peptides themselves are weakly immunogenic and such vaccine requires careful selection of an adjuvant. In the case of peptide vaccines salts and aluminum hydroxide, the adjuvants approved in all countries, are ineffective, whereas more effective adjuvants (for peptides) are not approved for clinical application in humans in most countries (e.g. they are forbidden for human use in the USA (Common Ingredients in U.S. Licensed Vaccines)). Nevertheless, deeper knowledge on structures of antigens of infectious agents, mechanisms of immune response formation, development of technologies for large-scale synthesis of long peptides, preparation of stabilized nanoparticles and the development of effective and safe adjuvants give hope that the effective peptide vaccines will be developed in the future.

7. Acknowledgements

The work on this chapter was supported with RFBR grant No. 09-04-12117 and the Federal program "Research and development on priority directions in scientific and technological complex of Russia in 2007-2012" contract No. 16.512.11.2069 (theme No. 2011-1.2-512-017-031).

8. References

Abbas, A.K. & Lichtman, A.H. (2011). *Basic Immunology: Functions and Disorders of the Immune System.* Saunders/Elsevier, ISBN 978-1-4160-5569-3, Philadelphia, PA, USA.

Aguilar, J.C. & Rodriguez, E.G. (2007) Vaccine Adjuvants Revisited. *Vaccine,* Vol. 25, No.19 (May 10, 2007), pp. 3752-3762, ISSN 0264-410X.

Ahmed, R.K. & Maeurer, M.J., (2009). T-Cell Epitope Mapping. In: *Methods Mol. Biol.,* Vol. 524, No. 4. *Epitope Mapping Protocols,* M. Schutkowski & Reineke, U. (Eds.), pp. 427-438, Humana Press, ISBN 978-1-59745-450-6_32.

Allison, A.C. & Byars, N.E. (1991) Immunological Adjuvants: Desirable Properties and Side-Effects. *Mol. Immunol.*, Vol. 28, No.3 (March 1991), pp. 279-284, ISSN 0161-5890.

Alvarez-Lajonchere, L., Shoukry, N. H., Gra, B., Amador-Canizares, Y., Helle, F., Bedard, N., Guerra, I., Drouin, C., Dubuisson, J., Gonzalez-Horta, E. E., Martınez, G., Marante, J., Cinza, Z., Castellanos, M. & Duenas-Carrera, S. (2009). Immunogenicity of CIGB-230, a Therapeutic DNA Vaccine Preparation, in HCV-Chronically Infected Individuals in a Phase I Clinical Trial. *J. Viral Hepat.*, 16, No. 2, (March 2009), pp.156-167, ISSN 1352-0504.

Amacker, M., Engler, O., Kammer, A.R., Vadrucci, S., Oberholzer, D., Cerny, A., & Zurbriggen, R., (2005) Peptide-Loaded Chimeric Influenza Virosomes for Efficient In Vivo Induction of Cytotoxic T Cells. *Int. Immunol.*, Vol. 17, No. 6, (June 2005), pp. 695-704, ISSN 0953-8178.

AMANET Launches Large-Scale Testing of Candidate Malaria Vaccine MSP3-LSP in Mali. Available at:
http://www.amanet-trust.org/ext/reports/newsletters/issue23June08.pdf

Badell, E., Oeuvray, C., Moreno, A., Soe, S., van Rooijen, N., & Bouzidi, A. (2000). Human Malaria in Immunocompromized Mice. An in Vivo Model to Study Defense Mechanisms against *Plasmodium falciparum*. *J. Exp. Med.*, Vol. 192, No. 11, (December 4, 2000), pp. 1653-1660, ISSN 0022-1007.

Barocchi, M.A., Censini, S., & Rappuoli, R. (2007) Vaccines in the Era of Genomics: the Pneumococcal Challenge. *Vaccine*, Vol. 25, No. 16 (April 20, 2007), pp. 2963-2973, ISSN: 0264-410X.

Barrett, A.D.T. & Stanberry, L.R. (Eds.). (2009). *Vaccines for Biodefense and Emerging and Neglected Diseases*, Elsevier Inc., ISBN 978-0-3-69408-9.

Ben-Yedidia, T. and Arnon, R., (1997) Design of Peptide and Polypeptide Vaccines. *Curr. Opin. Biotechnol.*, Vol. 8, No.4 (August, 1997), pp. 442-448, ISSN 0958-1669.

Bermúdes, A., Reyes, C., Guzmán, F., Vanegas, M., Rosas, J., Amador, R., Rodríguez, R., Patarroyo, M.A., & Patarroyo, M.E. (2007). Synthetic Vaccine Update: Applying Lessons Learned from Recent SPf66 Malarial Vaccine Physicochemical, Structural and Immunological Characterization. *Vaccine*, Vol. 25, No. 22 (May 30, 2007), pp. 4487-4501, ISSN: 0264-410X.

Bijker, M.S., Melief, C.J., Offringa, R., and van der Burg, S.H., (2007) Design and Development of Synthetic Peptide Vaccines: Past, Present and Future. *Expert Rev. Vaccines*, Vol. 6, No.4 (August, 2007), pp. 591-603, ISSN 1476-0584.

Bongartz, J., Bruni, N., & Or-Guil, M. (2009). Epitope Mapping Using Randomly Generated Peptide Libraries. In: *Methods Mol. Biol.*, Vol. 524, No. 4. *Epitope Mapping Protocols*, M. Schutkowski & Reineke, U. (Eds.), pp. 237-246, Humana Press, ISBN 978-1-59745-450-6_32.

Bouharoun-Tayoun, H., Oeuvray, C., Lunel, F., & Druilhe, P. (1995). Mechanisms Underlying the Monocyte-Mediated Antibody-Dependent Killing of *Plasmodium falciparum* Asexual Blood Stages. *J. Exp. Med.*, Vol. 182, No. 2, (August 1, 1995), pp. 409-418, ISSN 0022-1007.

Bruckdorfer, T, Marder, O., & Albericio, F. (2004). From Production of Peptides in Milligram Amounts for Research to Multi-tons Quantities for Drugs of the Future. *Curr. Pharm. Biotechnol.*, Vol. 5, No. 1, (February 2004), pp. 29-43.

van der Burg, S.H., Bijker, M.S., Welters, M.J., Offringa, R., & Melief, C.J. (2006) Improved Peptide Vaccine Strategies, Creating Synthetic Artificial Infections to Maximize Immune Efficacy. *Adv. Drug. Deliv. Rev.*, Vol. 58, No.8, (October 1, 2006), pp. 916-930, ISSN 0169-409X.

Castric, P.A. & Cassels, F.J. (1997) Peptide Epitope Mapping in Vaccines. *J. Ind. Microbiol. Biotechnol.*, Vol. 19, No.1 (July 1997), pp. 56-57.

Chua, B.Y., Eriksson, E.M., Brown, L.E., Zeng, W., Gowans, E.J., Torresi, J., & Jackson, D.C. (2008). A Self-Adjuvanting Lipopeptide-Based Vaccine Candidate for the Treatment of Hepatitis C Virus Infection. *Vaccine*, Vol. 26, No.31, (September 2, 2008), pp. 4866-4875, ISSN 0264-410X.

Chua, B.Y., Zeng, W., Lau, Y.F., & Jackson, D.C. (2007) Comparison of Lipopeptide-Based Immunocontraceptive Vaccines Containing Different Lipid Groups. *Vaccine,* Vol. 25, No. 1 (January 2, 2007), pp. 92-101, ISSN 0264-410X.

Collen, T., Dimarchi, D., & Doel, T.R. (1991) A T Cell Epitope in VP1 of Foot-and-Mouth Disease Virus is Immunodominant for Vaccinated Cattle. *J. Immunol.*, Vol. 146, No. 2 (January 15, 1991), pp. 749-755, ISSN 0022-1767.

Common Ingredients in U.S. Licensed Vaccines. (July, 2011). In: Vaccine Safety & Availability, 7.07.2011, Available from http://www.fda.gov/BiologicsBloodVaccines/SafetyAvailability/VaccineSafety/ucm187810.htm.

Cox, E., Verdonck, F., Vanrompay, D., & Goddeeris, B. (2006). Adjuvants Modulating Mucosal Immune Responses or Directing Systemic Responses towards the Mucosa. *Vet. Res.*, Vol. 37, No. 3, (May-June 2006), pp. 511-539, ISSN 0928-4249.

Deliyannis, G., Kedzierska, K., Lau, Y.F., Zeng, W., Turner, S.J., & Jackson, D.C. (2006) Intranasal Lipopeptide Primes Lung-Resident Memory CD8+ T Cells for Long-Term Pulmonary Protection against Influenza. *Eur. J. Immunol.*, Vol. 36, No. 3 (March, 2006), pp. 770-778, ISSN 0014-2980.

Dodoo, D., Theisen, M., Kurtzhals, J.A., Akanmori, B.D., Koram, K.A., Jepsen, S., Nkrumah, F.K., Theander, T.G. & Hviid, L. (2000). Naturally Acquired Antibodies to the Glutamate-Rich Protein are Associated with Protection against *Plasmodium falciparum* Malaria. *J. Infect. Dis.,*@ 2000, vol. 181, pp. 1202-1205, ISSN 0022-1899.

Druilhe, P., Spertini, F., Soesoe, D., Corradin, G., Mejia, P., Singh, S., Audran, R., Bouzidi, A., Oeuvray, C., & Roussilhon, C. (2005). A Malaria Vaccine that Elicits in Humans Antibodies Able to Kill *Plasmodium falciparum*. *PLoS Med.*, Vol. 2, No. 11, e344 . Available at http://www.plosmedicine.org/article/info%3Adoi%2F10.1371%2Fjournal.pmed.0020344.

Düesberg, U., von dem Bussche, A., Kirschning, C., Miyake, K., Sauerbruch, T., & Spengler, U. (2002). Cell Activation by Synthetic Lipopeptides of the Hepatitis C Virus (HCV)–Core Protein Is Mediated by Toll Like Receptors (TLRs). *Immunol. Lett.*, Vol. 84, No.2 (December 1, 2002), pp. 89-95, ISSN 0165-2478.

El Abd, Y.S., Tabll, A.A., Bader El Din, N.G., Hosny, A.E., Moustafa, R.I., El-Shenawy, R., Atef, K. & El-Awady, M.K. (2011). Neutralizing Activities of Caprine Antibodies towards Conserved Regions of the HCV Envelope Glycoprotein E2. *Virol. J.*, Vol. 8, No. 1, (August 5, 2011), p.391, ISSN 1743-422X.

El-Awady, M.K., Tabll, A.A., Yousif, H., El-Abd, Y., Reda, M., Khalil, S.B., El-Zayadi, A.R., Shaker, M.H. & Bader El Din, N.G. (2010). Murine Neutralizing Antibody Response and Toxicity to Synthetic Peptides Derived from E1 and E2 Proteins of Hepatitis C Virus. *Vacc ine,* Vol. 28, No. 52 (December, 6, 2010), pp. 8338-8344, ISSN 0264-410X.

Eldridge, J.H., Staas, J.K., Meulbroek, J.A., Tice, T.R., & Gilley, R.M. (1991). Biodegradable and Biocompatible Poly(DL-Lactide-co-Glycolide) Aicrospheres as an Adjuvant for Staphylococcal Enterotoxin B Toxoid which Enhances the Level of Toxin-Neutralizing Antibodies. *Infect. Immun.*, Vol. 59, No. 9, (September 1991), pp. 2978-2983, ISSN 0019-9567.

Elmowalid, G.A., Qiao, M., Jeong, S.H., Borg, B.B., Baumert, T.F., Sapp, R.K., Hu, Z., Murthy, K., Liang, T.J. (2007). Immunization with Hepatitis C Virus-Like Particles Results in Control of Hepatitis C Virus Infection in Chimpanzees. Proc. Natl. Acad. Sci. USA, Vol. 104, No. 20, (May 15, 2007), pp.8427-8432, ISSN 0027-8424.

Engler, O.B., Schwendener, R.A., Dai, W.J., W@lk, B., Pichler, W., Moradpour, D., Brunner, T., & Cerny, A. (2004). A Liposomal Peptide Vaccine Inducing CD8+ Cells in HLA-A2.1 Transgenic Mice, which Recognise Human Cells Encoding hepatitis C Virus (HCV) Proteins. *Vaccine,* Vol. 23, No. 1, (November 15, 2004), pp. 58-68, ISSN 0264-410X.

Epstein, J.E., Giersing, B., Mullen, G., Moorthy, V., & Richie, T.L.,(2007) Malaria Vaccines: Are We Getting Closer? *Curr. Opin. Mol. Ther.*, Vol. 9, No. 1, (February 2007), pp. 12-24, ISSN 1464-8431.

Firbas, C., Jilma, B., Tauber, E., Buerger, V., Jelovcan, S., & Lingnau, K., Buschle, M., Frisch, J., Klade, C.S. (2006) Immunogenicity and Safety of a Novel Therapeutic Hepatitis C Virus (HCV) Peptide Vaccine: a Randomized, Placebo Controlled Trial for Dose Optimization in 128 Healthy Subjects. *Vaccine,* Vol. 24, No. 20, (May 15, 2006), pp. 4343-4353, ISSN 0264-410X.

Felgner, P.L., Kayala, M.A., Vigil, A., Burk, C., Nakajima-Sasaki, R., Pablo, J., Molina, D.M., Hirst, S., Chew ,J.S.W., Wang, D., Tan, G., Duffield, M., Yang, R., Neel, J., Chantratita, N., Bancroft, G., Lertmemongkolchai, G., Davies, D.H., Baldi, P., Peacock, S., & Titball, R.W. (2009) A *Burkholderia pseudomallei* Protein Microarray Reveals Serodiagnostic and Cross-Reactive Antigens. *Proc. Natl. Acad. Sci. USA,* Vol. 106, No.32, (August 11, 2009), pp. 13499-13504, ISSN 0027-8424.

Freeman, A.J., Pan, Y., Harvey, C.E., Post, J.J., Law, M.G., White, P.A., Rawlinson, W.D., Lloyd, A.R., Marinos, G. & French, R.A. (2003). The Presence of an Intrahepatic Cytotoxic T Lymphocyte Response is Associated with Low Viral Load in Patients with Chronic Hepatitis C Virus Infection.*J. Hepatol.,* Vol. 38, No. 3, (March 2003), pp.349-356, ISSN 0168-8278.

Fritzer, A., Senn, B.M., Minh, D.B., Hanner, M., Gelbmann, D., Noiges, B., Henics, T., Schulze, K., Guzman, C.A., Goodacre, J., von Gabain, A., Nagy, E. & Meinke, A.L. (2010) Novel Conserved Group A Streptococcal Proteins Identified by the

Antigenome Technology as Vaccine Candidates for a non-M Protein-Based Vaccine. *Infect Immun.*, Vol.78, No.9, (September, 2010), pp. 4051-4067, ISSN 1098-5522.

Gal-Tanamy M., Walker C., Foung S., Lemon S.M. (2009). Hepatitis C. In: *Vaccines for Biodefence and Emerging and Neglected Diseases,* A.T. Barrett and L.R. Stanberry (Eds.). Academic Press, London-Amsterdam-Burlington-San Diego, pp. 413-440, ISBN 978-0-3-69408-9.

Garg, A.D, Nowis, D., Golab, J., Vandenabeele, P., Krysko, D.V., & Agostinis, P. (2010) Immunogenic cell death, DAMPs and anticancer therapeutics: an emerging amalgamation. *Biochim Biophys Acta,* Vol.1805, No.1 (January, 2010), pp.53-71, ISSN 0304-419X.

Glowalla, E., Tosetti, B., Krönke, M., & Krut, O. (2009) Proteomics-Based Identification of Anchorless Cell Wall Proteins as Vaccine Candidates against *Staphyllococcus aureus. Infect. Immun.*, Vol. 77, No. 7, (July, 2009), pp. 2719-2729, ISSN 1098-5522.

Graves, P. & Gelband, H. (2007). Vaccines for Preventing Malaria. *Cochrane Database Sys. Rev.*, No. 4, July 18, 2007. Available at http://onlinelibrary.wiley.com/doi/10.1002/14651858.CD000129.pub2/pdf.

Guévin, C., Lamarre, A., & Labonté, P. (2009). Novel HCV Replication Mouse Model Using Human Hepatocellular Carcinoma Xenografts.*Antiviral Res.,* Vol. 84, No. 1, (October 2009), @ 2009, pp. 14-22, ISSN 0166-3542.

Haro, I., Pérez, S., García, M., Chan, W.C., Ercilla, G. (2003). Liposome Entrapment and Immunogenic Studies of a Synthetic Lipophilic Multiple Antigenic Peptide Bearing VP1 and VP3 Domains of the Hepatitis A Virus: a Robust Method for Vaccine Design. *FEBS Lett.*, Vol. 540, No. 1-3, (April 10, 2003), pp. 133-140, ISSN .

He, Y., Rappuoli, R., De Groot, A.S. & Chen, R.T. (2010). Emerging Vaccine Informatics. *J. Biomed. Biotechnol.*, 2010; 2010: 218590 (June 15, 2011), ISSN 1110-7251.

Jackson, D.C., Lau, Y.F., Le, T., Suhrbier, A., Deliyannis, G., & Cheers, C. (2004). A Totally Synthetic Vaccine of Generic Structure that Targets Toll-Like Receptor 2 on Dendritic Cells and Promotes Antibody or Cytotoxic T Cell Responses. *Proc. Natl. Acad. Sci. USA,* Vol. 101, No. 43 (October 26, 2004), pp. 15440-15445, ISSN 0027-8424.

Jackson, D.C., Purcell, A.W., Fitzmaurice, C.J., Zeng, W., & Hart, D.N. (2002) The Central Role Played by Peptides in the Immune Response and the Design of Peptide-Based Vaccines against Infectious Diseases and Cancer. *Curr. Drug Targets,* Vol. 3, No.2, (April 2002), pp. 175-196, ISSN 1389-4501.

Kalyuzhny, A.E., (Ed.). (2005) *Handbook of ELISPOT. Methods and Protocols,* Humana Press, ISBN 978-1-58829-469-2.

Kaplun, A.P., Le Bang Shon, Krasnopolskii, Yu.M., & Shvets, V.I. (1999). Liposomes and Other Nanoparticles as Drug Delivery Means. *Vopr. Med. Khim.,* Vol. 45, No. 1, pp. 3-12, ISSN 0042-8809.

Khaitov, R.M. & Pinegin, B.V. (2005). Modern Views on the Polyoxidonium Mechanism of Action. *Immunologiya,* No. 4, (April 2005), pp. 197-205.

Kensil, C.R. (1996). Saponins as Vaccine Adjuvants. *Crit. Rev. Ther. Drug. Carrier. Syst.*, Vol. 13, No. 1-2, pp. 1-55, ISSN 0743-4863.

Klade, C.S. (2002) Proteomics Approaches towards Antigen Discovery and Vaccine Development. *Curr. Opin. Mol. Ther.*, Vol. 4, No. 3, (June, 2002), pp. 216-223, ISSN 1464-8431.

Klade, C.S., Wedemeyer, H., Berg, T., Hinrichsen, H., Cholewinska, G., Zeuzem, S., Blum, H., Buschle, M., Jelovcan, .S, Buerger, V., Tauber, E., Frisch, J., Manns, M.P. (2008) Therapeutic Vaccination of Chronic Hepatitis C Nonresponder Patients with the Peptide Vaccine IC41. *Gastroenterology*, Vol. 134, No. 5, (May 2008), pp. 1385-1395, ISSN 0016-5085.

Kolesanova, E.F., Farafonova, T.E., Moisa, A.A., Aleshina, E.Yu., Pyndyk, N.V., Sobolev, B.N. & Archakov, A.I. (2011). Development of Peptide Immunogens for Anti-HCV Vaccine. In: *Peptide Science 2010*, N. Fujii & Y. Kiso (Eds.), p.33, The Japanese Peptide Society, Osaka, ISBN 978-4-931541-11-5.

Kupriianova, M.A., Zhmak, M.N., Koroev, D.O., Chepurkin, A.V., Volpina, O.M., & Ivanov, V.T. (2000). Synthetic Peptide Designs Based on Immunoactive Fragments of the VP1 Protein of the Foot-and-Mouth Disease Virus Strain A22. *Bioorgan. Khim. (Russ.)*, Vol. 26, No.12 (December 2000), pp. 926-933.

Kuzmina, T.I., Olenina L.V., Sanzhakov, M.A., Farafonova, T.E., Abramikhina, T.V., Dubuisson, J., Sobolev, B.N., & Kolesanova, E.F. (2009). Antigenicity and B-Epitope Mapping of hepatitis C Virus Envelope Protein E2. *Biochemistry (Moscow) Supplement Series B: Biomedical Chemistry*, Vol. 3, No. 2, pp. 177–182, ISSN 1990-7508.

Lauer, G.M., Barnes, E., Lucas, M., Timm, J., Ouchi, K., Kim, A.Y., Day, C.L., Robbins, G.K., Casson, D.R., Reiser, M., Dusheiko, G., Allen, T.M., Chung, R.T., Walker, B.D., & Klenerman, P., (2004). High Resolution Analysis of Cellular Immune Responses in Resolved and Persistent Hepatitis C Virus Infection. *Gastroenterology*, Vol. 27, No. 3 (September, 2004), pp. 924-936, ISSN 0016-5085.

Law, M., Maruyama, T., Lewis, J., Giang, E., Tarr, A.W., Stamataki, Z., Gastaminza, P., Chisari, F.V., Jones, I.M., Fox, R.I., Ball, J.K., McKeating, J.A., Knellerman, N.M. & Burton, D.R. (2008). Broadly Neutralizing Antibodies Protect against Hepatitis C Virus Quasispecies Challenge. *Nat Med.*, Vol. 14, No. 1, (January 14, 2008), pp. 25-27, ISSN 1078-8956.

Liljeqvist, S. & Stahl, S.J. (1999).Recombinant Subunit Vaccines: Protein Immunogens, Live Delivery Systems or Nucleic Acid Vaccines. *J. Biotechnol.*, Vol.73, No.1, pp.1-33, ISSN 0168-1656.

Lin, H.H., Zhang, G.L., Tongchusak, S., Reinherz, E.L., & Brusic, V. (2008) Evaluation of MHC-II Peptide Binding Prediction Servers: Applications for Vaccine Research. *BMC Immunol.*, Vol. 9, No.8, (March 16, 2008), ISSN 1471-2172. Available at: http://www.biomedcentral.com/1471-2172/9/8.

Ling, E., Feldman, G., Portnoi, M., Dagan, R., Overweg, K., Mulholland, F., Chalifa-Caspi, V., Wells, J., & Mizrachi-Nebenzahl, Y. (2004). Glycolytic Enzymes Associated with the Cell Surface of *Streptococcus pneumoniae* are Antigenic in Humans and Elicit Protective Immune Responses in the Mouse. *Clin. Exp. Immunol.*, Vol. 138, No. 2, (November, 2004), pp. 290-298, ISSN 0009-9104.

Lloyd-Williams, P., Albericio, F., & Giralt, E. (1997). *Chemical Approaches to the Synthesis of Peptides and Proteins*, CRC Press LLC, New York, ISBN 978-0-84939-142-2.

Lu, X., DeFelippis, M.R., & Huang, L. (2009). Linear Epitope Mapping by Native Mass Spectrometry. *Anal. Biochem.,* Vol. 395, No.1 (December 1, 2009), pp. 100-107, ISSN 0003-2697.

Machiels, J.P., van Baren, N., and Marchand, M.(2002). Peptide-Based Cancer Vaccines. *Semin Oncol.,* Vol. 29, No.5 (October, 2002), pp. 494-502, ISSN 0093-7754.

MacNamara, A., Kadolsky, U., Bangham, C.R., & Asquith, B. (2009). T-cell Epitope Prediction: Rescaling Can Mask Biological Variation between MHC Molecules. *PLoS Comput. Biol.,* Vol. 5, No. 3, (March 2009), e1000327, eISSN 1553-7358.

Mäkelä, P.H. (2000) Vaccines, Coming of Age after 200 Years. FEMS Microbiol. Rev., Vol. 24, No. 1 (January, 2000), pp. 9-20, ISSN 0168-6445.

Male, D., Brostoff, J., Roth, D. & Roitt, I. (2006). *Immunology 7th Edition,* MOSBY Elsevier, ISBN 978-0-323-05448-5.

Målen, H., Søfterland, T., & Wiker, H.G. (2008). Antigen Analysis of *Mycobacterium tuberculosis* H37Rv Culture Filtrate Proteins. *Scand. J. Immunol.,* Vol. 67, No. 3, (March, 2008), pp. 245-252, ISSN 0300-9475.

Meinke, A., Henics, T., Hanner, M., Minh, D.B., & Nagy, E. (2005) Antigenome Technology: a Novel Approach for the Selection of Bacterial Vaccine Candidate Antigens. *Vaccine,*Vol. 23, No. 17-18, (March 18, 2005), pp. 2035-2041, ISSN: 0264-410X.

Mitsuaki, N., Shizuko, I., Satoshi, N., & Takuya, I. (1987). Peptide Synthesis by Fragment Condensation on a Soluble Polymer Support. 8. Maximum Peptide Chain Lengths of Carboxyl Component Peptides for Effective Coupling Reactions with Amino Component Peptides Anchored to Soluble and Cross-Linked Polystyrene Supports. *Macromolecules,* vol. 20, No.9, (September 1987), pp. 2306-2307, ISSN 0024-9297.

Moss, C.X., Tree, T.I., & Watts, C. (2007). Reconstruction of a Pathway of Antigen Processing and Class II MHC Peptide Capture. *EMBO J.,* Vol. 26, No.8, (April 18, 2007), pp. 2137-2147, ISSN 0261-4189.

Muhlradt, P.F., Kiess, M., Meyer, H., Sussmuth, R., & Jung, G.J. (1997) Isolation, Structure Elucidation, and Synthesis of a Macrophage Stimulatory Lipopeptide from *Mycoplasma fermentans* Acting at Picomolar Concentration. *J. Exp. Med.,* Vol. 185, No. 11, (June 2, 1997), pp. 1951-1958, ISSN 0022-1007.

Müller, M.R., Wiesmüller, K.H., Jung, G., Loop, T., Humar, M., Pfannes, S.D., Bessler, W.G., Mittenbühler, K. (2002). Lipopeptide Adjuvants: Monitoring and Comparison of P3CSK4- and LPS-induced Gene Transcription. *Int. Immunopharmacol.,* Vol. 2, No.8, (July 2002), pp. 1065-1077, ISSN 1567-5769.

Okitsu, S.L., Kienzl, U., Moehle, K., Silvie, O., Peduzzi, E., Mueller, M.S., Sauerwein, R.W., Matile, H., Zurbriggen, R., Mazier, D., Robinson, J.A., & Pluschke, G. (2007) Structure-Activity-Based Design of a Synthetic Malaria Peptide Eliciting Sporozoite Inhibitory Antibodies in a Virosomal Formulation. *Chem. Biol.,* Vol. 14, No. 5 (May 2007), pp. 577-587, ISSN 1074-5521.

Olenina, L.V., Nikolaeva, L.I., Sobolev, B.N., Blokhina, N.P., Archakov, A.I., & Kolesanova, E.F. (2002) Mapping and Characterization of B Cell Linear Epitopes in the Conservative Regions of Hepatitis C Virus Envelope Glycoproteins. *J. Viral Hepat.,* Vol. 9, No.3, (May 2002), pp. 174-182, ISSN 1352-0504.

Olenina, L.V., Kuzmina, T.I., Kuraeva, T.E., Sobolev, B.N., Kolesanova, E.F. & Archakov, A.I. (2003). Development of Laboratory Experimental Samples of Artificial Vaccine against Hepatitis C Virus. Immunogenicity of Highly Conserved Envelope Protein E2 Sites in Synthetic Constructs. *Novosti nauki i tehniki. Ser. Meditsina. Allergiya, astma i klinicheskaya immunologiya*, No. 9, pp. 51-53.

Olenina, L.V., Kuzmina, T.I., Sobolev, B.N., Kuraeva, T.E., Kolesanova, E.F. & Archakov, A.I. (2005). Identification of Glycosaminoglycan-Binding Sites within Hepatitis C Virus Envelope Glycoprotein E2. *J. Viral Hepat.*, Vol. 12, No. 6, (Novemder 2005), pp. 584-593, ISSN 1352-0504.

Palena, C., Abrams, S.I., Schlom, J., & Hodge, J.W. (2006). Cancer Vaccines: Preclinical Studies and Novel Strategies. *Adv. Cancer. Res.*, Vol. 95, pp. 115-145, ISSN 0065-230X.

Panina-Bordignon, P., Tan, A., Termijtelen, A., Demotz, S., Corradin, G., & Lanzavecchia, A.(1989). Universally Immunogenic T Cell Epitopes: Promiscuous Binding to Human MHC Class II and Promiscuous Recognition by T Cells. *Eur. J. Immunol.*, Vol. 19, No.12 (December 1989), pp. 2237-2242, ISSN 0014-2980.

Pereboeva, L.A., Pereboev, A.V., Wang, L.F., & Morris, G.E. (2000). Hepatitis C Epitopes from Phage-Displayed cDNA Libraries and Improved Diagnosis with a Chimeric Antigen. *J. Med. Virol.*, Vol. 60, No. 2 (February 2000), pp. 144-151, ISSN 0146-6615.

Perry, L.C., Jones, T.D., & Baker, M.P. (2008) New Approaches to Prediction of Immune Responses to Therapeutic Proteins during Preclinical Development. *Drugs R. D.*, Vol. 9, No.6, pp. 385-396, ISSN 1174-5886.

Rappuoli, R. (2001). Reverse vaccinology, a genome-based approach to vaccine development. *Vaccine*, Vol. 19, No. 17-19 (March 21), pp. 2688-2691, ISSN 0264-410X.

Rinnová, M., Lebl, M., Souček, M. (1999). Solid-Phase Peptide Synthesis by Fragment Condensation: Coupling in Swelling Volume. *Lett. Peptide Sci.*, Vol. 6, No. 1, (pp. 15-22, ISSN 0929-5666.

Rodriguez, L.L., Barrera, J., Kramer, E., Lubroth, J., Brown, F., & Golde, W.T. (2003). A Synthetic Peptide Containing the Consensus Sequence of the G-H Loop Region of Foot-and-Mouth Disease Virus Type-O VP1 and a Promiscuous T-helper Epitope Induces Peptide-specific Antibodies but Fails to Protect Cattle against Viral Challenge. *Vaccine*, Vol. 21, No. 25-26, (September 8, 2003), pp. 3751-3756, ISSN: 0264-410X.

Roestenberg, M., Remarque, E., de Jonge, E., Hermsen, R., Blythman, H., Leroy, O., Imoukhuede, E., Jepsen, S., Ofori-Anyinam, O., Faber, B., Kocken, C.H., Arnold, M., Walraven, V., Teelen, K., Roeffen, W., de Mast, Q., Ballou, W.R., Cohen, J., Dubois, M.C., Ascarateil, S., van der Ven, A., Thomas, A., & Sauerwein R. (2008). Safety and Immunogenicity of a Recombinant Plasmodium falciparum AMA1 Malaria Vaccine Adjuvanted with Alhydrogel™, Montanide ISA 720 or AS02. *PLoS One,* Vol. 3, No.12, (December 18, 2008), e3960,pp. 1-12, eISSN-1932-6203.

Roggen, E.L. (2006). Recent Developments with B-cell Epitope Identification for Predictive Studies. *J. Immunotoxicol.*, Vol. 3, No.3 (September 1, 2006), pp. 137-149, ISSN 1547-6901.

Sabatino, G. & Papini, A.M. (2008). Advances in Automatic, Manual and Microwave-Assisted Solid-Phase Peptide Synthesis. *Curr. Opin. Drug. Discov. Devel.*, Vol. 11, No.6, (November 2008), pp. 762-770, ISSN 1367-6733.

Scheerlinck, J.P. & Greenwood, D.L. (2008). Virus-Sized Vaccine Delivery Systems. *Drug. Discov. Today*, 2008, Vol. 13, No. 19-20, (October 2008), pp. 882-887, ISSN 1359-6446.

Scheerlinck, J.P. & Greenwood, D.L. (2006). Particulate Delivery Systems for Animal Vaccines. *Methods*, 2006, Vol. 40, No. 1, pp. 118-124, ISSN 1046-2023.

Schlaphoff, V., Klade, C.S., Jilma, B., Jelovcan, S.B., Cornberg, M., Tauber, E., Manns, M.P., & Wedemeyer, H. (2007). Functional and Phenotypic Characterization of Peptide-Vaccine-Induced HCV-Specific CD8+ T Cells in Healthy Individuals and Chronic Hepatitis C Patients. *Vaccine*, Vol. 25, No.37-38, (September 17, 2007), pp. 6793-6806, ISSN 0264-410X.

Schuler, M.M., Nastke, M.D. & Stevanovic, S. (2007) SYFPEITHI: Database for Searching and T-cell Epitope Prediction. In: *Methods Mol. Biol.* Vol. 409, No.1. *Immunoinformatics. Predicting Immunogenicity In Silico*, pp. 75-93, Flower, D.R. (Ed.), Springer, ISBN 978-1-60327-118-9.

Sesardic, D. J. (1993) Synthetic peptide vaccines. *J. Med. Microbiol.*, Vol. 39, pp. 241-242, ISSN 0022-2615.

Sieker, F., May, A., & Zacharias, M. (2009). Predicting Affinity and Specificity of Antigenic Peptide Binding to Major Histocompatibility Class I Molecules. *Curr. Protein. Pept. Sci.*, Vol. 10, No. 3, (March 2009), pp. 286-296, ISSN 1389-2037.

Singh, M., Kazzaz, J., Ugozzoli, M., Malyala, P., Chesko, J., & O'Hagan, D.T. (2006), Polylactide-co-Glycolide Microparticles with Surface Adsorbed Antigens as Vaccine Delivery Systems. *Curr. Drug. Deliv.*, vol. 3, No.1 (January 2006), pp. 115-120, ISSN 1567-2018.

Sirima, S.B., Tiono, A.B., Ouédraogo, A., Diarra, A., Ouédraogo, A.L., Yaro, J.B., Ouédraogo, E., Gansané, A., Bougouma, E.C., Konaté, A.T., Kaboré, Y., Traoré, A., Roma, C., Soulama, I., Luty, A.J., Cousens, S., & Nébié, I. (2009). Safety and Immunogenicity of the Malaria Vaccine Candidate MSP3 Long Synthetic Peptide in 12-24 Months-old Burkinabe Children. *PLoS One*, Vol. 4, No.10,e7549. Available at http://www.plosone.org/article/info%3Adoi%2F10.1371%2Fjournal.pone.0007549.

Sobolev, B.N., Olenina, L.V., Kolesanova, E.F., Poroikov, V.V., & Archakov, A.I. (2005) Computer Design of Vaccines: Approaches, Software Tools and Informational Resources. *Curr. Computer-Aided Drug Design*, Vol. 1, No.2, pp. 207-222, ISSN: 1573-4099.

Sobolev, B.N., Poroikov, V.V., Olenina, L.V., Kolesanova, E.F. & Archakov, A.I. (2000). Comparative Analysis of Amino Acid Sequences from Envelope Proteins Isolated from Different Hepatitis C Virus Variants: Possible Role of conservative and variable regions. *J. Viral Hepat.*, Vol.7, No. 4, (September 2000), pp. 368-374, ISSN 1352-0504.

Sobolev, B.N., Poroikov, V.V., Olenina, L.V., Kolesanova, E.F., & Archakov, A.I. (2003). Computer-Assiated Vaccine Design. *Biomed.Khim. (Russ).*, 2003, Vol. 49, No. 4, (July-August 2003), pp. 309-332.

Soe, S., Theisen, M., Roussilhon, C., Aye, K.S., & Druilhe, P. (2004). Association between Protection against Clinical Malaria and Antibodies to Merozoite Surface Antigens in an Area of Hyperendemicity in Myanmar: Complementarity between Responses to Merozoite Surface Protein 3 and the 220-Kilodalton Glutamate-Rich Protein. *Infect. Immun.*, vol. 72, No. 1, (January 2004), pp. 247-252, ISSN 0019-9567.

Solares, A.M., Baladron, I., Ramos T., Valenzuela, C., Borbon, Z., Fanjull, S., Gonzalez, L., Castillo, D., Esmir, J., Granadillo, M., Batte, A., Cintado, A., Ale, M., de Cossio, M.E.F., Ferrer, A., Torrens, I., Lopez-Saura, P. (2011). Safety and Immunogenicity of a Human Papillomavirus Peptide Vaccine (CIGB-228) in Women with High-Grade Cervical Intraepithelial Neoplasia: First-in-Human, Proof-of-Concept Trial. *ISRN Obstetrics and Gynecology*, Vol.2011, Article ID292951, 9 pp.

Stanekova, Z., Király, J., Stropkovská. A., Mikušková. T., Mucha. V., Kostolanský. F. & Varečková, E. (2011). Heterosubtypic Protective Immunity against Influenza A Virus Induced by Fusion Peptide of the Hemagglutinin in Comparison to Ectodomain of M2 Protein. *Acta Virol.*, Vol.55, No. 1, pp. 61-67, ISSN 0001-723X.

Strohmaier, K., Franze, R., & Adam, K.H. (1982) Location and Characterization of the Antigenic Portion of the FMDV Immunizing Protein. *J. Gen. Virol.*, Vol. 59, Pt.2, (April 1982), pp. 295-306.

Svirshchevskaya, E.V., Alekseeva, L.G., Reshetov, P.D., Phomicheva, N.N., Parphenyuk, S.A., Ilyina, A.V., Zueva, V.S., Lopatin, S.A., Levov, A.N. & Varlamov, V.P. (2009). Mucoadjuvant properties of lipo- and glycoconjugated derivatives of oligochitosans. *Eur. J. Med. Chem.*, Vol.44, No.5 , pp.2030-2037.

Takahashi, H., Takeshita, T., Morein, B., Putney, S., Germain, R.N., & Berzofsky, J.A. (1990). Induction of CD8+ Cytotoxic Cells by Immunization with Purified HIV-1 Envelope Protein in ISCOMs. *Nature*, Vol. 344, No. 6269 (April 26, 1990), pp. 873-875, ISSN 0028-0836.

Takala, S.L. & Plowe, C.V. (2009). Genetic Diversity and Malaria Vaccine Design, Testing and Efficacy: Preventing and Overcoming 'Vaccine Resistant Malaria'. *Parasite Immunol.*, Vol. 31, No. 9, (September 2009), pp. 560-573, ISSN 0141-9838.

Tam, J.P. (1988). Synthetic Peptide Vaccine Design: Synthesis and Properties of a High-Density Multiple Antigenic Peptide System. *Proc. Natl. Acad. USA*, Vol. 85, No.15, (August 1988), pp. 5409-5413, ISSN 0027-8424.

Tarradas, J., Monso, M., Muños, M., Rosell, R., Fraile, L., Frias, M.T., Domingo, M., Andreu, D., Sobrino, F. & Ganges, L. (2011). Partial Protection against Classical Swine Fever Virus Elicited by Dendrimeric Vaccine Candidate Peptides in Domestic Pigs. *Vaccine*, Vol 29, No. 26, (June10, 2011), pp.4422-4429, ISSN 0264-410X.

Tedeschi, G., Taverna, F., Negri, A., Piccinini, R., Nonnis, S., Ronchi, S., & Zecconi, A. (2009) Serological Proteome Analysis of *Staphylococcus aureus* Isolated from Sub-clinical Mastitis. *Vet. Microbiol.*, Vol. 134, No. 3-4, (March 2, 2009), pp. 388-391, 0378-1135.

Tester, I., Smyk-Pearson, S., Wang, P., Wertheimer, A., Yao, E., Lewinsohn, D.M., Tavis, J.E., & Rosen, H.R. (2005) Immune Evasion versus Recovery after Acute Hepatitis C Virus Infection from a Shared Source. *J. Exp Med*, Vol. 201, No. 11 (June 6, 2005), pp. 1725-1731, ISSN 0022-1007.

*The Methodical Recommendations 1/4.2.588-96,(*1998). Information-Editorial Center, Ministry of Public Health, Moscow, Russia.

The Sanitary Rules 3.3.2.015-94 (1995). Approved by State Sanitary and Epidemiologic Inspection, on 12.08.94, Ministry of Public Health of Russian Federation, Moscow, Russia.

The Sanitary Rules 3.3.2.561-96, approved by State Sanitary and Epidemiologic Inspection, on 31.10.96, Moscow: Information-Editorial Center, Ministry of Public Health, 1998.

Theisen, M., Dodoo, D., Toure-Balde, A., Soe, S., Corradin, G., Koram, K.K., Kurtzhals, J.A., Hviid, L., Theander, T., Akanmori, B., Ndiaye, M. & Druilhe, P.(2001) Selection of Glutamate-Rich Protein Long Synthetic Peptides for Vaccine Development: Antigenicity and Relationship with Clinical Protection and Immunogenicity. *Infect. Immun.*, Vol. 69, No. 9, (September 2001), pp. 11-17, ISSN 0019-9567.

Theisen, M., Soe, S., Jessing, S.G., Okkels, L.M., Danielsen, S., Oeuvray, C., Druilhe, P. & Jepsen, S. (2000) Identification of a Major B-Cell Epitope of the *Plasmodium falciparum* Glutamate-Rich Protein (GLURP), Targeted by Human Antibodies Mediating Parasite Killing. *Vaccine,* Vol. 19, No. 2-3 (September 15, 2000), pp.204-212, ISSN 0264-410X.

Thompson, F.M., Porter, D.W., Okitsu, S.L., Westerfeld, N., Vogel, D., Todryk, S., Poulton, I., Correa, S., Hutchings, C., Berthoud, T., Dunachie, S., Andrews, L., Williams, J.L., Sinden, R., Gilbert, S.C., Pluschke, G., Zurbriggen, R., Hill, A.V. Evidence of Blood Stage Efficacy with a Virosomal Malaria Vaccine in a Phase IIa Clinical Trial. *PLoS One,*Vol. 3 No. 1 (January 30, 2008). Available at http://www.plosone.org/article/info%3Adoi%2F10.1371%2Fjournal.pone.0001493 .

Tian, F., Yang, L., Lv, F., Yang, Q., & Zhou, P. (2009). In silico Quantitative Prediction of Peptides Binding Affinity to Human MHC Molecule: an Intuitive Quantitative Structure-Activity Relationship Approach. *Amino Acids,* Vol. 36, No.3, (March 2009), pp. 535-354, ISSN 1438-2199.

Torresi, J., Stock, O.M., Fischer, A.E., Grollo, L., Drummer, H., Boo, I., Zeng, W., Earnest-Silveira, L., & Jackson, D.C. (2007). A Self-Adjuvanting Multiepitope Immunogen that Induces a Broadly Cross-Reactive Antibody to Hepatitis C Virus. *Hepatology,* Vol. 45, No. 4, (April 2007), pp. 911-920, ISSN 0270-9139.

Tribbick, G. (2002) Multipin Peptide Libraries for Antibody and Receptor Epitope Screening and Characterization. *J. Immunol. Meth.,* Vol. 267, No. 1, (September 1, 2002), pp. 27-35, ISSN 0022-1759.

Uchaikin, V.G. & Shamsheva, O.V. (2001) Vaktsinoprofilaktika (Vaccine Prophylaxis), Moscow: Geotar-Med, 2001.

Urdaneta, M., Prata, A., Struchiner, C.J., Tosta, C.E., Tauil, P., & Boulos, M. (1998). Evaluation of SPf66 Malaria Vaccine Efficacy in Brazil. *Am. J. Trop. Med. Hyg.,* Vol. 58, No. 3, (March 1998), pp. 378-385, ISSN 0002-9637.

Van Regenmortel, M.H. & Muller, S. (1999). *Synthetic Peptides as Antigens,* Elsevier Science, Amsterdam, ISBN 0-444-82176-7.

Vogel, F.R., & Alving, C.R. (2002). Progress in immunologic adjuvant development: 1982 - 2002, In: *The Jordan Report, 20th Anniversary. Accelerated Development of Vaccines,* C. P.Heilman, P.McInnis, & S. Landry (Eds.), pp. 39-43, NIH/NIAID (USA).

Voisset, C. & Dubuisson, J. (2004). Functional Hepatitis C Virus Envelope Glycoproteins. Biol. Cell, Vol. 96, No. 6, pp. 413-420, ISSN 0248-4900.

Volpina, O.M., Gelfanov, V.M., Yarov, A.V., Surovoy, A.Yu., Chepurkin, A V., & Ivanov, V.T. (1993). New Virus-Specific T-Helper Epitopes of Foot-and-Mouth Disease Viral VP1 Protein. *FEBS Lett.,* vol. 333, No. 1-2, (October 25, 1993), pp. 175-178, ISSN 0014-5793.

Volpina, O.M., Surovoi A.Y., Zhmak, M.N., Kuprianova, M.A., Koroev, D.O., Toloknov, A.S., & Ivanov, V.T. (1999). A Peptide Construct Containing B-Cell and T-Cell Epitopes from the Foot-and-Mouth Disease Viral VP1 Protein Induces Efficient Antiviral Protection. *Vaccine,* vol. 17, No. 6, (February, 12, 1999), pp. 1375-1380, ISSN 0264-410X.

Vytvytska, O., Nagy, E., Blüggel, M., Meyer, H.E., Kurzbauer, R., Huber, L.A., & Klade, C.S. (2002). Identification of Vaccine Candidate Antigens of *Staphylococcus aureus* by Serological Proteome Analysis. *Proteomics,* Vol. 2, No.5, (May, 2002), pp. 580-590, ISSN 1615-9853.

Walker, J., Ghosh, S., Pagnon, J., Colantoni, C., Newbold, A., Zeng, W., Jackson, D.C. (2007). Totally Synthetic Peptide-Based Immunocontraceptive Vaccines Show Activity in Dogs of Different Breeds . *Vaccine,* Vol. 25, No.41, (October 10, 2007), pp. 7111-7119, ISSN 0264-410X.

Wang, T.T., Tan, G.S., Hai, R., Pica, N., Ngai, L., Ekiert, D.C., Wilson, I.A., Garsia-Sastre, A., Moran, T.M. & Palese, P. (2010). Vaccination with a Synthetic Peptide from the Influenza Virus Hemagglutinin Provides Protection against Distinct Viral Subtypes. *Proc. Natl. Acad. Sci. USA,* Vol. 107, No. 44, (November 2, 2010), pp.18979-18984, ISSN 0027-8424.

Wiwanitkit, V. (2009). Predicted Epitopes of Malarial Merozoite Surface Protein 1 by Bioinformatics Method: a Clue for Further Vaccine Development. *J. Microbiol. Immunol. Infect.,* Vol. 42, No. 1, (February 2009), pp. 19-21, ISSN 1684-1182.

Worm, M., Lee, H.H., Kleine-Tebbe, J., Hafner, R.P., Laidler, P., Healey, D., Buhot, C., Verhoef, A., Maillère, B., Kay, A.B. & Larché, M. (2011). Development and Preliminary Clinical evaluation of a Peptide Immunotherapy Vaccine for Cqt Allergy. J. Allergy Clin. Immunol. , Vol. 127, No. 1, (January 2011), pp. 89-97, ISSN 0091-6749.

Wulf, M., Hoehn, P., & Trinder, P. (2009). Identification and Validation of T-cell Epitopes Using the IFN-gamma ELISPOT Assay. In: *Methods Mol. Biol.* Vol. 524, No. 4. *Epitope Mapping Protocols,* M. Schutkowski & Reineke, U. (Eds.), pp. 361-367, Humana Press, ISBN 978-1-59745-450-6_32.

Yutani S., Komatsu, N. Shichijo, S., Yoshida, K., Hiroko Takedatsu, H., Minoru Itou, M., Kuromatu, R.,Ide, T., Tanaka, M., Sata, M., Yamada, A. & Itoh, K. (2009). Phase I Clinical Study of a Peptide Vaccination for Hepatitis C Virus-Infected Patients with Different Human Leukocyte Antigen-Class I-A Alleles. Cancer Sci., Vol. 100, No. 10, (October 13, 2009), pp.1935-1942, ISSN 1349-7006.

Zeng, W., Ghosh, S., Lau, Y.F., Brown, L.E., & Jackson, D.C. (2002). Highly Immunogenic and Totally Synthetic Lipopeptides as Self-Adjuvanting Immunocontraceptive Vaccines. *J. Immunol.,* Vol. 169, No. 9, (November 1, 2002),pp. 4905-4912, ISSN 0022-1767.

Zeng, W., Jackson, D.C., Murray, J., Rose, K., & Brown, L.E. (2000). Totally Synthetic Lipid-Containing Polyoxime Peptide Constructs are Potent Immunogens. *Vaccine,* Vol. 18, No. 11-12, (January 6, 2000), pp. 1031-1039, ISSN 0264-410X.

Zhu, Q., Oei, Y., Mendel, D.B., Garrett, E.N., Patawaran, M.B., Hollenbach, P.W., Aukerman, S.L., & Weiner, A.J. (2006). Novel Robust Hepatitis C Virus Mouse Efficacy Model. *Antimicrob. Agents Chemother.,* Vol. 50, No.10, (October 2006), pp. 3260-3268, ISSN 0066-4804.

Part 3

Environmental Epidemics in the Course of Therapeutic Outlook

12

Cytotoxicity of *Aspergillus* Fungi as a Potential Infectious Threat

Agnieszka Gniadek
Department of Medical and Environmental Nursing, Faculty of Health Sciences, Jagiellonian University Medical College, Kraków, Poland

1. Introduction

Moulds constitute the largest group of bacteria, prevailing both in the indoor and outdoor air. Approximately 200 000 species of moulds have been identified so far, where only a small group of around 200 may present a threat to human health. Fungi from *Aspergillus* species are among the moulds considered to be most pathogenic. They also constitute the group of most pathogenic moulds most frequently isolated from the environment. Over 250 types of this species are known; about 50 of them were precisely described before the year 2000 (Klich, 2009). Pathogenicity, due to their toxicity, was also documented in other species: *Aspergillus fumigatus, Aspergillus flavus, Aspergillus ochraceus, Aspergillus niger, Aspergillus versicolor, Aspergillus parasiticus. Aspergillus nidulans, Aspergillus ustus, Aspergillus glaucus, Aspergillus clavatus, Aspergillus sydowii* and *Aspergillus terreus*. Their taxonomic identification is still an open topic because of their morphological variability and ability to produce metabolites; new species which exhibit adverse health effects to humans are constantly being detected. *Aspergillus lentulus* is one of the recently detected species of considerable clinical importance; it reveals similarity to *Aspergillus fumigatus*, one of the most pathogenic fungus for humans (Balajee et al., 2005).Table 1 presents the classification of species of fungi pathogenic to humans from the *Aspergillus* species. The list has been created by the authors of "Atlas Grzybów Chorobotwórczych Człowieka" ("Atlas of Fungi Pathogenic to Humans") (Krzyściak et al., 2011).

2. Fungal metabolites of *Aspergillus* species present a threat for human health

In their metabolic process, moulds produce mycotoxins. Those natural products, poisonous to humans and animals, are created as the result of a secondary metabolic process of fungi, when grown on organic substrates. Chemical structure of these metabolites varies, however, they are largely of small molecular mass, which conditions their varied toxic characteristics. So far over 400 metabolites produced by moulds have been identified from different genus of fungi: *Aspergillus* sp., *Penicillium* sp., *Fusarium* sp., *Alternaria* sp. *Trichothecium* sp. or *Stachybotrys* sp. Secondary metabolites of fungi from *Aspergillus* species are: ochratoxin A, aflatoxin B1, aflatoxins G1 and M1, trichothecenes, sterigmatosystin, patulins, gliotoxins or cyclopiazonic acid. Table 2 presents metabolites produced by the selected, most pathogenic

Subtype	Section	Teleomorph	Species linked to infections in humans
Aspergillus	*Aspergillus*	*Eurotium*	A. *chevalieri (Eurotium chavalieri)* A. *glaucus (Eurotium herbariorum)* A. *hollandicus (Eurotium amstelodami)* A. *reptans (Eurotium repens)* A. *rubrobrunneus (Erotium rubrum)* A. *sejunctus*
	Restricti		A. *caesiellus* A. *conicus* A. *pencilliodes* A. *restrictus*
Fumigati	*Fumigati*	*Neosartorya*	A. *fischerianus (Neosartorya fischeri)* A. *fumigatus* A. *fumisynnematus* A. *lentulus* A. *spinosus (Neosartorya spinosa)* A. *thermomutans (Neosartorya pseudofischeri)* A. *viridinutans* *Neosartorya coreana* – no confirmation of pathogenicity in humans *Neosartorya fennelliae* - no confirmation of pathogenicity in humans *Neosartorya hiratsukae* *Neosartorya udagawae*
	Cervini		
Ornati	*Ornati*	*Neocarpentels*	
Clavati	*Clavati*	n.n.	*A. clavatoanicus* *A. clavtus*
Nidulantes	*Usti*		*A. calidoustus* *A. deflectus* A. *ustus*
	Versicolores		A. *granulosus* A. *janus* A. *sydowii* A. *versicolor*
	Terrei	*Fennellia*	A. *alabamensis* A. *terreus*
	Flavipedes	*Fennellia*	A. *carneus* A. *flavipes* A. *niveus (Fennellia nivea)*
	Nidulantes	*Emericella*	A. *nidulans (Emericella nidulans)* A. *quadrilineata A. tetrazonus (Emericella quadrilineata)* A. *unguius (Emericella unguis)*
Circumdati	*Circumdati*	*Neopetrmyces*	A. *alutaceus* (isolated from sputum, pathogenicity not confirmed in humans) A. *ochraceus* A. *sclerotiorum*
	Flavi	*Petromyces*	A. *alliaceus* A. *avenaceus* A. *beijingensis*

			A. *flavus* var. *oryzae (A. oryzae* teleomorph: *Eurotium oryzae)* A. *flavus* A. *tamarii*
	Nigri	*Petromyces, Saitoa*	A. *(niger* var.*) awamori* A. *aculeatus* A. *atroviolaceus* A. *japonicus* A. *niger*
	Candidi		A. *candidus*
	Wentii	*Chaetosartorya*	
	Cremei		
	Sparsi		A. *wangduanlii*
Stilbothamnium			
Ochraceoroseus			
n.n.	*n. n.*		A. *qizutongii* A. *ochraceopetaliformis*

Table 1. Classification of pathogenic to humans *Aspergillus* species.

to humans *Aspergillus* species . (Krzyściak et al., 2011; Bräse et al., 2009; Skaug et al., 2001; Pitt et al., 2000; Smith et al., 1995)

No	Species	Metabolites
1	*Aspergillus fumigatus*	gliotoxin, verruculogen, fumitremorgin A and B, fumitoxin, tryptoguivaline, fumigallin, helvolic acid , sphingofungins, brevianamide A, coumarin
2	*Aspergillus flavus*	kojic acid, 3-nitropropionic acid, cyclopiazonic acid, aflatoxin B1, B2, G1, G2, aspergillic acid, violaxanthin, aspertoxin
3	*Aspergillus niger*	naphto-g-pyrones, malformin, ochratoxin A, toxic oxalates, violaxanthin
4	*Aspergillus ochraceus*	penicillic acid, ochratoxin A and B, xanthomeganin, viomellein, violaxanthin, circumdatin A, B, C
5	*Aspergillus versicolor*	sterigmatocystin, nidulotoxin, antrachinons, anthraquinoid
6	*Aspergillus candidus*	kojic acid, terphenyllin, candidulin, xanthoascin, beta nitropropionic acid
7	*Aspergillus terreus*	terreic acid, patulin, citrinin, citreoviridin, lovastatin, gliotoxin, terrain, patulin
8	*Aspergillus nidulans*	sterigmatocystin, penicillin, cotanin, nidulotoxin
9	*Aspergillus clavatus*	patulin, cytochalasin E, tryptoguivaline, kojic acid, clavatol, kotanin
10	*Aspergillus lentulus*	gliotoxin, cyclopiazonic terreic acid, neosartorin, auranthine and pyripyropenes A, E
11	*Aspergillus parasiticus*	Aflatoxins A1, B1, G1, G2

Table 2. Metabolites of selected species of *Aspergillus* fungi.

Natural metabolites produced by fungi are for the most part cytotoxic to different cellular structures and depress their key processes such as RNA and DNA synthesis (Burr, 2001). Mycotoxins differ with respect to their nature, action towards target cells, cellular structures and their internal processes. Best described mycotoxins produced by fungi of the *Aspergillus* species are aflatoxins and ochratoxins. Aflatoxins are highly saturated heterocyclic compounds which contain elements of furan. Ochratoxins constitute a group of poliketides derived from isocoumarin, related to L-phenylalanine. Degradation of ochratoxin A within the human body produces (4-R)-4 hydroxyochratoxin A and ochratoxin α, which create an albumin bond in the plasma. Creation of such bond facilitates the substances` persistence in the human body for an extended period of time (Budak, 1998).

Influence on the health in exposed individuals exerted by secondary metabolites includes carcinogenic, teratogenic, mutagenic, hepatotoxic and nephrotoxic action (it particularly concerns aflatoxin A_1 and ochratoxin A) (Fischer & Dott 2003;Burr, 2001). Sterigmatocystin is one of the aflatoxin precursors on its biosynthesis pathway and its carcinogenic action is only slighly lower than that of aflatoxin itself. Gliotoxin is considered to be responsive to immunosuppression and cellular apoptosis; it is also a likely virulence factor in mycoses caused by *A. fumigatus*. Gliotoxin is a very frequently detected toxin in the serum of patients suffering from aspergillosis. (Bok et al., 2005). This toxin is present in the serum of animals with a natural *A. fumigatus* infection and in cancer patients with invasive aspergillosis (Lewis et al., 2005).

This was confirmed in the findings obtained by Kupfahl, in which analysis of gliotoxin was performed in 158 *Aspergillus* strains (100 *A. fumigatus*) originating from patients with invasive aspergillosis and from the environment. During analysis of the strains and their ability to produce gliotoxin he discovered that gliotoxin was detected in the majority of *A. fumigatus* strains isolated both from clinical materials and from the environment (98% and 96% respectively) (Kupfahl et al., 2008).

The variety of metabolites produced by fungi of the *Aspergillus* species (*A. fumigatus* produces as well fumigallin, helvolic acid, tryptoguivaline, *A. candidus* kojic acid, terphenyllin, *A. ochraceus* penicillic acid or viomellein, while *A. niger* produces malformin) equips the fungi with multiple options of invading the host`s body, at the same time limiting the therapeutic options resulting from targeted prophylaxis. As it turns out, applying targeted chemoprophylaxis does not always prove to be effective, as the medicine does not affect all of the metabolites produced just by one strain of fungi (Bräse et al., 2009; Domsch et al, 2007; Ribeiro et al., 2005; Raper & Fennell, 1965).

3. Epidemiology of infection and clinical health outcome, as caused by fungi of the *Aspergillus* species

Fungi of the *Aspergillus* species are typical isogenic opportunistic bacteria, which for the most part fail to trigger an infection with a healthy person; however, they constitute a threat predominantly to persons with immunity disorders. Factors which facilitate the conditions necessary for a fungal invasion are: disturbances in the functions of T lymphocytes, phagocytes as well as the reticuloendothelial system, chemo- and radiotherapy, skin incisions related surgery, therapy or care. Risk factors for developing an invasive aspergillosis are chronic neutropenia (exceeding 3 weeks), corticosteroid treatment, hematological neoplasms, cytotoxic treatment, AIDS- Acquired Immune Deficiency Syndrome and bone marrow transplant. Certain influence has also been attributed to cytomegalovirus (CMV) contraction. Treatment with infliximab, a monoclonal antibody against tumour necrosis (TNFα), has been described in literature as being a determining factor for aspergillosis. Mechanisms, through which the predisposition factors intensify invasiveness of fungi of the *Aspergillus* species, act through or directly at the host, or the fungus, or both. Factors which determine pathogenicity of the *Aspergillus* fungi are multiple polar or neutral lipids, phenolic compounds and heterocyclic toxins (mycotoxins). An additional factor intensifying the pathogenicity of the *Aspergillus* fungi is their capacity to produce various proteolytic enzymes e.g. protease, which assist fungal colonisation in the infected host tissues (Türel, 2011; Kurnatowski &Miśkiewicz, 2009; Macura, 1998).

A source of infection with *Aspergillus* fungi may be another infected person, in whose body the fungal process develops, but primarily it is the hospital environment: air, water pipe system, ventilation system, hospital food as well as the medical equipment. For isogenic fungi of the *Aspergillus* type the obvious portal of entry is the respiratory system of a sick person, as well as skin with lesions, e.g. a burn or damaged cornea. Infection within the respiratory system develops as a result of inhalation of the fungal spores present in the air. Very often, prior to development of aspergillosis, a patient`s oronasal cavity is subject to fungal spore colonization. A developing fungus located in the lungs (incubation period spans between 2 days to 3 months) results in haemorrhagic infarctions, which cause a further transmission of the infection through the bloodstream to the brain, liver, spleen, kidneys, pericardium or skin (Mortensen, 2011; Garczewska, 2008)

For patients with lymphopenia - where the number of CD4 cells is lower than 0.2 x 10e9/l - most of the cases where the respiratory tract is colonized with *Aspergillus,* aspergillosis may develop as a result. With immunosuppressed patients, e.g. those suffering from hematological neoplasms, the most predominant form of fungal infection is invasive aspergillosis in 70% of cases caused by *A. fumigatus*. A variant of aspergillosis a little less common is general aspergillosis which affects central nervous system, sinuses, kidneys, skin or bones. Observational studies (a five year period of observation carried out on 3228 patients who underwent HSCT (haematopoietic stem cell transplant) at 11 transplant wards in Italy, where fungal infection prophylaxis was implemented by means of use of fluconazole, fungal infections were observed in 121 patients (3.7%), where 75% of cases were invasive aspergillosis, mostly of *Aspergillus* aetiology (Asano-Mori, 2010; Pagano, 2007). Unfortunately, *Aspergillus* fungal infections display a high mortality rate. In untreated aspergillosis, mortality rate can soar as high as 100%, and in the cases where treatment is introduced it drops only slightly down to 60%. One of the patient groups highly susceptible to invasive fungal infections caused by *Aspergillus* is the hematooncologic patients, where mortality rate with chemotherapy patients is as high as 49.3%, and with patients who underwent a haematopoietic stem cell transplant it reaches 86.7%. It was also shown that invasive aspergillosis is prevalent more often with the allogeneic bone marrow transplant patients (2.9-16.0%), rather than with those who underwent the autologous bone marrow transplant (0.3-1.1%) (Butrym et al., 2011; Fraquet et al., 2004). Uncharacteristic symptoms and diagnostic difficulties represent a key reason for delayed diagnosis of the infections caused by the fungi of *Aspergillus* species and deferred commencement of adequate treatment. Chamilos et al. in their research showed that as many as 75% of fungal infection cases confirmed in post mortem analysis were not diagnosed when the patients were still alive (Chamilos et al., 2008). Very often symptoms of fungal infections caused by moulds, are misdiagnosed as bacterial infections. A success case of a 47-year old woman suffering from sarcoidosis, who had been treated with steroids, and for two years had a confirmed lung cavity, indicates that a successful treatment of aspergillosis is possible. In that case, major symptoms of the disease were high fever, chronic cough with sputum, weight loss and hemoptysis. After an ineffective course of antibiotic therapy, the patient was diagnosed with candidiasis and semi-invasive aspergillosis. A computer tomography (CT) scan revealed a mycetoma in the lung cavity, culture of the sputum revealed an *Aspergillus* infection, and a significant improvement after antifungal treatment confirmed the diagnosis of aspergillosis caused by fungi from *A. niger (*Kosacka et al., 2010).

At present, the most sensitive test able to confirm aspergillosis is a high resolution CT scan in conjunction with the galactomannan test, which detects the antigen peculiar to *Aspergillus*. Other molecular recognition techniques based on PCR reaction are also used in detecting nosocomial aspergillosis. Genetic material of a fungus in clinical materials can be isolated by certain starters, e.g. from the sequence of alkaline proteinase or on the basis of 26SrRNA (Kriengkauykiat et al., 2011; Garczewska, 2008, Kędzierska et al., 2007)

Most common forms of nosocomial infections with moulds from the *Aspergillus* species are as follows:

- aspergilloma located in the lungs, usually after tuberculosis
- invasive aspergilloma (usually the pulmonary variation - in immunocompromised patients, leukaemia and post-transplant patients, in children suffering from chronic granulomatous disease)
- paranasal sinus aspergillosis (in immunocompromised patients)
- central nervous system aspergillosis (accompanies its disseminated version or as a result of sinusitis)
- *Aspergillus* endocarditis and cardiac aspergillosis - (follow an open-heart surgery)
- eye aspergillosis, endophtalmitis (in patients with endocarditis and following an organ transplant, often as the result of eye injury or transmission via bloodstream)
- aspergillosis of the bone marrow (bone marrow aspergillosis) - in children with granulomatous disease
- disseminated aspergillosis - as oesophageal infection, infection of the intestines, or organ infection: liver, spleen or kidneys.
- chronic necrotising pulmonary aspergillosis - in patients with pulmonary diseases
- skin aspergillosis - in patients with catheters or as the result of transmission via bloodstream.
- allergic bronchopulmonary aspergillosis (asthma) - inhaling spores of fungus by persons allergic to its antigens (Garczewska, 2008).

As previously mentioned, fungi from *Aspergillus fumigatus* species bear most significant clinical relevance for humans. This fungal species may cause acute and chronic inhalatory respiratory tract infections (aspergillosis, aspergilloma) as well as infections of the hematopoietic system, digestive system, genitourinary tract, skeletal muscles, and nervous system. The primary focus of infection in such cases is usually located in the lungs. Another pathogenic species which causes infections of the respiratory system and which also may cause allergic aspergillosis is *Aspergillus flavus*. This fungus is also responsible for cases of chronic invasive sinusitis as well as deep fungal infections (of the kidneys, endocardium, and central nervous system). *Aspergillus ochraceus* may be the cause behind antromycosis, pulmonary invasion and onychomycosis. Fungi of the *Aspergillus niger* species may also cause infections of the inner and outer ear (otomycosis) as well as pulmonary aspergillosis. Similarly to other species of the *Aspergillus species*, it rarely is responsible for surface aspergillosis. *Aspergillus versicolor* may constitute an etiological factor for otomycosis, osteomylitis, skin lesions or pulmonary diseases. Recently, clinical significance has been attributed to infections caused by *Aspergillus terreus*. Its spores may cause an allergic reaction or invasive aspergillosis of the respiratory system, as well as infections of the skin, eye or liver. Aspergillosis in patients with compromised immunity has been attributed more frequently to this species. In retrospective research spanning over 10 years, carried out in Austria (Medical University Hospital of Innsbruck), for 67 cases of invasive aspergillosis, nearly half (32) were infections caused by *A. terreus*, while the remaining cases were attributed to other species of *Aspergillus* (Lass-Flörl et al., 2005).

4. Environmental factors facilitating development of fungi of the *Aspergillus* species

Environmental parameters adding up to microclimate of rooms which affect people`s physical state comprise: air temperature, relative humidity, airflow in the people zone, purity of the air - both with respect to chemical and microbiological cleanliness, intensity of smells, light and noise levels. Indoors, microclimate is made up of the following factors: outdoor climate, heating and ventilation, people in the room, technological processes which take place inside, thermal characteristics of the room (Kaiser, 2011).

Indoor environment is an active ecosystem which evolves as the time progresses, with changes in humidity, temperature, presence of other microorganisms. Humidity in the rooms designated for people should be between 30-70%. Excessively humid air encourages multiplication of microorganisms (bacteria, mould), decomposition and water condensation, which increases microbiological contamination of the air. Depending on their designation, temperature in hospital rooms is maintained at different levels, usually falling into the 22-25°C temperature brackets.

Moulds grow mainly in the environment where air humidity exceeds 45%, temperature is within the range of 5°C-35°C (optimum 18°-27°C), and water activity a_w exceeds 0.8. Such environment is conducive to production of secondary metabolites - mycotoxins. *Penicillium* and *Aspergillus* are dominating mould species in the rooms where water activity is around 0.85 (Jarviss, 2003). Coefficient of hygroscopic expansion a_w for fungi is lower than for bacteria, for the latter the prerequisite for development is the 0.99 to 0.995 range. Fungi of the *A.flavus* type belong to the group of fungi which require higher air and soil humidity. It requires a 0.902 a_w level, which constitutes an extremely humid environment (Zyska, 1999).

Development of fungi may be affected by light in many different ways. Depending on the species, light may inhibit spore development or cause its abundant growth. It has been found that with one of the *Alternaria* species light of wavelength of 0.415xm-0.49xm completely blocks spore development, while wavelength below 0.39xm and exceeding 0.5xm stimulates spore growth (Zyska, 2001).

Influence of hydrostatic pressure on fungi growth has not been adequately researched. Fungi show no sensitivity to hyperbaria. Fungal endospores display a unique resilience to high pressure. Osmotic pressure inside hyphae of some species may be as high as 4255 hPa (Kurnatowska, 1998). Mould conidia of *A.niger* do not show sensitivity to pressure of 1000MPa. Growth of most yeast is halted, however, at pressure levels of as little as 0.8 MPa. A considerable drop in the hydrostatic pressure - hypobaria, or even deep vacuum, do not pose a threat to cells of many types of fungi. Deep vacuum had little or no impact on fungal vegetative forms and endospores, e.g. those from the *Cheatomium globosum, Aspergillus oryzae,* and *Aspergillus terreus* species (Piotrowska, 2000).

From among external environmental chemical factors, the most important is acidity or alkalinity, which is measured in pH parameters. Lowest and highest values on the pH scale, within the boundaries of growth of a fungus, represent the scope characteristic for a given species. This factor ranging between 5 to 6 is appropriate for most fungi. As in the majority of cases fungi favour pH below 7, most may be labelled acidophilic. Many species of *Aspergillus, Penicillium,* and *Fusarium* may grow at pH close to 2. At the same time, species like *Penicillium variabilis i Fusarium oxysporum* thrive in the environment where pH reaches 11. It should also be added that fungi trigger a shift in pH levels in the soil they grow in (Haasum & Nielsen, 1998).

Fungi belong to aerobes or facultative anaerobes. An oxygen increase in the environment lowers the mycelium mass and starts a degenerative process, however, it does not destroy the fungus. An increase in carbon dioxide content also halts the growth of a fungus (Kurnatowska, 1998).

From among moulds, fungi of the *Aspergillus* species demonstrate highest pathogenicity; however, despite their prevalence in the environment, they produce fewer mycotoxins than the less prevalent mould of *Stachybotrys*. It is not a rule of the thumb for all fungi of the *Aspergillus* species, as sterigmatocystin produced by *Aspergillus versicolor* may produce approximately 1% of the total biomass of fungi from this species, with water activity at level 1. This fungus is rarely obtained from indoor environment, as the species occurs in colder regions, in mountain and polar climatic zones. Fungi most often isolated from the indoor air belong to *A. fumigatus* and *A. niger* species (Fog Nielsen, 2003).

Among all the microorganisms present in the indoor air, moulds are most prevalent, however, it is crucial to remember, that live microorganisms (bacteria and fungi) make up only 10% of the total microorganism mass. Survivability of bacteria and moulds in the air is contingent upon peculiar to species susceptibility to desiccation and to the impact of ultraviolet rays. Most susceptible to desiccation are the vegetative forms of bacteria, while the most resilient are fungal spores. Fungal spores measure between 1.5 to 20 µm. One of the largest spores are: *Rhizopus* 4- 6 µm, *Mucor* 4-8 µm, *Fusarium* 2.4-3.5 µm, *A. niger* 2.5-3.5 µm, *A. flavus* 3.5-4.5 µm, while the smallest spores belong to the most pathogenic species of the *Aspergillus* species: (*A. terreus* 1.5 – 2.5 µm, *A. fumigatus* 2.5 - 3 µm, or *A. versicolor* 2 -3.5 µm) (Krzyściak at al., 2011). Figures 1-3 present a scanning microscope image, showing conidiophores of fungi of the following species: *A. candidus, A. niger* and *A. flavus.* Images from author`s own collection.

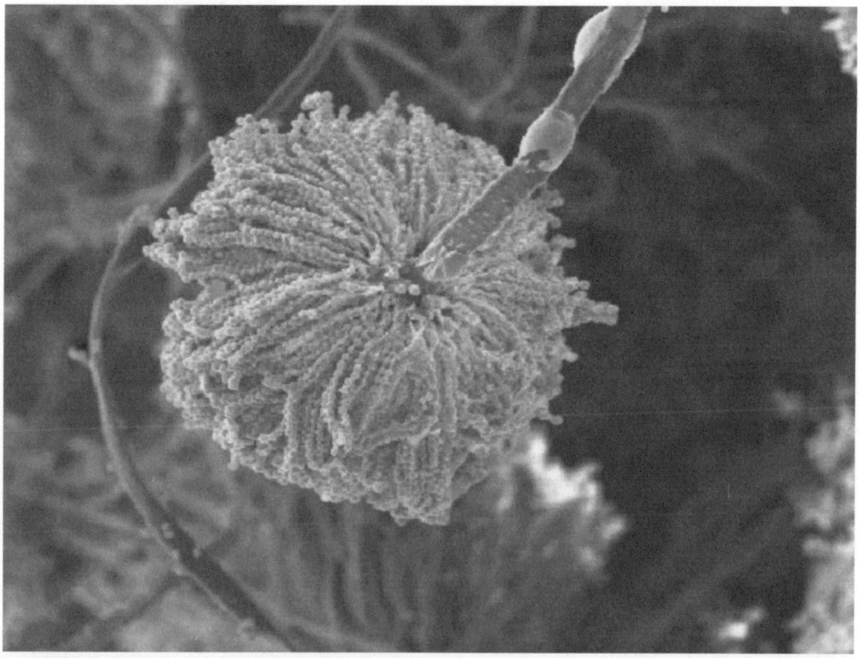

Fig. 1. *Aspergillus candidus* as seen under the scanning microscope; magnified by 1500x.

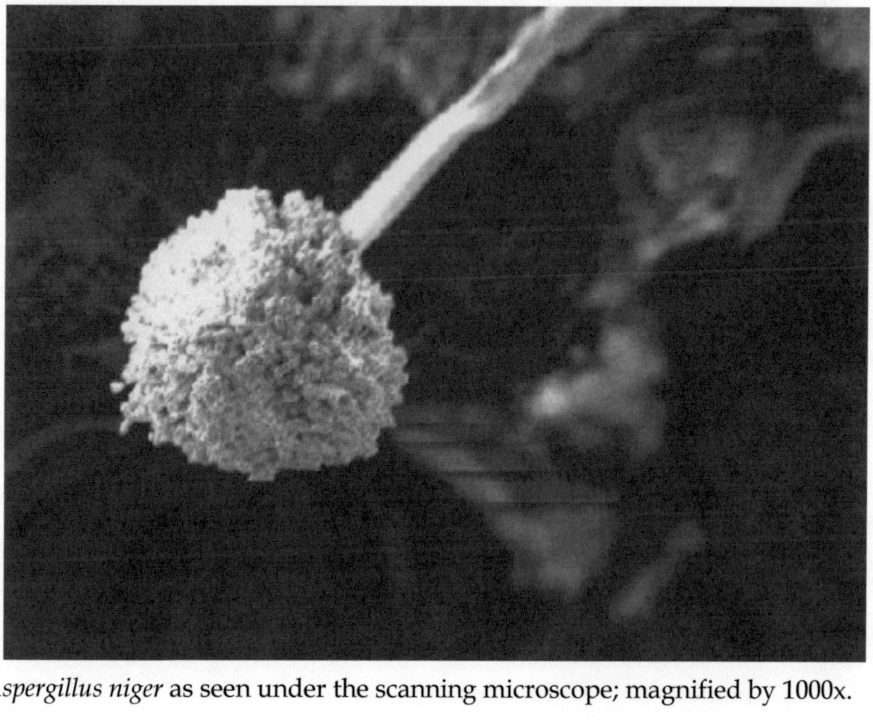

Fig. 2. *Aspergillus niger* as seen under the scanning microscope; magnified by 1000x.

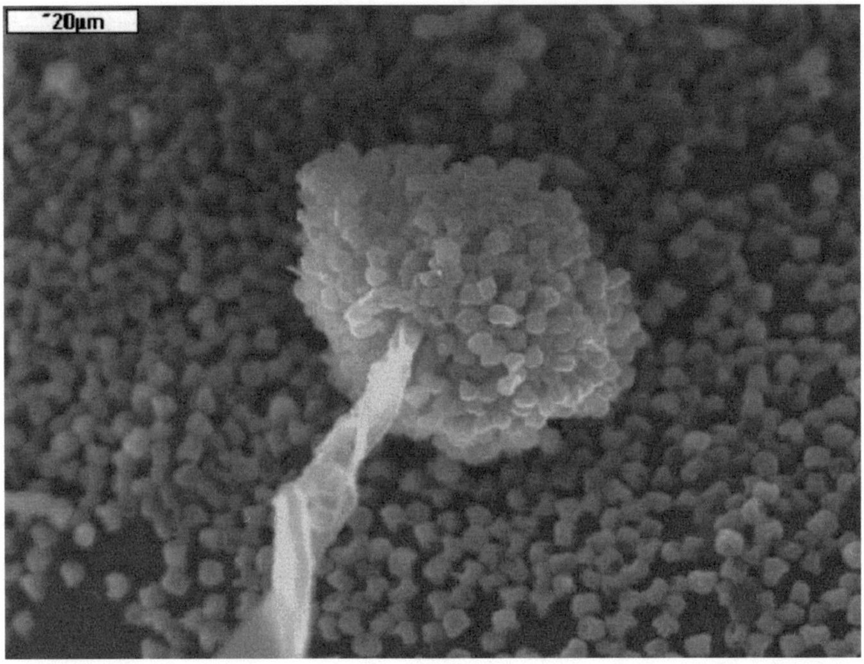

Fig. 3. *Aspergillus flavus* as seen under the scanning microscope; magnified by 1000x.

In contained rooms, not equipped with specialist ventilation systems and adequate air filtration, fungi and certain bacteria colonize places favourable to their development. Such areas are usually polluted places with increased humidity levels: ventilation shafts, air filters, noise reducing filters, insulation layers, air coolers, humidifier systems. Infected areas of such systems present a secondary source of microbiological contamination of the air. Ventilation and air-conditioning systems are more responsible for polluting the air with fungi than with bacteria. Most serious air infections happen in places where condensation is present. The risk increases if the systems are not properly utilised and if the air contains significant amounts of pollutants (Kaiser, 2011).

Required cleanliness level of air provided for indoors is achieved by filtration by means of air conditioning systems and ventilation equipped with proper filters. For indoor spaces with high hygienic standards it is crucial to implement the use of multi-tier filtration systems. A modern air-conditioning system contains a laminar flow ceiling cabinet. Such system for operating rooms (hospital rooms with high standards of microbiological cleanliness) should provide the necessary amount of fresh air and an adequate frequency of airflow changes per hour. A factor that may limit the occurrence of infections with patients who undergo surgery is creating an environment free from bacteria as well as keeping the surgery time as short as possible (Kremer et al., 2010). Knochen et al. in a study that compared environments of operating theatres, where floors were routinely disinfected after each surgery, with those where theatres were cleaned only when visible dirt appeared, and concluded that none of the procedures influences the number of infections occurring in patients undergoing surgery. Utilizing a laminar flow ceiling cabinet proves to be a sufficient bacteria limiting method (Knochen et al., 2010).

The problem of providing microbiological cleanliness inside hospital rooms is not exclusively related to observing the principles of air filter exchange in air conditioning systems according to manufacturer`s instructions. According to Kaiser (Kaiser, 2004), periodical ventilation of the air-conditioning system is necessary as well as drying the ventilation pipes and elements of the equipment. He also states that air-conditioning system should not be completely shut off . On the contrary, Dettenkofer et al. suggest that shutting off the ventilation systems in the operating rooms when they are not in use probably does not increase microbiological contamination of the indoor air shortly after the system is switched back on (Dettenkofer et al., 2003).

Proper utilisation of operating rooms also entails isolation of the inner environment from any possibility of contamination access from outside, by maintaining a pressure difference between the inner and outer rooms. Where proper ventilation systems are unavailable, limiting microbiological contamination from staff may result in an approximate twofold reduction in infections. Conclusions of research carried out by Lidwell suggest that with a drop in microbiological contamination concentration of the air below 10 c.f.u/m^3, the drop in risk of infection is minor (Lidwell, 1982). With such low levels of concentration of bacteria in the air, transmission of infectious pathogenic microorganisms this way becomes a less serious cause of infection.

4.1 Influence of physical and chemical factors on cytotoxicity of fungi

Fungi are not cytotoxic unless there are circumstances enabling them to produce metabolites. The factors conducive to toxin production include: culture medium, life cycle of the fungi, availability of nutrients, environmental conditions and/or the simultaneous presence of other moulds [Kelman et al., 2004; Pitt et al.,2000). It has been established that in laboratory settings fungal monocultures lose their toxin production potential (Jarvis & Miller, 2005). Environmental conditions considerably influence the synthesis of fungal virulence factors. When fungal receptors receive variations in such factors as moisture, temperature, water activity and the presence of nitrogen, a signal transduction cascade that controls effector genes expression may be activated, which results in toxin production. The processes of sporulation and mycotoxin production in the *Aspergillus* fungi are regulated by the protein G transduction signals pathway (Singh & Del Poeta, 2011). The investigations carried out by Watanabe et al. gave evidence that good environmental conditions, in this case oxygenation, stimulated the *A. fumigatus* fungi to gliotoxin production and were conducive to the increase of their general cytotoxicity (Watanabe et al., 2004).

The presence of the *Aspergillus* fungi in the human environment does not necessarily cause infection in risk group patients. Those fungi are opportunistic bacteria and are cleared away by means of natural defence mechanisms in healthy individuals, however, they produce severe invasive infections in immunosuppressed patients. So far, the threshold value establishing a requisite for opportunistic infection has not been determined. Therefore, the goal of preventive action should be to eliminate *Aspergillus* fungi from human environment. Such aim, however, is hard to attain as, obviously, among all bacteria in the air, moulds are most numerous. Methods of absolute elimination of mould spores from the environment have been known, though. Nevertheless, from a practical point of view it is not feasible. Bearing in mind immunosuppressed patients, the Airinspace Technologies system was created. It is based on creating a protective chamber around a patient, where air exchange takes place 60 times per hour, with the use of plasma as a bacteria killing agent, it is still very difficult to provide a patient with ultra-sterile air (Poirot et al., 2007).

Our own study on mycological cleanness of hospital rooms indoor air revealed that the *Aspergillus* species amounted to 20-38% of all of the moulds isolated, and the most frequently identified species was *A. fumigatus* [Gniadek et al., 2010; Gniadek et al., 2009). Domination of this species in the indoor air may be tantamount to a high risk of infection. The risk may be confirmed by the findings of *Aspergillus* cytotoxicity evaluation in such sites as adult intensive therapy ward, intensive neonatal care unit and chemotherapy and radiotherapy wards. The analysis was performed using an MTT test (3-(4.5-dimethylthiazol-2-yl) 2.5 diphenyltetrazolium bromide) in which general cytotoxicity was tested on swine kidney cells (SK), sensitive to most mycotoxins. The test is based on the reduction of yellow MTT tetrazolium salt to violet formazan, insoluble in water. The reduction occurs in the presence of intact SK, not damaged by mycotoxins. The intensity of reaction is proportional to the amount of metabolically active SK. When the SK are infected with moulds producing mycotoxins, their mitochondria fail to reduce tetrazolium salt into formazan. Therefore, when the SK are damaged by mycotoxins, the reaction is less intensive or does not occur, which can be measured photometrically as more or less intensive change of colour. Thus, the reduction or the absence of the reaction gives evidence of cytotoxicity of the fungal strain tested (Hanelt et al., 1994).

The analysis comprised the evaluation of a test sample (Petri dish with the moulds on Czapek medium) and a control sample (Petri dish with Czapek medium). The SK were grown in medium containing antibiotics (penicillin and streptomycin, Sigma Aldrich) and calf fetal serum (Sigma Aldrich) in the Hera Cell incubator with carbon dioxide, manufactured by Heraeus (5% CO2, 37°C, 98% humidity). The number of SK was 2.2×105. The ranges of testing concentrations were prepared in the ratio 1:2 and amounted from 31.251 to 0.061 cm^2/l. The value was expressed in terms of cm^2/ml, where the area of the Petri dish from which the moulds were extracted together with the medium, was measured in square centimetres.

The quantitative evaluation of cytotoxicity was performed using a microslide spectrophotometer (Elisa Digiscan reader, Asys Hitech GmbH, Austria) and the programme MikroWin 2000 (Mikrotek Laborsysteme GmbH, Germany). The readings were made at the wave-length of 510 nm. All of the absorption values below 50% of the threshold activity were considered as toxic. So, the borderline toxic concentration was evaluated on the basis of the dilution i.e. the mean inhibitory concentration IC50 was equal to the smallest sample (in cm2/ml) which was toxic to the SK. The cytotoxicity was considered as low (+) when the values were within the range of 31.251>15.625>7.813 [cm^2/ml], intermediate (++) for the values >3.906>1.953>0.977 [cm^2/ml], and high (+++) for >0.488>0.244>0.122>0.061. The lack of cytotoxicity was reported when the absorption value exceeded 31.251 [cm^2/ml] (Gareis, 1994).

In own researches for 57 isolated strains – *A. fumigatus, A. ochraceus, A. niger, A. flavus, A. versicolor* and *A. ustus*, as many as 48 (84%) were cytotoxic. It was also established that the *A. niger* species was considerably less cytotoxic than *A. ochraceus* and *A. fumigatus* ($p<0.05$) (Fig 4).

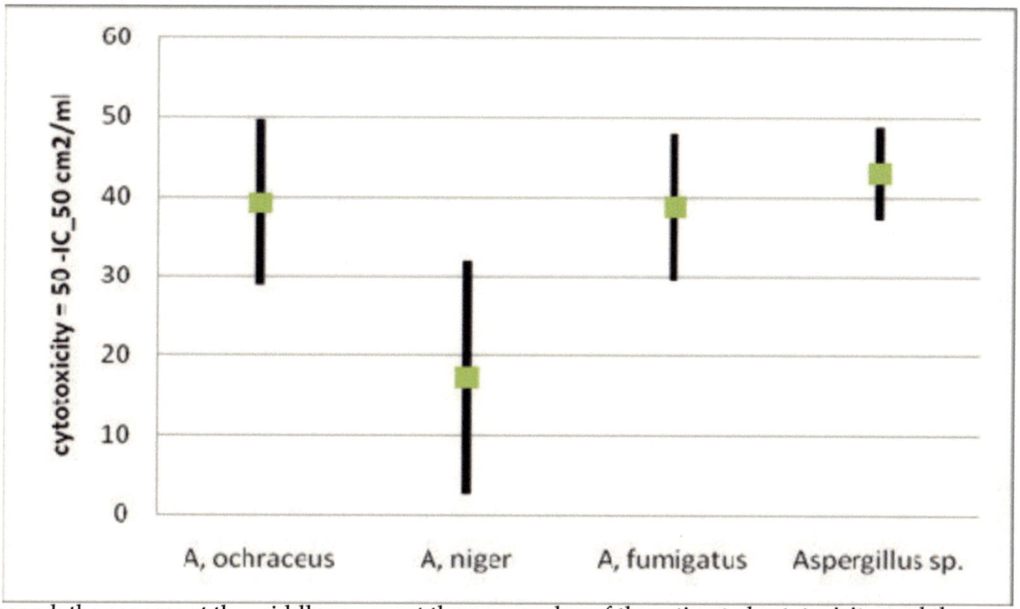

Legend: the squares at the middle represent the mean value of the estimated cytotoxicity, and the vertical lines represent the size of the confidence interval of the estimated cytotoxicity.

Fig. 4. Intervals of confidence 95% CI and mean value of *Aspergillus* cytotoxicity estimated as difference between reference level equal to 50 and measured value of IC 50 cm^2/ml.

Research has shown that among all of the examined strains the strains of *A. fumigatus*, but not of other species, were either of intermediate or high cytotoxicity (Gniadek et al., 2011). Particularly, eight out of nine strains isolated from indoor air in adult intensive care unit were cytotoxic. High cytotoxicity was found in the following species: *A. fumigatus, A. ochraceus* and *A. flavus*, while the cytotoxivity of *A. niger* was intermediate or lacked cytotoxicity altogether (Gniadek et al., 2009). A further confirmation of those findings was brought by another study in which the highest fungal virulence towards murine macrophages was found in *A. fumigatus*, while the lowest in *A. niger* and *A. terreus* (Kamei et al., 2002).

The considerable cytotoxicity of fungi isolated from the environment where immunocompromised patients are present encourages intensifying observations concerning the influence of environmental mycobiota on human health. Cases of aspergillosis caused by airborne infections were observed (a patient with aspergilosis infected two other patients in the same intensive therapy unit by airborne route). Recent literature does not provide evidence what level of exposure to toxin producing fungi may be dangerous to the health (Pegues et al., 2002). Nevertheless, there is a common opinion that moulds present indoors may be dangerous and the environmental conditions must be improved. The measurements of environmental occurrence of fungi indoors should include an evaluation of their cytotoxicity when the fungi are known to be toxic. Those measures should be habitual and preventive because evaluation after occurrence of infection will only reflect estimaton of risk at the initial stage of the disease and may not reflect the exposure to harmful substances in the course of the disease. It seems a fair policy that as preventive treatment for patients with compromised immunity, in order to contain the exposure, the mycological cleanliness of hospital environment should be monitored, inclusive of marking the cytotoxicity of fungi commonly labelled pathogenic.

5. Conclusion

From the epidemiological point of view, the results of exposure to a mix of mycotoxins and other noxious substances present in the air we breathe indoors remain unknown. Therefore, the adverse effect of fungi to human health may be evaluated by means of finding the relationship between the disease (predisposition) and exposure level (detection of pathogenic spores) in relation to symptoms typical for experimental conditions caused by myotoxins.

6. References

Asano-Mori, Y. (2010). Fungal infections after hematopoietic stem cell transplantation. *International Journal Hematology*, Vol. 91, No. 4, pp. 576-587, ISSN 0925-5710

Balajee, S.; Gribskov, J.; Hanley, E.; Nickle, D. & Marr K. (2005). *Aspergillus lentulus* sp. nov., a new sibling species of A. fumigatus. *Eukaryotic Cell*, Vol. 4, No. 3, pp. 625–632, ISSN 1535-9778

Bok, J.; Balajee, S.; Marr, K.; Andes, D.; Nielsen, K.; Frisvad, J. & Keller, N. (2005). LaeA, a regulator of morphogenetic fungal virulence factors. *Eukaryotic Cell*, Vol.4, No. 9, pp. 1574–1582, ISSN:1535-9778.

Bräse, S.; Encinas, A.; Keck, J. & Nising, C. (2009). Chemistry and biology of mycotoxins and related fungal metabolites. *Chemical Reviews*, Vo. 109, No. 9, pp. 3903-3990, ISSN 0009-2665

Budak, A. (1998). Mikotoksyny, In *Zarys mikologii lekarskiej*, E. Baran, (Ed.), 533 – 538,Volumed, ISBN 83- 85564-17-9, Wrocław, Poland

Burr, M. (2001). Health effects of indoor moldes. *Reviews on Environmental Health*, Vol. 16, No. 2, pp. 97-103, ISSN 0048-7554

Butrym, A.; Zywar, K.; Dzietczenia, J. & Mazur G. (2011). Invasive fungal infections in patients with hematological malignancies. *Mykologia Lekarska*, Vol. 18, No. 1, pp. 47-53, ISSN 1232-986X

Chamilos, G.; Luna, M.; Lewis, R.; Bodey, G.; Chemaly, R.; Tarrand, J.; Safdar, A.; Raad, I. & Kontoyiannis, D. (2006). Invasive fungal minfections in patients with hematologic malignancies in a tertiary care center: an autopsy study over a 15 year period (1989-2003). *Hematologica*, Vol. 91, No. 7, pp. 986-989, ISSN 0390-6078

Dettenkofer, M.; Scherrer, M.; Hoch, V.; Glaser, H.; Schwarzer, G.; Zentner, J. & Daschner, E. (2003). Shutting down operating theater ventilation when the theater is not in use: infection control and environmental aspects. *Infection Control Hospital Epidemiology, Vol.* 24, No. 8, pp.596-600, ISSN 0899-823X

Domsch, K.; Gams, W. &, Anderson, T. (2007). *Compedium of soli fungi* ed.2., IHW-Verlag, ISBN 978-3-930167-69-2, Eching, Germany

Fischer, G. & Dott, W. (2003). Relevance of airborne fungi and their secondary metabolites for environmental, occupational and indoor hygiene. *Archives of Microbiology*, Vol. 179, No. 2, pp. 75-82, ISSN 0302-8933

Fischer, G.; Müller, T.; Schwalbe, R.;Ostrowski,R. & Dott, W. (2000). Species-specific profiles of mycotoxins produced in cultures and associated with conidia of airborne fungi derived from biowaste. *International Journal of Hygiene and Environmental Health*, Vol. 203, No. 2, pp. 105 - 116, ISSN 1438-4639

Fog Nielsen, K. (2003). Mycotoxin production by indoor molds. *Fungal Genetics and Biology*, Vol. 39, No. 2, pp. 103-117, ISSN 1087-1845

Fraquet, T.; Gimenez, A. & Hidalgo, A. (2004). Imaging of opportunistic fungal infections in immunocompromised patient. *European Journal of Radiology*, Vol. 51, No. 2, pp. 130-138, ISSN 0720-048X

Garczewska, B. (2008). Szpitalne zakażenia grzybicze, In: *Zakażenia szpitalne*, D. Dzierżanowska, (Ed.), 409-425, α- medica press, ISBN 978-83-7522-022-3, Bielsko-Biała, Poland

Gareis, M. (1994). Cytotoxicity testing of samples originating from problem buildings, In: *Fungi and Bacteria in Indoor Air Environments: Health Effects, Detection and Remediation*, E. Johanning, (Ed.), 139 - 144, Eastern New York Occupational Health Program, Saratoga Springs, ISBN 0964730707, New York, USA,

Gniadek, A.; Macura, A.B.; Twarużek, M. & Grajewski, J. (2010). Cytotoxicity of Aspergillus strains isolated from the neonatal intensive care unit environment. *Advances in Medical Sciences*, Vol. 55, No. 2, pp. 242-249, ISSN 1896-1126

Gniadek, A.; Macura, A.B. & Twarużek, M. (2009). Characteristics fungi present in the intensive care unit environment. Part 2. Cytotoxicity of the isolated *Aspergillus* fungi. *Mikologia Lekarska*, Vol.16, No.1, pp. 15-18, ISSN 1232-986X

Gniadek, A.; Macura, A,B. & Górkiewicz, M. (2011). Cytotoxicity of *Aspergillus* fungi isolated from hospital environment. *Polish Journal of Microbiology*, Vol.60, No.1, pp. 59-63, ISSN 1733-1331

Haasum, I. & Nielsen, P. (1998). Ecophysiological characterization o common food -borne fungi in relation to pH and water activity under various atmospheric compositions. *Journal of Applied Microbiology*, Vol.84, No.3, pp. 451 - 460, ISSN 1364-5072

Hanelt, M.; Gareis, M. & Kollarczik, B.(1994). Cytotoxicity of mycotoxins evaluated by the MTT-cell culture assay. *Mycopathologia*, Vol. 128, No. 3, pp. 167 - 174, ISSN 0301-486X

Jarvis, B. (2003). Analysis for mycotoxins: the chemist's perspective. *Archives of Environmental Health*, Vo. 58, No. 8, pp. 479-483, ISSN 0003-9896

Jarvis, B. & Miller, J. (2005). Mycotoxins as harmful indoor air contaminants. *Applied Microbiology and Biotechnology*, Vol.66, No.4, pp. 367-372, ISSN 0175-7598

Kaiser, K. (2004). Wpływ zanieczyszczenia instalacji wentylacyjnych i klimatyzacyjnych podczas ich używania na jakość powietrza w obiektach szpitalnych. *Technika Chłodnicza i Klimatyzacyja* Vol. 98, pp.116-124, ISSN 1231-188X

Kaiser, K. (2011). Jakość powietrza wewnętrznego w szpitalach, In: *Profilaktyka zakażeń szpitalnych - bezpieczeństwo środowiska szpitalnego*, A. Pawińska, (Ed.), 57-87, α-medica press, ISBN 978-83-7522-068-1, Bielsko-Biała, Poland

Kamei, K.; Watanabe, A.; Nishimura, K. & Miyaji, M. (2002). Cytotoxicity of *Aspergillus fumigatus* culture filtrate against macrophages. *Nihon Ishinkin Gakkai Zasshi*, Vol.43, No.1, pp. 37-41, ISSN 0916-4804

Kelman, B.; Robbins, C.; Swenson, L. & Hardin, B. (2004). Risk from inhaled mycotoxins in indoor office and residential environments. *International Journal of Toxicology*, Vol.23, No.1, pp. 3-10, ISSN 1091-5818

Kędzierska, A.; Kochan, P.; Pietrzyk, A. & Kędzierska, J. (2007). Current status of fungal cell wall components in the immunodiagnostics of invasive fungal infections in humans: galactomannan, mannan and (1-->3)-beta-D-glucan antigens. *European Journal of Clinical Microbiology & Infectious Diseases*, Vol. 26, No. 11, pp. 755-766, ISSN 0934-9723

Klich, M. (2009). Health effects of *Aspergillus* in food and air. *Toxicology and Industrial Health*, Vol.25, No. 9-10, pp. 657-667, ISSN 0748-2337

Knochen, H.; Hübner, N.; Below, H.; Assadian, O.; Külpmann, R.; Kohlmann, T.; Hildebrand, K.; Clemens, S.; Bartels, C. & Kramer, A. (2010). Influence of floor disinfection on microbial and particulate burden measured under low turbulance air flow in ophthalmological operation theatres. *Klinische Monatsblätter für Augenheilkunde*, Vol. 227, No.11, pp.871-878, ISSN 0023-2165

Kosacka, M.; Nawrot, U.; Porębska, I.; Gostkowska A.; Dyła, T. & Jankowska R. (2010). The case of pulmonary semi-invasive aspergillosis and candidiasis of bronchi in patient with sarcoidosis. *Mikologia Lekarska*, Vol.17, No.4, pp. 244-247, ISSN 1232-986X

Kramer, A.; Külpmann, R.; Wille, F.; Christiansen, B.; Exner, M.; Kohlmann, T.; Heidecke, C.; Lippert, H.; Oldhafer, K.; Schilling, M.; Below, H.; Harnoss, J. & Assadian, O. (2010). Importance of displacement ventilation for operations and small surgical procedures from the infection preventive point of view. *Zentralblatt fur Chirurgie*, Vol.135, No. 1, pp.11-17, ISSN 0044-409X

Kriengkauykiat, J.; Ito, J. & Dadwal, S. (2011). Epidemiology and treatment approaches in management of invasive fungal infections. *Clinical Epidemiology*, Vol. 3, pp. 175–191, ISSN 1179-1349

Krzyściak, P.; Skóra, M. & Macura A.B. (2011). *Atlas grzybów chorobotwórczych człowieka*, MedPharm POLSKA, ISBN 978-83-60466-80-3, Wrocław, Poland

Kupfahl, C.; Michalka, A.; Lass-Flörl, C.; Fischer, G.; Haase, G.; Ruppert, T.; Geginat, G. & Hof, H. (2008). Gliotoxin production by clinical and environmental *Aspergillus fumigatus* strains. *International Journal of Medical Microbiology*, Vol. 298, No. 3-4, pp.319-327, ISSN 1438-4221

Kurnatowska, A. (1998). Biologia i ekologia grzybów chorobotwórczych, In: *Zarys mikologii lekarskiej*, E. Baran, (Ed.), 21 – 35,Volumed, ISBN 83-85564-17-9, Wrocław, Poland

Kurnatowski, P. & Miśkiewicz, S. (2009). Invasive aspergillosis among patients undergoing an transplantation. *Mikologia Lekarska*, Vol. 16, No.1, pp. 50-53, ISSN 1232-986X

Lass-Flörl, C.; Griff, K.; Mayr, A.; Petzer, A.; Gastl, G.; Bonatti, H,; Freund, M.; Kropshofer, G.; Dierich, M. & Nachbaur, D. (2005). Epidemiology and outcome of infections due to *Aspergillus terreus*: 10-year single centre experience. *British Journal of Haematology*, Vol. 131, No. 2, pp. 201-207, ISSN 0007-1048

Lewis, R.; Wiederhold, N.; Chi, J.; Han, X.; Komanduri, K.; Kontoyiannis, D. & Prince, R. (2005). Detection of gliotoxin in experimental and human aspergillosis. *Infection and Immunity*, Vol. 73, No. 1, pp. 635–637, ISSN 0019-9567

Lidwell, O.; Lowbury, E.; Whyte, W.; Blowers, R.; Stanley, S. & Lowe, D. (1982). Effect of ultraclean air in operating rooms on deep sepsis in the joint after total hip or knee replacement: a randomised study. *British Medical Journal* (*Clinical Research* ed), Vol. 285, No. 3, pp.10-14, ISSN 0267-0623

Macura, A.B. (1998). Czynniki sprzyjające zakażeniom grzybiczym. In *Zarys mikologii lekarskiej*, E. Baran, (Ed.), 289 - 295,Volumed, ISBN 83-85564-17-9, Wrocław, Poland

Mortensen, K.; Johansen, H.; Fuursted, K.; Knudsen, J.; Gahrn-Hansen, B.; Jensen, R.;. Howard, S. & Arendrup, M. (2011). A prospective survey of *Aspergillus* spp. in respiratory tract samples: prevalence, clinical impact and antifungal susceptibility. *European Journal of Clinical Microbiology & Infectious Diseases*, Epub ahead of print, DOI 10.1007/s10096-011-1229-7, ISSN 1435-4373

Pagano, L.; Caira, M.; Nosari, A.; Van Lint, M.; Candoni, A.; Offidani, M.; Aloisi, T.; Irrera, G.;Bonini, A.; Picardi, M.; Caramatti, C.; Invernizzi, R.; Mattei, D.; Melillo, L.; de Waure, C.; Reddiconto, G.; Fianchi, L.; Valentini, C.; Girmenia, C.; Leone, G. & Aversa, F. (2007). Fungal infections in recipients of hematopoietic stem cell transplants: results of the SEIFEM B-2004 study - Sorveglianza Epidemiologica Infezioni Fungine Nelle Emopatie Maligne. *Clinical Infectious Diseases*, Vol. 45, No.9, pp. 1161-1170, ISSN 1058-4838

Pegues, D.; Lasker, B.; McNeil, M.; Hamm, P.; Lundal, J. & Kubak, B. (2002). Cluster of cases on invasive aspergillosis in a transplant intensive care unit: evidence of person - to - person airborne tranmission. *Clinical Infectious Diseases*, Vol. 34, No. 3, pp. 412-416, . ISSN 1058-4838

Piotrowska, M. (2000). Grzyby strzępkowe, In: *Mikrobiologia techniczna*, Z. Libudzisz &., K. Kowal, (Ed.), 63-85, Politechnika Łódzka, ISBN 83-87198-5-1, Łódź, Polska

Pitt, J.; Basilico, J.; Abarca, M. & López L. (2000). Mycotoxins and toxigenic fungi. *Medical Mycology*, Vol. 38 (Suppl. 1), pp. 41-46, ISSN 1369-3786

Raper, K. & Fennell D. (1965). *The Genus Aspergillus*. The Williams & Wilkins Company. ISBN 978-1-904455-53-0, Baltimore, USA.

Ribeiro, S.; Santana, A,; Arriagada, G.; Martins, J. & Takagaki, T. (2005). A novel cause of invasive pulmonary infection in an immunocompetent patient: *Aspergillus candidus*. *The Journal of Infection*, Vol.51, No. 4, pp. 195-197, ISSN 0163-4453

Richardson, M. (2005). Changing patterns and trends in systemic fungal infections. *The Journal of Antimicrobial Chemotherapy*, Vol.56, Suppl. 1, pp. 5-11, ISSN 0305-7453

Poirot, J.; Gangneux, J.; Fischer, A.; Malbernard, M.; Challier, S.; Laudinet, N. & Bergeron, V. (2007). Evaluation of a new mobile system for protecting immune-suppressed patients against airborne contamination. *American Journal of Infection Control*, Vol.35, No. 7 pp.460-466, ISSN 0196-6553

Shelton, B.; Kirkland, K.; Flanders, W. & Morris G. (2002). Profiles of airborne fungi in buildings and outdoor environments in the United States. *Applied and Environmental Microbiology*, Vol.68, No. 4, pp. 1743–1753, ISSN 0099-2240

Singh, A. & Del Poeta, M. (2011). Lipid signalling in pathogenic fungi. *Cellular Microbiology*, Vol.13, No. 2, pp.177-185, ISSN 1462-5814

Skaug, M.; Eduard, W. & Stormer, F. (2001). Ochratoxin A in airborne dust and fungal conidia. *Mycopathologia*, Vo. 151, No. 2, pp. 93-98, ISSN 0301-486X

Smith, J.; Solomons, G.; Lewis, C. & Anderson, J. (1995). Role of mycotoxins in human and animal nutrition and health. *Natural Toxins*, Vol. 3, No. 4, pp.187-192, ISSN 1056-9014

Türel, O. (2011). Newer antifungal agents. *Expert Review of Anti-Infective Therapy*, Vol. 9, No. 3, pp.325-338, ISSN 1478-7210

Watanabe, A.; Kamei, K.; Sekine, T.; Higurashi, H.; Ochiai, E.; Hashimoto, Y. & Nishimura, K. (2004). Cytotoxic substances from *Aspergillus fumigatus* in oxygenated or poorly oxygenated environment. *Mycopathologia*, Vol. 158, No. 1, pp. 1-7, ISSN 0301-486X

Zyska, B. (1999). *Zagrożenia biologiczne w budynku*, Arkady, ISBN 83-213-4117-9, Warszawa, Poland

Zyska, B. (2001). *Katastrofy, awarie i zagrożenia mikrobiologiczne w przemyśle i budownictwie*, Politechnika Łódzka, ISBN 83-7283-018-5, Łódź, Poland

13

Expression and Characterization of Bovine Milk Antimicrobial Proteins Lactoperoxidase and Lactoferrin by Vaccinia Virus

Tetsuya Tanaka[1], Xuenan Xuan[2], Kozo Fujisaki[1] and Kei-ichi Shimazaki[3]
[1]*Laboratory of Emerging Infectious Diseases, Department of Frontier Veterinary Science, Faculty of Agriculture, Kagoshima University, Korimoto, Kagoshima,*
[2]*National Research Center for Protozoan Diseases, Obihiro University of Agriculture and Veterinary Medicine, Obihiro, Hokkaido,*
[3]*Laboratory of Dairy Food Science, Research Faculty Agriculture, Hokkaido University, Sapporo, Hokkaido,*
Japan

1. Introduction

Lactoperoxidase (LPO), a heme-containing oxidation-reduction enzyme present in milk and saliva, is part of an antimicrobial system, and converts thiocyanate to hypothiocyanate in a hydrogen peroxide-dependent reaction. The molecular weight of LPO is approximately 78 kDa, and the carbohydrate moiety comprises about 10% of the total weight (Mansson-Rahemtulla et al., 1988). LPO, myeloperoxidase (MPO), eosinophil peroxidase (EPO) and thyroid peroxidase (TPO) belong to the homologous mammalian peroxidase family and share 50 to 70% identity. Even higher homology can be found among their active site-related residues. These peroxidases can catalyze oxidation of halides and pseudohalides such as thiocyanate by hydrogen peroxide to form potent oxidant and bactericidal agents. MPO has been shown to inactivate influenza virus (Yamamoto et al., 1991) and HIV-1 virus (Klebanoff & Kazazi, 1995). Human recombinant MPO has been shown to have a virucidal effect on HIV-1 virus (Moguilevsky et al., 1992; Chochola et al., 1994) and cytomegalovirus (EI Messaoudi et al., 2002). However, few studies have examined whether LPO inhibits virus infection *in vitro* and *in vivo*.

Lactoferrin (LF), also called lactotransferrin, is an iron-binding protein present in milk, saliva, tears, mucus secretions and secondary granules of neutrophils. Each LF molecule can bind 2 Fe (III) ions tightly but reversibly. This binding is dependent on concomitant binding of anions such as bicarbonate and carbonate, which play an essential role in holding the metal firmly (Masson et al., 1968). Thus, LF can exist in an iron-free (apo) or iron-bound (holo) state. LF is a prominent antimicrobial component of mucosal surfaces prone to attack by microbial pathogens. LF is actively secreted by neutrophils in the inflammatory response (Gutteberg et al., 1984). As an anti-microbial component of colostrum and milk, LF may play significant roles in protection of neonates from infectious diseases (García-Montoya et al., 2011). The importance of LF in host defense is underlined by findings indicating that patients with congenital or acquired defects of LF production exhibit an abnormal predisposition to recurrent infections by bacteria, fungi and parasites (Venge et al., 1984; Tanaka et al., 1996). Patients with acute viral illnesses such as chickenpox, measles, rubella, hepatitis or Epstein-Barr virus infection have reduced plasma LF concentrations, although their total neutrophil numbers are similar to those of non-infected subjects (Bayners et al., 1986).

Vaccinia virus belongs to the family of poxviridae, and is the most intensively studied member of the poxvirus family (Moss et al., 1990). Poxviruses replicate in the cytoplasm of infected cells without using nuclear enzymes of the host cells for transcription or DNA synthesis. Vaccinia virus has circumvented the need for nuclear enzymes by encoding or packaging a complete enzyme system for transcription (Moss et al., 1990) and DNA synthesis, including a DNA-dependent DNA polymerase (Moss & Cooper, 1982), DNA topoisomerase (Shuman et al., 1987) and DNA ligase (Kerr et al., 1989). Consequently, the vaccinia virus is widely used as an expression system in molecular biotechnology. Recombinant vaccinia virus has been demonstrated to be an effective antigen delivery system for infectious diseases in many species, with rabies and rinderpest being notable examples (Ertl and Xiang, 1996; Tsukiyama et al., 1989). In addition recombinant vaccinia virus can give rise to long-term immunity (Inui et al., 1995). In previous studies, recombinant vaccinia virus has been used produce cytokines (e.g., IFN-β, IFN-γ) (Kohonen-Corish et al., 1989, 1990; Peplinski et al., 1996; Nishikawa et al., 2000, 2001), but it has not yet been used for expression of bovine LPO (bLPO) or bovine LF (bLF). In the present study, we constructed recombinant vaccinia viruses that express bLPO and bLF with antiviral activity, and characterized production of bLPO and bLF and replication of the recombinant virus. The present results indicate that expression of bLPO and bLF by recombinant vaccinia virus may be useful for treatment of infectious diseases in humans or animals (Tanaka et al., 2006).

2. Materials and methods

2.1 Cells and viruses

Rabbit kidney (RK13) cells were cultured in Eagle's minimum essential medium (EMEM, Sigma Chemicals Co., St. Louis, MO, USA) supplemented with 8% heat-inactivated fetal bovine serum (FBS). Vaccinia virus LC16mO (mO) strain and its recombinant were propagated in RK13 cells in EMEM supplemented with 8% FBS.

2.2 Construction of recombinant vaccinia virus that expresses bLPO and bLF

bLPO or bLF cDNA was amplified from mammary gland cells, using reverse polymerase chain reaction (RT-PCR) with primers designed from bLPO or bLF cDNA (Dull et al., 1990; Nakamura et al., 2001). The PCR products were blunted by T4 DNA polymerase and ligated with the vaccinia virus transfer vector pAK8 (Yasuda et al., 1990), which was cut with *Sal* I and then blunted. The plasmid (pAK/bLPO or pAK/bLF) was transfected into RK13 cells using a lipofectin reagent (Life Technologies Japan, Tokyo, Japan) for 1 h after infection with the mO strain. After 2 days of incubation, culture medium was collected. We isolated recombinant virus (vv/bLPO or vv/bLF) produced by homologous recombination between pAK8 and viral thymidine kinase (TK-) cells in the presence of 100 μg/ml 5-bromo-2'-deoxyuridine, selecting TK- viruses by plaque isolation.

2.3 Immunofluorescence test (IFAT)

RK13 cells were infected with mO, vv/bLPO and vv/bLF (5 plaque-forming units [PFU]/cell, 48 h), and subjected to indirect immunofluorescence assay test (IFAT). The infected RK13 cells were fixed with acetone, and incubated with mouse anti-bLPO monoclonal antibody (anti-bLPO mAb) or mouse anti-bLF monoclonal antibody (anti-bLF mAb); these antibodies were produced by the present authors (Shimazaki et al., 1998; Watanabe et al., 1998). The cells were then stained with fluorescein-conjugated goat anti-mouse antibody (Southern Biotechnology Associates Inc., Birmingham, AL, UK) or fluorescein-conjugated sheep anti-rabbit antibody (Waco Pure Chemical, Osaka, Japan). The cells were observed using fluorescence microscopy.

2.4 Sodium dodecylsulfate-polyacrylamide gel electrophoresis (SDS-PAGE) and western blot analysis

RK13 cells in tissue culture (colony diameter, 15 mm) were infected with the mO strain or the recombinant vaccinia virus at a multiplicity of infection (moi) of 5 for 1 h at 37°C. Then, the cells were washed with EMEM and cultured in 500 μl of EMEM at 37°C for 48 h. The cell extracts and culture supernatants were subjected to SDS-PAGE (Laemmli, 1970) under reducing conditions, followed by electrical transfer of proteins to a PVDF membrane (Osmonics Inc., Westborough, MA, USA). The membrane was immersed in blocking buffer (phosphate-buffered saline [PBS] containing 3% bovine serum albumin) at 4°C overnight, incubated with rabbit anti-bLPO polyclonal antibody (anti-bLPO Ab) or anti-bLF mAb (diluted in the blocking buffer) at 37°C for 1 h, washed 3 times with PBS, and then incubated with alkaline phosphatase-conjugated goat anti-rabbit IgG antibodies (Promega Co., Madison, WI, USA) or horseradish peroxidase-conjugated goat anti-mouse IgG antibodies (Waco Pure Chemical, Osaka, Japan) (diluted in the blocking buffer) at 37°C for 1 h. The membrane was visualized by incubation with BCIP/NBT color substrate (Promega Co.) or 0.5 mg/ml diaminobenzidine and 0.005% H_2O_2.

2.5 Tunicamycin treatment

Recombinant vaccinia virus-infected RK13 cells (5 PFU/cell) were incubated in EMEM containing 1 μg/ml tunicamycin (Sigma Chemical Co.), which prevents synthesis of N-linked sugars, for 1 to 48 h post-infection (pi). The cells were then harvested, and the cell lysate was subjected to Western blot analysis to assay for expression of recombinant proteins.

2.6 Virus growth analysis

RK13 cells were infected with mO or recombinant viruses at a moi of 5 PFU/cell. After 1 h, the infected cells were washed with EMEM and cultured for 12-72 h after viral infection. Virus titers were determined by plaque titration according to Nishikawa et al. (2000). Data from this experiment were evaluated using Student's t-test. The 95% level of significance was used in the analysis.

3. Results

3.1 Expression of bLPO and bLF by recombinant vaccinia virus in RK13 cells

Vaccinia virus mO strain and pAK/bLPO or pAk/bLF were allowed to infect RK13 cells, and virus-containing medium of the infected RK13 cells was collected and analyzed by IFAT or Western blotting for the presence of recombinant bLPO or bLF. A recombinant bLPO or bLF-expressing clone was selected by the plaque-assay technique. vv/bLPO-infected cells were examined by IFAT and reacted with anti-bLPO mAb (Fig. 1B). Anti-bLF mAb reacted with vv/bLF-infected RK13 cells (Fig. 1C). mO-infected cells served as negative reference and were labeled with both antibody reagents (Fig. 1A). Recombinant bLPO and bLF were detected in cell extracts by Western blot analysis using anti-bLPO Ab and anti-bLF mAb (Fig. 2A, C lane 4). Recombinant bLPO and bLF were secreted into supernatants, as indicated by recombinant bLPO bands at 88 and 90 kDa and bLF band at 80 kDa (Fig.2B, D lane 4). The apparent molecular weight of these recombinant bLPO molecules (88 and 90 kDa) was greater than that of native bLPO (78 kDa), but apparent molecular weight of the bLF molecules (80 kDa) was equal to that of native bLF (80 kDa). To test whether the increase of molecular weights in recombinant bLPO was due to glycosylation, the infected cells were treated with tunicamycin. As a result, no protein was secreted into the supernatant by infected cells treated with tunicamycin (data not shown). In the cell extracts, the apparent molecular weight of bLPO was reduced to 80 kDa (Fig. 3 lane 4), indicating that recombinant bLPO were modified by N-linked sugars. The 90 kDa molecule would be a proprotein. Recombinant bLF was not detected in cell extracts from infected cells treated with tunicamycin, suggesting that tunicamycin treatment completely abolished production of recombinant bLF (data not shown).

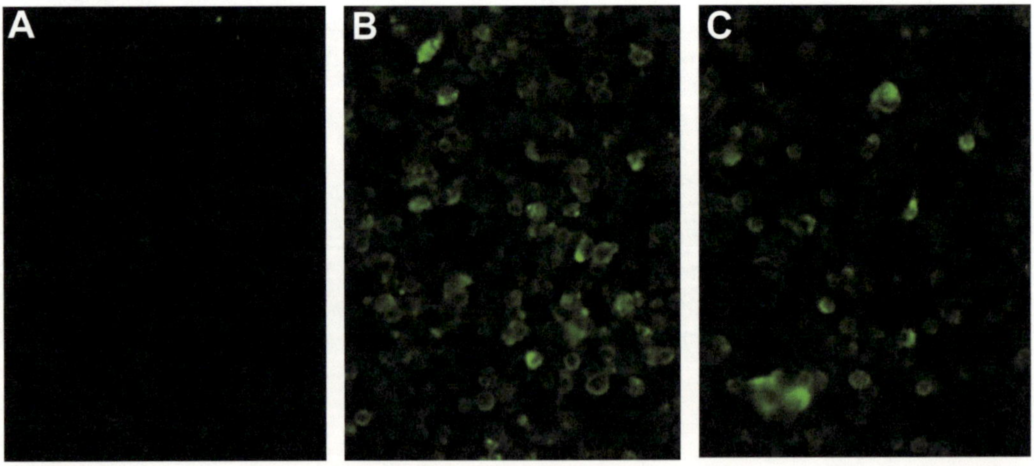

Fig. 1. Immunofluorescence analysis of vv/bLPO and vv/bLF expressed in RK 13 cells. (A) mO-infected RK13 cells reacted with anti-bLPO mAb and anti-bLF mAb. (B) vv/bLPO-infected RK13 cells reacted with anti-bLPO mAb. (C) vv/bLF-infected RK13 cells reacted with anti-bLF mAb.

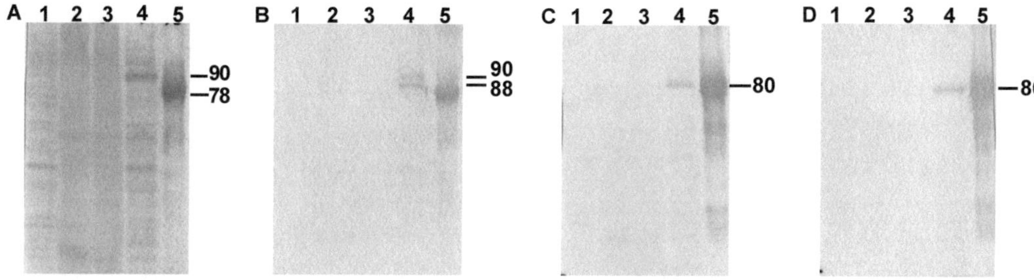

Fig. 2. Western blot analysis of bLPO (A, B) and bLF (C, D) in RK13 cells. Cell extracts (A, C) and culture supernatants (B, D) of RK13 cells infected with recombinant vaccinia virus were analyzed using anti-bLPO Ab or anti-bLF mAb. Lane 1, RK13 cells; lane 2, mO-infected RK13 cells; lane 3, vv/green florescence protein-infected RK13 cells; lane 4, vv/bLPO- or vv/bLF-infected RK13 cells; lane 5, native bLPO or bLF (2 μg). Molecular weights of marker proteins are given in kDa.

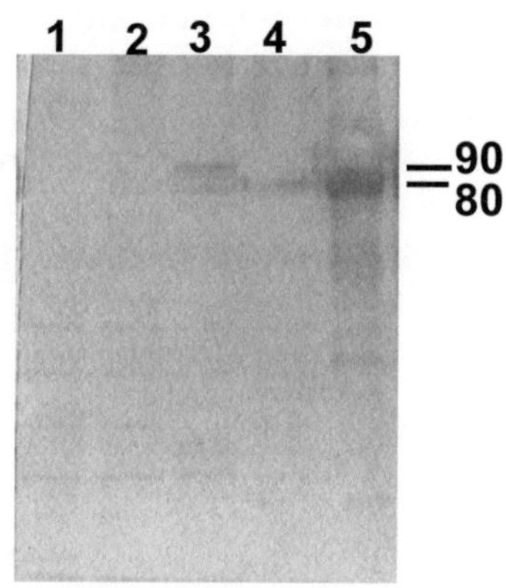

Fig. 3. Western blot analysis of bLPO in RK13 cells treated with tunicamycin. Cell extracts of RK13 cells infected with recombinant vaccinia virus were analyzed using anti-bLPO Ab. Lane 1, mO-infected RK13 cells; lane 2, mO-infected RK13 cells treated with tunicamycin; lane 3, vv/bLPO-infected RK13 cells; lane 4, vv/bLPO-infected RK13 cells treated with tunicamycin; lane 5, native bLPO (2 μg). Molecular weights of marker proteins are given in kDa.

3.2 Time course of bLPO and bLF production in the recombinant vaccinia virus system

To analyze the kinetics of expression of bLPO and bLF gene products, culture supernatants from RK13 cells infected with vv/bLPO and vv/bLF were collected from 12-72 h pi. Recombinant bLPO and bLF were first detectable in culture supernatant at 24 h pi (Fig. 4 lane 2). The amount of recombinant bLPO and bLF increased from 36 to 48 h pi, and reached plateau levels by 72 h pi (Fig. 4 lane 3-6).

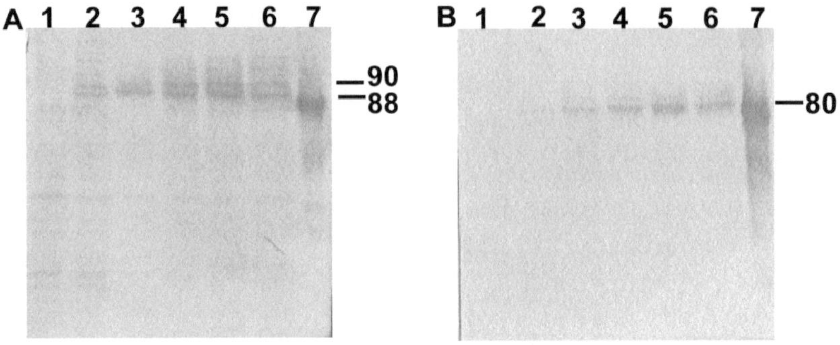

Fig.4. Kinetics of rbLPO (A) and rbLF (B) synthesis. RK13 cells were infected with recombinant vaccinia virus and harvested at 12 (lane 1), 24 (lane 2), 36 (lane 3), 48 (lane 4), 60 (lane 5) and 72 hours pi (lane 6). Lane 7, native bLPO or bLF (2 μg). Culture supernatants of infected RK13 cells were analyzed by Western blotting using anti-bLPO Ab or anti-bLF mAb. Molecular weights of marker proteins are given in kDa.

3.3 Growth analysis of vv/bLPO and vv/bLF in RK13 cells

The growth curves of mO, vv/bLPO and vv/bLF are compared in Fig. 5. Peak titers (reached at 48 h pi) of mO, vv/bLPO and vv/bLF were 1.6×10^5, 1.6×10^5 and 0.2×10^5 PFU/ml, respectively. These results indicate that bLF, but not bLPO, inhibits growth of recombinant virus in infected RK13 cells. There were no significant differences in growth between mO and vv/bLPO until 72 h pi ($P>0.05$, Student's t test mO vs. vv/bLPO). However, there were significant differences in growth between mO and vv/bLPO on one side and vv/bLF on the other side 48h pi through 72 h pi ($P<0.05$, Student's t test mO or vv/bLPO vs. vv/bLF).

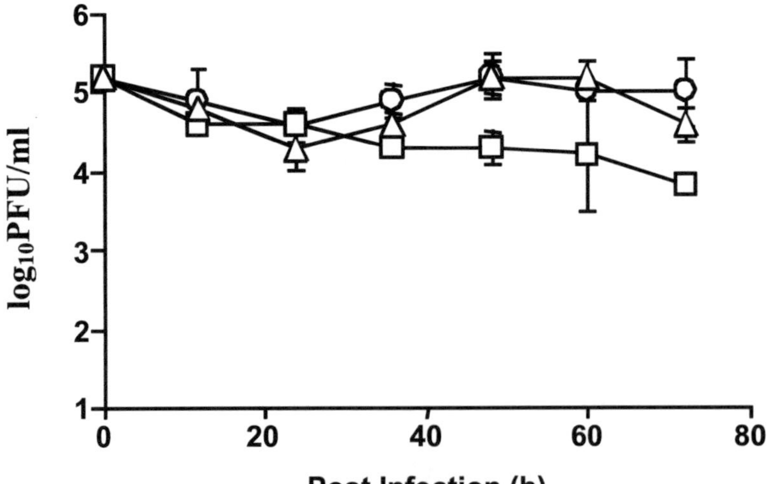

Fig. 5. Virus growth analysis. RK13 cells were infected with mO (○), vv/bLPO (△) and vv/bLF (□) at a moi of 5. Samples were harvested at the indicated time points, and progeny virus of RK13 cells was titered in triplicate.

4. Discussion

The expression systems using recombinant baculovirus or Chinese hamster ovary cells have been used to express bLPO (Tanaka et al., 2003; Watanabe et al., 1998). However, there have been no previous reports of use of vaccinia virus to express bLPO and bLF. The available evidence suggests that growth of vaccinia virus is inhibited by expression of bLPO and bLF. In the present study, recombinant vaccinia viruses expressing bLPO or bLF (vv/bLPO and vv/bLF, respectively) were constructed. RK13 cells were infected with vv/bLPO or vv/bLF, and we characterized virus growth and post-translation modifications of the resultant product.

Recombinant bLPO extracted from cell extracts and culture supernatants had an apparent molecular weight of 88 and 90 kDa, which is greater than that of native bLPO (78 kDa) in Western blot analysis. These size differences may be due to a difference in glycosylation level and differences in processing between RK13 cells and the mammary gland. When the infected RK13 cells were treated with tunicamycin, the apparent molecular weight of recombinant bLPO in the cells was 80 kDa, suggesting that recombinant bLPO is modified by N-linked glycosylation. Tunicamycin treatment completely abolished secretion of bLPO, indicating that N-linked glycosylation is essential for bLPO secretion. Therefore, recombinant bLPO was differentially processed during synthesis and secretion from RK13 cells compared with the mammary gland. A similar situation was previously reported for recombinant bLPO expressed in insect cells (Tanaka et al., 2003). Interestingly, the molecular weight of recombinant bLPO produced in RK13 cells was higher than that expressed in insect cells. The carbohydrate structure analysis of purified recombinant bLPO expressed in insect cells and native bLPO found different reactivity with PHA-E4, PNA, and RCA120 by using lectin assay (Tanaka et al., 2003). Therefore, the glycosylation level of recombinant protein might also be different between RK13 cells and insect cells. Most of the bLPO extracted from milk showed Asp-101 as the N-terminal amino acid residue (Dull et al., 1990; Watanabe et al., 2000). However, Watanabe et al. (2000) found also that different preparations of bLPO showed a different N-terminal amino acid residue. These variations may result from differences in the disk-electrophoresis and ion-exchange chromatography methods used for analysis (Carlström, 1969). Thus, it might be possible that the 90 kDa form of recombinant bLPO did not undergo proteolysis, whereas the 88 kDa form of recombinant bLPO be the result of proteolysis of some N-terminal amino acid residues during synthesis and secretion by RK 13 cells as observed for bLPO synthesized by the mammary gland.

Bovine Lactoferrin is a 80 kDa iron-binding glycoprotein found in physiological fluids of mammals. bLF has also an antimicrobial activity as bLPO, and presumably contributes to the protective functions of milk against infectious diseases. In RK13 cells infected with vv/bLF, recombinant bLF was detected in both cell extracts and culture supernatants. However, the replication of vv/bLF at a moi of 5 PFU/cell was inhibited by the antiviral activity of recombinant bLF, suggesting that vv/bLF has an antiviral effect against vaccinia virus. On the other hand, the expression of bLPO was also detected in cell extracts and culture supernatants of the vv/bLPO-infected cells as well as vv/bLF-infected cells. However, the replication of vv/bLPO at a moi of 5 PFU/cell was not inhibited by antiviral activity of recombinant bLPO, because LPO catalyzes oxidation of endogenous thiocyanate

(SCN^-) to produce hypothiocyanate ($OSCN^-$) only in the presence of hydrogen peroxide (H_2O_2). These products have a broad-spectrum antimicrobial and antiviral activity (Shin et al., 2001, 2005). Therefore due to the absence of thiocyanate (SCN^-) and/or hydrogen peroxide (H_2O_2) the replication of recombinant virus is not inhibited by recombinant bLPO.

Studies indicate that gene therapy using viral vectors containing the bLPO gene can produce anti-microbial and anti-tumor activity (Odajima et al., 1996; Stanislawski et al., 1989). The major problem with such viral vectors is their attenuation. The recombinant vaccinia viruses in this report are TK^- in phenotype that may reduce pathogenicity *in vivo* (Buller et al., 1985) because of insertion of the bLPO gene into the TK gene. Our results demonstrate the attenuation of the viral pathogenicity by introduction of the bLPO gene into vaccinia virus. Thus fine tuning of bLPO activity, may allow the control of virulence of vaccinia virus vector necessary for medical and veterinary applications *in vivo*.

5. Conclusion

Lactoperoxidase (LPO) is a 78 kDa heme-containing oxidation-reduction enzyme present in milk, and lactoferrin (LF) is an 80 kDa iron-binding glycoprotein found in physiological fluids of mammals. LPO and LF have antimicrobial activity, and presumably contribute to the protective functions of milk against infectious diseases. In this study, recombinant vaccinia viruses expressing bovine lactoperoxidase (vv/bLPO) or bovine lactoferrin (vv/bLF) were constructed. In rabbit kidney (RK13) cells infected with vv/bLPO or vv/bLF, recombinant bLPO or bLF was detected in both cell extracts and supernatants. Growth of vv/bLPO at a multiplicity of infection was not inhibited by antiviral activity of recombinant bLPO, indicating that this recombinant virus could be used as a suicide viral vector. Unfortunately, growth of vv/bLF at a multiplicity of infection was inhibited by antiviral activity of recombinant bLF, suggesting that vv/bLF has an antiviral effect against vaccinia virus. These results indicate that a combination of bLPO and vaccinia virus vector may be useful for medical and veterinary applications *in vivo*.

6. Acknowledgments

This work was supported by grants from the Hokuto Foundation and the Food Science Institute Foundation (Ryoshoku-kenkyukai, Odawara). The first author is supported by Postdoctoral Fellowships for Research Abroad of the Japan Society for the Promotion of Science.

7. References

Baynes, R.; Bezwoda, W.; Bothwell, T.; Khan, Q. & Mansoor, N. (1986). The non immune inflammatory response: serial changes in plasma iron, iron binding capacity, lactoferrin, ferritin and C reactive protein. *Scandinavian Journal of clinical and Laboratory Investigation,* Vol.46, No.7, (November 1986), pp.695-704, ISSN 0036-5513

Buller, RM.; Smith, GL.; Cremer, K.; Notkins, AL. & Moss, B. (1985). Decreased virulence of recombinant vaccinia virus expression vectors is associated with thymidine kinase-negative phenotype. *Nature,* Vol.317, No.6004, (October 1985), pp.813-815, ISSN 0028-0836

Carlström, A. (1969). Lactoperoxidase. Identification of multiple molecular forms and their interrelationships. *Acta Chemica Scandinavica,* Vol. 23, No.1, (1969), pp.171-184, ISSN 0001-5393

Chochola, J.; Yamaguchi, Y.; Moguilevsky, N.; Bollen, A.; Strosberg, D.A. & Stanislawski, M. (1994). Virucidal effect of myeloperoxidase on human immunodeficiency virus type-1 infected cells. *Antimicrobial Agents and Chemotherapy,* Vol.38, No.5, (May 1994), pp.969-972, ISSN 0066-4804

Dull, TJ.; Uyeda, C.; Strosberg, AD.; Nedwin, G. & Seilhamer, J.J. (1990). Molecular cloning of cDNA encoding bovine and human lactoperoxidase. *DNA and Cell Biology,* Vol.9, No.7, (September 1990), pp.499-509, ISSN 1557-7430

El Messaoudi, K.; Verheyden, AM.; Thiry, L.; Fourez, S.; Tasiaux, N.; Bollen, A. & Moguilevsky, N. (2002). Human recombinant myeloperoxidase antiviral activity on cytomegalovirus. *Journal of Medical Virology,* Vol.66, No.2, (February 2002), pp.218-223, ISSN 1096-9071

Ertl, HC. & Xiang, Z. (1996). Novel vaccine approaches. *Journal of Immunology,* Vol. 156, No.10 , (May 1996), pp.3579-3582, ISSN 0022-1767

García-Montoya, IA.; Cendón, TS.; Arévalo-Gallegos, S. & Rascón-Cruz, Q. (2011) Lactoferrin a multiple bioactive protein: An overview. *Biochim Biophys Acta (BBA) - General Subjects,* (In press), ISSN 0304-4165

Gutteberg, T.; Haneberg, B. & Jorgenson, T. (1984). Lactoferrin in relation to acute phase proteins in sera from newborn infants with severe infections. *European Journal of Pediatrics,* Vol.142, No.1, (April 1984), pp.37-39, ISSN 0340-6199

Inui, K.; Barrett, T.; Kitching, RP. & Yamanouchi, K. (1995). Long-term immunity in cattle vaccinated with a recombinant rinderpest vaccine. *Veterinary Record,* Vol.137, No.26 , (December 1995), pp.669-670, ISSN 0042-4900

Kerr, SM. & Smith, GL. (1989). Vaccinia virus encodes a polypeptide with DNA ligase activity. *Nucleic Acids Research,* Vol.17, No.22, (November 1989), pp.9039-9050, ISSN 0305-1048

Klebanoff, SJ. & Kazazi, F. (1995). Inactivation of human immunodeficiency virus type 1 by the amine oxidase-peroxidase system. *Journal of Clinical Microbiology,* Vol.33, No.8 , (August 1995), pp.2054-2057, ISSN 0095-1137

Kohonen-Corish, MR.; Blanden, RV. & King, N. (1989). Induction of cell surface expression of HLA antigens by human IFN-gamma encoded by recombinant vaccinia virus. *Journal of Immunology,* Vol.143, No.2 , (July 1989), pp.623-627, ISSN 0022-1767

Kohonen-Corish, MR.; King, NJ.; Woodhams, CE. & Ramshaw, IA. (1990). Immunodeficient mice recover from infection with vaccinia virus expressing interferon-gamma. *European Journal of Immunology,* Vol.20, No.1, (January 1990), pp.157-161, ISSN 1521-4141

Laemmli, UK. (1970). Cleavage of structural proteins during the assembly of the head of bacteriophage T4. *Nature,* Vol.227, No.5259, (August 1970), pp.680-685, ISSN 0028-0836

Masson, PL. & Heremans, JF. (1968). Presence of an iron binding protein (lactoferrin) in the genital tract of the female. I. its immunohistochemical localization in the endometrium. *Fertility and Sterility* Vol.19, No.5, (September 1968), pp.679-689, ISSN 0015-0282

Mansson-Rahemtulla, B.; Rahemtulla, F.; Baldone, DC.; Pruitt, KM. & Hjerpe, A. (1988). Purification and characterization of human salivary peroxidase. *Biochemistry,* Vol.27, No.1, (January 1988), pp.233-239, ISSN 0006-2960

Moguilevsky, N.; Steens, M.; Thiriart, C.; Prieels, J. P.; Thiry, L. & Bollen, A. (1992). Lethal oxidative damage to human immunodeficiency virus by human recombinant myeloperoxidase. *FEBS Letter,* Vol.302, No.3, (May 1992), pp.209-212, ISSN 0014-5793

Moss, B. (1990). Regulation of vaccinia virus transcription. *Annual Review of Biochemistry,* Vol.59, (July 1990), pp.661-688, ISSN 1545-4509

Moss, B. & Cooper, N. (1982). Genetic evidence for vaccinia virus-encoded DNA polymerase: isolation of phosphonoacetate-resistant enzyme from the cytoplasm of cells infected with mutant virus. *Journal of Virology,* Vol.43, No.2, (August 1982), pp. 673-678, ISSN 0022-538X

Nakamura, I.; Watanabe, A.; Tsunemitsu, H.; Lee, N-Y.; Kumura, H.; Shimazaki, K. & Yagi, Y. (2001). Production of recombinant bovine lactoferrin N-lobe in insect cells and its antimicrobial activity. *Protein Expression and Purification,* Vol.21, No.3, (April 2001), pp.424-431, ISSN 1046-5928

Nishikawa, Y.; Iwata, A.; Katsumata, A.; Xuan, X.; Nagasawa, H.; Igarashi, I.; Fujisaki, K.; Otsuka, H. & Mikami, T. (2001). Expression of canine interferon-γ by a recombinant vaccinia virus and its antiviral effect. *Virus Research,* Vol.75, No.2, (June 2001), pp.113-121, ISSN 0168-1702

Nishikawa, Y.; Iwata, A.; Xuan, X.; Nagasawa, H.; Fujisaki, K.; Otsuka, H. & Mikami, T. (2000). Expression of canine interferon-β by a recombinant vaccinia virus. *FEBS Letters,* Vol.466, No.1, (January 2000), pp.179-182, ISSN 0014-5793

Odajima, T.; Onishi, M.; Hayama, E.; Motoji, N.; Momose. Y. & Shigematsu, A. (1996). Cytolysis of B-16 melanoma tumor cells mediated by the myeloperoxidase and lactoperoxidase systems. *Biological Chemistry,* Vol.377, No.11, (November 1996), pp.689-693, ISSN 1431-6730

Peplinski, G.R.; Tsung, K.; Meko, J.B. & Norton, J.A. (1996). Prevention of murine breast cancer by vaccination with tumor cells modified by cytokine-producing recombinant vaccinia viruses. *Annals of Surgical Oncology,* Vol.3, No.1, (January 1996), pp.15-23, ISSN 1068-9265

Shimazaki, K.; Kamio, M.; Nan, M.S.; Harakawa, S.; Tanaka, T.; Omata, Y.; Saito, A.; Kumura, H.; Mikawa, K.; Igarashi, I. & Suzuki, N. (1998). Structure and immunochemical studies on bovine lactoferrin fragments. *Advances in Experimental Medicine and Biology,* Vol.443, (1998), pp. 41-48, ISSN 0065-2598

Shin, K.; Hayasawa, H. & Lönnerdal, B. (2001). Inhibition of *Escherichia coli* respiratory enzymes by the lactoperoxidase-hydrogen peroxidase-thiocyanate antimicrobial system. *Journal of Applied Microbiology,* Vol.90, No.4, (April 2001), pp.489-493, ISSN 1365-2672

Shin, K.; Wakabayashi, H.; Yamauchi, K.; Teraguchi, S.; Tamura, Y.; Kurokawa, M. & Shiraki, K. (2005). Effects of orally administered bovine lactoferrin and lactoperoxidase on influenza virus infection in mice. *Journal of Medical Microbiology,* Vol.54, No.8, (August 2005), pp.717-723, ISSN 0022-2615

Shuman, S. & Moss, B. (1987). Identification of a vaccinia virus gene encoding a type I DNA topoisomerase. *Proceedings of the National Academy of Sciences of the United States of America,* Vol.84, No.21, (November 1987), pp.7478-7482, ISSN 1091-6490

Stanislawski, M.; Rousseau, V.; Goavec, M. & Ito, H. (1989). Immunotoxins containing glucose oxidase and lactoperoxidase with tumoricidal properties: In vitro killing effectiveness in a mouse plasmacytoma cell model. *Cancer Research,* Vol.49, No.20, (October 1989), pp.5497-5540, ISSN 0008-5472

Tanaka, T.; Murakami, S.; Kumura, H.; Igarashi, I. & Shimazaki, K. (2006). Parasiticidal activity of bovine lactoperoxidase against *Toxoplasma gondii*. *Biochemstry and Cell Biology,* Vol.84, No.5, (October 2006), pp.774-779, ISSN 0829-8211

Tanaka, T.; Omata, Y.; Saito, A.; Shimazaki, K.; Igarashi, I. & Suzuki, N. (1996). Growth inhibitory effects of bovine lactoferrin to *Toxoplasma gondii* parasites in murine somatic cells. *The Journal of Veterinary Medical Science,* Vol.58, No.1, (January 1998), pp.61-65, ISSN 0916-7250

Tanaka, T.; Sato, S.; Kumura, H. & Shimazaki, K. (2003). Expression and characterization of bovine lactoperoxidase by recombinant baculovirus. *Bioscience Biotechnology and Biochemistry,* Vol.67, No.10, (October 2003), pp.2254-2261, ISSN 1347-6947

Tsukiyama, K.; Yoshikawa, Y.; Kamata, H.; Imaoka, K.; Asano, K.; Funahashi, S.; Maruyama, T.; Shida, H.; Sugimoto, M. & Yamanouchi, K. (1989). Development of heat-stable recombinant rinderpest vaccine. *Achieves Virology,* Vol.107, No.3-4, (September 1989), pp.225-235, ISSN 0304-8608

Venge, P.; Foucard, T.; Henrickson, J.; Hakansson, L. & Kreuger, A. (1984). Serum-levels of lactoferrin, lysozyme and myeloperoxidase in normal, infection-prone and leukemic children. *Clinica Chimica Acta,* Vol.136, No.2-3, (January 1984), pp.121-130, ISSN 0009-8981

Watanabe, S.; Murata, S.; Kumura, H.; Nakamura, S.; Bollen, A.; Moguilevsky, N. & Shimazaki, K. (2000). Bovine lactoperoxidase and its recombinant: comparison of structure and some biochemical properties. *Biochemical and Biophysical Research Communications,* Vol.274, No.3, (August 2000), pp.756-761, ISSN 0006-291X

Watanabe, S.; Varsalona, F.; Yoo, Y. C.; Guillaume, JP.; Bollen, A.; Shimazaki, K. & Moguilevsky, N. (1998). Recombinant bovine lactoperoxidase as a tool to study the heme environment in mammalian peroxidases. *FEBS Letters,* Vol.441, No.3, (December 1998), pp.476-479, ISSN 0014-5793

Yamamoto, K.; Miyoshi-Koshio, T.; Utsuki, Y.; Mizuno, S. & Suzuki, K. (1991). Virucidal activity and viral protein modification by myeloperoxidase: a candidate for defense factor of human polymorphonuclear leukocytes against influenza virus infection. *Journal of Infectious Diseases,* Vol.164, No.1, (July 1991), pp.8-14, ISSN 0022-1899

Yasuda, A.; Kimura-Kuroda, J.; Ogimoto, M.; Miyamoto, M.; Sata, T.; Sato, T.; Takamura, C.; Kurata, T.; Kojima, A. & and Yasui, K. (1990). Induction of protective immunity in animals vaccinated with recombinant vaccinia viruses that express PreM and E glycoproteins of Japanese encephalitis virus. *Journal of Virology*, Vol.64, No.6, (June 1990), pp.2788-2795, ISSN 0022-538X

14

Three Cases of *Mycobacterium tuberculosis* Infection Initially Recognized by Focus Changing Examination in Gram Staining

Yoshiko Atsukawa[1], Sayoko Kawakami[1], Yasuo Ono[3], Ryuichi Fujisaki[2], Yukihisa Miyazawa[1] and Hajime Nishiya[2]
[1]*Department of Central Clinical Laboratory, Teikyo University Hospital, Tokyo;*
[2]*Department of Internal Medicine, Teikyo University School of Medicine, Tokyo;*
[3]*Department of Microbiology, Teikyo University School of Medicine, Tokyo, Japan*

1. Introduction

Patients with fever and pulmonary symptoms with consolidation shadows on chest X-ray are assumed to have pneumonia, which in most cases is bacterial-induced, and their sputa are first stained with gram stain. In patients with pneumonia, aside from cases with shadows typical of tuberculosis, the first empiric therapy is usually antimicrobial agents.

On gram staining of sputum, *Mycobacterium tuberculosis* either is weakly gram-positive or appears as colorless rods or "ghosts" (Hinson et al.,1981;Trifito et al.,1990). However, there is no description of Gram staining as useful staining for *M. tuberculosis* in the textbooks.

If tubercle bacilli could be easily detected in clinical samples with gram staining, it would be possible to detect tuberculosis more promptly and easily, which may contribute to tuberculosis control. In this paper, we present three infective tuberculosis cases in which gram staining easily detected tubercle bacilli before Ziehl-Neelsen (Z-N) staining and diagnosed by polymerase chain reaction (PCR) or culture.

Case 1

A 67-year-old man with hypertension, hyperlipidemia and atrial fibrillation visited our hospital because of lumbago, fever of approximately 38°C and an increased serum CRP level. Five years earlier, he had undergone resection of a prostate tumor. Two years prior to the current admission, thymectomy was performed because of myasthenia gravis and he was administered 20 mg/day prednisolone and 150 mg/day cyclophosphamide. One month earlier, he developed swelling on the back of the right hand. Gram staining of pus from the back of the hand showed many neutrophils with no bacteria when focus was adjusted on the nucleus of neutrophil, but contained gram-positive granular rods with slightly longer focus and brightening colorless rods with slightly shorter focus, suggesting the presence of *M. tuberculosis*.

The bacilli were positive (2+) on Z-N staining(Fig.1,2,3,4). The presence of *M. tuberculosis* was confirmed by PCR.

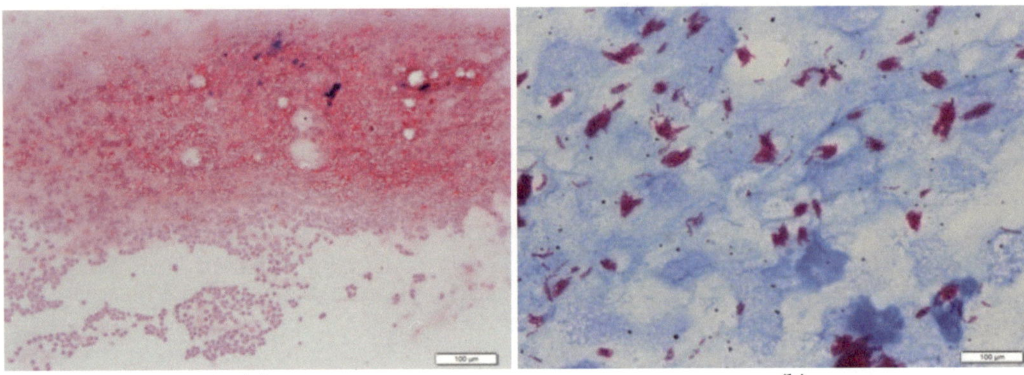

(a) (b)

Fig. 1. Gram staining and Ziehl-Neelsen staining of the pus in case 1. Gram staining of pus under a hundred-fold focus (a) and Ziehl-Neelsen staining of the pus (b). The sample contained 2+ bacilli on Ziehl-Neelsen staining(X 1000). The presence of *M. tuberculosis* was confirmed by PCR.

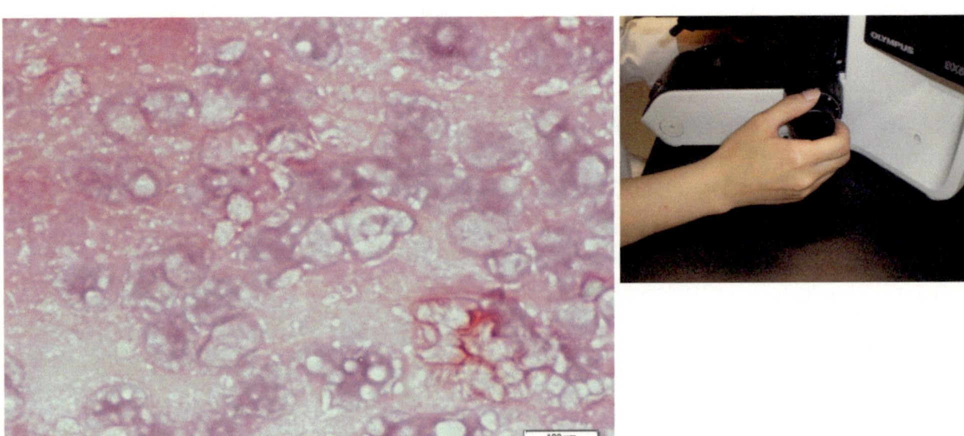

Fig. 2. Gram staining of pus under ordinary focus in case1. Gram staining of pus (X 1000) under ordinary focus in case 1. The purulent samples contained abundant of neutrophils without any causative bacteria. The small right upper figure shows left hand catching dial at ordinary style.

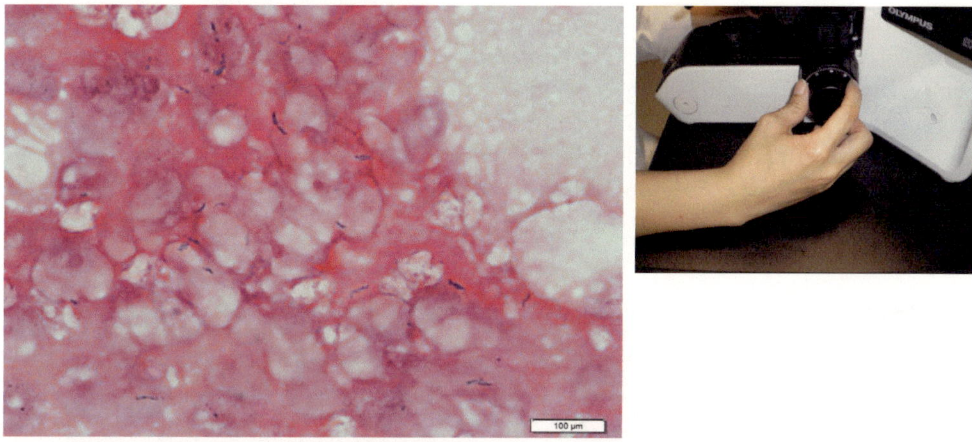

Fig. 3. Gram-positive cord-like bacilli in Gram stain in case 1. Turning the dial to adopt a slightly longer focus distance clearly showed gram-positive cord-like bacilli. The small right upper figure of hand catching dial showed position of the hand making longer focus.

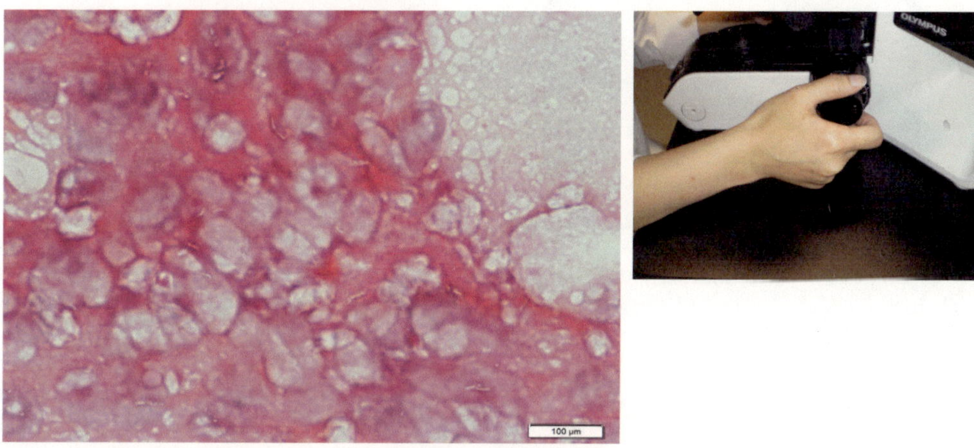

Fig. 4. Brightened rods and colorless bacilli in Gram stain in case 1. A slightly shorter focus distance revealed brightened rods and colorless bacilli in Gram stain. The small right upper figures of hand catching dial showed position of the hand making shorter focus.

Case 2

A 62-year-old man with type II diabetes mellitus presented to our hospital because of fatigue and loss of appetite. Five months earlier, he had undergone surgery for cancer at the base of the oral cavity (T4N0M0). Fifty days prior to the current admission, he noticed general malaise, loss of appetite, and fever. He was seen in our hospital, at which time the serum sodium level was 115 mEq/l. His temperature was 38.1°C. He had hypoxemia and hypoalbuminemia. Antimicrobial therapy was started. On the fourth hospital day, bilateral pleural effusion was detected, and pneumonia and congestive heart failure were suspected. On the fifth hospital day, he gradually lost consciousness. Gram staining of his sputum revealed many gram-positive cocci and gram-negative bacilli, with large numbers of neutrophils and oral epithelial cells. With small changes in focus under the microscope, some bacilli showed a change in staining pattern from gram-positive to unstained neutral. The sample contained 3+ bacilli on Z-N staining, and the presence of *M. tuberculosis* was confirmed by PCR and culture(Fig. 5,6,7). Electrocardiogram and laboratory data suggested the existence of ischemic heart disease, and he died after a decrease in blood pressure. However, the exact cause of death was unclear. Autopsy revealed the existence of miliary tuberculosis with no myocardial infarction.

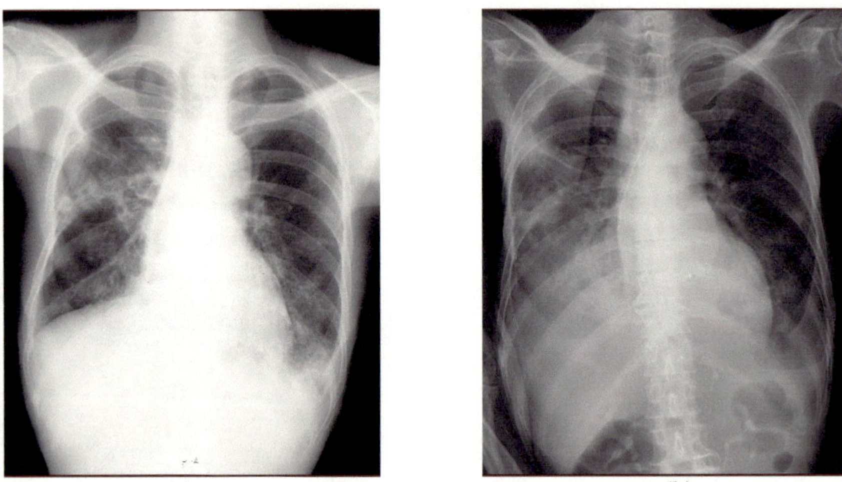

(a) (b)

Fig. 5. Chest X-rays in case 2. On admission consolidation was detected in the right lung (a). Consolidation shadows and pleural effusion were detected in the right lung on the sixth hospital days (spine position) (b).

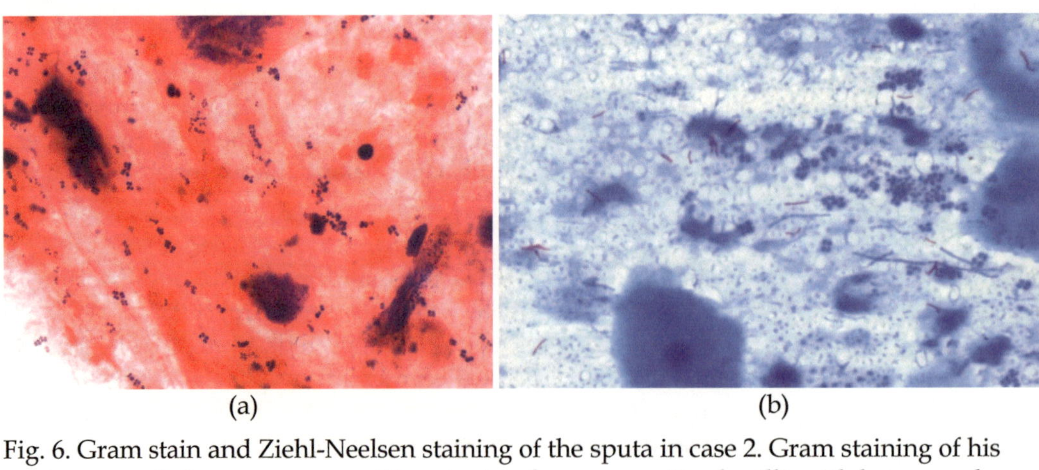

(a) (b)

Fig. 6. Gram stain and Ziehl-Neelsen staining of the sputa in case 2. Gram staining of his sputum revealed many gram-positive cocci and gram-negative bacilli, with large numbers of neutrophils and oral epithelial cells (X 1000) (a). The sample contained 3+ bacilli on Ziehl-Neelsen staining(X 1000) (b), and the presence of *M. tuberculosis* was confirmed by PCR and culture.

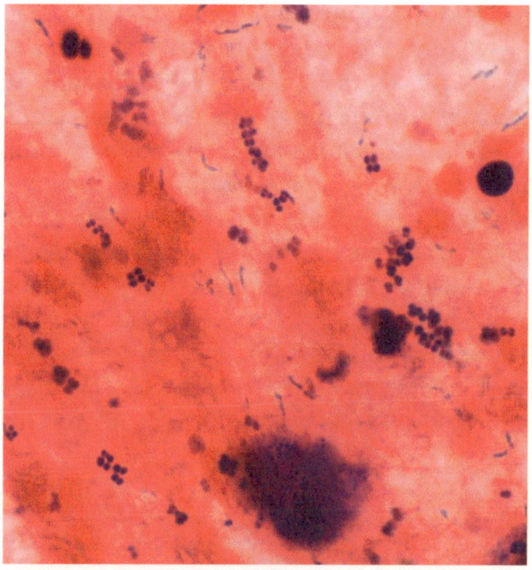

(a)

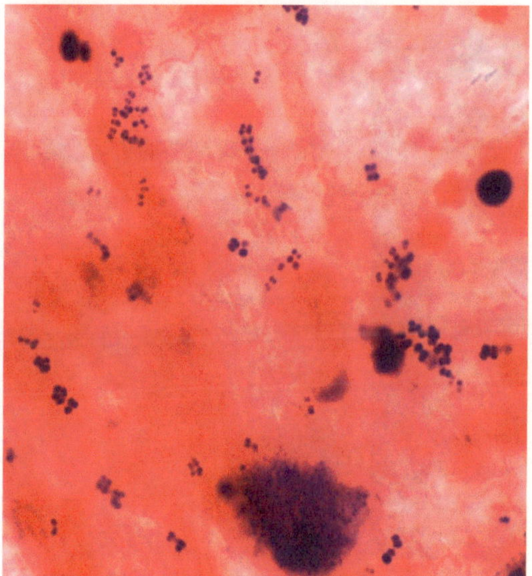

(b)

Fig. 7. Changing focus examination of sputa in case 2. Gram staining of pus in case 2 (X 1000). Turning the dial to adopt a slightly longer focus distance clearly showed gram-positive cord-like bacilli (a) and to adopt a slightly shorter focus distance revealed brightened rods and colorless bacilli (b).

Case 3

A 75-year-old man was transferred to our hospital to receive additional therapy for pneumonia that was treated unsuccessfully at another hospital. He had been treated with home oxygen therapy for chronic obstructive pulmonary disease for the past 19 years. Thirteen days earlier, he was admitted to another hospital because of pneumonia in the left lung. Several antimicrobial agents (meropenem, ciprofloxacin, imipenem/cilastatin, and vancomycin) were successively administered, but were ineffective. After being transferred to our hospital, he was administered biapenem in addition to minocycline and micafungin. Z-N staining of his sputum, done only once on admission, was negative. His inflammatory laboratory data improved slightly, but thirteen days later, the data showed abnormal levels again and hypoxemia emerged. Biapenem was changed to tazobactam/piperacillin. Gram staining of the sputum showed a large number of gram-negative rods with many neutrophils; the bacteria were confirmed to be *Burkholderia cepacia*. However, the sputum contained gram-positive granular rods, which were observed as brightened rods with a change in focus, suggesting the presence of *M. tuberculosis*. The bacilli were recognized to be positive (2+) for Z-N staining(Fig. 8,9). The presence of *M. tuberculosis* in the sputum was later confirmed by PCR.

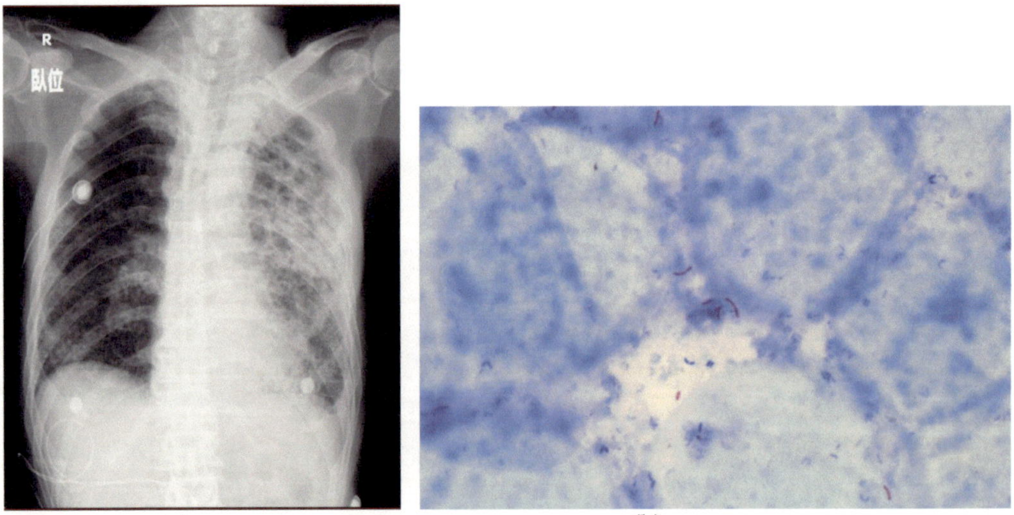

(a) (b)

Fig. 8. Chest X-rays and Ziehl-Neelsen staining of the sputa in case 3. On the seventh hospital days the part of consolidation in the upper of the left lung with emphysematous lung was persisted after successively and ineffectively administration of broad spectrum antimicrobial agents (a). Ziehl-Neelsen staining of the sputum were recognized to be positive (2+). The presence of *M. tuberculosis* was later confirmed by PCR.

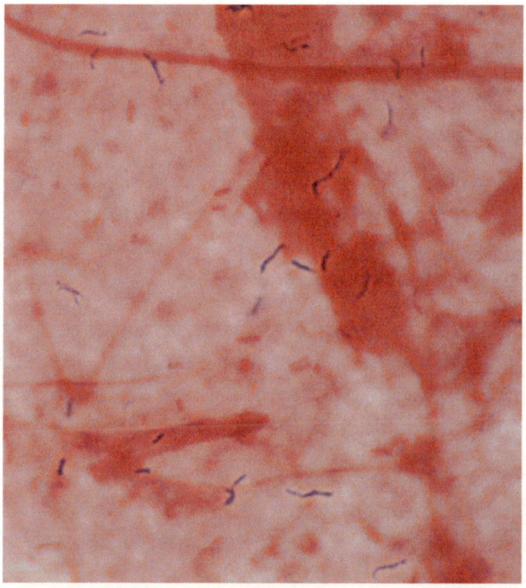

(a)

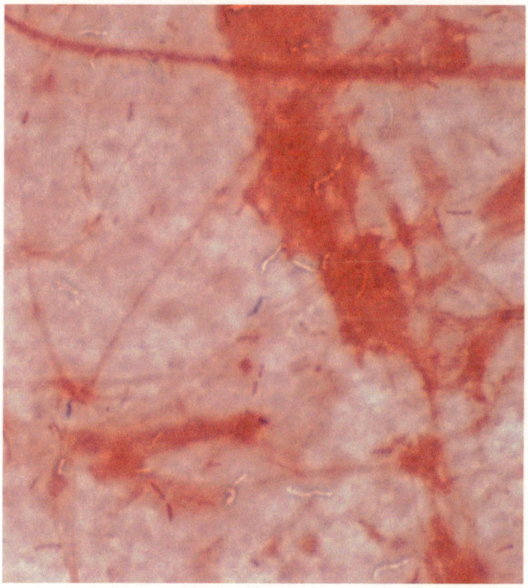

(b)

Fig. 9. Changing focus examination of sputa in case 3. Gram staining of pus in case 3 (X 1000). Turning the dial to adopt a slightly longer focus distance clearly showed gram-positive cord-like bacilli (a) and to adopt a slightly shorter focus distance revealed brightened rods and colorless bacilli (b).

2. Discussion

Gram staining is a useful technique for detecting bacteria in infectious diseases. But when infections with tuberculosis is probable, special staining, such as Ziehl-Neelsen staining is essential in detecting of *Mycobacterium tuberculosis* .

Hinson (Hinson et al., 1981) and Trifiro et al. (Trifiro et al. ,1990) observed tubercle bacilli as ghost mycobacteria in Gram staining of clinical samples.

In some textbooks one and/or two patterns of gram-stained tubercle bacilli have been described. *M. tuberculosis* often shows neutral staining (Raviglione & O'Brien,2008) , often appears as beaded gram-positive bacilli or fails to stain at all (Inderlied, 2004), or shows weak gram-positive staining and appears as colorless rods or "ghosts" (Fitzgerald,2005).

We presented a technique of Gram staining for detecting infective tuberculosis in clinical samples, the focus chaining technique (Atsukawa et al., 2011). It is a very useful procedure as an easy and rapid initial diagnostic tool to recognize highly infective tuberculosis because it can be directly applied to clinical specimens, such as sputum and pus.

Recently, we experienced a case with tuberculosis meningitis, in which Gram staining of cerebrospinal fluid with predominantly neutrocytic pleocytosis was useful as an initial adjunct to the diagnosis of tuberculous meningitis(Kawakami et al., 2012).

There are two types of samples for which the changing focus procedure on Gram staining is useful. One is purulent samples including pus without any causative bacteria. In the samples search for tubercle bacilli should be made. In an usual fixed focus, we might miss the ghost bacilli (Figure 2). The changing focus procedure is done in three steps as follows. 1) Firstly, in the ordinary focus, weakly stained gram-positive long bacilli or no conspicuous bacilli are found in samples(Fig. 2,6a), 2) with a slightly longer focus distance the gram-positive thin cord-like bacilli can be clearly observed(Fig. 3,7a,9a), and 3) with shorter focus distance the gram-positive bacilli have changed into the brightened, colorless or ghost bacilli(6)(Fig. 4,7b,9b).

The other is the samples with various amounts of gram-negative and/or gram-positive organism. Especially in purulent sputum, the existence of abundant of organisms with neutrophils usually leads a diagnosis of bacterial pneumonia. In the case2, the Gram staining showed many gram-positive cocci (Fig. 6a) and in the case3, it showed many gram-negative rods, which were confirmed to be *Burkholderia cepacia* by culture. The diagnosis of these cases by the clinicians were bacterial pneumonia and antimicrobial agents were administered.

In the ordinary procedure of Gram staining of purulent sputa, neutrophils firstly are brought into focus to check the adequacy of the safranin-staining and after once setting a focus, there is no need to change it. In the focus gram-negative and/or -positive organisms usually being also brought into focus and only we have to do is to investigate phagocytosed bacteria to catch causative organisms. However, in the focus, tubercle bacilli are weakly stained as unclear thin cord-like positive rods or sometimes inconspicuous neutral crystal-like fragments among abundant of gram-negative and/or gram-positive organism. In addition, the number of tubercle bacilli is far less than the other gram-negative and/or -positive organisms. These facts may explain why tubercle bacilli are most likely to be missed so far in Gram stained purulent sputum with various organisms and the staining have been recognized as useless one in detecting pulmonary tuberculosis. In pulmonary tuberculosis with atypical features as in case 2 and 3, sometimes the delay of Z-N staining of sputum, which is sometimes done after the first antimicrobial agent's therapy has proven unsuccessful, lead to the delay in diagnosis of pulmonary tuberculosis. The delay of Z-N staining is partly due to the complexity of the staining and the need for trained staff. However, with the repeated changing focus procedure, in a slightly longer focus distance, the weekly stained gram-positive cord-like rod had changed into clear conspicuous gram positive thin bacilli though the other organism were out of focus. And with shorter focus distance brightened and colorless bacilli, "gram-neutral" or "gram-ghost", were revealed.

Our experience has shown that, even when the sample contains various amounts of organisms, repeated changing the focus of the microscope slightly longer and shorter during the examination of the slide is indispensable in searching for tubercle bacilli. The staining characteristics of the tubercle bacilli in Gram stain , biphasic stain patterns as conspicuous thin long gram-positive bacilli changing into gram-neutral, is only noticeable by changing the focus.

The patients in case1and 2 had previous surgery for cancers. The patient in case 1 also had been administered prednisolone and cyclophosphamide and the patient in case 2 had type II diabetes mellitus. The patient in case 3 had been successively and ineffectively administered many antimicrobial agents with the broad spectrum. The patients in the case 1 and 2 dead. If their tuberculosis had been diagnosed earlier, a more rapid start of anti-tubercle therapy might save their lives.

Especially, when patients have predisposing factors to active tuberculosis, such as diabetes mellitus, liver cirrhosis, hemo-dialysis, and administration of immune-suppressive drugs, careful examination on gram staining is needed along with Z-N staining. The present study showed that gram staining is an effective initial test to check for infective tuberculosis. Considering that the clinical diagnosis of tuberculosis begins with a high index of suspicion , we should always check samples of Gram staining with the focus changing procedure.

There are certain types of images to which attention must be paid to avoid misidentification on Gram staining. Crystal-like fragments are sometimes visualized as thin, brightened neutral rods. However, when changing the focus, the brightened neutral rods never change into long gram-positive bacilli as tubercle bacilli.

The tuberculosis epidemic is far from over and is aggravated by multi-drug resistant tubercle bacilli and the even more dangerous form, extensively drug-resistant tubercle bacilli.

This study showed that gram staining represents an easy and rapid procedure for recognizing highly infective *M. tuberculosis*. The ease of the procedure and the rapidity of staining will contribute greatly to initial testing for tuberculosis, not only in developing countries but also developed countries where the number of immune-suppressed patients have increased in hospitals. Further studies are needed to clarify the usefulness of gram staining in finding infectious tuberculosis in various clinical fields or situations.

3. References

Atsukawa,Y., Kawakami,S., Asahara, M., Ishigaki, S.,Tanaka, T., Ono,Y., Hishiya, H., Fujisaki, R., Koga, I., Ota, Y.& Miyazawa, Y. (2011). The usefulness of changing focus during examination using Gram staining as initial diagnostic clue for infective tuberculosis. J Infec Chemother Vol 17: 571-574.

Fitzgerald, D. & Haas, D.(2005) Mycobacterium tuberculosis, in chapter 248 of Mandell, Bennett & Dolin (ed),*Principles and Practice of Infectious Disease 6th ed* , Elsevir Churchill Livingstone, Philadelphia, Pennsylvania, pp.2853.

Hinson, M., Bradsher,W. & Bodner, J. (1981). Gram-stain neutrality of Mycobacterium tuberculosis. Am Rev Respir Dis Vol 123: 365-366.

Inderlied, B.(2004). Mycobacteria, in chapter 233 of Cohen & Powderly (ed), *Infectious Diseases 2ed ed.* Mosby Elsevir Limitted, Edinburgh London ,pp.2297.

Kawakami, S., Kawamura, Y., Nishiyama, K., Hatanaka, H., Fujisaki, R., Ono, Y., Miyazawa, Y. & Nishiya, H. (2012). Case of *Mycobacterium tuberculosis* meningitis: Gram staining as a useful initial diagnostic clue for tuberculous meningitis. J Infec Chemother (accepted)

Raviglione MC, O`Brien RJ. Tuberculosis (chapter 158) In; Harrison`s Principal of Internal Medicine 17th ed. New York; The McGraw-Hill Companies, Inc.: 2008.p.1006

Trifiro, S., Bourgault, M. & Lebel, F. (1990). Ghost mycobacteria on Gram stain. J Clin Microb Vol 28:146-147.

15

Temperature Sensitivity of the Diphtheria Containing Vaccines

Ümit Kartoğlu
World Health Organization
Switzerland

1. Introduction

Immunization managers can improve the efficiency of immunization programmes through enhancing their knowledge of a vaccine's stability.

Vaccine management is basically all the actions related to handling of vaccines at the country level from the moment they arrive until the moment they are used. These include arrival and acceptance procedures, appropriate temperature monitoring, ensuring sufficient storage volume, maintaining standards of buildings, equipment and vehicles, effective stock management, vaccine delivery systems as well as effective use of policies such as the multi-dose vial policy (MDVP) and the use of vaccine vial monitors (VVM).

The World Health Organization (WHO) and UNICEF offer standard tools to effectively monitor management performance of vaccine stores and the vaccine management system in a country (World Health Organization, 2010).

Assessments conducted in various countries on effective vaccine management (EVM) indicate that maintaining equipment at the temperature range recommended by the WHO is not always observed (Milstien J et al., 2006). Moreover, in case of such violations, no proper follow-up actions are taken. Many countries still lack appropriate temperature monitoring tools for vaccine stores and refrigerators. Among the studies documenting temperature violations there are some that indicate that temperature violations may affect the diphtheria containing vaccines (Bishai et al., 1992; Burgess & McIntyre, 1999; Hanjeet et al., 1996; Lugosi & Battersby, 1990; Jeremijenko et al., 1996; Milhomme, 1993; Thakker & Woods, 1992; Wawryk et al., 1997; Wirkas et al., 2006). It has been observed that cold chain practices tend to rather prioritize protecting vaccine from heat damage, thus often creating the risk of exposure to freezing temperatures. As a result, inadvertent freezing of vaccines is a largely overlooked problem all over the world. In a recent systematic review, comparison of the occurrence of freezing temperatures during storage and transport were found to be a global problem occurring both in the resource-rich as well as the resource-limited settings (Matthias et al., 2007).

2. Stability of diphtheria containing vaccines

National regulatory authorities (NRA) establish the expiry dates for diphtheria toxoid vaccines through a licensing process applicable for each vaccine. In this licensing process, the manufacturer provides data to support the claimed shelf life, although vaccine may still be efficacious beyond the claimed shelf life at 2-8°C.

2.1 Analysis of vaccine stability

2.1.1 Exposure to high temperatures

The stability of diphtheria toxoid is similar to that of any simple polypeptide, that is, unaffected by rising temperatures up to the point where secondary structure is lost: generally well above 50°C (Milstien et al., 2006). In monovalent or combination vaccines diphtheria toxoid is always adsorbed onto aluminium-based adjuvants. They are stable at elevated temperatures even at long periods of storage. On the contrary, diphtheria toxoid containing vaccines may change their appearance and lose potency when frozen due to freezing destroying the gel structure of the adjuvant. The shelf-life, at the temperature usually recommended by manufacturers (2-8°C), depends on the nature of the vaccine. Monovalent toxoid and combined diphtheria and tetanus toxoid vaccines have longer shelf life (usually three years) compared to DTP and DTP combination vaccines (18-24 months). In DTP and DTP combinations, the pertussis is the least stable component compared to both diphtheria and tetanus toxoids, therefore limiting the shelf-life.

Diphtheria toxoids exposed to 60°C are destroyed in three to five hours (Sporzynska, 1965).

2.1.2 Exposure to freezing temperatures

Adsorbed diphtheria vaccines, whether monovalent or combined, alter their physical appearance after freezing changes the structure and morphology of the aluminium adjuvant. Changes in pH and storage at higher temperatures have no influence on the structure of aluminium gel, but freezing causes extensive morphological changes that are visible under the phase-contrast microscope (PCM) and scanning electron microscope (SEM) (Aleksandrowicz et al., 1990; Kartoğlu et al., 2010a). The development of heavy conglomerates, floccules or other granular matter produces an increase in sedimentation rates (Shmelyova, 1976; World Health Organization, 1980; Aleksandrowicz et al., 1990; Kartoğlu et al, 2010a). The size of the granules seems to increase on repeated freezing and thawing. The time required to freeze diphtheria containing vaccines as well as all other freeze-sensitive vaccines depend on the number of doses in the vial (the greater the volume, the longer the time) and on the temperature exposed. Studies conducted by the WHO indicate that to freeze diphtheria containing vaccines around 110-130 minutes are required at -10°C, 25 to 45 minutes at -20°C, and 9 to 11 minutes at -70°C. Because of supercooling, the temperature in diphtheria containing vaccine vials falls to well below zero (-1.6°C to -2.6°C when the outside temperature is -4.2°C to -4.6°C) before reaching an unstable threshold. At the moment of solidification the temperature in the frozen vaccine rises to the scientific freezing point, which is about -0.5°C (World Health Organization, 1990). Phase change in freezing is also affected by the vibration where the vials are resting mainly by accelerating the friction among the molecules to trigger the crystallization.

The physical changes induced by freezing can be detected by the "shake test", which is the only test that can detect freezing in all aluminium adjuvanted vaccines (World Health Organization, 1980; Kartoğlu et al., 2010a). A learning guide in Box 1 under section 3.3

explains how to do a shake test. WHO has also produced an educational video explaining how to conduct a shake test (Kartoğlu, 2010c).

The amount of antigen in a frozen non-homogeneous vaccine can vary greatly, and the administration of such a vaccine may be associated with a reduced immune response. Similarly, it may also be linked an increased incidence of local reactions due to an increased amount of aluminium adjuvant in the dose drawn for injection.

In diphtheria containing combination vaccines, reduction of the potency of different components evidently varies slightly depending on the composition of the vaccine. The tetanus toxoid component in two of five DTP vaccines stored for 12 hours at -30°C showed a decrease in potency of about 30%, while there was no such decrease in vaccines kept at -5°C to -10°C. However, the potency of the tetanus toxoid component in adsorbed DT vaccine was reduced after freezing at both -5°C and -30°C (World Health Organization, 1980). This difference is undoubtedly due to the aluminium adjuvant effect of the pertussis component in the DTP vaccines when the potency is tested by animal assay. The relevance of this observation to protective efficacy is not known. Since it would be unethical to conduct studies with known frozen vaccines, real efficacy data are difficult to get as each product has its own particular threshold for freeze damage. This also shows that there is a difference between exposure to freezing temperatures and actual freezing to destroy the potency. That is why the shake test is so important to decide whether vaccines are affected by freezing.

A study performed by Serum Institute of India Ltd. on their own DT, Td, and DTP vaccines using three freeze-thaw cycles gave the results presented in Fig 1 (Serum Institute of India, 2005).

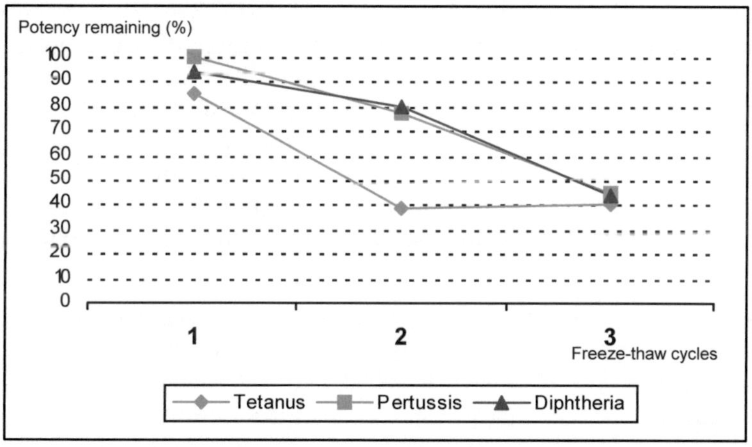

Fig. 1. Results of freeze-thaw cycles on potency of adsorbed DTP vaccine from Serum Institute of India.

3. Ensuring the optimal potency of vaccine

3.1 Temperature control requirements for diphtheria containing vaccines

To ensure the optimal potency of vaccines, careful attention is needed in vaccine handling practices at the country level. These include storage and transport of vaccines from the primary vaccine store down to the end-user at the health facility, and further down at the outreach sites. The WHO recommended conditions for storing the diphtheria containing vaccines used in immunization programmes are shown in Table 1. This Table also indicates the maximum storage periods and temperatures in each case.

	Primary vaccine store	Intermediate vaccine store		Health centre	Health post
		Province	District		
Storage temperature	+2°C to +8°C	+2°C to +8°C	+2°C to +8°C	+2°C to +8°C	+2°C to +8°C
Maximum storage period	6-12 months	3 months	1-3 month	1 month	According to session plan

Table 1. WHO recommended storage temperatures and maximum storage periods of diphtheria containing vaccines in a country cold chain system (World Health Organization, 2011).

Since the diphtheria containing vaccines are sensitive to freezing, the vaccines should be protected from being exposed to freezing temperatures both during storage and transport. Use of frozen icepacks is the major source of freezing in transport. Although for years, organizations recommended conditioning of icepacks as the best practice to prevent freezing in cold boxes, serious compliance problems have been observed and reported in the field. In principle, if used with freeze-sensitive vaccines, icepacks should be fully conditioned before being placed in the cold box with the vaccines (World Health Organization, 2002a). In order to do so, the frozen icepacks should be kept at room temperature until the icepack temperature has reached 0°C, that is, when the icepack contains a mixture of ice and water. The only way to check whether this is the case is to shake the icepack and verify whether the ice moves about slightly inside its container through listening to a slush noise. Conditioning requires both space and, more importantly, time, therefore patience. An area of approximately 1 m^2 is needed to condition 25 icepacks, a number usually required for loading one large cold box. This practice is generally found to be impractical and unrealistic because it requires more than one hour at an ambient temperature of +20°C. The practice of wrapping the freeze-sensitive vaccines to protect them from frozen icepacks and avoid freezing is found to be ineffective and no longer recommended by WHO (World Health Organization, 2004).

Although conditioning of frozen icepacks is said to be followed in the field, in a recent systematic review the occurrence of freezing temperatures during transport was found to be 16.7% in developed countries compared to 35.3% in developing countries. This difference is not statistically significant, potentially indicating that the current transport practice common to all countries - vaccines placed with frozen ice packs inside of insulated carriers - is placing vaccines at risk, regardless of the resource setting in which it is conducted (Matthias et al., 2007). In the six studies that analyzed the exposure of vaccine shipments to freezing temperatures as they travelled through both shipment and storage segments of the cold chain from either national or regional stores all the way to peripheral health centres, the findings were even more striking. In these studies, between 75% and 100% of the vaccine shipments were exposed to freezing temperatures at least once during the distribution process (Matthias et al., 2007). These comprehensive studies suggest that the risk of damaging freeze-sensitive vaccines is present in virtually every stage of the cold chain.

Between 2002 and 2004, WHO conducted a series of controlled laboratory studies and field tests (Nepal, Myanmar, Turkey and Zimbabwe) to assess the impact of using cool water packs (pre-cooled to a temperature between +2°C to +8°C) on the cold life of the vaccine transportation boxes and on the shelf life of the vaccines (Kartoğlu et al., 2009). Evaluations were conducted to verify the assumption that cool water packs can safely replace the use of icepacks for the transport of vaccines and, thus prevent the freezing of vaccines. Based on the recorded temperatures, the remaining shelf life of the vaccines were calculated through vaccine vial monitor (VVM) reactions using the Arrhenius equation[1]. Based on the results, investigators defined "cool life" (+2°C to +20°C) as a safety margin such that all vaccines except OPV can safely be transported with cool water packs even in hot climates and up to a repetition of four times (Kartoğlu et al., 2009). Fig 2 illustrates the impact of temperatures to vaccine shelf life calculated based on VVM reaction.

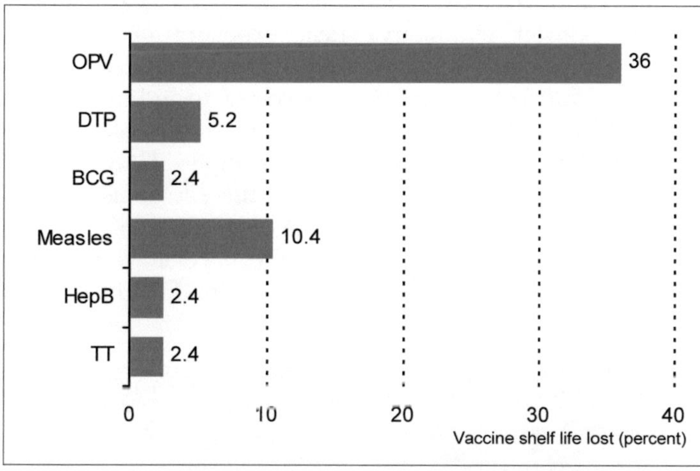

Fig. 2. Temperature impact on life loss of vaccines calculated on the basis of VVM reaction (Each transportation is assumed to be done at a continuous ambient temperature of +43°C for a period of 48 hours with a minimum temperature reading inside the vaccine transport box recorded as 11.5°C, a maximum of 25.3°C, and an average of 18.9°C throughout each journey. This scenario was repeated four times.)

Following this study, the Performance, Quality and Safety project at WHO has included the definition of "cool life" in passive cooling equipment performance specifications and now requires additional testing for cool life in prequalification of passive containers (World Health Organization, 2011a). Cool life *(with cool water-packs at +5°C)* is measured from the moment when the container is closed, until the temperature of the warmest point inside the vaccine storage compartment first reaches +20°C, at a constant ambient temperature of +43°C (World Health Organization, 2011a).

[1] The Arrhenius equation gives the quantitative basis of the relationship between the activation energy and the rate at which a reaction proceeds. Both VVM and vaccine degradation due to time and temperature exposure follow Arrhenius equation. For details on how a VVM works, please refer to section 3.2 Vaccine vial monitors and diphtheria containing vaccines.

The above results demonstrate that the use of cool water packs is a safe practice for vaccines, including diphtheria containing formulations. This clearly indicates that water packs can safely replace frozen icepacks without any damage to the vaccine potency or any major impact on vaccine shelf life. Successful implementation of this vaccine transport system has been observed in Moldova during an assessment (Babalioğlu & Kartoğlu, 2004). One drawback to the use of cool water packs could be the refrigeration volume required to store water packs to cool for use when needed. Therefore, volume requirements for introduction of cool water packs should be carefully calculated. Countries may consider conducting a temperature monitoring study in their vaccine cold chain before introducing cool water packs. Special study protocols should be used for this particular purpose (World Health Organization, 2005).

3.2 Vaccine vial monitors (VVM) and diphtheria containing vaccines

A vaccine vial monitor (VVM) is a label containing a heat-sensitive material which is placed on a vaccine vial to register cumulative heat exposure over time (World Health Organization, 2002, 2011b, 2011c). The VVM, which was introduced in 1996 for Oral Polio Vaccine (OPV), became available for all other vaccines including diphtheria containing vaccines in 1999 (World Health Organization, 2005). Today, all diphtheria containing presentations come with VVM through the United Nations (UN) procurement agencies. VVM clearly indicates to health workers whether a vaccine can be used. VVM is designed to meet the vaccine's heat stability curve, allowing a margin of safety (World Health Organization, 2011b, 2011c). Correlation between the vaccine vial monitor and vaccine potency was tested with OPV and good correlation was found (World Health Organization, 1999b).

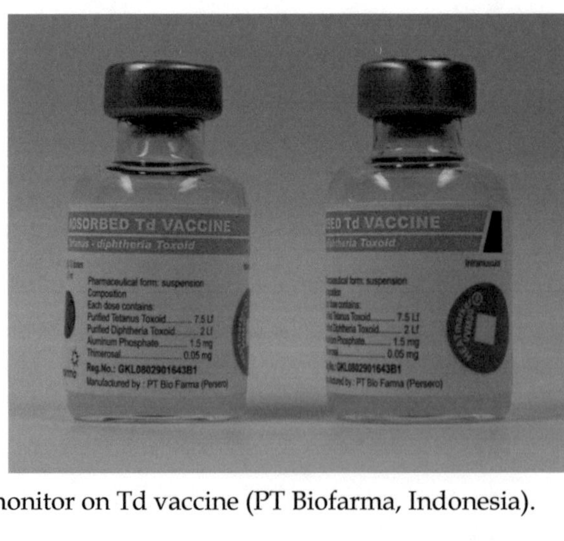

Photograph: PT Biofarma, Indonesia

Fig. 3. Vaccine vial monitor on Td vaccine (PT Biofarma, Indonesia).

The inner square of the VVM is made of heat sensitive material (monomer) that is light at the starting point and becomes darker with the combined effect of time and heat exposure. This change (polymerization) is cumulative and irreversible. Until the temperature and/or duration of heat reaches a level known to degrade the vaccine beyond acceptable limits, the inner square remains lighter than the outer circle. At the discard point, the inner square reaches the same color as the outer circle. This reflects that the vial has been exposed to an unacceptable level of heat and the vaccine degraded beyond acceptable limits. The inner square will continue to darken with heat exposure until it is much darker than the outer circle. Whenever the inner square matches or is darker than the outer circle, the vial must be discarded.

The below Fig 4 explains the interpretation of VVM.

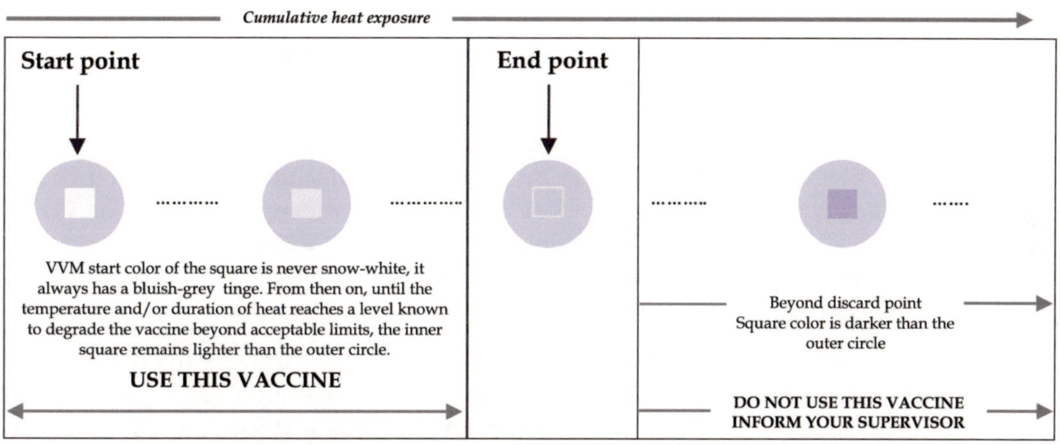

Fig. 4. VVM interpretation guidelines (Milstien et al., 2006).

A direct relationship exists between the rate of color change and temperature:

- The lower the temperature, the slower the color change.
- The higher the temperature, the faster the color change.

VVMs are located either on the label or on the top of the cap or on the neck of the ampoule depending on the following conditions. Diphtheria containing vaccines fall in the first category and VVMs in these vaccines are applied to their labels (World Health Organization, 2011b, 2011c):

- For multi-dose vials containing a vaccine that can be used in subsequent sessions: regardless of the vaccine presentation (liquid, freeze-dried or two vial combinations of liquid and freeze-dried), the VVM must be permanently attached to the label of the vaccine vial and must remain readily observable before, during, and after use, until the entire contents of the vial have been used.
- For vaccines that must be discarded at the end of the session or within 6 hours, whichever comes first: the VVM must be attached to the vaccine vial or ampoule and must remain readily observable until the vial or ampoule is opened, but not observable after opening. In order to achieve this requirement, the VVM must be located on the flip-off top of a vial or on the neck of an ampoule.

There are four different types of VVMs designed for different stability profiles (Table 2). Reaction rates are specific to four different models of VVM, relating to four groups of vaccines according to their heat stability at minimum two specific temperature points.

Category (Vaccines)	No. of days to end point at +37°C	No. of days to end point at +25°C	Time to end point at +5°C
VVM 30: High Stability	30	193	> 4 years
VVM 14: Medium Stability	14	90	> 3 years
VVM 7: Moderate Stability	7	45	> 2 years
VVM 2: Least Stable	2	N/A*	225 days

*VVM (Arrhenius) reaction rates determined at two temperature points

Table 2. VVM reaction rates by category of heat stability (World Health Organization, 2011b).

The above table does not give specific references to vaccine products, and only refer to the stability profile. Same type vaccines made by different manufacturers may have different heat stability characteristics and may therefore be assigned to different categories by WHO. In general, DT and Td combinations are either with VVM14 or VVM30 depending on their stability characteristics. DTP combination vaccines are usually with VVM14 mainly due to limiting component of pertussis.

Vaccines with VVMs including diphtheria containing ones can be taken out of the cold chain if health workers and others persons handling the vaccines have been trained to interpret VVM readings correctly and to discard any vial bearing a VVM that has reached its discard point. Although most of the out-of-cold chain studies are conducted with HepB vaccine and OPV, recent studies show that taking vaccines with VVMs out of the cold chain can successfully be implemented without compromising vaccine potency (Guthridge et al., 1996; Halm et al., 2010; Hipgrave et al., 2006; Huong et al., 2006; Lixia et al., 2007; Nelson et al., 2004; Otto et al., 2000; Zipursky et al., 2011). WHO recommends all Member States to consider adoption of policies permitting the use of vaccines beyond the cold chain where warranted for routine immunization activities or on a limited basis in certain areas or under special circumstances, such as (World Health Organization, 2007a):

- national immunization days;
- hard-to-reach geographical areas;
- immunizations provided at home - including hepatitis B vaccine birth dose;
- cool seasons;
- storage and transportation of freeze-sensitive vaccines (DTP, TT, DT, Td, hepatitis B and Hib vaccines) where the risk of freezing is greater than the risk of heat exposure.

In 2007, WHO has celebrated the 10 year anniversary of VVM introduction. Detailed information on the event as well as many other visuals and documents on VVM can be reached at http://www.who.int/immunization_standards/vaccine_quality/vvm_10years/en/index.html (World Health Organization, 2007b).

3.3 Shake test: detecting freeze-damage to diphtheria containing vaccines

Practices inadvertently exposing vaccines to sub-zero temperatures are widespread in both developed and developing countries and at all levels of health systems. (Bishai et al.,

1992; Burgess & McIntyre, 1999; Hanjeet et al., 1996; Lugosi & Battersby, 1990; Jeremijenko et al., 1996; Milhomme, 1993; Thakker & Woods, 1992; Wawryk et al., 1997; Wirkas et al., 2006). The most recent systematic literature review of vaccine freezing practices showed that inadvertent freezing occurs across all parts of the cold chain (Matthias et al., 2007). Between 14% and 35% of refrigerators or transport shipments were found to have exposed vaccines to freezing temperatures. In studies that all segments of the distribution chain were studied, between 75% and 100% of the vaccine shipments were exposed to sub-zero temperatures.

When a vaccine containing an antigen adsorbed to an aluminium adjuvant (e.g. hepatitis B, diphtheria toxoid, ..) is damaged by freezing, the loss of potency can never be restored, the damage is permanent (Dimayuga et al., 1995; World Health Organization, 1980).

Freezing affects the adsorbed vaccines by changing their physical form. Freezing does not affect non-potency parameters (such as acid content, pH; flocculating ability (Lf); ratio of free aluminium to aluminium phosphate; free formaldehyde; and thiomersal content). After freezing, the lattice (made up of bonds between the adsorbent and the antigen) in a vaccine is broken, whether monovalent or combined. Separated adsorbent tends to form larger, heavier granules that gradually settle at the bottom of the vial when this is shaken. It has been observed that ice crystals formed during freezing force aluminium particles to overcome repulsion, thereby producing strong inter-particle attraction resulting in aluminium particle coagulation/agglomeration. Thus the particles become bigger and heavier. As a simple physics rule, these heavy particles sediment faster than particles in never frozen vaccines. The size of the granules seems to increase on repeated freezing and thawing cycles.

As shown in Fig 5, diphtheria containing vaccines kept at the optimal temperature (+2°C to +8°C) show a fine-grain structure under PCM. In contrast, large conglomerates of massed precipitates with a crystalline structure are observed in vaccines affected by freezing (Kartoğlu et al., 2010a). Vaccines that are exposed to subzero temperatures without freezing show identical physical characteristics to vaccines that are kept at optimum conditions. These vaccines were also found to be in full liquid state despite being exposed to -2°C over a 24 hour period.

In this study, under PCM, particles in the non-frozen samples measured from 1 µm (DTP and DTP-HepB) to 20 µm (DT). By contrast, aggregates in the freeze-damaged samples measured up to 700 µm (DTP) and 350 µm on average (Kartoğlu et al., 2010a).

Scanning electron microscopy and X-ray analysis results in frozen and non-frozen diphtheria containing vaccines are illustrated in Fig 6, 7 and 8 (With permission from Kartoğlu, U., World Health Organization, Geneva, Switzerland and Kurzatkowski, W., Institute of Hygiene, Warsaw, Poland). Scanning electron microscopy of vaccines kept at +2°C to +8°C showed uniform flocculent structure either dense or dispersed (Fig 6A). Scanning electron microscopy of vaccines damaged by freezing (exposed to -25 °C for 24 hours) exhibited conglomerates either with rough or smooth surfaces (Fig 7A and B). Phosphate content was found to be related with formation of the precipitates, lower values are mostly resulted in rough surfaces with sharp edges while higher phosphate content affected precipitates' surfaces to be more smooth. As shown in Fig 6B and 8B, X-ray analysis

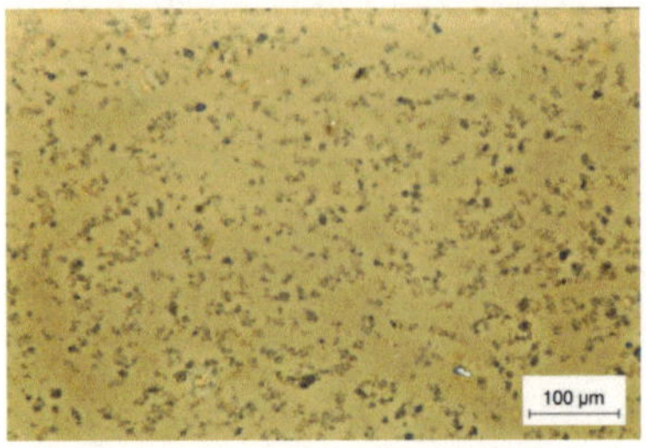

Fine-grain structure of dT vaccine kept between +2°C to +8°C temperature

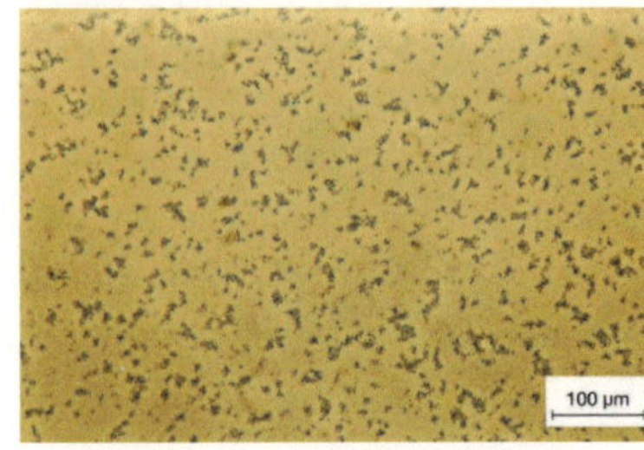

Fine-grain structure of DTP-HepB vaccine kept between +2°C to +8°C temperature

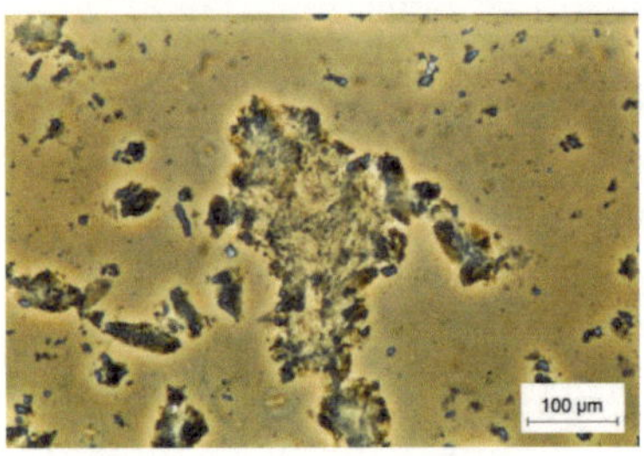

dT vaccine affected by freezing (-25°C) showing large conglomerates of large precipitates with crystalline structure

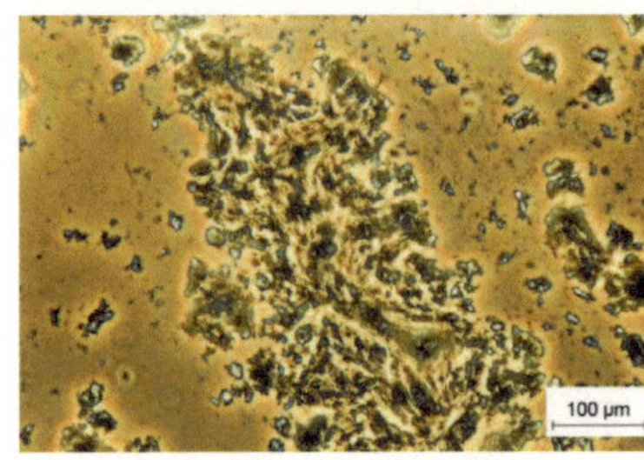

DTP-HepB vaccine affected by freezing (-25°C) showing large conglomerates of large precipitates with crystalline structure

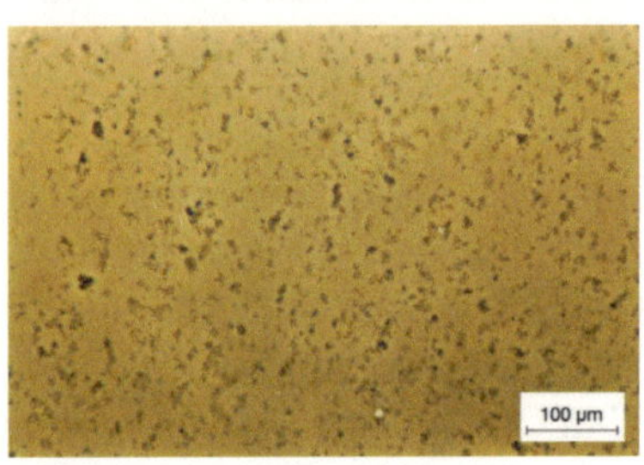

Fine-grain structure in dT vaccine exposed to -2°C for 24 hrs

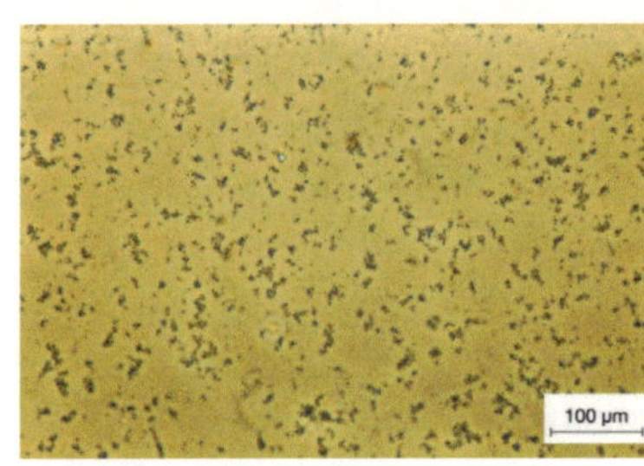

Fine-grain structure in DTP-HepB vaccine exposed to -2°C for 24 hrs

Fig. 5. Phase contrast microscopy of various vaccines kept at different temperatures (Kartoğlu et al., 2010a).

of precipitates in vaccines affected by freezing showed high aluminum content, indicating that the conglomerates are mainly aluminium clutters.

The physical changes initiated by freezing can be detected by the shake test simply by naked eyes. The shake test is designed to understand whether the vaccines are damaged by freezing based on the difference in sedimentation rates of freeze-sensitive vaccines in frozen and non-frozen vials (Fig 9). Shake test is validated by a WHO study against PCM with a 100% positive predictive value (Kartoğlu et al., 2010a, 2010b). In a typical demonstration of the shake test, two identical vials of a vaccine (i.e. from the same batch and the same manufacturer) that is suspected of having been exposed to freezing temperatures are selected; one of the two vials is purposely frozen and then thawed as the "negative control", while the second vial serves as the vial to be "tested" against this negative control. The two

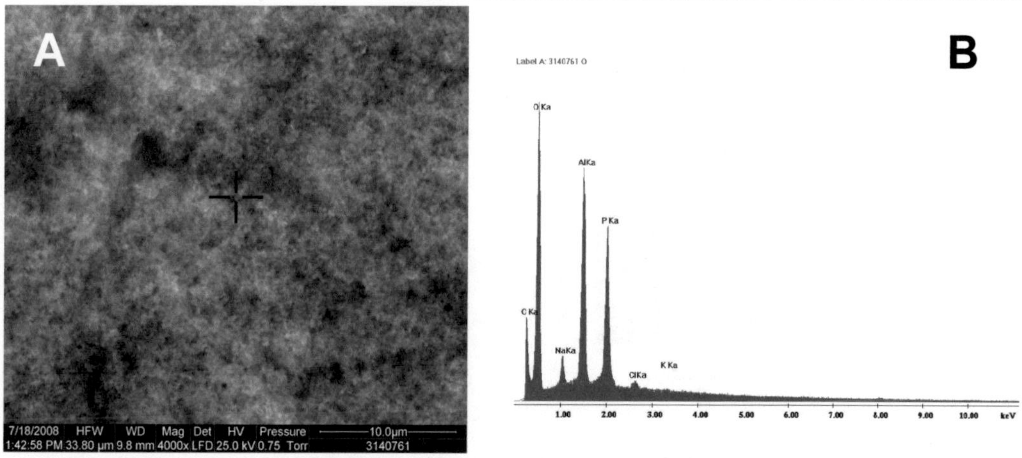

DTP-HepB vaccine with dispersed structure

X-ray analysis of the precipitate (marked with + sign in A) with high phosphate content in DTP-HepB vaccine

Fig. 6. Scanning electron micrograph (A) and X-ray analysis of the elements (B) of non-frozen DTP-HepB vaccine (kept at +2°C to +8°C at all times).

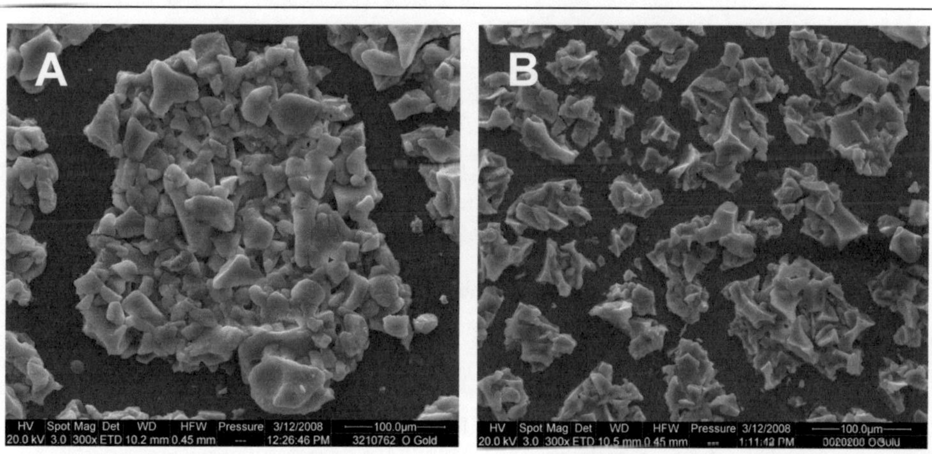

DTP-HepB vaccine with smooth surfaces of precipitate

DT vaccine with rough/smooth surfaces of precipitate

Fig. 7. Scanning electron micrographs of gold coated conglomerates of frozen DTP-HepB (A) and DT vaccines (B) exposed to -25°C for 24 hrs

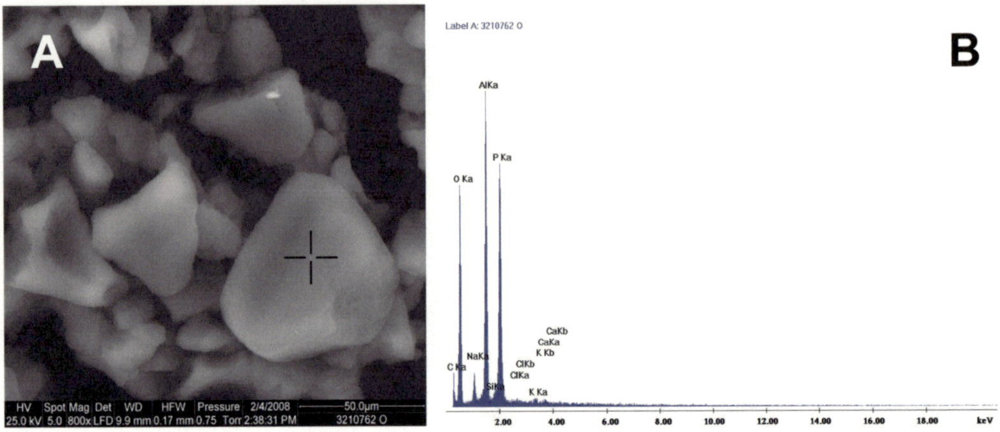

DTP-HepB vaccine with smooth surfaces of precipitate

X-ray analysis of the precipitate (marked with + sign in A) showing high phosphate content in DTP-HepB vaccine

Fig. 8. X-ray analysis of the elements of frozen DTP-HepB vaccine exposed to -25°C for 24 hrs.

vials are held together in one hand and shaken; they are then placed side by side on a flat surface. Provided the test vial has not been frozen, sedimentation is slower in the test vial than in the control vial that has been frozen and thawed. If the test vial has been frozen, the test and control vials will have similar sedimentation rates.

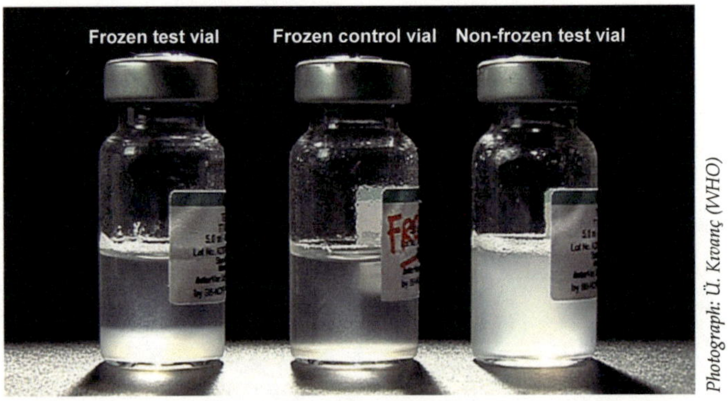

Fig. 9. Visual difference in sedimentation rates after shake test for detecting freeze damage to adsorbed DTP vaccine (Kartoğlu et al., 2010a).

The shake test correctly identifies if a vaccine has been affected by freezing 100% of the time (95% confidence interval, CI: 0.97–1.00) and it also correctly identifies if a vaccine has not been frozen 100% of the time (95% CI: 0.99–1.00). Sensitivity and specificity of the shake test for slushy vaccines were both calculated as 100% (sensitivity 95% CI: 0.86–1.00; specificity 95% CI: 0.93–1.00). In addition to the article (Kartoğlu et al., 2010a), WHO has produced a video article illustrating all steps of the validation study. This can be viewed at http://vimeo.com/8381355 (Kartoğlu et al., 2010b).

The shake test should not be conducted under the following circumstances and vials should be discarded immediately, without the need for any confirmatory shake test (Milstien et al., 2006):

- When a solid frozen vaccine vial(s) has been found
- With a vial for which a homogeneous solution CANNOT be obtained after vigorous shaking as seen in Fig 10. In such cases, the white lump/sediment cannot be separated from the walls of the glass vial. This happens only with DTP vials that are exposed to subzero temperatures without freezing (due to P component).

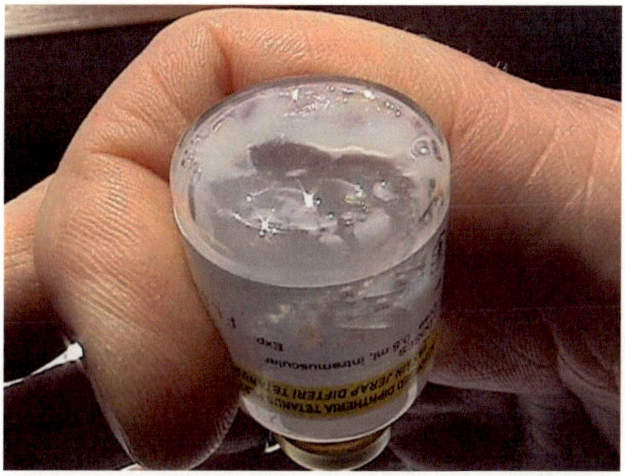

Photograph: Ü. Kartoğlu (WHO)

Fig. 10. Sub-zero temperature effect on DTP vaccine (after 10 minutes of vigorous shaking)

A learning guide to conduct the shake test is given in Box 1.

4. Summary

Diphtheria toxoids are some of the most stable vaccines in common use. They are stable at temperatures of 2 to 8°C for years, at room temperature for months, and at 37°C for weeks. At the temperature of 45°C the degradation of diphtheria toxoid is accelerated and its potency can decline during few weeks. At 53°C diphtheria toxoid lose its potency after few days, and at 60°C potency lost occurs within few hours. Freezing can reduce the potency of adsorbed diphtheria toxoid containing vaccines, however, it does not seem to affect the immunogenicity of unadsorbed products. The freezing point for adsorbed toxoids is between -5°C and -10°C. Adsorbed diphtheria toxoids containing vaccines should never be frozen.

As recommended by the WHO, all diphtheria toxoid containing vaccine products should be stored at +2°C to +8°C at all levels of any cold chain. Use of frozen icepacks at transport increases the risk of freezing the diphtheria containing vaccines. It has been observed and reported that the conditioning of icepacks for the purpose of preventing freezing during transport is not practiced in the field. Today WHO recommends to remove ice and introduce cool water packs (pre-cooled to a temperature between + 2°C to + 8°) for in-country transport of freeze-sensitive products including diphtheria containing vaccines.

Name of health staff: ____

Performance assessment scale:

1. Insufficient: Health staff performs the shake test incorrectly, or not in the right order or skips it altogether.

2. Competent: Health staff performs the shake test correctly and in the right order but either misses some points or needs to be reminded and encouraged by the study coordinator.

3. Proficient: Health staff performs the shake test correctly, in the right order, and without hesitating.

NOTES:		Practice no.		
□ **This protocol must not be altered**. There is only one correct way to conduct a Shake Test. □ The test procedure described below should be repeated with all suspect batches. In the case of international arrivals, the shake test should be conducted on a random sample of vaccine. However, if there is more than one lot in the shipment, the random sample must include a vial taken from each and every lot.		**1**	**2**	**3**
1. Take a vial of vaccine of the same type and batch number as the vaccine you want to test, and made by the same manufacturer.				
2. Clearly mark the vial as **"FROZEN"**.				
3. Freeze the vial in a freezer or the freezing compartment of a refrigerator until the contents are completely solid.				
4. Let it thaw. Do <u>**NOT**</u> heat it!				
5. Take your **"TEST"** vial from the batch that you suspect has been frozen.				
6. Hold the **"FROZEN"** vial and the **"TEST"** vial together in one hand.				
7. Shake both vials vigorously for 10-15 seconds.				
8. Place both vials on a flat surface side-by-side and start continuous observation of the vials until test is finished. *(NOTE: If the vials have large labels, which conceal the vial contents, turn both vials upside down and observe sedimentation in the neck of the vial.)*				
9. Use an adequate source of light to compare the sedimentation rates between vials. **IF,**				
10. The TEST vial sediments slower than the FROZEN vial, **THEN,**	10. Sedimentation is similar in both vials **OR** The TEST vial sediments faster than the FROZEN vial **THEN,**			
11. Use the vaccine batch.	11. <u>Vaccine damaged</u>: Notify your supervisor. Set aside all affected vaccine in a container marked "DAMAGED VACCINE FOR DISPOSAL- DO NOT USE"			
	12. Discard all affected vaccine once you have received permission to do so.			
	13. Fill in the Loss/Adjustment Form.			

Box 1. Shake test learning guide.

Heat impact on vaccines is cumulative. The VVM, which was introduced in 1996 for Oral Polio Vaccine (OPV), became available for all other vaccines in 1999. Today, all diphtheria containing products procured by the United Nations procurement agencies come with VVM. At any time in the process of distribution and at the time a vaccine is administered, the VVM indicates whether the vaccine has been exposed to a combination of excessive temperature over time and whether it is likely to have been damaged. It clearly indicates to health workers whether a vaccine can be used. With the help of VVM, vaccines can be taken beyond the cold chain under special circumstances defined by the WHO. These include national immunization days, hard-to-reach geographical areas; immunizations provided in the home - including hepatitis B vaccine birth dose; cool seasons; storage and transportation of freeze-sensitive vaccines (DTP, TT, DT, Td, hepatitis B and Hib vaccines) where the risk of freezing is greater than the risk of heat exposure.

Freezing of vaccines is a widespread problem across the world. When a vaccine containing an antigen adsorbed to an aluminium adjuvant is damaged, the loss of potency can never be restored. Freezing affects the physical form of the adsorbed vaccines through breaking the lattice structure that is made up of bonds between the adsorbent and the antigen. Separated aluminium adjuvant tends to form larger, heavier granules that gradually settle at the bottom of the vial when the latter is shaken. The shake test can demonstrate these facts and is the only test to determine whether freeze-sensitive adsorbed vaccines have been affected by freezing.

5. References

Aleksandrowicz, J.; Drozdz, M., Fieka, M. & Kurzatkowski, W. (1990). Evaluation of the physico-chemical state of aluminium hydroxide in biopreparations stored at various conditions. *Medycyna doswiadczalna i mikrobiologia,* Vol. 42, No.3-4, pp. 163-170, ISSN. 0025-8601

Babalioğlu, N. & Kartoğlu, U. (2004). *EVSM assessment: Chisinau primary vaccine store,* Republic of Moldova. 6-10 December 2004 (unpublished EVSM external assessment report)

Bishai, D.M.; Bhatt, S., Miller, L.T. & Hayden, G.F. (1992). Vaccine storage practices in pediatric offices. *Pediatrics* Vol. 89, No. 2, pp. 193–196, ISSN. 0031-4005

Burgess, M.A. & McIntyre, P.B. (1999). Vaccines and the cold chain: is it too hot... or too cold? *Med J Aust,* Vol. 171, No. 2, pp. 82, ISSN 0025-729X

Dimayuga, R.; Scheifele, D. & Bell, A. (1995). Effects of freezing on DTP and DTP-IPV vaccines, adsorbed. *Can Commun Dis Rep* Vol. 21, pp. 101–103, ISSN. 1188-4169

Guthridge, S.L. & Miller, N.C. (1996). Cold chain in a hot climate. *Australian and New Zealand Journal of Public Health.* Vol. 20, No. 6, pp. 657-660, ISSN. 1326-0200

Halm, A.; Yalcouyé, I., Kamissoko, M., Keïta, T., Modjirom, N., Zipursky, S., Kartoğlu, U. & Ronveaux, O. (2010). Using oral polio vaccine beyond the cold chain: a feasibility study conducted during the national immunization campaign in Mali. *Vaccine.* Vol. 28, No. 19, pp. 3467-3472.

Hanjeet, K.; Lye, M.S., Sinniah, M. & Schnur, A. (1996). Evaluation of cold chain monitoring in Kelantan, Malaysia. *Bull World Health Organ* Vol. 74, No. 4, pp. 391–397, ISSN. 0042-9686

Hipgrave, D.B.; Maynard, J.E. & Biggs, B.A. (2006). Improving birth dose coverage of hepatitis B vaccine. *Bulletin of the World Health Organization,* Vol. 84, No. 1, pp. 65–71, ISSN. 0042-9686

Huong, V.M.; Hipgrave, D., Hills, S., Nelson, C., Hien, D.S. & Cuong, N.V. (2006). *Out-of-Cold-Chain Delivery of the Hepatitis B Birth Dose in Four Districts of Vietnam.* PATH. October 2006 (unpublished study)

Jeremijenko, A.; Kelly, H., Sibthorpe, B. & Attewell, R. (1996). Improving vaccine storage in general practice refrigerators. *BMJ* Vol. 312, No.7047, pp. 1651–1652, ISSN. 0959-8138

Kartoğlu, U. (2007). Five senses, 14 September 2011, Available from: http://vimeo.com/8373523

Kartoğlu, U.; Ganivet, S., Guichard, S., Aiyer, V., Bollen, P., Maire, D. & Altay, B. (2009). Use of cool water packs to prevent freezing during vaccine transportation at the country level. *PDA Journal of Pharmaceutical Science and Technology.* Vol. 63, No. 1, pp. 11-26, ISSN. 1079-7440

Kartoğlu, U.; Ozguler, N.K., Wolfson, L.J. & Kurzątkowski, W. (2010). Validation of the shake test for detecting freeze damage to adsorbed vaccines. *Bull World Health Organ* Vol. 88, No. 8, pp. 624-631, ISSN. 0042-9686

Kartoğlu, U.; Ozguler, N.K. & Wolfson, L.J. (2010). Shake and tell Tell - video article. 14 September 2011, Available from: http://vimeo.com/8381355

Kartoğlu, U. (2010). Step-by-step how to conduct a shake test - educational video. 15 September 2011, Available from http://vimeo.com/8389435

Lixia, W.; Junhua, L., Haiping, C., Fangjun, L., Gregory, L.A., Carib, N., Wenyuan, Z. & Craig, N.S. (2007). Hepatitis B vaccination of newborn infants in rural China: evaluation of a village-based, out-of-cold-chain delivery strategy. *Bulletin of the World Health Organization,* Vol.85, No. 9, pp.688–694, ISSN. 0042-9686

Lugosi, L. & Battersby, A. (1990). Transport and storage of vaccines in Hungary: the first cold chain monitor study in Europe. *Bull World Health Organ* Vol. 68, No. 4, pp. 431–439, ISSN. 0042-9686

Matthias, D.M.; Robertson, J., Garrison, M.M., Newland, S. & Nelson, C. (2007). Freezing temperatures in the vaccine cold chain: a systematic literature review. *Vaccine* Vol. 25, No.20, pp. 3980–3986, ISSN. 0264-410X

Milhomme, P. (1993). Cold chain study: danger of freezing vaccines. *Can Commun Dis Rep* Vol. 19, No. 5, pp. 33–38, ISSN. 1188-4169

Milstien, J.; Kartoğlu, U. & Zaffran, M. (2006). *Temperature sensitivity of vaccines.* World Health Organization, WHO/IVB/06.10, Geneva, Switzerland

Nelson, C.M.; Wibisono, H., Purwanto, H., Manssur, I., Moniaga, V. & Widjaya, A. (2004). Hepatitis B vaccine freezing in the Indonesian cold chain: evidence and solutions. *Bulletin of the World Health Organization,* Vol. 82, No. 2, pp. 99-105, ISSN. 0042-9686

Otto, B.F.; Suarnawa, I.M., Steward, T., Nelson, C., Ruff, T.A., Widjaya, A. & Maynard, J.E. (2000). At-birth immunisation against hepatitis B using a novel pre-filled immunisation device stored outside the cold chain. *Vaccine.* Vol. 18, No. 5-6, pp. 498-502, ISSN. 0264-410X

Serum Institute of India. (2005). Personal communication.

Shmelyova, E.I. (1976). Study of stability of physical properties and biological activity of liquid and freeze dried adsorbed pertussis-diphtheria-tetanus vaccines. *Proceedings of the symposium on stability and effectiveness of measles, poliomyelitis and pertussis vaccines.* Yugoslav Academy of Sciences and Arts, pp. 159-179, Zagreb, Yugoslavia

Sporzynska, Z. (1965). Studies on the stability of toxoids. I. The effect of temperature on the immunogenic properties of diphtheria toxoid. *Experimental medicine and microbiology*, Vol. 17, pp. 130-139.

Thakker, Y. & Woods, S. (1992). Storage of vaccines in the community: weak link in the cold chain? *BMJ* Vol. 304, No. 6829, pp. 756–758, ISSN. 0959-8138

Wawryk, A.; Mavromatis, C. & Gold, M. (1997). Electronic monitoring of vaccine cold chain in a metropolitan area. *BMJ* Vol. 315, No. 7107, pp. 518, ISSN. 0959-8138

World Health Organization. (1980). The effects of freezing on the appearance, potency, and toxicity of adsorbed and unadsorbed DTP vaccines. *Wkly Epidemiol Rec* Vol. 55, No. 50, pp. 385–392, ISSN. 0049-8414

World Health Organization. (1990). Tests of the freezing point of vaccines. *Cold chain newsletter*, 90.3, pp.5

World Health Organization. (1999). *Quality of the cold chain: WHO-UNICEF policy statement on the use of vaccine vial monitors in immunization services.* WHO/V&B/99.18, World Health Organization, Geneva, Switzerland

World Health Organization. (1999). *Testing the correlation between vaccine vial monitors and vaccine potency.* World Health Organization, WHO/V&B/99.11, Geneva, Switzerland.

World Health Organization. (2002). *Guideline for establishing or improving primary and intermediate vaccine stores.* WHO/V&B/02.34, World Health Organization, Geneva, Switzerland

World Health Organization. (2022). *Getting started with Vaccine Vial Monitors.* WHO/V&B/02.35, World Health Organization, Geneva, Switzerland

World Health Organization. (2004). *Immunization in Practice.* WHO/IVB/04.06, World Health Organization, Geneva, Switzerland

World Health Organization. (2005). *Study protocol for temperature monitoring in the vaccine cold chain.* WHO/IVB/05.01, World Health Organization, Geneva, Switzerland

World Health Organization. (2007). *WHO-UNICEF policy statement on the implementation of vaccine vial monitors: The role of vaccine vial monitors in improving access to immunization.* WHO/IVB/07.04, World Health Organization, Geneva, Switzerland

World Health Organization. (2007). WHO celebrates 10 years of VVM implementation, In: Immunization standards, 14 September 2011, Available from: http://www.who.int /immunization_standards/vaccine_quality/vvm_10years_index/en/index.html

World Health Organization. (2010). Effective vaccine management (EVM) initiative, In: *EVM - setting standards for the Immunization Supply Chain*, 14 September 2011, Available from: http:// www.who.int/immunization_delivery/systems_policy/logistics/ en/index6.html

World Health Organization. (2011). *Performance Quality and Safety Devices Catalogue*, (version 2 August 2011), pp. 1-234, Geneva, Switzerland, Retrieved from http://www.who.int/entity/immunization_standards/vaccine_quality/pqs_devices_catalogue_02aug2011.pdf

World Health Organization. (2011). *PQS performance specification for vaccine vial monitor.* Retrieved from WHO/PQS/E06/IN05.2, http://www.who.int/entity/immunization_standards/vaccine_quality/who_pqs_e06_in05_rev_july2011.pdf

World Health Organization. (2011). *PQS independent type-testing protocol for vaccine vial monitors.* Retrieved from WHO/PQS/E06/IN05.VP2, http://www.who.int/ entity/ immunization_standards/vaccine_quality/who_pqs_e06_in05_vp_rev_may2011.pdf

Wirkas, T.; Toikilik, S., Miller, N., Morgan, C. & Clements, C.J. (2006). A vaccine cold chain freezing study in PNG highlights technology needs for hot climate countries. *Vaccine* Vol. 25, No. 4, pp. 691–697, ISSN. 0264-410X

Zipursky, S.; Boualam, L., Cheikh, D.O., Fournier-Caruana, J., Hamid, D., Jannsen, M., Kartoğlu, U., Waeterlos, G. & Ronveaux, O. (2011). Assessing the potency of oral polio vaccine kept outside of the cold chain during national immunization campaign in Chad. *Vaccine.* Vol. 29, No.34 , pp. 5662-5656, ISSN. 0264-410X

16

Iron and Microbial Growth

Argiris Symeonidis[1] and Markos Marangos[2]
[1]*Hematology Division and*
[2]*Division of Infectious Diseases,*
Dept of Internal Medicine, University of Patras Medical School, Patras,
Greece

1. Introduction

Iron is an essential element for the growth and development of all the scale of living organisms, and acquiring iron is crucial for the development of any pathogen. Iron participates in a large number of cellular processes, the most important of which are oxygen transport, ATP generation, cell growth and proliferation, and detoxification. It is a co-enzyme or enzyme activator of ribonucleotide reductase, a key enzyme for DNA synthesis, which catalyzes the conversion of ribonucleotides to deoxyribonucleotidides and particularly of deoxyuridine to thymidine.[1]

Iron is essential for both, the pathogen and the host, and complex mechanisms have evolved that illustrate the longstanding battle between pathogens and hosts for iron acquisition. The host has developed mechanisms to withhold iron from the microorganisms, thus preventing their growth, while the microorganisms have the capacity to adapt to the iron restricted environment by several strategies. Furthermore, iron modulates immune effector mechanisms, such as cytokine activities, nitric oxide (NO) formation or immune cell proliferation, and consequently, host immune surveillance.[2] High levels of free iron may damage or destroy the natural resistance. It catalyzes the formation of highly reactive compounds, such as hydroxyl radicals, that cause damage to the macromolecular components of the cells, including DNA and proteins.[3,4] Most environmental iron is in the Fe^{3+} state, which is almost insoluble at neutral pH. To overcome the virtual insolubility and potential toxicity of iron, ingenious transport systems and related proteins have evolved, to mediate balanced and regulated acquisition, transport, and storage of iron in a soluble, biologically useful, non-toxic form. The various proteins involved in mammalian iron transport and metabolism are presented in Table I.

2. The role of iron in normal cell growth

Iron holds an important metabolic role on the regulation of the cell cycle. It activates the cyclin/cyclin-dependent kinase complexes, favouring the progression to the S phase. Normally, all eukaryotic cells, entering the S-phase, upregulate transferrin receptor-1 expression, to obtain iron from the extracellular environment. Low levels of intracellular Fe^{3+} increase cyclin-dependent kinase inhibitor $p21^{CIP1/WAF1}$ levels, delaying or inhibiting the transition to the S-phase. As a result, Bcl-2 is down-regulated and Bax levels are increased, conditions that activate caspase-3, caspase-8, and caspase-9, and lead to apoptotic cell

Protein	Function
Duodenal Cytochrome B	Reduces Fe^{3+} to Fe^{2+} in the intestinal lumen, to facilitate iron absorbtion
Nramp1 (Natural resistance-macrophage protein-1	Divalent iron transporter expressed in phagocytes. Participates in intracellu- associated lar iron recycling.
DMT1 (Nramp2 or DCT1)	Associates and transports Fe^{2+} from intestinal lumen – Intracellular iron transporter – receives and delivers endosomal iron
HFE protein	Binds to Tf Receptor - antagonizes Tf binding
Ferroportin	Cell membrane iron transporter, both importer and exporter
Hepcidin	Allosteric inhibitor of Fp – Induces Fp internalization and degradation
Ceruloplasmin	Bivalent metal iron transporter mainly for copper and iron
Hephaestin	Facilitates iron efflux by the enterocyte
Hemojuvelin	GPI-linked membrane protein – Upregulates hepcidin gene expression
Transferrin	Main iron transporter in the systemic circulation
Transferrin Receptor-1	Main cellular receptor for iron internalization
Transferrin Receptor-2	Mainly expressed in the liver – Binds only holotransferrin
Matriptase-2	Membrane-bound serine protease - Downregulates hepcidin gene expression
Iron Regulatory Protein-1	Regulates intracellular iron homeostasis by binding to various iron regulatory elements – Cytosolic aconitase activity
Iron Regulatory Protein-2	RNA-binding protein – Regulates translation of iron protein mRNA
PCBP1	Cytosolic chaperone – Trafficks iron from endosomes to cytosolic ferritin
Lactoferrin	Tissue iron-binding protein with pleiotropic activity
Ferritin	High molecular weight protein-complex – Main iron storage protein
Mitoferrin	Inner mitochondrial membrane protein – Importer of iron to mitochondria
Frataxin	Mitochondrial iron-storage protein. Mediates iron transport to Iron-Sulfur cluster-containing proteins and iron export from the mitochondrion
ABCB7	Main mitochondrial iron exporter
Mitochondrial Ferritin	High H-Ferritin molecule with higher affinity for iron than ferritin found in the intramitochondrial space – Storage protein

Table 1. Proteins involved in iron transportation and metabolism.

death.[5] Therefore, unavailability of extracellular iron, and consequently intracellular iron deprivation, results in impaired DNA synthesis, and the cell cycle progression is arrested at the transition from G1 to S phase. Studying gene expression profile alterations in the HL-60 cell line, it has been demonstrated that, under iron-deprived conditions 11 of 43 genes are >50% inhibited. These genes are Rb, $p21^{WAF1/CIP1}$, bad, cdk2, cyclin-A, -D3, -E1, c-myc, egr-1, iNOS and FasL, all of which are essential for cell-cycle regulation and apoptosis.[6] Apoptosis of the HL-60 cells, induced by iron deprivation, was not attributed to decreased bcl-2 or c-myc expression, but to the activation of the cyclin-dependent inhibitor $p21^{WAF1/CIP1}$.[5,7] However, although this metabolic step has long ago been recognized, it appears that additional key-points of cellular growth and development, exist, still vaguely known, which are controlled by intracellular iron and iron-containing proteins, since in some cases cell cycle arrest may also occur at the transition from the G2 to M phase.[7]

Iron is highly toxic for biologic substrates, due to its high oxidative potential and its ability to generate Reactive Oxygen Species (ROS) according to the Haber-Weiss reaction: ($O_2^- + H_2O_2 \Rightarrow HO + O_2 + HO^-$).[8] The major amount of intracellular iron is stored in ferritin, and the major cellular part of active iron implementation is the mitochondria. Iron is transported in the endomitochondrial space, with the assistance of the specific transporter mitoferrin and is stored in a specific type of ferritin, the mitochondrial ferritin.[9] In the mitochondria, iron participates as coenzyme in the respiratory chains enzynes, the cytochromes, and in the formation of heme, which is incorporated in the other heme-containing proteins, hemoglobin and myoglobin. In the cytoplasm iron is usually found in the endosomes, loosely bound with transferrin, and ready to be transported to specific substrates, in various as yet poorly-defined proteins and molecules and is stored in ferritin. All the sources of non-ferritin bound iron are collectively defined by the term intracellular labile iron.[10,11,12]

Iron is a major regulator of the cell cycle, by intervening with the formation and activity of the cyclin/cyclin-dependent kinase complexes. Depletion of intracellular iron by various iron chelators leads to cell cycle arrest, particularly in the G1 and the S phase, by producing an allosteric inhibition of cyclin-A, cyclin-E, and of cdc2 and cdk2. Moreover, it decreases intracellular levels of cyclin-D and cdk4 and changes retinoblastoma protein phosphorylation.[13] In neuroepitheliomatous cells iron depletion reduces the expression particularly of the group D cyclins, and affects also negatively the expression of other cyclins.[14] Iron chelators enhance the expression of several genes, involved in the down-regulation of cell cycle progression, such as WAF1 and GADD45, in a p53-independent mechanism.[15] In addition, cdc2 (p34) protein levels, which regulate the checkpoint of the G2/M phase transition, are decreased following incubation with iron chelators.[16] A group from Sydney, Australia, specialized on iron metabolism has reported that iron depletion with deferroxamine (DFO) is associated with substantial decrease of cyclin D1 levels, through post-transcriptional modification of the protein, in a ubiquitin-independent manner, in contrast to what happens under normal conditions, in which cyclin D1 is cleared through proteasomal degradation.[17] However, the expression of other cyclins, such as cyclin-E may be induced by iron deprivation, but since this cyclin form complex with cdk2, whose expression is down-regulated, the final result is again cell cycle arrest.[16]

Excluding cyclins and cdks, many other cytoplasmic biological pathways are severely modified in relation to the concentration of intracellular iron. One of this is the retinoblastoma gene protein (pRb), which is a major regulator of the cell cycle. Under iron-deplete conditions pRp is hypophosphorylated, an effect probably mediated by lactoferrin (Lf), and cell cycle is arrested. Lf is also a cell cycle regulator. In MCF-7 cells it induces Akt phosphorylation, which is followed by phosphorylation of pRb and of two G1-checkpoint Cdk inhibitors, $p21^{Cip1/WAF1}$ and $p27^{kip1}$.[18] Hence the two inhibitors cannot cross nuclear membrane, remain in the cytoplasm and are degraded, whereas E2F transcription factor, the final inducer of the PI3K/Akt pathway, promotes the S phase entry. Lf-induced higher cytoplasmic localization of $p21^{Cip1/WAF1}$ levels are abolished when cells are treated with the PI3K inhibitor LY294002. Thus Lf behaves as an antagonist of the Cdk inhibitors.[19]

Other cell regulators, whose expression is influenced by the intracellular iron levels are p53 and Hypoxia-Inducing Factor-1α (HIF-1α). Iron is a cofactor of the enzyme HIF-1α prolyl hydroxylase, which down-regulates HIF-1α activity. Under iron-deprived conditions intracellular HIF-1α levels are increased, resulting in phosphorylation and stabilization of p53, whose levels are also increased. p53 in turn, induces transcription of the Cdk inhibitor $p21^{Cip1/WAF1}$, with the previously mentioned consequences.[20] Quercetin, a flavonoid antioxidant, strong metal chelator, increases and stabilizes HIF-1α levels in normoxia and inhibits cell proliferation, predominantly by decreasing the concentration of intracellular iron.[21] An additional cell cycle control system, influenced by the intracellular iron levels is accomplished by the cytochromes. In cells without a functional mitochondrial respiratory chain, and also in normal cells, quenching of mitochondrial ROS synthesis with MitoQ, the proliferation rate is delayed. In both cases important cell-cycle regulators such as cyclin D3, cdk6, $p18^{INK4C}$, $p27^{KIP1}$ and $p21^{CIP1/WAF1}$are reduced. Therefore, functional loss of mitochondrial electron transport chain inhibits cell-cycle progression, and this may occur through the decreased concentration of ROS, leading to down-regulation of $p21^{CIP1/WAF1}$.[22]

Finally iron appears to influence also the mRNA translational process. A Japanese group investigated the interaction of the multifactorial Y-box-binding protein (YB-1), with the iron-regulatory protein-2 (IRP2) on translational regulation. Direct interaction of YB-1 and IRP2 is taking place in the presence of high iron concentration. YB-1 reduces the formation of the IRP2-mRNA complex, and both, YB-1 and IRP2 inhibit mRNA translation. However, co-administration of both proteins, abrogate the inhibitory effect of each protein alone. IRP2 binds to YB-1, in the presence of iron and a proteasome inhibitor. The interaction of these two proteins demonstrate the involvement of YB-1 and of an iron-related protein in the translational regulation.[23] The various intracellular signal pathways in which there is a known implication of iron are depicted in Table 2.

Activity	Mediator	Result
Inactivation of $p21^{CIP1/WAF1}$and $p27^{kip1}$	Uknown	Cell cycle progression, bcl-2 upregulation
Stabilization of cyclin D1 and -E	Uknown	Cell cycle progression, Bax downregulation
Stabilization of cdc2 (p34)	Uknown	G2 M phase progression
Activation of cyclin-A	Uknown	G1 S phase progression
P33/cdk2 complex formation	Uknown	G0 G1 phase progression
Phosphorylation of Rbp	Lactoferrin/Akt	Cell cycle progression
HIF-1α down-regulation	HIF-1α hydroxylase	Inactivation of p53
Stabilization of mitochondrial electron transport chain	Frataxin	ROS production, cell growth
TB-1/IRP2 complex formation	Uknown	mRNA translation enhancement
Ribonucleotide Reductase	Direct action	Deoxyribonucleotide formation
PI3K/Akt phosphorylation	Uknown	Cell cycle progression, differentiation
NFκ-B nuclear maintenance/activation	Uknown	Transcriptional activation
Upregulation of IRF-1 gene expression	Uknown	Cytokines' gene expression
Upregulation of c-myc gene expression	Uknown	Cell proliferation

Table 2. Intracellular signal transduction pathways in which iron is implicated.

3. The role of iron in immune function

Since the majority of the effector functions of the immune system rely on the rapid development and fast proliferation of the immunocompetent cells, and taking into account the strong influence of cell growth, proliferation and differentiation by intracellular iron levels, it is self-evident that iron would exert significant regulatory role on the immune system. Moreover, since iron plays also a crucial role for the growth and development of many pathogens, a large variety of cellular mechanisms, dedicated to both, microbial growth and host defense, are orchestrated, upon a combat for iron acquisition or iron deprivation.[24]

The most primitive and less specific antimicrobial mechanisms of innate immunity are based on the development of proteins with high affinity to trivalent iron, such as transferrin (Tf) and Lf. These proteins are excreted by many cell types, but particularly by the neutrophils, to the extracellular space, bind iron from the circulating blood and tissues, thus creating an environment not favoring pathogens' growth. On the other hand, all pathogens elaborate specific iron-picking mechanisms from their environment, and in many instances also from the iron transporting proteins of the hosts, by synthesizing very high-affinity low molecular weight iron-chelators, the siderophores.

Lf, in addition to its iron-depriving properties, exerts various direct antimicrobial, antiviral, antifungal and antiparasitic activities. By directly interacting with the cellular surface, Lf inhibits microbial and viral adhesion, and consequently prevents the entrance to the host cells, probably by interfering to various glycosaminoglycan-type receptors and viral particles. It also acts at later phases, impairing viral DNA insertion and replication.[25] Degradation of Lf by some proteolytic enzymes, leads to the formation of lactoferricin, which shares stronger antimicrobial activity and inhibits the growth of many pathogens, included multiresistant strains of bacteria and fungi. Both, Lf and lactoferricidin can prevent bacteremia, following food contamination of milk-fed animals with strong pathogenic bacteria or fungi (*E.coli, Staph.aureus, C.albicans*) and protect the intestinal mucosa from injury.[26] Lf is also protective against the development of insult-induced *Systemic Inflammatory Response Syndrome* (SIRS) and its progression towards septic shock. This is accomplished through reduction or almost complete inhibition of the generation of intracellular and tissue oxidative stress, following LPS exposure, as measured by mitochondrial ROS expression, in a dose-dependent way. In vivo administration of Lf to experimental animals, significantly lowered LPS-induced mitochondrial dysfunction, estimated by decreased H_2O_2 release and mitochondrial DNA damage.[27]

More striking was the clarification of the ability of stress hormones and inotropes, to stimulate the growth of pathogenic bacteria. Using electron paramagnetic resonance spectroscopy and chemical iron-binding analyses it was demonstrated that catecholamines form direct complexes with Fe^{3+}, found within Tf and Lf. The formation of such complexes results in the reduction of Fe^{3+} to Fe^{2+} and the loss of protein-complexed iron. Both forms of iron, released from Tf or Lf is thereafter used as bacterial nutrient sources. Therapeutically relevant concentrations of stress hormones and inotropes in human serum could directly affect iron binding by Tf, so that the normally highly bacteriostatic tissue fluids may become significantly more supportive of the bacterial growth. The relevance of these catecholamine-Tf/Lf interactions to the infectious disease process is under ongoing research.[28]

Lf is also a very potent immunomodulator and anti-inflammatory protein.[29] It recognizes specific microbial molecules/receptors, named *Pathogen-Associated Molecular Patterns* (PAMPs), which are LPS from the gram-negative cell wall, and bacterial unmethylated CpG DNA, acting either as a competitor for these receptors, or as a partner molecule, depending on the physiological status of the organism. By interacting with proteoglycans and membrane receptors of many cells of the innate- and adaptive immune system (lymphocytes, antigen-presenting cells, endothelial cells), Lf modulates the migration, maturation and function of these cells, and thus influences both arms of immunity.[30] Bovine Lf attenuated Staphylococcal Enterotoxin B (SEB)-induced proliferation, IL-2 production and CD25 expression by transgenic mouse T-cells, an effect not induced through iron-deprivation of staphylococci, but by lactoferricin. Cytokine secretion, following SEB-stimulation by T-cell lines and by normal peripheral blood mononuclear cells, was also inhibited by Lf, suggesting a possible therapeutic applicability of this protein.[31] When given orally, Lf is easily uptaken by enterocytes, but also by the CD3+ lymphocytes of the lamina propria and the small intestinal submucosal tissue, and is mainly distributed in the cytosol. However, occasionally, it may also be distributed in the nucleus, suggesting that it might exert a direct regulatory role.[32]

Similar immunoregulatory properties have been postulated for Tf, which plays an essential role for normal T-lymphocyte growth and early differentiation. The absolute number of T-cells has been found substantially reduced in hypotransferrinemic $Trf^{hpx/hpx}$ mice, and this could not be attributed to increased apoptosis. Moreover, the differentiation of CD4-CD8-CD3-CD44-CD25+TN3 into CD4-CD8-CD3-CD44-CD25-TN4 cells was impaired, and a similar impairment of early T-cell differentiation was observed in mice with reduced levels of Tf receptor.[33]

The iron chelator DFO arrests cell cycle progression in activated T lymphocytes in the late G1 phase, before the G1/S border, by inhibiting transcription of the cdc2 gene, but has no effect on accumulation of cdk2, cdk4, or IL-2-transcripts. p34/cdc2 protein complex becomes undetectable, whereas synthesis of the p33/cdk2 protein begins and is activated as an H1 histone kinase, but this complex is insufficient to complete the G1 phase. Synthesis and early accumulation of cyclin E and cyclin E-dependent kinase are not affected by DFO, but cyclin A and cyclin A-dependent kinase are inhibited, although cyclin-A mRNA levels remain normal. Thus, DFO blocks cell cycle progression, through inhibition of cyclin A appearance, which is a major component of the p33/cdk2 complex.[34] DFO but not ferrioxamine (iron saturated DFO) inhibits growth and proliferation of the Jurkat T-cell line at the G0/G1 transition and induces apoptosis. However, iron-loaded Jurkat cells are not arrested. Silybin, a flavonoid antioxidant, free radical scavenger, acting also as iron chelator, shows a bimodal effect, inducing cell proliferation at low-, and DNA synthesis inhibition and apoptosis at high concentrations. The effect of silybin on the growth and viability of iron-loaded cells was similar to that of its iron complex, implying that the biological effects of silybin are different than those of DFO, and it probably shares pro-oxidant effect, via iron-catalyzed oxidation and generation of ROS.[35]

The high frequency of infections, reported in hemodialysis patients, when receiving intravenous (IV) iron preparations, revealed that IV iron administration is associated with time-dependent increases of the intracellular oxidative stress in many immunocompetent cell populations, resulting in dysfunctional cellular immunity. The CD4+ lymphocytes are mainly affected, with a statistically significant reduction in their survival after incubation with all doses of iron preparations. IV iron products induce also various deleterious effects on CD16+ lymphocyte populations, which may also be mediated by intracellular ROS formation.[36]

Iron tetrakis (N-methyl-4'-pyridyl-porphyrinato: FeTMPyP) is a potent antiinflammatory and scavenger of ROS. Treatment of thymocytes with FeTMPyP results in the inhibition of various mitogen-or cytokine-induced proliferation signals, and of the DNA-binding activity of NF-κB and IL-2 secretion. Inhibitors of p38-MAPK and of the ERK protein block the growth and proliferation of ConA-stimulated thymocytes, the NF-κB activation and IL-2 secretion.[37] Interferon regulatory factor-1 (IRF1) regulates the expression of genes involved in the inflammatory response and cell cycle control. IRF1 expression is transcriptionally mediated by TNF-α or IFN-γ, via iron-dependent pathways and is inhibited when cells are pretreated with iron chelators. Addition of exogenous iron reconstitutes cytokine responsiveness, indicating that iron is the target for the chelator effect.[38]

In addition to Lf, ferroportin (Fp), an iron efflux protein, strongly influences host response to infection. Murine macrophages overexpressing Fp show impaired intracellular *M.tuberculosis* killing at early stages of infection. When challenged with LPS or *M.tuberculosis* infection, control macrophages increase NO synthesis, but macrophages overexpressing Fp had significantly reduced NO and iNOS mRNA and protein production, thus limiting the bactericidal activity of these macrophages. IFN-γ reversed the inhibitory effect of Fp on NO production, findings suggesting a role for Fp in attenuating macrophage-mediated immune response.[39] Hepcidin, the allosteric inhibitor of Fp, regulates intracellular iron levels by interacting with, and promoting Fp degradation. All immunoregulatory cells express hepcidin mRNA; hepcidin mRNA expression increases after T-lymphocyte activation and in response to holotransferrin (Fe-Tf) or ferric citrate challenge. Therefore, low hepcidin expression impairs normal lymphocyte proliferation.[40]

Normal tissue macrophages are polarized, through the action of cytokines, into classically- (M1) and alternatively-activated (M2). M1 macrophages have low IRP-1 and -2 binding activity, express high levels of H-ferritin, low levels of Tf receptor-1 and internalize iron, only at high extracellular concentrations. Conversely, M2 macrophages have high IRP-binding activity, larger intracellular labile iron pool, express low levels of H-ferritin and high levels of Tf receptor-1, and effectively internalize and release iron, even at low concentrations. Iron export correlates with Fp expression, which is higher in M2 macrophages. In the absence of iron, only M1 macrophages are effectively activating antigen-specific, MHC class II-restricted T cells. Thus finally, cytokines control iron handling, by differentiating macrophages into a subset with relatively-low intracellular iron content (M1), or a relatively-high iron containing subset, endowed with the ability to recycle iron (M2).[41] Besides the classical mechanisms of antimicrobial activity (peptidic antibiotics, induction of oxidative stress, leading to respiratory burst) macrophages can deprive intracellular pathogens of necessary nutrients, and most importantly of iron. Moreover, according to the type of phagocytized pathogen, they can modulate, even the extracellular environment, impeding pathogens the access to essential nutrients. Thus various membrane transporters may remove nutrients from vacuolar compartments, degrade growth factors, and sequester other molecules, important for microbial growth, in a way similar to iron deprivation.[42]

Iron deficiency has been associated with various immune abnormalities, and particularly with impaired lymphocyte proliferation. T-cells from iron deficient mice exhibit poorer monocyte stimulatory activity following Con-A activation, as estimated by CD80 and CD86 expression on antigen presenting cells. The addition of DFO increased the expression of both markers on resting B and T cells. Lymphocyte proliferative responses to mitogens correlated positively with CD80 and CD86 expression, but negatively with the percentage of CD80+ cells. Therefore, the impaired lymphocyte proliferation of iron deficiency cannot be attributed to reduced CD80 and CD86 expression.[43]

The immunoregulatory properties of ferritin include binding to T lymphocytes, suppression of the delayed-type hypersensitivity and of antibody production by B lymphocytes, and impairment of phagocytosis by the granulocytes.

4. The role of iron in inflammatory and neoplastic diseases

Iron plays a major role in the generation and perpetuation of inflammatory processes. Many chronic inflammatory diseases are directly influenced by the intracellular and extracellular iron concentrations. Disease activity, and particularly the manifestation of serositris and various hematological disturbances in rheumatoid arthritis, systemic lupus erythematosous, Still's disease, dermatomyositis, and other collagen diseases are strongly correlated with serum and tissue ferritin levels.[44,45] Ferritin and iron homeostasis are implicated in the pathogenesis of many other disorders, including atherosclerosis, Parkinson's disease, Alzheimer disease, and restless leg syndrome. Iron contributes to the synthesis of myelin, and severely iron deficient patients exhibit impaired myelin formation. In patients with multiple sclerosis, serum and cerebrospinal fluid levels of Tf and ferritin levels have been found significantly elevated only during progressive active disease.[46] Brain tissue of patients with multiple sclerosis exhibits abnormal distribution of Tf and ferritin.[47] Ferritin binding to the inflammatory lesion and the immediate periplaque region within the white matter is practically absent, but returns to normal as the distance from the lesion increases. Therefore, the loss of ferritin binding is correlated with demyelination, accompanying multiple sclerosis.[48] Reactive Oxygen Species participate in the pathogenesis of allergic encephalomyelitis, whereas the infusion of apoferritin in experimental animals may induce a remission status.[49] Thyroid hormone upregulates ferritin genes' expression, and elevated serum ferritin levels have been reported in patients with subacute thyroiditis, which were correlated with disease activity. These levels were higher, as compared to patients with Graves' disease and Hashimoto's thyroiditis.[50]

Ferritin synthesis is regulated by the main proinflammatory cytokines (TNF-α, and IL-1α) at various levels (transcriptional, post-transcriptional, translational) during cellular development, differentiation and inflammation. Cytokine-induced cellular response to infection by various pathogens includes the upregulation of ferritin genes. Translation of ferritin is induced by IL-1β, IL-6 and TNFα, and iron is required for this regulation. Ferritin is accumulated in macrophages during various inflammatory conditions, when serum iron levels are decreased, leading to the formation of ferritin molecules with high content of iron.[51]

High heme oxygenase-1 (HO-1) expression, elevated ferritin accumulation in renal tubules and increased iron deposition in renal proximal tubules have been reported in patients with immunohemolytic anemia.[52] HO-1 degrades heme to biliverdin, carbon monoxide and free iron. HO-1 expression is induced among others, by proinflammatory cytokines and high intracellular ROS levels. This enzyme appears to have significant immunoregulatory properties, acting as inhibitor of immune reactions and participating in the pathogenesis of many inflammatory, infectious, allergic and autoimmune diseases and conditions, and has been proposed as a possible target inducing immunosuppression in allogeneic stem cell transplantation.[53]

Besides the stimulatory role on DNA synthesis, iron interferes with cell proliferation, by enhancing c-myc expression. Regulation of c-myc expression is crucial for the maintenance of cellular homeostasis. Overexpression or abnormal intracellular localization of c-myc results in the activation and deregulation of this oncogene. Surprisingly, when added to Burkitt's lymphoma cell lines, iron markedly inhibits cell proliferation, through cell cycle arrest in the G2/M transition, followed by a significant decrease in c-myc expression. A similar effect is not observed in cell lines with constitutive c-myc expression. Down-regulation of c-myc, which is independent from cell cycle blockade, leads to apoptotic cell death, implying the existence of another iron-dependent cell cycle regulatory mechanism, involving modulation of c-myc expression.[54]

Antisense oligodeoxynucleotide treatment against H- and L-ferritin chains increased the steady-state labile iron pool and the production of ROS after oxidative challenges and down-regulated Tf receptors, whereas it had no effect on the long-term growth of the cells. However, repression of ferritin synthesis facilitated renewal of the growth and proliferation of cells pre-arrested at the G1/S phase. Renewed cell growth was significantly less dependent on external iron supply, when ferritin synthesis was repressed, and its degradation was inhibited by lysosomal antiproteases.[55]

5. Iron and bacterial infections

Bacteria are confronted with a low availability of iron owing to its insolubility of the Fe^{3+} form, or its binding to host proteins. Free iron concentration in the host environment is about, or lower than 10^{-15}M and in some instances as low as 10^{-24}. Bacteria and other microorganisms need powerful and sophisticated mechanisms to acquire iron. Iron availability is a signal, alerting pathogenic bacteria, when they enter the hostile environment. When bacterial pathogens infect a host, cytotoxins damage the host cells releasing ferritin, hemolytic toxins lyse erythrocytes releasing hemoglobin, and Lf is produced by neutrophils and epithelial cells. The bacteria cope with the iron deficiency, by developing various uptaking systems: siderophores (low-molecular weight substances, with very high affinity for iron), systems for free heme and heme bound to hemoproteins (hemoglobin, hemoglobin-haptoglobin, heme-albumin, heme-hemopexin) and siderophore-based mechanisms to acquire iron from the iron-binding proteins Tf and Lf.

Pathogens encounter a period of iron starvation, upon entering their host and they sense alterations of the iron status, via the *Ferric Uptake Regulator* (FUR). The FUR protein plays a key role in the transcriptional response to iron of *Escherichia coli* and other gram-negative bacteria. The mechanism of action of FUR is repression of siderophore production and iron transport promoters. When iron is limiting, FUR protein is inactive as a repressor. This results in derepressed transcription of genes, involved in siderophore synthesis, and high-affinity iron uptake. FUR homologues are present in many bacteria.[56] In addition heme-sensing systems have been evolved by many pathogens, like *Staphylococcus aureus*, *Bacillus anthracis*, and *Corynebacterium diphtheriae*. For instance, *S. aureus* is able to sense heme through the heme sensing system (HssRS), two-component system that detect the presence of toxic levels of exogenous heme. Upon sensing heme, HssRS directly regulates the expression of the heme-regulated ABC transporter HrtAB, which alleviates heme toxicity.[57] In some halophilic bacteria, such as *Chromohalobacter salexigens*, iron homeostasis is coupled to the reaction to osmotic stress, through the activity of FUR. A decrease in iron and histidine requirements and a lower level of siderophore synthesis were observed at high salinity.[58]

Siderophores (named after the Greek word for iron carriers) are low molecular weight iron-binding complexes, produced and secreted by bacteria, fungi and plants. These molecules target ferric iron (Fe^{3+}), the form of iron found in well oxygenated environment in the host. Based on the metal chelating group, there are three major classes of microbial siderophores, the catecholate, the hydroxycarboxylate and the hydroxamate class. These substances exhibit extremely high affinity for iron, and hold it with three bidentate bonds. The high affinity is specific for iron, and does not extend to other bivalent cations. Siderophore production is enhanced in conditions of iron starvation, and many metabolic steps of their biosynthesis have been characterized. Siderophores have higher binding constants for iron, than do Tf and Lf, and thus are capable of detaching iron from these proteins. Their biosynthesis is confined to bacterial and fungal cells, and their expression increases the virulence of these species.[59] The most commonly encountered siderophores are described in Table 3.

Citrate
Hydroxamate class of siderophores
N,N'N''-triacetylfusarinine C
Rhodorotulic acid
Brucebactin (*Brucella abortus*)
Dihydrobenzoic acid (2,3-DHBA, *Brucella spp*)
Enterobactin (Dihydroxybenzoylserine, *E.coli*)
Enterochelin (*E.coli)*
Salmochelin (*Salmonella enteritidis, E.Coli spp, Klebsiella spp*)
Acinetobactin (*Acinetobacter baumannii*)
Pyoverdin *(Pseudomonas aeruginosa)*
Pyochelin *(Pseudomonas aeruginosa)*
Quinolobactin *(Pseudomonas aeruginosa)*
Bacillibactin (*Bacillus Anthacis, B.subtilis, other Bacillus spp)*
Petrobactin (*Bacillus Anthacis)*
Amphibactins
Agrobactin
Synechobactin
Ochrobactin
α-Hydroxycarboxylate and carboxylate class of siderophores
Aerobactin (*Vibrio spp)*
Anguibactin (*Vibrio anguillarum)*
Achromobactin *(Pseudomonas spp, marine microorganisms)*
Vibriobactin
Acinetoferrin (*Acinetobacter spp*)
Staphyloferrin (*Staph. aureus*)
Rhizoferrin
Vibrioferrin (*Marinobacter spp*)
Vanchrobactin (*Vibrio anguillarum*)
Amonabactin (*Aeromonas hydrophila)*
Mycobactin-T (*Mycobacterium Tuberculosis)*
Carboxymycobactin (*M. Tuberculosis* and other *Mycobactrerium spp)*
Yersiniabactin (*Yersinia enterocolitica)*
Rhizobactin (*Sinorhizobium meliloti)*
Desferrioxamines (A, B, C, D1, E, F, G)(*Actinomycetes spp*)
Ferric complexes of β-hydroxyaspartate
Aquachelins
Loihichelins
Marinobactins
Alterobactins
Ferrichrome class of siderophores (*Aspergillus, Ustilago, Penicillium etc*)
Ferricrocin
Ferrirubin
Ferrichrysin
Ferrirhodin
Ferredoxin
Rubredoxin
Asperchromes
Ferrichrome
Fusigen
Coprogen

Table 3. The major microbial sideropophores.

Iron loaded siderophores bind to cognate receptors, expressed at the bacterial surface. In gram negative bacteria, there is an outer membrane, external to a very thin (1-nm) peptidoglycan layer. Peptidoglycan is the structure that confers cell wall rigidity and resistance to osmotic lysis, in both, gram positive- and gram negative bacteria. In gram positive bacteria peptidoglycan is the only layered structure external to the cell membrane and is thick (20-80 nm). In gram negative bacteria the ferric-siderophores use outer membrane transporters, because they are large enough to pass through the porins (the small pores in the bacterial outer membrane that allow passive diffusion of molecules with molecular weight <600 Da).[60] The energy for the transport of these ligands across the outer membrane is delivered from the inner membrane, by a complex of three cytoplasmic membrane proteins TonB, ExbB, and ExbD.[61,62] TonB spans the periplasm, contacts outer membrane transporters by its C-terminal domain, and transduces energy from the proton motive force to the transporters. There is no need for TonB-ExbB-ExbD complex and outer membrane trasporters in gram-positive bacteria, as there is no outer membrane. Each class of siderophore is shuttled by a specific periplasmic binding protein (PBP) to the inner membrane. For example, FhuD is a siderophore binding PBP with a well-determined structure, found in gram negative and gram positive bacteria.[63] When iron-replete siderophores arrive at the microbial cytoplasmic membrane, they are taken up across the membrane by periplasmic binding protein-dependent ABC transporters in an ATP-dependent process. ABC trasporters comprise of two transmembrane domains forming a channel for the siderophore, to pass through and two nucleotide binding domains that hydrolyse ATP. The complex is internalised into the bacterium and the iron is released by proteolysis or by the action of enzymes that reduce Fe^{3+}. Fe^{2+} is incorporated into metalloenzymes or stored in bacterioferritin or in the related Dps proteins. The genes for siderophore biosynthesis and transport are usually under transcriptional control in response to the cellular pool of iron.

At the site of infection, leukocytes secrete siderocalin (also called lipocalin-2, neutrophil gelatinase-associated lipocalin). Siderocalin is also produced by epithelial cells and macrophages. Upon encountering invading bacteria, the Toll-like receptors on immune cells stimulate the transcription, translation and secretion of siderocalin. Secreted siderocalin then binds to ferric-siderophore complexes, participating in the antibacterial iron depletion strategy of the innate immune system.[64,65,66] However, pathogens produce structurally modified enterobactin-type siderophores, that are resistant to siderocalin and are known as stealth siderophores.[67] The first glucosylated siderophore described was salmochelin, a C-glucosylated enterobactin produced by *Salmonella* species, uropathogenic *Escherichia coli* strains, and some *Klebsiella* strains.[68]

Except of siderophores, gram positive and gram negative bacteria may use free heme or heme bound to host hemoproteins as iron source.[69,70] Like siderophores, this iron uptake pathway includes a TonB-dependent outer membrane receptor, while the transport across the cytoplasmic membrane requires periplasmic and inner membrane proteins comprising the ABC systems, which utilize the energy derived from ATP hydrolysis.[71] In addition, bacteria elaborate hemophores which are molecules that can remove heme from host hemoproteins. Bacterial hemophores are secreted to the extracellular medium, where they scavenge heme from various hemoproteins, due to their higher affinity for this compound, and return it to their specific outer membrane receptor.[72] An example is *Serratia marcescens,* that secretes a heme-binding protein, HasA, which functions as a hemophore that catches heme and shuttles it to a cell surface specific outer membrane receptor, HasR. The HasR receptor belongs to the TonB-dependent family of outer membrane receptors. HasAp, a gene from *Pseudomonas aeruginosa* has been isolated. HasAp is an iron-regulated extracellular heme-binding protein that shares about 50% identity with HasA and is required for *P. aeruginosa* utilization of hemoglobin iron.[73]

Pathways analogous to those described above are also utilized in gram-negative bacteria, for the uptake of iron from the iron-binding proteins Tf and Lf. Lf and Tf receptors are present in pathogenic bacteria.[74] Iron must be stripped away from Lf and ferritin prior to be transported into the bacterial cell. Two proteins, Tf-binding protein A (TbpA) and Tf-binding protein B (TbpB), function like the Tf receptor in many pathogenic bacteria, such as *Neisseria meningitides*. The expression of these genes is induced along with several other proteins under iron-restricted conditions.[70] Lf-binding protein A (LbpA) and Lf-binding protein B (LbpB) have been identified as outer membrane receptors for Lf. The extracted iron is then transfered into the periplasm. Within the periplasm, the ferric ion is complexed by ferric ion-binding protein A (FbpA). FbpA shuttles the iron to an inner membrane complex consisting of two proteins, the inner transmembrane FbpB and the cytoplasmic ATPase FbpC, finally transported into the cytoplasm.

Pseudomonas aeruginosa produces 2 siderophores under iron-limiting conditions, pyoverdine and pyochelin. Vanadium a rare metal, and probably other metallic ions, form complexes with both of these siderophores and strongly inhibit *P.aeruginosa* growth. Pyoverdin-deficient mice were more sensitive to vanadium, whereas pyochelin-negative mutants were more resistant. V-pyochelin strongly inhibits pseudomonas growth, increasing the activity of Superoxide Dismutase by about two times. Therefore, it appears that V-pyochelin catalyses a Fenton-type reaction, in which superoxide anion O^{2-} is generated, and vanadium compromises pyoverdin utilization.[75] However, in some pyoverdin deficient strains another siderophore molecule was identified, and this is quinolobactin. Its receptor is the 75-kDa iron-repressed outer membrane protein (IROMP) and the quinolobactin-mediated iron uptake system functions only in the absence of pyoverdine, and is repressed by pyoverdine.[76] Multicopper ferroxidases are enzymes that oxidize Fe^{2+} to Fe^{3+} in the microbial environment, so that iron will be transformed in a less active form, easily uptakable by microbial siderophores. *Ps. aeruginosa* possesses such an enzyme. Mutant strains are unable to grow with Fe^{2+} as iron source, because they cannot uptake iron. Thus multicopper ferroxidase represents another iron acquisition mechanism, important for virulence and pathogenicity of many bacteria.[77]

Some strains of *Vibrio anguillarum* produce a catechol-type siderophore named vanchrobactin, whose biosynthesis is under complex regulation, in an effort to adjust its production according to environmental iron concentrations.[78]

Although iron is important for all the scale of microorganisms, some types are less strictly dependent on iron than others. Moreover, growth characteristics and virulence of intracellular pathogens may vary, according to the type of infected cells. *Chlamydia pneumoniae* is an intracellular bacterium, causing chronic inflammatory disease in humans. When endothelial cells and monocytes were infected with *C.pneumoniae*, supplemented with iron and then stimulated with IFN-γ, iron had no significant effect on *Chlamydia* growth within monocytes, whereas on endothelial cells iron enhanced its proliferation and differentiation, and IFN-γ had an inhibitory effect. *C.pneumoniae* infection induced a pro-inflammatory immune response in monocytes, but not in endothelial cells and *Chlamydia* remains in a persistent-latent form within monocytes but it differentiates and proliferates within endothelial cells.[79]

Various drugs may interfere with the microbial-host battle for iron acquisition. The calcium channel blocker nifedipine enhances host resistance against intracellular pathogens, by restricting iron availability. In a murine macrophage cell line, nifedipine significantly reduced intracellular bacterial survival of *Salmonella Typhimurium* and *Chlamydophila pneumoniae*. Moreover, in mouse models of iron overload, nifedipine was capable of mobilizing tissue iron. When these mice were infected intraperitoneally with *Salmonella,* and subsequently treated with nifedipine for 3 consecutive days, bacterial counts in livers and spleens were significantly reduced and survival was prolonged, compared with placebo-treated animals. Nifedipine increased Fp expression in the spleen, whereas splenic levels of ferritin and serum iron concentrations were reduced. Therefore, nifedipine, and probably other drugs, may induce Fp expression, export iron from macrophages and thus restrict iron availability for intracellular pathogens.[80]

The *Brucella* spp are facultative intracellular pathogens. The two predominant host cell types inhabited by *Brucella* are macrophages and placental trophoblasts. These bacteria produce 2,3-dihydroxybenzoic acid (2,3-DHBA) in response to iron limitation *in vitro,* which functions as a siderophore.[81] In addition, *Brucella abortus* strain 2308 produces brucebactin, a more complex 2,3-DHBA-based siderophore.[82] It has been showed that these siderophores are not required for wild-type replication of *B. abortus* in cultured murine macrophages. Paulley et al showed that heme is an important iron source for the bacterium, during chronic infection. Heme has a key role during the stationary phase, allowing *Brucella* to maintain intracellular residence in host macrophages. Recent analysis of the known *Brucella* genome sequences revealed a homolog of the heme transporter *shuA* gene of *Shigella dysenteriae* and has been given the designation *bhuA* (Brucella heme utilization).[83,84] The gene encodes a TonB-dependent outer membrane heme transporter. In *Brucella* spp the genes involved in the transport of heme across the cytoplasmic membrane are located in an operon distant from the *bhuA* locus.[85] In other gram negative bacteria, the genes for the periplasmic binding protein-dependent ABC transporter, responsible for the transportation of heme across the cytoplasmic membrane, are located in an operon with the gene for the TonB-dependent outer membrane transporter.

6. Iron and mycobacterial infections

Mycobacterium tuberculosis (Mtb) has developed various means of attacking the host system. One such crucial strategy is the exploitation of the iron resources of the host system. When Mtb evade the mammalian immune system, it resides within macrophages in an early phagosome, whose maturation to the late phagosome and phagolysosome stages is blocked. The control of the intraphagosomal environment is crucial. Macrophages digest senescent erythrocytes and degrade heme, thus accumulating iron. Iron mainly egresses the macrophage bound to Tf, although a part of it is incorporated into ferritin in the cytosol. Other main iron sources for the macrophage are the hemoglobin-haptogobin complex, taken up via the hemoglobin scavenger receptor CD163 during hemolysis, and iron bound to Tf and Lf that enters macrophages, via the transferrin-transferrin receptor and lactoferrin receptor pathway, respectively.[71] Iron is exported from the cell via Fp-1 which is the receptor for hepcidin. In the presence of inflammation serum hepcidin is high and the binding to Fp induces conformational changes to this molecule, resulting in allosteric inhibition of its function, thus halting iron egress, and promoting internalization and degradation of Fp.[86,87]

Within its phagosome, Mtb acquires iron from the cytoplasmic sources or from the Tf/Tf-receptor complex.[88] By the time Mtb faces the low-iron environment of the phagosome, several Mtb genes, involved in the biosynthesis of siderophores, are induced. There is a dual mycobacterial siderophore system, made of mycobactins, the water-soluble carboxymycobactin, and the lipophilic mycobactin-T, which transfers iron captured by the hydrophilic carboxymycobactin, across the cell wall.[89] Mycobactin, except from participating in iron internalization, it prevents sudden influx of excess iron, when the metal becomes available. For the transportation across the cell membrane, a reductase converts Fe^{3+}-mycobactin to the Fe^{2+} form. The ferrous ion, possibly complexed with salicylic acid, is then shuttled across the membrane, either for direct incorporation into various porphyrins and apoproteins, or for storage of iron within the bacterial cytoplasm. The overall process of iron acquisition and utilization requires the activation of a number of mycobacterial genes. Mtb contains four potential iron-dependent regulators, belonging to two different families of metalloregulatory proteins. Two genes, *furA* and *furB*, encode proteins, belonging to the FUR family. The other two genes, IdeR and SirR are members of the DtxR (diphtheria toxin repressor) family. IdeR is an essential regulator with a major role in controlling iron metabolism, by repressing siderophore production, activating iron storage genes and positively regulating oxidative stress responses.[90] In Mtb-infected macrophages an upregulation of IdeR was found as part of the bacterial protective mechanism against iron-mediated oxidative stress.

Immune cell derived mediators control systemic and cellular iron homeostasis. On the other hand, iron affects the activity of transcription factors related to immune responses, and therefore, the secretion of cytokines.[91] Iron, directly inhibits the action of IFN-γ, which is crucial for the control of intracellular infections. In iron-loaded macrophages, an inhibition of IFN-γ mediated pathways is noted while intraphagosomal Mtb growth is stimulated.[92] However, IFN-γ activation of human monocytes decreases iron availability to Mtb.[93] Sow et al. examined the expression of hepcidin in macrophages, infected with Mycobacterium avium and Mtb and found that IFN-γ induced high levels of hepcidin mRNA and protein by pathways involving STAT1 activation and Toll-like receptors TLR2 and TLR4.[94,95]

Dietary iron overload, mainly in rural populations in sub-Saharan Africa, causing iron overload of macrophages and hepatocytes may increase the risk of tuberculosis. The incidence of tuberculosis has markedly increased the last decades, primarily as a result of the infection with the human immunodeficiency virus (HIV). Acquired immunodeficiency syndrome (AIDS) patients exhibit alterations in iron metabolism that lead to increased deposition of this element in the tissues. Such alterations may underlie the increased susceptibility of AIDS patients to mycobacterial infections. Many ongoing studies are aiming to investigate the Mycobacterial iron-acquisition pathways and their role in the treatment of tuberculosis e.g. synthesizing selective inhibitors of iron metabolism that may be helpful as chemotherapeutic agents. Table 4 resumes the most commonly encounterd iron uptaking mechanisms, during bacterial growth.

— Expression of receptors for iron containing proteins of the host (Transferrin, Lactoferrin, Hemoglobin)
— Adaptation of the expression of a polymorphic Tf receptor according to host's Tf structure
— Non-enzymatic reduction of Fe^{2+} to Fe^{3+} by 3-hydroxylanthranilic acid or melanin (*C.neoformans*)
— Enzymatic oxidation of the Fe^{2+} to Fe^{3+} out of bacteria in the surroundings (various ferroxidases)
— Production and release of iron-depleted siderophores and uptake of iron-saturated siderophores
— Expression of specific siderophore ligands in the outer surface of the bacterial membrane
— Production, release and uptake of heme-picking substances (ABC transporter HrtAB)
— Oxidation of heme by heme oxygenase and uptaking of the iron from the porphyrin ring
— Production and release of hemophores (removing heme from hemoproteins, for example HasA)
— Expression of specific hemophore ligands in the outer surface of the bacterial membrane (HasR)
— Elaboration of iron permease-ferroxidase complex (Ftr1-Fet3, Aft1-Aft2, CIR1, HapX/Php4)
— Production, release and uptake of specific protein iron transporters (Sit1 in *C. Glabrata*)
— Induction of iron-starving conditions in the host and upregulation of Tf receptor (Intracellular pathogens)
— Modulation of the IRPs and/or the IRE of critical genes of the host cells (Intracellular pathogens)

Table 4. Summary of the most common iron upatking mechanisms elaborated by pathogens.

7. Iron and fungal infections

The larger proportion of systemic fungal infections are opportunistic i.e. an important factor for their occurrence is a background of primary or secondary (in the majority of cases iatrogenic) immunosuppression. For all fungal pathogens iron is essential for many metabolic processes and the most intelligent and complex systems of iron acquisition from the host cells and tissues, is found among various fungal strains. Particularly for fungi, iron is a major virulence factor.[96] Many if not all, host-developed mechanisms of host defence against pathogenic fungi are orchestrated through iron deprivation. Lf, produced and released mainly by neutrophils and monocytes, represents the major fungistatic factor of human serum, milk and other fluids.[97]

Fungal pathogens require 10^{-7} to 10^{-6} M iron for their growth, and, therefore, serum and other biological fluids and tissues, containing $<10^{-15}$ and as low as 10^{-24} M of iron are normally fungistatic for all species, including Candida, Aspergillus and Zygomycetes.[98] The fungistatic properties of human serum are completely abolished by the in vitro addition of exogenous iron, and Candida albicans can grow in serum cultures with Tf saturation >90%, but not in serum with normal Tf saturation. Diseases and conditions, accompanied by a high iron burden have been associated with increased susceptibility to fungal infections. Among these are tissue hypoxia, diabetic ketoacidosis, acidosis of any other cause, tissue damage and necrosis, post-traumatic states or those induced by chemotherapy, hemochromatosis, liver disease and cancer. Patients with acute myelogenous leukemia or other hematologic malignancies have commonly an excess of iron, and particularly, non-transferrin-bound iron, which is further increased following chemotherapy,[99] either because of tissue damage or, in some cases, as a result of circulating iron complexes. Such complexes are produced by the leukemic cells and are liberated following their death, induced by chemotherapy. All the above, render leukemic neutropenic patients particularly vulnerable to fungal infections. Liver iron overload, in patients undergoing orthotopic liver transplantation, is also a predisposing factor for the development of invasive fungal infections, and such infections occur almost three times more commonly among transplanted patients with elevated levels of iron in the liver.[100]

Iron uptake by fungi is accomplished by specific transport systems, in which an initially Fe^{3+} form is reduced to Fe^{2+} iron, through the action of specific cell surface reductases (ferroxidases). Ferrous iron is then internalized by three different mechanisms. The first is achieved thank to the high affinity of the iron-containing ferroxidases for a specific type of fungal transport proteins, named permeases. The iron permease-ferroxidase complexes (Ftr1-Fet3) easily transverse the fungal wall and cell membrane, and iron is thereafter provided intracellularly. There are three types of specific transcriptional activators or repressors of the genes encoding ferroxidases and permeases, which modulate their expression under iron-deprived conditions: the Aft1 and Aft2 activators in *Saccharomyces cerevisiae* and other yeast, or the Cryptococcus iron regulator gene (CIR1) in *Cryptococcus neoformans*, the GATA-type repressors, such as Sfu-1, present in many fungal species and the HapX/Php4 in *Schizosaccharomyces pombe* and *Aspergillus* species. A second mechanism or iron acquisition involves the production of siderophores, which are excreted through the fungal wall in the deferric form, bind iron, and then are taken up by the fungi. Finally, a third mechanism is related to a fungal heme oxygenase, which takes up iron from heme.[101,102]

C. albicans possesses two high-affinity iron permease genes that are essential for its virulence. Iron permeases are encoded by iron-responsive genes, which are regulated by the specific transcriptional activator Hap43 and the repressor Sfu1. Deletion of these genes renders mutant strains non-virulent.[103] Various iron overload conditions enhance *C. albicans* growth and increase the mortality rate of infected mice. Elevated serum iron levels have been documented among patients with urogenital candidiasis. In *C. albicans* CIR1 is a gene regulating iron homeostasis, as well as calcium and cAMP signaling, cell wall integrity, and the expression of all virulence functions, including capsule and melanin formation and growth at host temperature. Hap43 protein is essential for the growth and virulence of *C.albicans* under low-iron conditions, and is accumulating in the nucleus. Hap43 is not required for iron acquisition, but it is responsible for repression of genes encoding iron-dependent proteins involved in mitochondrial respiration and iron-sulfur cluster formation. There is an association between Hap43 and the global corepressor Tup1 in response to iron deprivation.[104]

Sit1 is a combined siderophore-iron transporter, found in *C. glabrata*. For this yeast iron acquisition is necessary, not only for the growth and virulence, but also for maintaining its survival against the fungicidal activities of macrophages. Within the Sit1 transporter, a conserved extracellular *SIderophore Transporter Domain* (SITD) has been identified, that is critical for the ability of *C. glabrata* to resist macrophage killing. *C. glabrata* senses altered iron levels within the phagosomal compartment and Sit1 functions as a determinant of survival in a way that is dependent on the iron status inside the macrophage.[105]

Non-enzymatic reduction of ferric iron by 3-hydroxylanthranilic acid and melanin has been documented in *Cryptococcus neoformans*.[106] The expression of permease genes in *Aspergillus* and *zygomycetes* is upregulated during their growth and virulence.[107] The growth, survival and virulence of *Aspergillus fumigatus* and other mold species in serum is associated with the removal of iron from Tf and other iron-containing proteins.[108] This is accomplished by siderophores. HapX, a bZIP-type transcriptional regulator, is a very important gene, which sets up the adaptation mechanism to iron starvation in *A. fumigatus*. HapX represses all iron-dependent and mitochondrial-orchestrated metabolic activities, including respiration, TCA cycle, amino acid metabolism, iron-sulfur cluster formation and heme biosynthesis. Iron starvation induces significant modulation of the amino acid pool and HapX coordinates the production of siderophores and their precursor amino acid ornithine. HapX activity is restricted to iron-deplete conditions, therefore, HapX-deficiency causes significant attenuation of virulence in a murine model of aspergillosis.[109]

Fungal species are capable of synthesizing many different siderophores; however, the most important and most commonly found in *Aspergillus* and zygomycetes are N'',N', N-triacetylfusarinine C and ferricrocin. *Aspergillus* uses two iron uptake mechanisms, the reductase-permease complex and the siderophore-assisted mechanism.[110] The latter has been demonstrated in vitro, as holotransferrin, but not apotransferrin, supports the growth of *Aspergillus spp.* in iron-depleted serum culture systems. In such systems, siderophore production becomes evident following 10 h of incubation and reaches a peak at 20 h.[105] Nevertheless, not all species and strains produce siderophores. Some fungi use ferric reductases or low molecular mass iron reductants, to reduce ferric to ferrous iron, and extract it from the extracellular environment. Such mechanisms have been documented in *C. albicans*, *Histoplasma capsulatum*,[111] and in *Cryptococcus neoformans*.[112]

7.1 Iron metabolism in Zygomycetes

Zygomycosis is a difficult-to-treat systemic fungal infection, caused by the *zygomycetes*, and is associated with a high mortality rate, ranging from 50% to 100%. *Rhizopus oryzae* is the most common cause of zygomycosis. The disease is usually presented with the rhinocerebral form and is characterized by the propensity of *zygomycetes* for vascular invasion and dissemination, commonly resulting in thrombosis and tissue necrosis. The infection can rapidly extend from the paranasal sinuses to the oral cavity, to the orbit and intracranially, sometimes producing cavernous sinus thrombosis.[113] Zygomycosis almost always occurs among patients with a pre-existing immune defect, although rare cases have been reported among apparently normal individuals.[114] In the majority of cases, the course is rapidly progressive and eventually fatal, unless prompt treatment with high doses of liposomal amphotericin B (LAmB), in association with careful and may be repeated surgical debridement, can change the otherwise dismal clinical course.

Since the spectrum of diseases for which the use of immunosuppressive treatments, such as corticosteroids, cyclosporine, purine analogs (fludarabine, cladribine, nelarabin, pentostatin), rapamycin and mTOR inhibitors, various monoclonal antibodies (rituximab, bevacizumab, infliximab, basiliximab, Campath, etc) and allogeneic hematopoietic stem-cell transplantation has enlarged,[115] and since the use of systemic antifungal prophylaxis with agents that are ineffective against *zygomycetes*, mainly azole derivatives has increased, zygomycosis appears to be an emerging threat the last two decades.[116] Well-recognized predisposing factors for zygomycosis are diabetes mellitus (especially when complicated by ketoacidosis), treatment with corticosteroids, immunosuppression, prolonged leukopenia (neutropenia and lymphopenia), recent chemotherapy and tissue damage, history of allogeneic stem cell transplantation, chronic graft-versus-host-disease, and prolonged treatment with broad spectrum antibiotics and azole-type antifungal prophylaxis.

However, a common denominator of almost all of these conditions is the presence of excessive iron overload, either as high tissue iron burden, or as elevated serum Tf, and also as increased non-transferrin-bound iron.[117] In particular, it has been suggested that diabetic ketoacidosis and acidoses of any aetiology predispose to zygomycosis by facilitating the dissociation of iron from iron-carrying proteins, thus providing increased available free iron.[118] Elevated serum and tissue iron have a tremendous impact on the growth and development of *zygomycetes*.[119] There are reports of fast *Mucor* growth, with formation of intra-arterial thrombi, among immunocompromised patients with iron overload.[120,121] In a retrospective analysis of 263 allotransplanted patients, all five cases of invasive zygomycosis had significantly higher serum ferritin levels, Tf saturation, and number of previously transfused red blood cell units, as compared with matched controls. *Zygomycetes* possess a specific high-affinity iron permease gene (RFTR1), which has been characterized and cloned.[122] Analysis of the polymorphisms of this gene, has recently been proposed as a tool for the molecular identification of the different *zygomycete* species.[123] FTR1 is expressed during infection in diabetic ketoacidosis (DKA) and is required for full virulence of R.oryzae in mice. Disrupted FTR1 in multinucleated *R. oryzae* resulted in the inability of the fungus to segregate to a homokaryotic null allele. However, reduction of the relative copy number of FTR1-mRNA and inhibition of FTR1 expression by RNAi compromised the ability of *R. oryzae* to acquire iron in vitro and reduced its virulence in DKA mice. Importantly, passive immunization with anti-Ftr1p immune sera protected DKA mice from infection with *R. oryzae*.[124]

The well-documented and repeatedly reported increased susceptibility to zygomycosis of haemodialysis patients, during treatment with DFO, an iron chelator that is capable of removing tissue iron, initially appeared to be a paradox.[125,126] It became clear, however, that although DFO chelates iron, from the perspective of *zygomycetes* it is a xenosiderophore, as fungal siderophores have higher affinity for iron than DFO and therefore, are capable of easily and effectively detaching iron from it and providing it to the fungi.[101,126] This ability is particularly prominent in *zygomycetes*, and these species can remove 8–40 times greater amounts of iron from DFO than *A. fumigatus* and *C. albicans*, respectively. The rapid and effective iron uptake by *zygomycetes* results in rapid growth in serum. The growth of *Rhizopus rhizopodiformis* spores, isolated from a dialysis patient with zygomycosis while on DFO therapy, was studied in an iron-deficient medium, containing human serum at increasing concentrations, enriched with different concentrations of ferrioxamine. A serum concentration of 40% inhibited fungal growth by >50%. However, in the presence of serum, ferrioxamine produced significant growth stimulation at 24 h that persisted at 48 h (Figure 1).[127] Data from animal models emphasize the exceptional requirement of iron for *Rhizopus* pathogenicity, since administration of DFO or free iron worsens the survival of animals infected with *Rhizopus*, but not with *Candida*.[128] DFO can act as a xenosiderophore in *Rhizopus*, other members of the *Mucorales*, and probably other pathogenic fungi. It is assumed that fungal enzymes or siderophores are able to specifically bind to ferrioxamine and, because they have higher affinity for iron, strip iron from ferrioxamine and facilitate iron uptake by the fungi. A similar phenomenon does not take place with deferiprone.[129] The susceptibility of dialysis patients, treated with DFO, to zygomycosis could be attributed to the fact that uraemia results in significant retention of the iron-loaded ferrioxamine in the circulation, and that this is removed during dialysis, causing patients' serum to lose its fungistatic power and be transformed to a favourable culture medium for *zygomycetes*.[130]

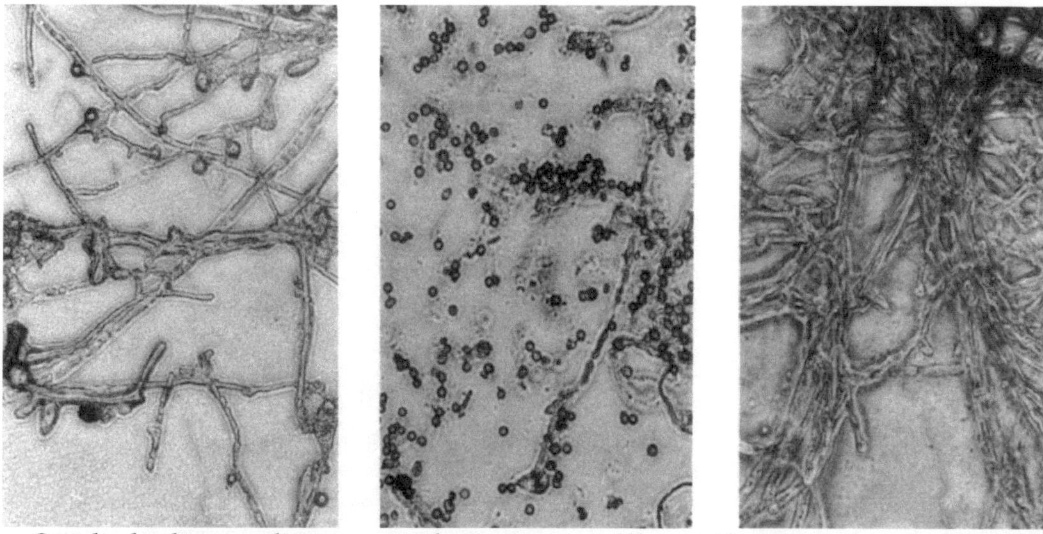

Fig. 1. Spores of Rhizopus were cultivated for 24 h at 370C in standard culture medium BDM alone (A), in BDM with 40% human serum (B) or in BDM with 40% serum + 1 MM Fe.DFO (C). Lugol stain x 500. Reprinted from Boelaert J et al. *J.Clin.Invest.* 1993; 91: 1979-1986.

7.2 The role of newer iron chelators

Since the mid-90's additional orally administered iron chelators are available. There are two newer molecules, deferiprone (DFP, Ferriprox, Apotex), which was introduced in the 1990s, and deferasirox (DFX, Exjade, Novartis), which was introduced more recently.[131] Both drugs are effective in clinical practice, but their use has not been associated with increased numbers of fungal infections and particularly, of zygomycosis. The reason for this discrepancy, as compared with DFO, may be the different chemical structure and chelating affinities of the three drugs. DFO is an exadentate chelator, has a higher molecular weight and shows a chelating relationship with the ferric iron of 1 : 1, which implies that each DFO molecule chelates one ferric ion. DFP is a bidentate chelator, and its chelating relationship is 3 : 1, meaning that each ferric iron is chelated by three molecules of DFP. DFX is a tridentate chelator, and its chelating relationship is 2 : 1, meaning that each ferric iron is chelated by two molecules of DFX.[132] The chemical structures of the three iron chelators are shown in Figure 2.

The two newer iron chelators do not act as xenosiderophores, apparently because the fungal iron uptake systems are incapable of detaching iron from them. This could be due, either to inadequate molecular access, since they are smaller molecules than DFO, or to their higher affinity for iron, which means that DFP and DFX might form more stable chemical structures with iron, that are not destabilized in the presence of fungal enzymes or siderophores. Moreover, the demonstration of clear inhibitory activity of the two newer chelators on fungal growth suggests that these molecules are probably capable of detaching iron from the fungal iron uptake molecules and holding it more strongly.[133] This has been proven in vivo, using animal models of zygomycosis, in which treatment of *Rhizopus*-

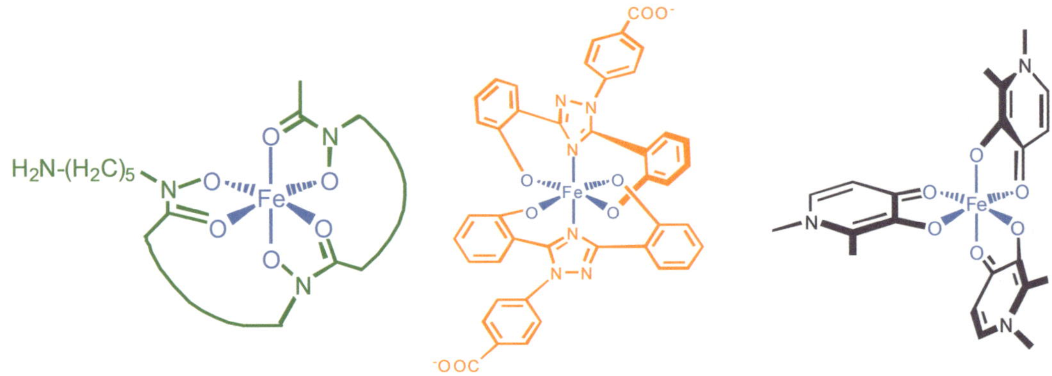

Deferroxamine (DFO) Deferasirox (DFX) Deferiprone (DFP)

Fig. 2. Stereochemical structure and mocecular chelating relationship of the three available iron chelators. Deferroxamine (DFO) has higher molecular weight (MW) and is a hexadentate, i.e. each molecule holds one ferric iron (chelating ratio 1:1). Deferasirox (DFX) has lower MW and it is a tridentate, i.e. 2 DFX molecules hold each ferric iron (chelating ratio 2:1). Deferiprone (DFP) has even lower MW and it is a bidentate, i.e. 3 DFP molecules chelate each ferric iron (chelating ratio 3:1).

infected mice or guinea pigs with DFP markedly improved survival.[133] In cultures of *Rhizopus oryzae*, DFP has fungistatic activity at 24 h, confirmed at 48 h.[129] The introduction of DFX and the recognition of the safety and efficacy profile of the drug encouraged its use in sporadic cases of systemic zygomycosis and in experimental animal studies. DFX induces an iron-starvation response in *R. oryzae* and activates RFTR1 expression. Addition of DFX to cultures of different members of the *Mucorales* produced a fungicidal effect, which was reversed by the addition of iron. The MIC90s of DFX against various *Mucor spp.* were much lower than the levels achieved by the administration of the usual daily dose of 20 mg/kg. Treatment with routine doses of DFX of diabetic ketoacidotic mice, infected with spores of *R. oryzae* led to significantly improved survival, as compared with controls, and resulted in a more than ten-fold reduction of brain and kidney fungal burden as compared with placebo-treated animals. The kidneys of DFX-treated mice had no visible hyphae and there was an effective neutrophil inflammatory reaction, whereas kidneys of placebo-treated mice had extensive filamentous fungi and manifested a poor or complete absence of a neutrophil inflammatory response.[134] In another experiment, mice infected intranasally with 10^7 spores of *R. oryzae* were treated for 7 days, starting 24 h post-infection, with either DFX 10 mg/kg twice daily or placebo. Similar to controls, infected or uninfected mice were treated with DFO 50 mg/kg. DFX was significantly more protective than placebo or DFO. As expected, DFO worsened the survival of infected mice, although it had no effect on uninfected mice. Treatment with DFX resulted in significantly increased Th1 and Th2 splenocyte subpopulations, and in significantly higher splenic and kidney levels of the proinflammatory cytokines TNF-α and IFN-γ, than those in mice treated with saturating iron or placebo.[134,135]

8. Iron, protozoan and parasitic infections

For the most intracellular protozoa, survival, growth and replication within the phagolysosomes of the macrophages is almost entirely relied on their successful iron acquisition from the host cells. These microorganisms elaborate elegant mechanisms for obtaining iron and transfer it into the iron-poor endophagosomal environment.

Legionella pneumophila requires iron for optimal extracellular and intracellular growth. Some mutants are both, sensitive to the iron chelators and resistant to streptonigrin, an antibiotic which requires high levels of intracellular iron to exert microbicidal activity. These mutants were about 100-fold more sensitive than the wild type to treatment with DFO, indicating that they have defective intracellular iron acquisition and assimilation. This strain was unable to mediate any cytopathic effect and was impaired for infectivity of an amoebal host.[136] *L.pneumophila* is engulfed into macrophages by macropinocytosis, and is not digested but proliferates intracellularly. Proliferation can be blocked by the Nramp1 protein, an iron transporter that reduces endolysosomal iron and confers resistance against invasive pathogens. However, inactivation of the PI3K pathway enhances *Legionella* infection and suppresses the protective activity of Nramp1. *L.pneumophila* abrogates phosphoinositide-dependent fusion of macropinosomes with acidic vesicles, without affecting Nramp1 recruitment. Thus *Legionella* escapes fusion with acidic vesicles and Nramp1-induced resistance to pathogens.[137]

For any protozoan pathogen iron is an absolutely necessary nutrient to effectively grow and multiply. On the other hand many antiparasistic immune effector mechanisms of innate and adaptive immunity are orchestrated through iron deprivation. Incubation of human enterocyte cell lines with IFN-γ and in vitro infection with the protozoan enteropathogen *Cryptosporidium parvum* resulted in the upregulation of IFN-γ receptors and was followed by inhibition of the parasite growth and development. IFN-γ mediated its action by inhibition of parasite invasion and by modification of intracellular Fe^{++} concentration, and this effect was partially reversed by inhibition of the JAK/STAT signaling pathway. IFN-γ directly induces enterocyte resistance against *C.parvum* infection.[138]

Toxoplasma gondii is an obligate intracellular parasite and a common opportunistic pathogen in HIV positive patients, and macrophage early nonspecific response is an important part of host defense. About 18 h following infection of mouse macrophages with a high burden of *T.gondii* tachyzoites, a strong down-regulation of the macrophage Tf receptor levels was observed. Stimulation of the mouse cells with toxoplasma lysate antigen had no effect on Tf receptor expression.[139] IFN-γ alone or in combination with IL-1, IL-6 or TNF-α significantly inhibited *T.gondii* growth in murine astrocytes. However this inhibition appear not to be mediated through induction of ROS expression, or iron deprivation, but by other, as yet unclear mechanisms.[140]

The in vitro growth of Pneumocystis Carinii can be easily suppressed by daphnetin (7,8-dihydroxycoumarin) a well-known iron chelator, through iron deprivation in a dose-dependent way. The inhibitory activity is not exerted when iron-repleted daphnetin is added to the culture system. Inhibition of *P.carinii* growth by daphnetin is associated with morphological changes, clearly determined by transmission electron microscopy.[141]

Leishmania donovani uses another mechanism to obtain iron from the labile iron pool of the macrophages. As a consequence, intracellular macrophage iron is depleted, iron sensor, through IRP-1 and -2 is activated, mRNA of the Tf receptor-1 is stabilized and is transcribed, Tf receptor expression is upregulated and Tf uptake is increased. Then Leishmania easily retrieves iron from holotransferrin.[142] *L. donovani* itself expresses a Tf receptor and their in vitro growth is inhibited by iron chelators. Moreover, in vivo administration of DFO in mice infected with Leishmania leads to a slight delay in the development of cutaneous lesions. Unexpectedly however, systemic iron delivery at early time points of infection, decreased parasite load at the site of parasite inoculation, the regional lymph node, the liver and spleen. The protective effect of iron correlated with lower IL-4 and IL-10, but higher type-1 cytokine transcripts (IFN-γ and inducible NO synthase) at the site of inoculation, as well as by increased serum levels of IgG2a.[143] An iron-dependent superoxide dismutase from *Leishmania Chagas* is expressed at low levels in the early logarithmic stage of development and increases at later stages of growth. The parasite demonstrates significant growth reduction when endogenous superoxide levels are increased, following the addition of paraquat in culture. There is a protective gene, LcFeSODB, which plays an important role in the parasite growth and survival by protecting the glycosomes from superoxide toxicity.[144]

Malnutrition alters the innate immune response against *L.donovani*. Thus, diets deficient in calories, protein, and in the metal elements zinc and iron represent a risk factor for the development of visceral leishmaniasis, and in malnourished mice, a greater parasite burden is found in the spleen and liver, which is attributed to a failure of lymph node barrier function. Lymph node cells from the malnourished group produced increased levels of PGE_2 and decreased levels of IL-10 and inducible NO synthase activity.[145] Iron deficiency may finally favor the host and impair *L.donovani* growth. When iron availability is restricted the parasite's growth may be reduced and the infection attenuated.[146]

Another *Leishmania spp, Leishmania amazonensis,* elaborates an inducible ferrous iron transport system through LIT1, a novel parasitic membrane protein. LIT1 is only detectable upon intracellular invasion of the parasite and its expression is accelerated under iron-deprived conditions. *L. amazonensis* lacking LIT1 protein abolishes its virulence and its replicating capacity within macrophages.[147]

Trichomonas vaginalis is the most common non viral pathogen, transmitted sexually and is highly-dependent on iron. *T. vaginalis* is adhered to vaginal epithelial cells, through specific surface proteins (AP65, AP51, AP33 and AP23) named adhesins. Free iron, heme and hemoglobin induce AP65 mRNA and protein expression on the parasistic membrane, thus favoring virulence. Heme-induced AP65 expression was about 10-fold higher in a low-iron culture medium, indicating that *T. vaginalis* can use heme as an alternative source of iron, important to its growth and regulation of expression of the adhesin genes.[148] An iron-responsive promoter and other iron regulatory elements (IRE) in the 5'-UTR of the ap65-1 gene, as well as two IRE-like hairpin-loop structures in mRNAs of TVCP4 and TVCP12 cysteine proteinases, have been identified in *T.vaginalis,* suggesting the existence of a post-transcriptional iron regulatory mechanism of critical genes by an IRE/IRP-like system in this protozoon.[149] DFO killed all *T.vaginalis* isolates with a minimum lethal concentration of 30 μM after 48 h of exposure, and a potent and persistent inhibitory effect of DFO on the parasite viability and growth was observed, with lower drug concentration and shorter time of exposure.[150]

Tritrichomonas foetus is a protozoan pathogen of cattle, and its growth and virulence is greatly influenced by the iron concentration of the culture medium. In iron-restricted media both, Lf and Tf support *T.foetus* growth. However, a specific binding to the outer parasitic membrane has been demonstrated only for Lf, whose uptake at 37^{0} C is about 3.5-fold higher, a finding indicating a mechanism of receptor-mediated endocytosis. In contrast, Tf binding is nonspecific, and iron retrieval is achieved via extracellular release and siderophore assistance.[151] Many microbial siderophores can also support *T. foetus* growth under iron-limited conditions, providing iron to ferredoxin, the major siderophore of the parasite. Iron uptake is not mediated by previous extracellular reduction, although *T.foetus* possesses some ferrireductase activity. Siderophores are pinocytosed by the parasites in small vesicles, exhibiting a very acidic environment. Hemin also supports *T. foetus* growth, probably with the involvement of heme oxygenase.[152] Parasites grown in iron-depleted media exhibit reduced capability to destroy epithelial cell monolayers and reduced activity of several cysteine proteases, indicating that iron is an extracellular signal, modulating T.foetus' ability to interact with host epithelial cells.[153] In one study, mice inoculated intraperitoneally with a moderately- or a highly-virulent strain of *T.foetus* and treated with ferric citrate exhibited high mortality rate by the moderately-virulent strain up to the level of the highly-virulent strain. Peritoneal cultures showed that iron overload was associated with stimulation of parasite replication, which was strongly suppressed in untreated mice, and the less virulent strains showed lower efficiency for iron acquisition from Tf and other sources.[154]

The greatest experience about the influence of iron metabolism on parasite growth has emerged from the study of malaria infection. *Plasmodium* grows up fluently in the intraerythrocyte environment, where plenty of iron, contained in hemoglobin, can be easily accessed and uptaken. Since about 3 decades ago there has been emerging evidence that, iron deprivation might represent an important mechanism in the battle of man against malaria.[155] Asymptomatic parasitemia has been associated with the existence of hypochromic anemia, in the absence of a prominent acute phase reaction. These patients exhibit higher serum hepcidin concentration, higher ferritin, lower iron and transferrin levels, and lower transferrin saturation, and consequently have impaired intestinal iron absorption and dietary iron utilization. On the other hand malaria commonly coexists with a background of frank iron deficiency. Antimalarial treatment partly restores low-grade inflammation and decreases serum hepcidin, ferritin, and other indeces of inflammation, and should be preceded of any effort for anemia correction with iron. Clearance of parasitemia increases dietary iron absorption but did not affect systemic iron utilization. Therefore, in areas of high prevalence of malaria, since asymptomatic parasitemia has a protracted course, careful clinical evaluation of anemic patients is mandatory, because the unjustified or mistimed iron supplementation will be ineffective and may even be hazardous and render malaria symptomatic.[156, 157] Among pregnant women in areas with high malaria prevalence, malaria parasitemia, hookworm infection, gravidity and advanced gestational age were associated with lower hemoglobin and iron deficiency. Malaria parasitemia, *Ascaris lumbricodes* and *Trichuris trichiura* infections and older age were associated with lower serum ferritin levels.[158]

Intraerythrocytic malaria parasites digest hemoglobin to obtain the amino acids needed for their own protein synthesis. Hemoglobin degradation and total parasite protein content increase in parallel with parasite maturation, but the rate of hemoglobin degradation is higher, than the utilized amount of amino acids.[159] Hemoglobin degradation yields also large quantities of ferriprotoporphyrin IX and iron, which create a highly oxidative erythrocyte environment and high requirements for detoxification. Redox-active iron released inside the erythrocyte, mediate the conversion of H_2O_2 to hydroxyl radical $[HO]^-$ which is more reactive. Superoxide dismutase (SOD) and nitroxide SOD detoxifies the erythrocyte and acts similarly to the antimalarial drug 4-OH,2,2,6,6,tetramethyl piperidine-N-oxyl (Tempol) in *P.falciparum* growth. Tempol inhibits parasite growth, and induces accelerated mortality in a SOD-overexpressing mouse model of malaria.[160] SOD has therefore a protective role for the erythrocytes, and transgenic copper/zinc superoxide dismutase$^{- -}$ (CuZnSOD) mouse strains show higher sensitivity to infection by *Plasmodium berghei*. Moreover, treatment of infected erythrocytes, either SOD transgenic or normal, with oxidative stress inducers, reduces parasite viability. Therefore, CuZnSOD does not support plasmodium development, and impairment of its activity results in higher oxidative stress, favoring malaria growth.[161]

Iron deficiency modulates *Plasmodium yoelii* development in hepatocytes, by inactivating hepatic xanthine-oxidase. Iron-deficient mice infected with *Pl. yoelii* sporozoites, exhibited enhanced development of hepatic stage, resulting in the earlier appearance of blood parasites. An iron-starving diet increased penetration of sporozoites into liver cells, whereas inactivation of hepatic xanthine-oxidase inhibited both, sporozoite penetration and schizont maturation. Moreover, inhibition of heme synthesis also results in inhibition of parasite development.[162] Another mechanism, favorably influencing the clinical course of *Pl.falciparum* infection in iron deficient subjects, is the faster clearance of infected erythrocytes. Iron deficiency accelerates unifected erythrocyte death and enhances death and removal of infected erythrocytes by phagocytosis, which is evident from phosphatidylserine exposure. Indeed, parasitized iron deficient erythrocytes are more susceptible to phagocytosis in vitro, than normal erythrocytes.[163,164] The importance of iron in plasmodium growth has shifted antimalarial treatment strategies and research towards the identification and application of new drugs intervening with the parasite iron metabolism. More details on the topic are mentioned in the following paragraphs.

Trypanosomiasis or Chagas' disease has been associated with iron overload. *Trypanosoma* possesses a unique mechanism of adaptation and iron acquisition from the host environment. *Trypanosoma brucei* escapes destruction by the host immune system, by regularly replacing its *Variant Surface Glycoprotein* (VSG) coat. The VSG is expressed together with expression site associated genes, encoding the heterodimeric Tf receptor. There are about 20 VSG expression sites and trypanosomes can change the active site, according to environmental conditions. Since the various Tf receptor genes, localized in different expression sites, differ somewhat in sequence, expression site switching results in the production of a slightly different Tf receptor. Trypanosomes can adapt the expression site of its Tf receptor to achieve the highest affinity for the host Tf molecule.[165]

Hypochromic anemia is a dominant characteristic of this disease and its severity is correlated with the severity of trypanosomiasis. The parasite induces a strong type-I immune response, activating bone marrow and tissue macrophages and establishing an imbalance between erythropoiesis and erythrophagocytosis or erythroblastic apoptosis, which is the typical pathogenetic mechanism of anemia of chronic disease.[166] In a murine model of trypanosomiasis, erythrophagocytosis by cytokine-activated M1 macrophages was the main initial cause of aggressive anemia during the acute phase of infection. Persistence of type I cytokine production in the chronic phase of infection perpetuates and deteriorates anemia. Meanwhile, iron homeostasis is perturbed and there is increased iron sequestration by macrophages, resulting after upregulation of Fp, Tf and ceruloplasmin genes, indicating that iron export is reduced. In the chronic phase of trypanosomiasis, iron sequestration worsens, while the enhanced uptake of iron-containing molecules is maintained.[167]

Entamoeba histolytica trophozoites can grow in vitro within culture media, containing ferrous or ferric iron, and they can use hemoglobin, holotransferrin, hololactoferrin and ferritin as iron sources. Iron-binding proteins are specifically bound to the amoeba surface, are uptaken by endocytosis, traffick through the endosomal/lysosomal route and are degraded by neutral and acidic cysteine-proteases. Tf and ferritin are mainly uptaken as clathrin-coated vesicles. However, apolactoferrin bound to membrane lipids and cholesterol, induces cell death. In vivo trophozoites secrete products capable to destroy enterocytes, erythrocytes and hepatocytes, releasing Tf, hemoglobin, ferritin and other iron-containing proteins, which, together with Lf derived from neutrophils and acinar cells, can be used as iron supplies by amoebas.[168] Many biological functions and pathogenicity of the free-living amoeba *Naegleria fowleri* are dependent on the composition of the culture medium. The iron-containing porphyrins hemin or hematin or the iron-free protoporphyrin IX, can support *N.fowleri* growth in serum free media, whereas iron-binding proteins, including hemoglobin cannot.[169] Some growth-promoting factors for *Entamoeba* species are low molecular weight substances, found in cellular fractions of various cells, and are probably siderophores, such as ferredoxins and rubredoxin.[170]

Hookworm infection has been associated with growth delay and iron deficiency anemia. In a mouse model of this disease, infected animals, fed with a standard diet exhibited significant growth delay and reduced hemoglobin levels, compared to uninfected controls, whereas no significant difference in weight or hemoglobin concentration was observed between infected and uninfected animals, fed with an iron-restricted diet. Moreover, iron-restricted animals exhibited reduced intestinal worm burden, compared to animals fed with the standard diet. Finally, infected animals fed with intermediate-iron containing diet exhibited greater weight loss and anemia, than animals fed with iron-restricted- or high-iron diets. Mortality was also higher in the intermediate-iron containing diet. Therefore, severe dietary iron restriction impairs hookworm development, but moderate iron restriction enhances host susceptibility to severe disease.[171]

The human blood fluke *Schistosoma japonicum* is responsible for significant morbidity and mortality in tropical areas. For this fluke and some other invertebrates, an additional role for iron has been postulated, and this concerns the stabilization of the extracellular matrix. *Schistosoma* requires iron for its development and stores abundant iron in the vitelline (eggshell-forming) cells of the female system, in the form of yolk ferritin that is upregulated in females and is also expressed at low levels in egg-stages and adult males. Iron concentrations have been found higher in the female- than the male adult parasite, but also in the parasite eggs and purified eggshell, whose matrix is composed of heavily cross-linked eggshell precursor proteins.[172]

9. Clinical considerations - infections in iron overloaded patients

As previously noted, iron is crucial for the growth and proliferation of all microorganisms, due to its role in mitochondrial respiration and DNA synthesis. Iron starvation and oxidative stress are the hurdles that bacteria must overcome to establish an infection. In some cases there is excess iron available and specific infections are more common. Iron overload may be secondary to lysis of red cells from free heme compounds, as a result of trauma and due to altered metabolism (hemochromatosis, hepatic disease or post chemotherapy).

In the presence of hemolytic disorders, caused by malaria or *Bartonella bacilliformis* (in cases of Oroya fever) *salmonella* infections are noted.[173] The presence of free hemoglobin or heme may effectively impair or completely destroy the mechanism of natural resistance. Bullen et al. showed that ferric citrate, hematin hydrochloride, lysed guinea-pig red cells and crystalline human hemoglobin greatly enhanced *E. coli* virulence, when injected intraperitoneally into normal guinea-pigs.[174]

Blood transfusions may increase the free hemoglobin. Red blood cell transfusions should be used sparingly, keeping in mind the potential risks of infection and poor outcomes in critically ill patients. In a prospective, observational cohort study by Taylor et al. the posttransfusion nosocomial infection rate was 14.3% in 428 evaluable patients, significantly higher than that observed in nontransfused patients (5.8%; $p < 0.0001$).[175] In a multivariate analysis controlling for patient age, maximum storage age of red blood cells, and number of red blood cell transfusions, only the number of transfusions was independently associated with nosocomial infection (odds ratio 1.097; $p = 0.005$). In addition mortality and length of stay (in intensive care unit and hospital) were significantly higher in transfused patients, even when corrected for illness severity.[176] Secondary analysis of a multicentered, prospective observational study of transfusion practice in intensive care units in the United States showed that transfusion of packed red blood cells increases the risk of developing VAP (ventilator associated pneumonia). The effect of transfusion on late-onset VAP was more pronounced (odds ratio 2.16; 95% CI, 1.27-3.66) and demonstrated a positive dose-response relationship.[177] To determine whether blood transfusion influences infection after trauma, Agarwal et al. analyzed data on 5366 consecutive patients, hospitalized for more than 2 days. Even when patients were stratified by Injury Severity Score, the infection rate increased significantly with the higher numbers of transfused blood units. Blood transfusion in the injured patients is an important independent statistical predictor of infection. Its contribution cannot be attributed to age, sex, or the underlying mechanism of severity of injury.[178] Both, modified and native human hemoglobin may promote infection.[179] They showed that pyridoxalated polymerised human hemoglobin promotes fulminant *E. coli* septicemia in mice, which draws attention to the potential danger of such products in the clinic.

Hereditary hemochromatosis is the prototype disease for primary iron overload. *Vibrio vulnificus* has been linked to primary sepsis, which usually occurs in patients with underlying liver disease (cirrhosis or hemochromatosis).[180] Although this pathogen can be destroyed by human plasma, it multiplies rapidly when free iron is available. After eating raw sea food, like oysters, the patient develops high fever, prostration, hypotension and in most cases characteristic cutaneous manifestations (initially erythematous patches followed by ecchymoses, vesicles and bullae) with a mortality rate up to 50% without the prompt therapy. Primary hemochromatosis was the commonest underlying disease in patients with liver abscesses caused by *Yersinia enterocolitica*.[181] Some *Yersinia* strains are unable to synthesize siderophores but they can exploit host-chelated iron stores and the drug DFO. As a result, iron overload appears to be independent risk factor for *Y. enterocolitica* bacteremia, mainly by the serotypes O:3 and O:9. *Yersinia* bacteremia must be considered as an indicator of possible iron overload and *Yersinia* infection must be suspected in febrile hemochromatosic patients. In the past, patients with chronic renal failure, undergoing dialysis received multiple transfusions and frequent parenteral iron preparations. In a study by Boelaer *Yersinia* bacteremias (*Y. enterocolitica* and *Y. pseudotuberculosis*) were detected more often when ferritin levels were >500 ng/ml.[182] *Y. enterocolitica* has also been identified as a causative agent of posttransfusion septic shock. *Yersinia* bacteremias complicate the transfusions of blood that has been stored for more than 3 weeks.[183,184] The high-pathogenicity island (HPI), present in pathogenic *Yersinia* and encoding the siderophore yersiniabactin, has been found in *E. coli* pathotypes, responsible for bacteremias, neonatal meningitis and urosepsis.[185]

The spleen, an important part of the reticuloendothelial system, acts as a filter for circulating debris, including bacteria and as an important source of lymphoid cells and antibody production. Splenectomy may alter the ability to prevent or suppress some infections. There appears to be a high risk of severe bacterial infections when splenectomy is performed in patients with thalassaemia major, hepatitis, cirrhosis, histocytosis or inborn errors of metabolism.[186,187] Seventy three patients with β-thalassemia/HbE were studied 1-28 years after splenectomy. Serum ferritin levels in both, HbH and β-thalassemia/Hb E patients were higher than normal. They were higher in β-thalassemia/HbE than HbH disease. Most striking was the significantly higher serum ferritin levels in splenectomized patients with β-thalassemia/HbE disease than in the nonsplenectomized ones. After splenectomy, in patients with β-thalassemia/HbE disease, there was an increase of the Tf saturation in addition to increased circulating non-trasferrin bound iron.[188]

Levels of serum iron are elevated in patients undergoing hematopoietic stem cell transplantation (HSCT), as a result of disturbed iron metabolism, pre-transplantation blood transfusions, or cytotoxic therapy, for conditioning before HSCT. The complications of iron overload in HSCT patients include bacterial and fungal infections, mucositis, chronic liver disease (fibrosis progression), sinusoidal obstruction syndrome, and other regimen-related toxicities. Iron overload can be considered as an independent adverse prognostic factor in allogeneic HSCT. Screeneing for iron overload at various time points before and after transplantation may be beneficial especially in patients with thalassemia and myelodysplastic syndromes.[189]

Singh et al, assessed the role of hepatic explant iron overload as a risk factor for *Staph. aureus* bacteremia in liver transplant recipients. Noncarriers (patients without *S. aureus* nasal carriage) who developed *S. aureus* bacteremia were more likely to have hepatic iron overload. A quantifiable assessment of hepatic iron in patients without carriage at the time of transplantation can potentially identify those who may be at risk for early *S. aureus* bacteremia.[190] In healthy humans the lower respiratory tract as well as all mucosa, contains a very low free iron concentration (10^{-18} M), while in cystic fibrosis (CF) patients, sputum iron concentration is very high, showing a median value of 63×10^{-6} M. Accumulation of catalytic reactive iron contributes to subsequent clinical complications in the lung disorders by the production of ROS and increases bacterial growth and virulence. The iron-overload of the sputum of CF patients induces nonmotile forms, aggregation and biofilm formation both in *Pseudomonas aeruginosa* and *Burkholderia cenocepacia* which are the main pathogens in these patients, facilitating the penetration of host epithelial barriers and contributing to the establishment of infection, colonization, persistence and systemic spread of these pathogens.[191]

In human plasma, a fall in Eh (oxidation-reduction potential) or pH results in the abolition or marked reduction of its bactericidal properties. This is highly relevant to infection after trauma, where a fall in Eh and pH frequently accompanies tissue damage. Hypoxia interferes with the oxidative killing of many bacteria by polymorphonuclear leukocytes. In addition it produces a fall in tissue Eh and as a result free ferrous iron is produced, leading to overwhelming growth of bacteria. If the Eh is lowered, the ferric iron is reduced to the ferrous form, no longer bound to Tf.

The bactericidal power of fresh human plasma against *Klebsiella pneumoniae* and *E. coli* is extremely sensitive to changes in Eh and pH. At a high Eh (approx. +200 mV) the bacteria were destroyed, but rapid regrowth was observed when the Eh was lowered to -400 mV. Abolition of the bactericidal effect was also produced by adding ferric iron at a high Eh (approx. +200 mV). Lowering the pH to 6.5 reduced or prevented the bactericidal effect. Rising the Eh from –400 to +200 mV restored the bactericidal effect.[192] Some bacteria like *Cl. Perfringens* or *E. coli* have developed reducing systems. They may take advantage of a reduction in skin Eh and they are capable of lowering the Eh of tissue fluids to a level where Fe^{2+} is freely available. These results are probably related to the availability of iron for bacterial growth, and could be important for understanding the development of infection in injured or diseased tissue. Iron supplementation to treat anemia is controversial, since it may promote the progression of the underlying infectious disease but existing data are insufficient to support this hypothesis.[193]

10. Iron chelators as adjuvant treatment in systemic fungal and protozoan infections

It is self-evident if we take into consideration all the above, that an important weapon in the war against the various infectious microorganisms might be iron deprivation. Many efforts have been performed for this task, in targeting the appropriate microbial pathway, identifying the ideal compound for each microorganism, evaluating its efficacy, confirming its safety and testing its clinical usefulness. The usually acute clinical course of bacterial infections, the abundance of antibiotics and the relative satisfactory handling has restricted research programs testing iron chelators for fungal and protozoan infections and infestations.

Among fungal infections the most challenging is zygomycosis, for which effective treatment is still unavailable. Many studies, elaborating animal models for this disease have tried to address the efficacy of iron chelating agents, against this mycosis. In a mouse model of zygomycosis, animals were infected with *R. oryzae* spores, and 24 h later were treated with DFP at dose levels of 50, 100 or 200 mg/kg every day or every other day. The dose of 100 mg/kg every other day resulted in a significant survival advantage of DFP-treated mice, as compared with placebo-treated animals. The other dose schedules were either ineffective or toxic. The survival advantage was comparable to, although lower than, that of Liposomal Amphotericin-B (LAmB)-treated mice. Both drugs significantly reduced the brain fungal burden as compared with placebo. The beneficial effect of DFP was abrogated when animals were given ferric chloride.[133] In a similar mouse model of established zygomycosis, the administration of DFX was associated with comparable efficacy to that of LAmB. DFX has shown efficacy in neutropenic and diabetic ketoacidotic mice with zygomycosis. In these experiments, DFX at a daily dose of 20 mg/kg, starting 24 h after infection was synergistic with LAmB at a high-dose schedule of 15 mg/kg daily, in the reduction of fungal burden from the brain and the kidney. Moreover, the combination of the two drugs significantly improved survival time as compared with placebo or each drug separately.[134] Similar results have been obtained with the combination treatment in a mouse model of aspergillosis.[135]

The use of iron chelators as adjuvant treatment in systemic zygomycosis and other mycoses appears to be rational, and has been shown to be effective in sporadic cases. Reed et al. reported a case of a 40-year-old diabetic patient with aggressive rhinocerebral zygomycosis and progressive central nervous system involvement, despite combination treatment with high-dose LAmB plus caspofungin and surgical debridement. As brain magnetic resonance imaging (MRI) showed new parenchymal lesions and left cavernous sinus thrombosis, he was given a 7-day salvage treatment with DFX 1000 mg daily. A new brain MRI scan showed significant improvement, and treatment with LAmB was discontinued. The patient, 4 months later, remained in good condition without any neurological deficit. This is the first reported case of zygomycosis being successfully treated with a combination of classical antifungal treatment and an iron chelator.[194] We have recently treated two patients with acute lymphoblastic leukemia in remission (one of them following allogeneic transplantation) with zygomycosis (one with concurrent rhinocerebral and pulmonary form, the second with classical rhinocerebral form) with a combination of LAmB 10 mg/kg, posaconazole and DFX 20 mg/kg daily. Restricted intranasal and intrasinus surgical debridement was also applied repeatedly. Both patients responded very well, with rapid defervescence, resolution of pain and chymosis, and disappearance of the dense pulmonary and sinonasal infiltrates (unpublished data). Some more published cases have also shown encouraging results[195] however in other cases, iron chelation treatment was unsuccessful.[196]

Therefore, the possible benefit of iron chelation as adjuvant treatment in systemic mycoses, and particularly in zygomycosis, had to be tested in a prospective randomized trial. Such a clinical trial, the DEFEAT mucor study, investigated the existence of synergy between the classical treatment plus or minus DFX. Twenty patients with proven or probable zygomycosis were randomized to receive LAmB plus DFX (20 mg/kg/day for 14 days) or LAmB plus placebo. Surprisingly, death was more frequent in the DFX than in the placebo arm and global success was worse for the DFX arm, since patients of this arm had higher mortality rate at 90 days. This was attributed to population imbalances between the two arms, and therefore, make generalizable conclusions cannot be drawn.[197]

DFO, although is a xenosiderophore for *Zygomycetes*, may have direct and irreversible toxic effects on *P.carinii*, independently of iron chelation. This direct and irreversible damage of *P.carinii* by DFO was confirmed in vivo, in an animal model, in which a once-a-week aerosol treatment of PCP with DFO was effective in 100% of the animals, both as a prophylactic and as a curative treatment.[198]

All the available iron chelators can inhibit the growth of malaria parasites. Using a flow cytometric method for testing in vitro drug susceptibility of *Pl.falciparum* to hydroxypyridinone derivatives and to DFO, it has been found that both classes of chelators exhibited dose-dependent inhibition of parasite growth, but DFO demonstrated a stronger inhibitory effect. The MIC required for the parasite growth, correlated with observed abnormal microscopic morphology, and sensitivity to iron chelators was shown for both, chloroquine- and pyrimethamine-resistant parasites.[199] In another study, comparing the efficacy of DFO and DFX at 30 μM/l or 60 μM/l, added in cultures of *Pl. falciparum* in human erythrocytes, it was observed that DFX had marked antimalarial activity by 6 h after exposure, and over 48 h of culture, and although the IC50s were similar for DFX and DFO, malarial growth was significantly lower with DFX than with DFO at both concentrations (P=0.001).[200]

Dexrazoxane is an iron chelating prodrug, used for the protection of anthracyclin-induced cardiotoxicity, which must undergo intracellular hydrolysis to bind iron. Investigating the antimalarial properties of dexrazoxane on *Pl. falciparum* cultured in human erythrocytes, and on *P.yoelii* cultured in mouse hepatocytes, it was found that dexrazoxane inhibited *P. falciparum* growth, only at suprapharmacologic concentrations. In contrast, pharmacologic concentrations of dexrazoxane inhibited *P.yoelli* growth by 45-69%, implying the presence of a dexrazoxane-hydrolyzing enzyme in hepatocytes but not in erythrocytes or malaria parasites.[201] Novel aroylhydrazone and thiosemicarbazone iron chelators exhibit strong inhibitory activity on cultured tumor cells. These compounds were tested as antimalarials on chloroquine-sensitive- and -resistant strains of *Pl. falciparum*, and were significantly more active in both strains than DFO. The anti-malarial activity correlated with anti-proliferative activity against neoplastic cells. This class of lipophilic chelators may be potentially useful agents as anti-malarials.[202] Among various other synthetic siderophores the most promising profile (low MIC for plasmodia and minimum toxicity to mammalian cells) was demonstrated by an acylated monocatecholate or a triscatecholate as substituent.[203] To examine the site of action of antimalarial iron chelators, Loyevsky et al. have shown that specific fluorescence indicating the presence of iron chelators was observed within the parasites, implying that iron chelators bind labile iron within the plasmodium.[204]

The antimalarial activity of zinc-desferrioxamine (Zn-DFO) was found to be superior to that of DFO in vitro. A possible explanation is that the complex Zn-DFO might be more easily permeable into parasitized erythrocytes, exchange zinc for ferric ions due to higher affinity and deprive iron from the parasite. Parasites treated with Zn-DFO were less likely to recover at a later stage, in comparison to parasites treated with DFO, therefore, the complex Zn-DFO, which is more effective in vitro, should be examined for its in vivo activity.[205]

Many iron chelators are very effective in the treatment of trypanosomiasis and almost as effective as benznidazole, the classical drug used for the treatment of this disease. Some of them inhibit *T.Cruzi* growth at very low concentrations, thanks to their ability to interfere with and disrupt essential steps of epimastigote iron, copper or zinc metabolism at intracellular sites.[206] Eleven out of 13 other iron chelators inhibited trypanosoma growth in vitro, but many of these chelators were also cytotoxic for human HL-60 cells and therefore were not further tested. Newer, more specific, lipophilic iron-chelators may serve as lead compounds for novel anti-trypanosomal drug development.[207] Bloodstream forms of *T.brucei* are 10 times more sensitive than mammalian cells to iron depletion, and treatment with DFO inhibits parasite proliferation, inducing inhibition of DNA synthesis and decrease in oxygen consumption, findings implying that DFO impairs ribonucleotide reductase and alternative oxidase activity, apparently by chelating cellular iron and preventing its incorporation into the newly synthesized apoproteins. DFO treatment for 24 h has no effect on superoxide dismutase activity.[208] Three compounds of an aminothiol family of iron chelators were tested against *Trypanosoma Cruzi*. BAT-TE completely arrested the growth of trypomastigote forms in mouse blood, while BAT-TM arrested growth in *T.cruzi*-infected mice. These results render BAT derivatives potential candidates for the clearing of donated blood from trypomastigotes in endemic areas.[209]

11. References

[1] Thelander L, Graslund A, Thelander M. Continual presence of oxygen and iron required for mammalian ribonucleotide reduction: Possible regulation mechanism. Biochem Biophys Res Commun 1983; 110:859-865.

[2] Weiss G. Modification of iron regulation by the inflammatory response. Best Pract Res Clin Haematol 2005; 18: 183-201.
[3] Aisen P, Enns C, Wessling-Resnick M. (2001) Chemistry and biology of eukaryotic iron metabolism. Int. J. Biochem. Cell Biol. 2001; 33:940-959.
[4] Imlay JA, Chin SM, Linn S. Toxic DNA damage by hydrogen peroxide through the Fenton reaction in vivo and in vitro. Science 1988; 240:640-642.
[5] Gazitt Y, Reddy SV, Alcantara O, Yang J, Boldt DH. A new molecular role for iron in regulation of cell cycling and differentiation of HL-60 human leukemia cells: iron is required for transcription of p21(WAF1/CIP1) in cells induced by phorbol myristate acetate. J Cell Physiol. 2001; 187(1):124-135.
[6] Alcantara O, Kalidas M, Baltathakis I, Boldt DH. Expression of multiple genes regulating cell cycle and apoptosis in differentiating hematopoietic cells is dependent on iron. Exp Hematol. 2001; 29(9):1060-1069.
[7] Dong Fu, Richardson DR. Iron chelation and regulation of the cell cycle: 2 mechanisms of inhibitor p21CIP1/WAF1 by iron depletion post-transcriptional regulation of the universal cyclin-dependent kinase. Blood 2007; 110: 752–761.
[8] Kehrer JP. The Haber-Weiss reaction and mechanisms of toxicity. Toxicology 2000; 149(1):43-50.
[9] Shaw GC, Cope JJ, Li L, Corson K, Hersey C, Ackermann GE et al. Mitoferrin is essential for erythroid iron assimilation. Nature 2006; 440:96-100.
[10] Hentze MW, Muckenthaler MU, Andrews NC. Balancing acts: Molecular control of mammalian iron metabolism. Cell 2004; 117:285-297.
[11] Hentze MW, Kuhn LC. Molecular control of vertebrate iron metabolism: mRNA-based regulatory circuits operated by iron, nitric oxide, and oxidative stress. Proc Natl Acad Sci USA 1996; 93:8175-82.
[12] Napier I, Ponka P, Richardson DR. Iron trafficking in the mitochondrion: Novel pathways revealed by disease. Blood 2005; 105:1867-1874.
[13] Renton FJ, Jeitner TM. Cell cycle-dependent inhibition of the proliferation of human neural tumor cell lines by iron chelators. Biochem Pharmacol 1996; 51:1553-61.
[14] Gao J, Richardson DR. The potential of iron chelators of the pyridoxal isonicotinoyl hydrazone class as effective antiproliferative agents, IV: The mechanisms involved in inhibiting cell-cycle progression. Blood 2001; 98:842-50.
[15] Darnell G, Richardson DR. The potential of analogues of the pyridoxal isonicotinoyl hydrazone class as effective antiproliferative agents, III: the effect of the ligands on molecular targets involved in proliferation. Blood. 1999; 94:781-792.
[16] Kulp KS, Green SL, Vulliet PR. Iron deprivation inhibits cyclin-dependent kinase activity and decreases cyclin D/CDK4 protein levels in asynchronous MDA-MB-453 human breast cancer cells. Exp Cell Res 1996; 229:60-8.
[17] Nurtjahja-Tjendraputra E, Fu D, Phang JM, Richardson DR. Iron chelation regulates cyclin D1 expression via the proteasome: A link to iron deficiency-mediated growth suppression. Blood 2007; 109:4045-54.
[18] Wang G, Miskimins R, Miskimins WK. Regulation of p27(Kip1) by intracellular iron levels. Biometals. 2004; 17(1):15-24.
[19] Lee SH, Pyo CW, Hahm DH, Kim J, Choi SY. Iron-saturated lactoferrin stimulates cell cycle progression through PI3K/Akt pathway. Mol Cells. 2009; 28(1):37-42.
[20] Le NT, Richardson DR. The role of iron in cell cycle progression and the proliferation of neoplastic cells. Biochim Biophys Acta. 2002; 1603(1):31-46.
[21] Triantafyllou A, Liakos P, Tsakalof A, Chachami G, Paraskeva E, Molyvdas PA, Georgatsou E, Simos G, Bonanou S. The flavonoid quercetin induces hypoxia-

inducible factor-1alpha (HIF-1alpha) and inhibits cell proliferation by depleting intracellular iron. Free Radic Res. 2007; 41(3):342-56.
[22] Schauen M, Spitkovsky D, Schubert J, Fischer JH, Hayashi J, Wiesner RJ. Respiratory chain deficiency slows down cell-cycle progression via reduced ROS generation and is associated with a reduction of p21CIP1/WAF1. J Cell Physiol. 2006; 209(1):103-12.
[23] Ashizuka M, Fukuda T, Nakamura T, Shirasuna K, Iwai K, Izumi H et al. Novel translational control through an iron-responsive element by interaction of multifunctional protein YB-1 and IRP2. Mol Cell Biol. 2002; 22(18):6375-6383.
[24] Nevitt T. War-Fe-re: iron at the core of fungal virulence and host immunity. Biometals. 2011; 24(3):547-558.
[25] Berlutti F, Pantanella F, Natalizi T, Frioni A, Paesano R, Polimeni A, Valenti P. Antiviral properties of lactoferrin-a natural immunity molecule. Molecules. 2011; 16(8):6992-7018.
[26] Yen CC, Shen CJ, Hsu WH, Chang YH, Lin HT, Chen HL, Chen CM. Lactoferrin: an iron-binding antimicrobial protein against Escherichia coli infection. Biometals. 2011; 24(4):585-94.
[27] Kruzel ML, Actor JK, Radak Z, Bacsi A, Saavedra-Molina A, Boldogh I: Lactoferrin decreases LPS-induced mito-chondrial dysfunction in cultured cells and in animal endotoxemia model. Innate Immun. 2010; 16(2):67-79.
[28] Sandrini SM, Shergill R, Woodward J, Muralikuttan R, Haigh RD, Lyte M, Freestone PP. Elucidation of the mechanism by which catecholamine stress hormones liberate iron from the innate immune defense proteins transferrin and lactoferrin. J Bacteriol. 2010; 192(2):587-594.
[29] Actor JK, Hwang SA, Kruzel ML. Lactoferrin as a natural immune modulator. Curr Pharm Des. 2009; 15:1956-1973
[30] Legrand D, Mazurier J. A critical review of the roles of host lactoferrin in immunity. Biometals. 2010; 23(3):365-376.
[31] Hayworth JL, Kasper KJ, Leon-Ponte M, Herfst CA, Yue D, Brintnell WC et al: Attenuation of massive cytokine response to the staphylococcal enterotoxin B superantigen by the innate immunomodulatory protein lactofer-rin. Clin Exp Immunol. 2009; 157(1):60-70.
[32] Nielsen SM, Hansen GH, Danielsen EM. Lactoferrin targets T cells in the small intestine. J Gastroenterol. 2010; 45(11):1121-1128.
[33] Macedo MF, de Sousa M, Ned RM, Mascarenhas C, Andrews NC, Correia-Neves M. Transferrin is required for early T-cell differentiation. Immunology 2004; 112(4):543-549.
[34] Lucas JJ, Szepesi A, Domenico J, Takase K, Tordai A, Terada N, Gelfand EW. Effects of iron-depletion on cell cycle progression in normal human T lymphocytes: selective inhibition of the appearance of the cyclin A-associated component of the p33cdk2 kinase. Blood. 1995; 86(6):2268-2280.
[35] Gharagozloo M, Khoshdel Z, Amirghofran Z. The effect of an iron (III) chelator, silybin, on the proliferation and cell cycle of Jurkat cells: a comparison with desferrioxamine. Eur J Pharmacol. 2008; 589(1-3):1-7.
[36] Gupta A, Zhuo J, Zha J, Reddy S, Olp J, Pai A. Effect of different intravenous iron preparations on lymphocyte intracellular reactive oxygen species generation and subpopulation survival. BMC Nephrol. 2010; 11:16.
[37] Kang JL, Lee HS, Jung HJ, Kim HJ. Iron tetrakis (N-methyl-4'-pyridyl) porphyrinato inhibits proliferative activity of thymocytes by blocking activation of p38 mitogen-

activated protein kinase, nuclear factor-kappaB, and interleukin-2 secretion. Toxicol Appl Pharmacol. 2003; 191(2):147-155.
[38] Gira AK, Casper KA, Otto KB, Naik SM, Caughman SW, Swerlick RA. Induction of interferon regulatory factor 1 expression in human dermal endothelial cells by interferon-gamma and tumor necrosis factor-alpha is transcri-ptionally regulated and requires iron. J Invest Dermatol. 2003; 121(5):1191-1196.
[39] Johnson EE, Sandgren A, Cherayil BJ, Murray M, Wessling-Resnick M. Role of ferroportin in macrophage-mediated immunity. Infect Immun. 2010; 78(12):5099-5106.
[40] Pinto JP, Dias V, Zoller H, Porto G, Carmo H, Carvalho F, de Sousa M. Hepcidin messenger RNA expression in human lymphocytes. Immunology. 2010; 130(2):217-230.
[41] Corna G, Campana L, Pignatti E, Castiglioni A, Tagliafico E, Bosurgi L et al. Polarization dictates iron handling by inflammatory and alternatively activated macrophages. Haematologica 2010; 95(11):1814-1822.
[42] Appelberg R. Macrophage nutriprive antimicrobial mechanisms. J Leukoc Biol. 2006; 79(6):1117-1128.
[43] Kuvibidila SR, Porretta C. Differential effects of iron deficiency on the expression of CD80 and CD86 co-stimulatory receptors in mitogen-treated and untreated murine spleen cells. J Cell Biochem. 2002; 86(3):571-582.
[44] Yildirim K, Karatay S, Melikoglu MA, Gureser G, Ugur M, Senel K. Associations between acute phase reactant levels and disease activity score (DAS28) in patients with rheumatoid arthritis. *Ann Clin Lab Sci* 2004; 34:423-426.
[45] Lim MK, Lee CK, Ju YS, Cho YS, Lee MS, Yoo B, Moon HB. Serum ferritin as a serological marker of activity in systemic lupus erythematosus. *Rheumatol Int* 2001; 20:89-93.
[46] Sfagos C, Makis AC, Chaidos A, Hatzimichael EC, Dalamaga A, Kosma K, Bourantas KL. Serum ferritin, transferrin and soluble transferring receptor levels in multiple sclerosis patients. *Mult Sclerosis* 2005; 11:272-275.
[47] Izawa T, Yamate J, Franklin RJ, Kuwamura M.Abnormal iron accumulation is involved in the pathogenesis of the demyelinating dmy rat but not in the hypomyelinating mv rat. Brain Res. 2010; 1349:105-114.
[48] Hulet SW, Powers S, Connor JR. Distribution of transferring and ferritin binding in normal and multiple sclerotic human brains. J Neurol Sci 1999; 165:48-55.
[49] Levine SM, Maiti S, Emerson MR, Pedchenko TV. Apoferritin attenuates experimental allergic encephalomyelitis in SJL mice. Dev Neurosci 2002; 24:177-183.
[50] Sakata S, Nagai K, Maekawa H, Kimata Y, Komaki T, Nakamura S, Miura K. Serum ferritin concentration in subacute thyroiditis. Metabolism 1991; 40:683-688.
[51] Tran TN, Eubanks SK, Schaffer KJ, Zhou CY, Linder MC. Secretion of ferritin by rat hepatoma cells and its regulation by inflammatory cytokines and iron. Blood 1997; 90(12): 4979-4986.
[52] Fervenza FC, Croatt AJ, Bittar CM, Rosenthal DW, Lager DJ, Leung N et al. Induction of heme oxygenase-1 and ferritin in the kidney in warm antibody hemolytic anemia. Am J Kidney Dis. 2008; 52(5):972-977.
[53] Blancou P, Tardif V, Simon T, Rémy S, Carreño L, Kalergis A, Anegon I. Immunoregulatory properties of heme oxygenase-1. Methods Mol Biol. 2011; 677:247-268.

[54] Habel ME, Lemieux R, Jung D. Habel M, Lemieux R, Jung D. Iron specific growth inhibition of Burkitt's lymphoma cells in vitro, associated with a decrease in translocated c-myc expression. J Cell Physiol. 2005; 203(1):277-285.

[55] Kakhlon O, Gruenbaum Y, Cabantchik ZI. Repression of ferritin expression increases the labile iron pool, oxidative stress, and short-term growth of human erythroleukemia cells. Blood 2001; 97(9):2863-2871.

[56] Kadner R. Regulation by Iron: RNA rules the rust. J Bacteriol 2005; 187(20): 6870-6873

[57] Stauff DL, Skaar EP. The heme sensor system (HssRS) of Staphylococcus Aureus. Contrib Microbiol 2009;16: 210-135.

[58] Argandoña M, Nieto JJ, Iglesias-Guerra F, Calderón MI, García-Estepa R, Vargas C. Interplay between iron homeostasis and the osmotic stress response in the halophilic bacterium Chromohalobacter salexigens. Appl Environ Microbiol. 2010; 76(11):3575-3589.

[59] Neiland JB. Siderophores: structure and function of microbial iron transport compounds. J Biol Chem 1995; 270: 26723-26726.

[60] Ferguson AD, Chakraborty R, Smith BS, Esser L, van der Helm D, Deisenhofer J. Structural basis of gating by the outer membrane transporter FecA. Science 2002;295:1715-1719

[61] Ferguson A, Deisenhofer J. Metal import through microbial membrane.Cell 2004; 116: 15-24.

[62] Krewulak KD, Vogel HJ. Structural biology of bacterial iron uptake. Biochim Biophys Acta. 2008 ;1778(9):1781-804.

[63] Clarke TE, Ku SY, Dougan DR, Vogel HJ, Tari LW. The structure of the ferric siderophore binding protein FhuD complexed with gallichrome. Nat Struct Biol 2000; 7: 287-291.

[64] Goetz M, Bubert A, Wang G, Chico-Calero I, Vazquez-Boland JA, Beck M et al. Microinjection and growth of bacteria in the cytosol of mammalian host cells. Proc Natl Acad Sci U S A. 2001; 98(21):12221-12226.

[65] Borreqaard N, Cowland JB. Neutrophil gelatinase-associated lipocalin, a siderophore-binding eukaryotic protein. Biometals 2006; 19:211-215.

[66] Flo TH, Smith KD, Sato S, Rodriguez DJ, Holmes MA, Strong RK, Akira S, Aderem A. Lipocalin 2 mediates an innate immune response to bacterial infection by sequestrating iron. Nature 2004; 432:917-921.

[67] Fischbach MA, Lin H, Liu DR, Walsh CT. How pathogenic bacteria evade mammalian sabotage in the battle for iron. Nat Chem Biol 2006;2: 132-138.

[68] Müller SI, Valdebenito M, Hantke K. Salmochelin, the long-overlooked catecholate siderophore of Salmonella. Biometals 2009; 22(4):691-695.

[69] Wandersman C, Delepelaire P. Bacterial iron sources: from siderophores to hemophores. Annu Rev Microbiol 2004; 58:611-647.

[70] Perkins-Balding D, Ratliff-Griffin M, and Stojiljkovic I. Iron Transport Systems in *Neisseria meningitides.* Microbiol Mol Biol Rev 2004; 68(1):154-171.

[71] Nielsen MJ, Møller HJ, Moestrup SK. Hemoglobin and heme scavenger receptors. Antioxid Redox Signal. 2010; 12(2):261-273.

[72] Cescau S, Cwerman H, Létoffé S, Delepelaire P, Wandersman C, Biville F. Heme acquisition by hemophores. Biometals 2007; 20:603-613.

[73] Létoffé S, Redeker V, Wandersman C. Isolation and characterization of an extracellular haem-binding protein from Pseudomonas aeruginosa that shares function and sequence similarities with the Serratia marcescens HasA haemophore. Mol Microbiol. 1998; 28(6):1223-1234.

[74] Gray-Owen SD, Schryvers AB. Bacterial transferrin and lactoferrin receptors. Trends Microbiol 1996; 4:185-191.

[75] Baysse C, De Vos D, Naudet Y, Vandermonde A, Ochsner U, Meyer JM et al. Vanadium interferes with siderophore-mediated iron uptake in Pseudomonas aeruginosa. Microbiology 2000; 146 (Pt 10):2425-2434.

[76] Mossialos D, Meyer JM, Budzikiewicz H, Wolff U, Koedam N, Baysse C, Anjaiah V, Cornelis P. Quinolobactin, a new siderophore of Pseudomonas fluorescens ATCC 17400, the production of which is repressed by the cognate pyoverdine. Appl Environ Microbiol. 2000; 66(2):487-492.

[77] Huston WM, Jennings MP, McEwan AG. The multicopper oxidase of Pseudomonas aeruginosa is a ferroxidase with a central role in iron acquisition. Mol Microbiol. 2002; 45(6):1741-1750.

[78] Balado M, Osorio CR, Lemos ML. Biosynthetic and regulatory elements involved in the production of the siderophore vanchrobactin in Vibrio anguillarum. Microbiology 2008; 154(Pt 5): 1400-1413.

[79] Bellmann-Weiler R, Martinz V, Kurz K, Engl S, Feistritzer C, Fuchs D et al. Divergent modulation of Chlamydia pneumoniae infection cycle in human monocytic and endothelial cells by iron, tryptophan availability and interferon gamma. Immunobiology 2010; 215(9-10):842-848.

[80] Mair SM, Nairz M, Bellmann-Weiler R, Muehlbacher T, Schroll A, Theurl I et al. Nifedipine affects the course of Salmonella enterica serovar Typhimurium infection by modulating macrophage iron homeostasis. J Infect Dis. 2011; 204(5):685-694.

[81] López-Goñi I, Moriyón I. Production of 2,3-dihydroxybenzoic acid by *Brucella* species. Curr. Microbiol 1995; 31:291-293.

[82] González-Carreró MI, Sangari FJ, Agüero J, García Lobo JM. *Brucella abortus* 2308 produces *brucebactin*, a highly efficient catecholic siderophore. Microbiology 2002; 148:353-360.

[83] Halling SM, Peterson-Burch BD, Bricker BJ, Zuerner RL, Zing Z, Li LL, Kapur V, Alt DP, Olsen SC. Completion of the gene sequence of *Brucella abortus* and comparison to the highly similar genomes of *Brucella melitensis* and *Brucella suis*. J Bacteriol 2005; 187:2715-2726.

[84] Mills M, Payne SM. Identification of *shuA*, the gene encoding the heme receptor of *Shigella dysenteriae*, and analysis of invasion and intracellular multiplication of a *shuA* mutant. Infect Immun 1997; 65:5358-5363.

[85] Paulley JT, Anderson ES, Martin Roop II R. *Brucella abortus* requires the heme transporter BhuA for maintenance of chronic infection in BALB/c Mice Infect Immun 2007; 75:5248-5254.

[86] Hentze MW, Muckenthaler MU, AndrewsNC. Balancing acts: molecular control of mammalian iron metabolism. Cell 2004; 117:285-297.

[87] Nemeth E, Tuttle MS, Powelson J, Vaughn MB, Donovan A, Ward DM, Ganz T, Kaplan J. Hepsidin regulates cellular iron efflux by binding to ferroportin and inducing its internalisation. Science 2004; 306:2090-2093.

[88] Appelberg R. Macrophage nutriprive antimicrobial mechanisms. J Leukoc Biol 2006; 79:1117-1128.

[89] Ratledge C. Iron, mycobacteria and tuberculosis.Tuberculosis 2004; 84:110-130.

[90] Rodriguez GM, Voskuil MI, Gold B, Schoolnik GK, Smith I. *ideR*, an essential gene in *Mycobacterium tuberculosis*: role of IdeR in iron-dependent gene expression, iron metabolism, and oxidative stress response. *Infect Immun 2002;* 70:3371-3381.

[91] Ludwiczek S, Aigner E, Theuri I, Weiss G. Cytokine-mediated regulation of iron transport in human monocyte cells. Blood 2003; 101:4148-4154.
[92] Gomes MS, Boelaert JR, Appelberg R. Role of iron in experimental Mycobacterium avium infection. J Clin Virol. 2001; 20:117-122.
[93] Kahnert A, Seiler P, Sein M, et al. Alternativeactivation deprives macrophages of a coordinated defense program to *Mycobacterium tuberculosis*. Eur J Immunol 2006; 36:631-647.
[94] Sow FB, Florence WC, Satoskar AR, Schlesinger LS, Zwilling BS, Lafuse WP. Expression and localization of hepcidin in macrophages: a role in host defense against tuberculosis. J Leukoc Biol 2007; 82:934-945.
[95] Sow FB, Alvarez GR, Gross RP, Satoskar AR, Schlesinger LS, Zwilling BS, Lafuse WP. Role of STAT1, NF-kappaB and C/EBPbeta in the macrophage transcriptional regulation of hepsidin by mycobacterial infection and IFN-gamma. J Leukoc Biol 2009;86: 1247-1258.
[96] Weinberg ED. Iron availability and infection. Biochim Biophys Acta. 2009; 1790(7):600-605.
[97] Andersson Y, Lindquist S, Lagerqvist C, Hernell O. Lactoferrin is responsible for the fungistatic effect of human milk. Early Hum Dev 2000; 59: 95-105.
[98] Bullen JJ, Griffiths E. Iron binding proteins and host defence. In: Bullen JJ, Griffiths E, eds. 'Iron and infection.' Molecular, physiological and clinical aspects, 2nd ed. Chichester: Wiley, 1999; 327-368.
[99] Halliwell B, Aruoma OI, Mufti G, Bomford A. Bleomycin detectable iron in serum from leukaemic patients before and after chemotherapy. FEBS Lett 1988; 241: 202–204.
[100] Alexander J, Limaye AP, Ko CW, Bronner MP, Kowdley KV. Association of hepatic iron overload with invasive fungal infection in liver transplant recipients. Liver Transpl 2006; 12: 1799–1804.
[101] de Locht M, Boelaert JR, Schneider YJ. Iron uptake from ferrioxamine and from ferrirhizoferrin by germinating spores of Rhizopus microsporus. Biochem Pharmacol 1994; 47: 1843–1850.
[102] Nyilasi I, Papp T, Tako´ M, Nagy E, Vagvolgyi C. Iron gathering of opportunistic pathogenic fungi. A mini review. Acta Microbiol Immunol Hung 2005; 52: 185–197.
[103] Ramanan N, Wang Y. A high-affinity iron permease essential for Candida albicans virulence. Science 2000; 288: 1062–1064.
[104] Hsu PC, Yang CY, Lan CY. Candida albicans Hap43 is a repressor induced under low-iron conditions and is essential for iron-responsive transcriptional regulation and virulence. Eukaryot Cell. 2011; 10(2):207-225.
[105] Nevitt T, Thiele DJ. Host iron withholding demands siderophore utilization for Candida glabrata to survive macrophage killing. PLoS Pathog. 2011; 7(3):e1001322.
[106] Tangen KL, Jung WH, Sham AP, Lian T, Kronstad JW. The iron- and cAMP-regulated gene SIT1 influences ferrioxamine B utilization, melanization and cell wall structure in C. neoformans. Microbiology 2007; 153(Pt 1): 29–41.
[107] Hissen AHT, Wan AN, Warwas ML, Pinto LJ, Moore MM. The Aspergillus fumigatus siderophore biosynthetic gene sidA, encoding L-ornithine N5-oxygenase, is required for virulence. Infect Immun 2005; 73:5493–5503.
[108] Hissen AH, Chow JM, Pinto LJ, Moore MM. Survival of Aspergillus fumigatus in serum involves removal of iron from transferrin: the role of siderophores. Infect Immun 2004; 72:1402–1408.

[109] Schrett M, Beckmann N, Varga J, Heinekamp T, Jacobsen ID, Jöchl C et al. HapX-mediated adaption to iron starvation is crucial for virulence of Aspergillus fumigatus. PLoS Pathog. 2010 Sep 30;6(9):e1001124.
[110] Schrett M, Bignell E, Kragl C et al. Distinct roles for intra- and extracellular siderophores during Aspergillus fumigatus infection. PLoS Pathog 2007; 3: 1195–1207.
[111] Timmerman MM, Woods JP. Potential role for extracellular glutathione-dependent ferric reductase in utilization of environmental and host ferric compounds by Histoplasma capsulatum. Infect Immun 2001; 69: 7671–7678.
[112] Nyhus K, Wilborn AT, Jacobson ES. Ferric iron reduction by Cryptococcus neoformans. Infect Immun 1997; 65: 434–438.
[113] Anand VK, Alemar G, Griswold JA Jr. Intracranial complications of mucormycosis: an experimental model and clinical review. Laryngoscope 1992; 102: 656-662.
[114] Petrikkos G, Skiada A, Sambatakou H et al. Mucormycosis: ten-year experience at a tertiary-care center in Greece. Eur J Clin Microbiol Infect Dis 2003; 22: 753-756.
[115] Maertens J, Demuynck H, Verbeken EK et al. Mucormycosis in allogeneic bone marrow transplant recipients: report of five cases and review of the role of iron overload in the pathogenesis. Bone Marrow Transplant 1999; 24: 307-312.
[116] Spellberg B, Edwards JJ, Ibrahim A. Novel perspectives on mucormycosis: pathophysiology, presentation, and management. Clin Microbiol Rev 2005; 18: 556-569.
[117] Symeonidis A. The role of iron and iron chelators in zygomycosis. Clin Microbiol Infect. 2009; 15(s5): 26-32.
[118] Artis WM, Fountain JA, Delcher HK, Jones HE. A mechanism of susceptibility to mucormycosis in diabetic ketoacidosis: transferrin and iron availability. Diabetes 1982; 31: 1109-1114.
[119] McNab AA, McKelvie P. Iron overload is a risk factor for zygomycosis. Arch Ophthalmol 1997; 115: 919-921.
[120] Kubota N, Miyazawa K, Shoji N et al. A massive intraventricular thrombosis by disseminated mucormycosis in a patient with myelodysplastic syndrome during deferoxamine therapy. Haematologica 2003; 88: EIM13.
[121] Miyata Y, Kajiguchi T, Saito M, Takeyama H. Development of arterial thrombus of Mucorales hyphae during deferoxamine therapy in a patient with aplastic anemia in transformation to myelodysplastic syndrome [in Japanese]. Rinsho Ketsueki 2000; 41: 129-134.
[122] Fu Y, Lee H, Collins M et al. Cloning and functional characterization of the Rhiz. oryzae high affinity iron permease (rFTR1) gene. FEMS Microbiol Lett 2004; 235: 169-176.
[123] Nyilasi I, Papp T, Csernetics A, Krizsa´n K, Nagy E, Va´gvlgyi C. High-affinity iron permease (FTR1) gene sequence-based molecular identification of clinically important Zygomycetes. Clin Microbiol Infect 2008; 14: 393-397.
[124] Ibrahim AS, Gebremariam T, Lin L, Luo G, Husseiny MI, Skory CD et al. The high affinity iron permease is a key virulence factor required for Rhizopus oryzae pathogenesis. Mol Microbiol. 2010; 77(3):587-604.
[125] Boelaert JR, Fenves AZ, Coburn JW. Deferoxamine therapy and mucormycosis in dialysis patients: report of an international registry. Am J Kidney Dis 1991; 18: 660–667.

[126] Kaneko T, Abe F, Ito M, Hotchi M, Yamada K, Okada Y. Intestinal mucormycosis in a hemodialysis patient treated with desferrioxamine. Acta Pathol Jpn 1991; 41: 561-566
[127] Boelaert JR, de Locht M, van Cutsem J et al. Mucormycosis during deferoxamine therapy is a siderophore mediated infection: in-vitro and in-vivo animal studies. J Clin Invest 1993; 91: 1979-1986.
[128] Verdonck AK, Boelaert JR, Gordts BZ, Van Landuyt HW. Effect of ferrioxamine on the growth of Rhizopus. Mycoses 1993; 36: 9-12.
[129] Boelaert JR, Van Cutsem J, de Locht M, Schneider YJ, Crichton RR. Deferoxamine augments growth and pathogenicity of Rhizopus, while hydroxypyridinone chelators have no effect. Kidney Int 1994; 45: 667-671.
[130] Verpooten GA, D'Haese PC, Boelaert JR, Becaus I, Lamberts LV, De Broe ME. Pharmacokinetics of aluminoxamine and ferrioxamine and dose finding of deferrioxamine in haemodialysis patients. Nephrol Dial Transplant 1992; 7: 931-938.
[131] Neufeld EJ. Oral chelators deferasirox and deferiprone for transfusional iron overload in thalassemia major: new data, new questions. Blood 2006; 107: 3436-3441.
[132] Symeonidis A. The role of iron and iron chelators in zygomycosis. Clin Microbiol Infect. 2009; 15(s5): 26-32.
[133] Ibrahim AS, Edwards JE Jr, Fu Y, Spellberg B. Deferiprone iron chelation as a novel therapy for experimental mucormycosis. J Antimicrob Chemother 2006; 58: 1070-1073.
[134] Ibrahim AS, Gebermariam T, Fu Y et al. The iron chelator deferasirox protects mice from mucormycosis through iron starvation. J Clin Invest 2007; 117: 2649-2657.
[135] Ibrahim AS, Gebremariam T, French SW, Edwards JE Jr, Spellberg B. The iron chelator deferasirox enhances liposomal amphotericin B efficacy in treating murine invasive pulmonary aspergillosis. J Antimicrob Chemother. 2010; 65(2):289-292.
[136] Pope CD, O'Connell W, Cianciotto NP. Legionella pneumophila mutants, that are defective for iron acquisition and assimilation and intracellular infection. Infect Immun. 1996; 64(2):629-636.
[137] Peracino B, Balest A, Bozzaro S. Phosphoinositides differentially regulate bacterial uptake and Nramp1-induced resistance to Legionella infection in Dictyostelium. J Cell Sci. 2010; 123(Pt 23): 4039-4051.
[138] Pollok RC, Farthing MJ, Bajaj-Elliott M, Sanderson IR, McDonald V. Interferon-γ induces enterocyte resistance against infection by the intracellular pathogen Cryptosporidium parvum. Gastroenterology 2001; 120(1):99-107.
[139] Dziadek B, Dytnerska-Dzitko K, Długońska H. The modulation of transferrin receptors level on mouse macropha-ges and fibroblasts by Toxoplasma gondii. Pol J Microbiol. 2004; 53 Suppl:75-80.
[140] Halonen SK, Weiss LM. Investigation into the mechanism of gamma interferon-mediated inhibition of Toxoplasma gondii in murine astrocytes. Infect Immun. 2000; 68(6):3426-3430.
[141] Ye B, Zheng YQ, Wu WH, Zhang J. Iron chelator daphnetin against Pneumocystis carinii in vitro. Chin Med J (Engl). 2004; 117(11):1704-1708.
[142] Das NK, Biswas S, Solanki S, Mukhopadhyay CK. Leishmania donovani depletes labile iron pool to exploit iron uptake capacity of macrophage for its intracellular growth. Cell Microbiol. 2009; 11(1):83-94.

[143] Bisti S, Konidou G, Papageorgiou F, Milon G, Boelaert JR, Soteriadou K. The outcome of Leishmania major expe-rimental infection in BALB/c mice can be modulated by exogenously delivered iron. Eur J Immunol. 2000; 30(12):3732-3740.
[144] Plewes KA, Barr SD, Gedamu L. Iron superoxide dismutases targeted to the glycosomes of Leishmania chagasi are important for survival. Infect Immun. 2003; 71(10):5910-5920.
[145] Anstead GM, Chandrasekar B, Zhao W, Yang J, Perez L, Melby PC. Malnutrition alters the innate immune response and increases early visceralization following Leishmania donovani infection. Infect Immun 2001; 69(8):4709-4718.
[146] Malafaia G, Marcon Lde N, Pereira Lde F, Pedrosa ML, Rezende SA. Leishmania chagasi: effect of the iron deficiency on the infection in BALB/c mice. Exp Parasitol. 2011; 127(3):719-723.
[147] Huynh C, Sacks DL, Andrews NW. A Leishmania amazonensis ZIP family iron transporter is essential for parasite replication within macrophage phagolysosomes. J Exp Med. 2006; 203(10):2363-2375.
[148] Alderete JF, Nguyen J, Mundodi V, Lehker MW. Heme-iron increases levels of AP65-mediated adherence by Trichomonas vaginalis. Microb Pathog. 2004; 36(5):263-271.
[149] Torres-Romero JC, Arroyo R. Responsiveness of Trichomonas vaginalis to iron concentrations: evidence for a post-transcriptional iron regulation by an IRE/IRP-like system. Infect Genet Evol. 2009; 9(6):1065-1074.
[150] Mahmoud MS. Effect of the iron chelator deferoxamine on Trichomonas vaginalis in vitro. J Egypt Soc Parasitol. 2002; 32(3):691-704.
[151] Tachezy J, Kulda J, Bahníková I, Suchan P, Rázga J, Schrével J. Tritrichomonas foetus: iron acquisition from lactoferrin and transferrin. Exp Parasitol. 1996; 83(2):216-228.
[152] Sutak R, Chamot C, Tachezy J, Camadro JM, Lesuisse E. Siderophore and haem iron use by Tritrichomonas foetus. Microbiology. 2004; 150(Pt 12):3979-3987.
[153] Melo-Braga MB, da Rocha-Azevedo B, Silva-Filho FC. Tritrichomonas foetus: the role played by iron during parasite interaction with epithelial cells. Exp Parasitol. 2003; 105(2):111-120.
[154] Kulda J, Poislová M, Suchan P, Tachezy J. Iron enhancement of experimental infection of mice by Tritrichomonas foetus. Parasitol Res. 1999; 85(8-9):692-699.
[155] Weinberg ED, Moon J. Malaria and iron: history and review. Drug Metab Rev. 2009; 41(4):644-662.
[156] de Mast Q, Syafruddin D, Keijmel S, Riekerink TO, Deky O, Asih PB et al. Increased serum hepcidin and alterations in blood iron parameters associated with asymptomatic P.falciparum and P.vivax malaria. Haematologica 2010; 95(7):1068-1074.
[157] Cercamondi CI, Egli IM, Ahouandjinou E, Dossa R, Zeder C, Salami L et al. Afebrile Plasmodium falciparum parasitemia decreases absorption of fortification iron but does not affect systemic iron utilization: a double stable-isotope study in young Beninese women. Am J Clin Nutr. 2010; 92(6):1385-1392.
[158] Ndyomugyenyi R, Kabatereine N, Olsen A, Magnussen P. Malaria and hookworm infections in relation to hemoglobin and serum ferritin levels in pregnancy in Masindi district, western Uganda. Trans R Soc Trop Med Hyg. 2008; 102(2):130-136.
[159] Krugliak M, Zhang J, Ginsburg H. Intraerythrocytic Plasmodium falciparum utilizes only a fraction of the amino acids derived from the digestion of host cell cytosol for the biosynthesis of its proteins. Mol Biochem Parasitol. 2002; 119(2):249-256.
[160] Schwartz E, Samuni A, Friedman I, Hempelmann E, Golenser J. The role of superoxide dismutation in malaria parasites. Inflammation 1999; 23(4):361-370.

[161] Golenser J, Peled-Kamar M, Schwartz E, Friedman I, Groner Y, Pollack Y. Transgenic mice with elevated level of CuZnSOD are highly susceptible to malaria infection. Free Radic Biol Med. 1998; 24(9):1504-1510.

[162] Goma J, Renia L, Miltgen F, Mazier D. Effects of iron deficiency on the hepatic development of Plasmodium yoelii. Parasite 1995; 2(4):351-356.

[163] Koka S, Föller M, Lamprecht G, Boini KM, Lang C, Huber SM, Lang F. Iron deficiency influences the course of malaria in Plasmodium berghei infected mice. Biochem Biophys Res Commun. 2007; 357(3):608-614.

[164] Matsuzaki-Moriya C, Tu L, Ishida H, Imai T, Suzue K, Hirai M et al. A critical role for phagocytosis in resistance to malaria in iron-deficient mice. Eur J Immunol. 2011; 41(5):1365-1375.

[165] Gerrits H, Mussmann R, Bitter W, Kieft R, Borst P. The physiological significance of transferrin receptor variations in Trypanosoma brucei. Mol Biochem Parasitol. 2002; 119(2):237-247.

[166] Weiss G, Goodnough LT. Anaemia of chronic disease. N Eng J Med 2005; 352:1011-1023.

[167] Stijlemans B, Vankrunkelsven A, Brys L, Magez S, De Baetselier P. Role of iron homeostasis in trypanosomiasis-associated anemia. Immunobiology 2008; 213(9-10):823-835.

[168] López-Soto F, León-Sicairos N, Reyes-López M, Serrano-Luna J, Ordaz-Pichardo C, Piña-Vázquez C, Ortiz-Estrada G, de la Garza M. Use and endocytosis of iron-containing proteins by Entamoeba histolytica trophozoites. Infect Genet Evol. 2009; 9(6):1038-1050.

[169] Bradley SG, Toney DM, Zhang Y, Marciano-Cabral F. Dependence of growth, metabolic expression, and pathogenicity of Naegleria fowleri on exogenous porphyrins. J Parasitol. 1996; 82(5):763-768.

[170] Khalifa SA, Imai E, Kobayashi S, Haghighi A, Hayakawa E, Takeuchi T. Growth-promoting effect on iron-sulfur proteins on axenic cultures of Entamoeba dispar. Parasite 2006; 13(1):51-58.

[171] Held MR, Bungiro RD, Harrison LM, Hamza I, Cappello M. Dietary iron content mediates hookworm pathogenesis in vivo. Infect Immun. 2006; 74(1):289-295.

[172] Jones MK, McManus DP, Sivadorai P, Glanfield A, Moertel L, Belli SI, Gobert GN. Tracking the fate of iron in early development of human blood flukes. Int J Biochem Cell Biol. 2007; 39(9):1646-1658.

[173] Mabey DCW, Brown A, Greenwood BM. *Plasmodium falciparum* malaria and *Salmonella* infections in Gambian children. J Infect Dis 1987; 155:1319-1321.

[174] Bullen JJ, Leigh LC, Rogers HJ. The effect of iron compounds on the virulence of *Escherichia coli* for guinea-pigs. Immunology 1986; 15:581-588.

[175] Taylor RW, Manganaro L, O'Brien J, Trottier SJ, Parkar N, Veremakis C. Impact of allogenic packed red blood cell transfusions on nosocomial infection rates in the critically ill patient. Crit Care Med 2002; 30:2249-2254.

[176] Taylor RW, O'Brien J, Trottier SJ, Manganaro L, Cytron M, Lesko MF et al. Red blood cell transfusions and nosocomial infections in critically ill patients Crit Care Med. 2006;34(9): 2302-2308.

[177] Shorr, AF, Duh MS, Kelly KM, Kolief MH. Red blood cell transfusion and ventillator-associated pneumonia, a potential link? Crit Care Med 2004; 32:666-674.

[178] Agarwal N, Murphy JG, Cayten CG Stahl WM. Blood transfusion increases the risk of infection after trauma. Arch Surg 1993; 128:171-176.

[179] Griffiths E, Cortes A, Gilbert N, Stevenson P, MacDonald S, Pepper D. Haemoglobin-based blood substitutes and sepsis. Lancet 1995; 345:158-160.
[180] Chart H, Griffiths E. The availability of iron and the growth of *Vibrio vulnificus* in sera from patients with haemochromatosis. FEMS Microbiol Lett 1985; 26:227-231
[181] Vadillo M, Corbella X, Pac V, Fernandez-Viladrich P, Pujol R. Multiple liver abscesses due to *Yersinia enterocolitica* discloses primary hemo chromatosis: three case reports and review. Clin Infect Dis 1994; 18: 938-941.
[182] Boelaert JR, van Landuyt HW, Valcke YJ, et al. The role of iron overload in *Yersinia enterocolitica* and *Yersinia pseudotuberculosis* bacteremia in hemodialysis patients. J Infect Dis 1987; 156:384-387.
[183] Leclercq A, Martin L, Vergnes ML, Ounnoughene N, Laran JF, GiraudP, Carniel E. Fatal Yersinia enterocolitica biotype 4 serovar O:3 sepsis after red blood cell transfusion. Transfusion 2005; 45:814-818.
[184] Beresford AM. Transfusion reaction due to Yersinia enterocolitica and review of other reported cases. Pathology 1995; 27(2):133-135.
[185] Clermont O, Bonacorsi S, Bingen E. The Yersinia high-pathogenicity island is highly predominant in virulence-associated phylogenetic groups of Escherichia coli. FEMS Microbiol Lett. 2001; 196:153-157.
[186] Eraklis AJ, Brammer SR, Diamond LK, Gross RE. Hazard of overwhelming infection after splenectomy in childhood. N Engl J Med 1967; 267:1225-1229.
[187] Bishard N, Omari H, Lavi I Raz R. Risk of infection and death among post-splenectomy patients. J Infect 2001; 43(3):182-186.
[188] Pootrakul P, Rugkiatsakul R, Wasi P. Increased transferrin iron saturation in splenectomized thalassaemic patients. Br J Haematol. 1980; 46(1):143-145.
[189] de White T. The role of iron in patients after bone marrow transplantation. Blood Rev 2008; 22(suppl2): S22-28.
[190] Singh N, Wannstedt C, Keyes L, Mayher D, Tickerhoof L, Akoad M et al. Hepatic iron content and the risk of Staphylococcus aureus bacteremia in liver transplant recipients. Prog Transplant 2007; 17(4):332-336.
[191] Berlutti F, Morea C, Battistoni A, Sarli S, Cipriani P, Superti F et al. Iron availability influences aggregation, biofilm, adhesion and invasion of Pseudomonas aeruginosa and Burkholderia cenocepacia. Int J Immunopathol Pharmacol 2005; 18(4): 661-670.
[192] Bullen JJ, Spalding PB, Ward CG, Rogers HJ. The role of Eh, pH, and iron in the bactericidal power of human plasma. FEMS Microbiol Lett 1992; 94: 47-52.
[193] Weiss G. Modification of iron regulation by the inflammatory response. Best Pract Res Clin Haematol 2005;18: 183-201.
[194] Reed C, Ibrahim A, Edwards JE Jr, Walot I, Spellberg B. Deferasirox, an iron-chelating agent, as salvage therapy for rhinocerebral mucormycosis. Antimicrob Agents Chemother 2006; 50: 3968-3969.
[195] Ting JY, Chan SY, Lung DC, Ho AC, Chiang AK, Ha SY et al. Intra-abdominal Rhizopus microsporus infection successfully treated by combined aggressive surgical, antifungal, and iron chelating therapy. J Pediatr Hematol Oncol. 2010; 32(6):e238-240.
[196] Soummer A, Mathonnet A, Scatton O et al. Failure of deferasirox, an iron chelator agent, combined with antifungals in a case of severe zygomycosis. Antimicrob Agents Chemother 2008; 52:1585-1586.
[197] Spellberg B, Ibrahim AS, Chin-Hong PV, Kontoyiannis DP, Morris MI, Perfect JR et al. The Deferasirox-AmBisome Therapy for Mucormycosis (DEFEAT Mucor) study: a

randomized, double-blinded, placebo-controlled trial. J Antimicrob Chemother. 2011 (in press).
[198] Clarkson AB Jr, Turkel-Parrella D, Williams JH, Chen LC, Gordon T, Merali S. Action of deferoxamine against Pneumocystis carinii. Antimicrob Agents Chemother. 2001; 45(12):3560-3565.
[199] Pattanapanyasat K, Thaithong S, Kyle DE, Udomsangpetch R, Yongvanitchit K, Hider RC, Webster HK. Flow cytometric assessment of hydroxypyridinone iron chelators on in vitro growth of drug-resistant malaria. Cytometry 1997; 27(1):84-91.
[200] Goudeau C, Loyevsky M, Kassim OO, Gordeuk VR, Nick H. Assessment of antimalarial effect of ICL670A on in vitro cultures of Plasmodium falciparum. Br J Haematol. 2001; 115(4):918-923.
[201] Loyevsky M, Sacci JB Jr, Boehme P, Weglicki W, John C, Gordeuk VR. Plasmodium falciparum and Plasmodium yoelii: effect of the iron chelation prodrug dexrazoxane on in vitro cultures. Exp Parasitol. 1999; 91(2):105-114.
[202] Walcourt A, Loyevsky M, Lovejoy DB, Gordeuk VR, Richardson DR. Novel aroylhydrazone and thiosemicarbazone iron chelators with anti-malarial activity against chloroquine-resistant and -sensitive parasites. Int J Biochem Cell Biol. 2004; 36(3):401-407.
[203] Rotheneder A, Fritsche G, Heinisch L, Möllmann U, Heggemann S, Larcher C, Weiss G. Effects of synthetic siderophores on proliferation of Plasmodium falciparum in infected human erythrocytes. Antimicrob Agents Chemother. 2002; 46(6):2010-2013.
[204] Loyevsky M, John C, Dickens B, Hu V, Miller JH, Gordeuk VR. Chelation of iron within the erythrocytic Pl. falciparum parasite by iron chelators. Mol Biochem Parasitol. 1999; 101(1-2):43-59.
[205] Chevion M, Chuang L, Golenser J. Effects of zinc-desferrioxamine on Plasmodium falciparum in culture. Antimicrob Agents Chemother. 1995; 39(8):1902-1905.
[206] Rodrigues RR, Lane JE, Carter CE, Bogitsh BJ, Singh PK, Zimmerman LJ et al. Chelating agent inhibition of Trypanosoma cruzi epimastigotes in vitro. J Inorg Biochem. 1995; 60(4):277-288.
[207] Merschjohann K, Steverding D. In vitro growth inhibition of bloodstream forms of Trypanosoma brucei and Trypanosoma congolense by iron chelators. Kinetoplastid Biol Dis. 2006; 5:3.
[208] Breidbach T, Scory S, Krauth-Siegel RL, Steverding D. Growth inhibition of bloodstream forms of Trypanosoma brucei by the iron chelator deferoxamine. Int J Parasitol. 2002; 32(4):473-479.
[209] Deharo E, Loyevsky M, John C, Balanza E, Ruiz G, Muñoz V, Gordeuk VR. Aminothiol multidentate chelators against Chagas disease. Exp Parasitol. 2000; 94(3):198-200.

Part 4

Molecular Epidemiology and Mitigation Strategy

17

Diphtheria Disease and Genes Involved in Formation of Diphthamide, Key Effector of the Diphtheria Toxin

Shanow Uthman[1], Shihui Liu[2], Flaviano Giorgini[1], Michael J. R. Stark[3], Michael Costanzo[4] and Raffael Schaffrath[1,5]
[1]*Department of Genetics, University of Leicester, Leicester,*
[2]*Laboratory of Bacterial Diseases, NIAID, NIH, Bethesda, MD,*
[3]*Wellcome Trust Centre for Gene Regulation & Expression, University of Dundee,*
[4]*The Donnelly Centre, University of Toronto, Toronto, Ontario,*
[5]*Institut für Biologie, Mikrobiologie, Universität Kassel, Kassel,*
[1]*UK*
[2]*USA*
[3]*Scotland*
[4]*Canada*
[5]*Germany*

1. Introduction

Within shared ecological niches, secretion of lethal protein toxins by microorganisms is a common strategy to ensure positive selection and survival of the toxin producing killer strains amongst other microbial competitors including bacteria, yeast and fungi (Schmitt & Schaffrath, 2005). Frequently, toxin production and secretion are traits that are genetically associated with extrachromosomal elements such as linear DNA killer plasmids and double-stranded RNA mycoviruses from yeast and fungi or episomal and prophage DNA integrated into the chromosome of the microbial toxin producer (reviewed by Meinhardt et al., 1997; Schaffrath & Meinhardt, 2005; Leis et al., 2005). The latter scenario is predominantly found in bacterial species and accounts for lysogenic conversions, phenomena in which phenotypes of the microbial host including pathogenicity, growth performance and production of virulence factors and toxins can be significantly affected by expression of prophage encoded genes. Prominent examples for phage-dependent toxin expression and disease formation include exotoxin-associated scarlet fever by *Streptocoocus pyogenes* (Johnson et al., 1986; Broudy et al., 2001), dysentery causing Shiga toxins Stx1 and Stx2 from *Shigella dysenteriae* (Newland et al., 1985; Willshaw et al., 1985; Huang, et al., 1986), phage CTXφ encoded cholera toxin from *Vibrio cholera* (Waldor & Mekalanos, 1996; Faruque & Nair, 2002) and diphtheria toxin encoded on a beta prophage from lysogens of *Corynebacterium diphtheriae* (Holmes & Barksdale, 1969; Bishai & Murphy 1988). Together with tRNase ribotoxins and anticodon nucleases from prokaryal and eukaryal microbes that have been shown to be encoded by transposable elements as well as circular and non-conventional linear DNA plasmids (Tokunaga et al., 1990; Kaufmann, 2000; Schaffrath & Meinhardt, 2005; Schaffrath et al., 1999), all of these genetic constellations implicate scenarios in which killer phenotypes have been evolved and spread by way of viral DNA transduction pathways or other forms of horizontal gene transfer. In support of this notion, certain cytoplasmic killer plasmids and their associated toxin phenotypes can be transferred between distinct yeast genera by means of cytoduction (Gunge 1983; Sugisaki et al., 1985) and horizontal transfer of the diphtheria toxin encoding *tox* gene from phages has been assigned to *in situ* lysogenic conversion of non-toxigenic to virulent corynebacteria (Freeman, 1951).

With regards to individual toxin response pathways in sensitive target cells, the specific cellular components being targeted by individual microbial protein toxins, not surprisingly, vary significantly depending on the nature of the essential cellular process that is targeted by the toxin in question (Schmitt & Schaffrath, 2005). For instance, microbial toxins capable of inhibiting the process of protein biosynthesis not only have been shown to target individual steps of mRNA translation (e.g. initiation, elongation and termination) but also to attack different components of the ribosomal machinery or associated factors required for mRNA translation (e.g. proteins, mRNAs, tRNAs and rRNAs). In this review, we will focus on one such microbial protein toxin that targets the essential process of mRNA translation and protein biosynthesis: diphtheria toxin (DT) from the Gram-positive bacterium *Corynebacterium diphtheriae* (for previous reviews, see Pappenheimer, 1977, 1984; Murphy, 1996). For DT to unfold its lethal action, the toxin needs to hijack a post-translationally modified residue known as diphthamide in its target protein EF2 (eukaryotic translation elongation factor 2). Next and by virtue of its enzymatic activity, DT ADP-ribosylates its target protein, an irreversible modification that inactivates the essential function of EF2 in mRNA translation. Eventually, EF2 inactivation by DT causes depletion of *de novo* protein biosynthesis and results in the death of the target cell including the model eukaryote and budding yeast *Saccharomyces cerevisiae* (reviewed by Collier, 2001; Todar 2004; Ratts & Murphy, 2005). Here, we review recent advances in the molecular biology of DT and present new insights into DT mode of action and DT response pathway components. An attractive idea emerging from research into DT mode of action is to take its basic molecular biology and apply it to biomedical intervention schemes against tumour cells, microbial pathogens or other biomedically and biotechnically relevant cell systems whose proliferation heavily relies on mRNA translation and protein biosynthesis (White-Gilbertson et al., 2009; Uthman et al., 2011). Such strategies are particularly informed by the use of chimeric DT fusion proteins that combine the lethal ADP-ribosylation activity of DT with a specific cell surface receptor domain for target cell or tissue specificity (Kreitman, 2006, 2009).

2. History and discovery of the diphtheria pathogen

Since the discovery in 1884 by German bacteriologists and physicists Edwin Klebs (1834–1912) and Friedrich Löffler (1852–1915), that *Corynebacterium diphtheriae* (also known as the *Klebs-Löffler* bacillus) is the causative agent of diphtheria (Fig. 1), diphtheria has arguably developed into one of the prototypic, toxigenic and infectious human diseases. Soon after Löffler speculated that organ damage during diphtheria was the consequence of a bacterial toxin, French Pierre-Paul-Émile Roux (1853-1933) and Swiss-French Alexandre Émile Jean Yersin (1863-1943) showed elegantly at the Pasteur Institute that the major bacterial virulence factor was indeed a potent exotoxin (Roux & Yersin, 1888). Upon sterile-filtration of *C. diphtheriae* cultures, they injected toxin-containing, cell free supernatants into laboratory animals and found that disease symptoms (including the eventual death of the animals) were developed in a manner indistinguishable from animals infected with the bacterium alone or even from infected humans. In addition, they proved that toxin-containing urine obtained from children infected with *C. diphtheriae* was sufficient to induce the disease symptoms seen in the above laboratory animals.

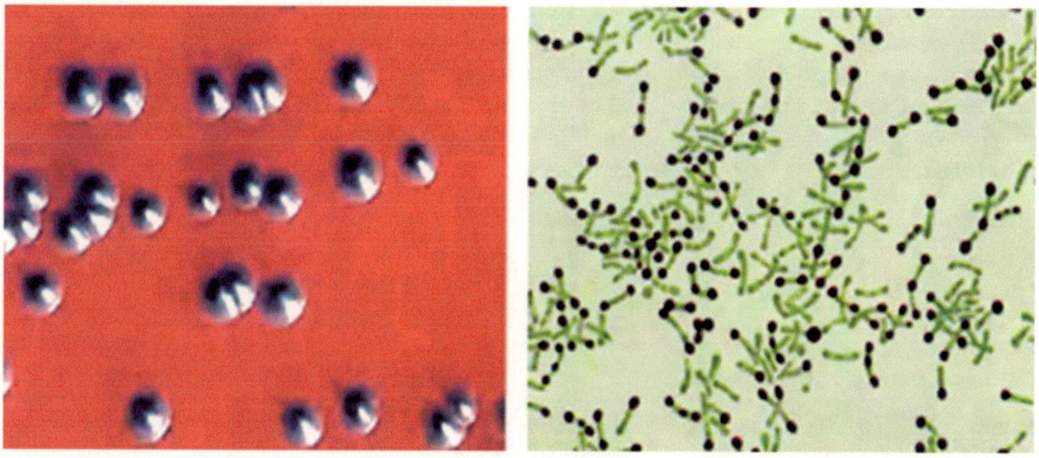

Fig. 1. *Corynebacterium diphtheriae*, the causative agent of the diphtheria disease. Formation of *C. diphtheriae* colonies is shown on blood agar (left panel) according to the CDC (Centers for Disease Control and Prevention, USA). Stained cells of *C. diphtheriae* (right panel). Their barred appearance is due to metachromatic granules which contain polyphosphate. Permission by Professor Kenneth Todar, University of Wisconsin, USA, to show the photographs (Todar, 2004) is gratefully acknowledged by the authors.

Löffler was the first to show that the pathogen could selectively be cultured from nasopharyngeal infections, indicating that diphtheria spreads within the upper respiratory tract. The disease causes a sore throat, low fever and an adherent green-grey membrane on the tonsils, pharynx, and nasal cavities. This thick and fibrinous pseudomembrane, which can severely obstruct airways and suffocate patients, is the result of a combination of bacterial and host effects in response to pathogen cell growth and toxin production as well as the host's immune response and necrosis of the underlying host cell tissue. In 1890, German scientists Emil Adolf von Behring (1854–1917) and Paul Ehrlich (1854–1915) began to study the immunization of horses against diphtheria in order to generate a serum for medical use in humans. Considered to be Ehrlich's first bacteriological achievement attracting world-wide renown, the transformation of diphtheria antitoxin into an effective protective preparation was successfully used during an epidemic in Germany. Rather controversially, however, only von Behring was awarded the first Nobel Prize in Medicine in 1901 for developing a serum therapy against diphtheria.

3. Manifestations, pathogenesis and epidemiology of diphtheria

There are two disease forms, cutaneous and nasopharyngeal diphtheria (Fig. 2). The latter may vary from mild pharyngitis to hypoxia and suffocation with symptoms including fever of more than 39.5°C (~103°F) and profound swelling of the neck upon cervical lymph node infections (also known as bull neck diphtheria). Ultimately, diphtheria may cause life-threatening complications including loss of motor function and difficulty in swallowing and/or congestive heart failure as a result of diphtheria toxin (DT) induced myocarditis (~20% of cases) and peripheral motor neuropathy (~10% of cases) (Fig. 2) (Solders et al., 1989; Havaldar et al., 2000). Diphtheritic skin lesions in the milder form of cutaneous diphtheria are also covered by the typical pseudomembrane (see above). Eventually, DT distribution by way of the circulatory system may reach distant organs and cause paralysis (Fig. 2). Asymptomatic nasopharyngeal carriage is common in regions where diphtheria is endemic. In susceptible individuals, toxigenic strains cause disease by multiplying and secreting DT in either nasopharyngeal or skin lesions (Fig. 2). The diphtheritic lesion is often covered by the pseudomembrane which is composed of fibrin, bacteria, and inflammatory cells (Fig. 2).

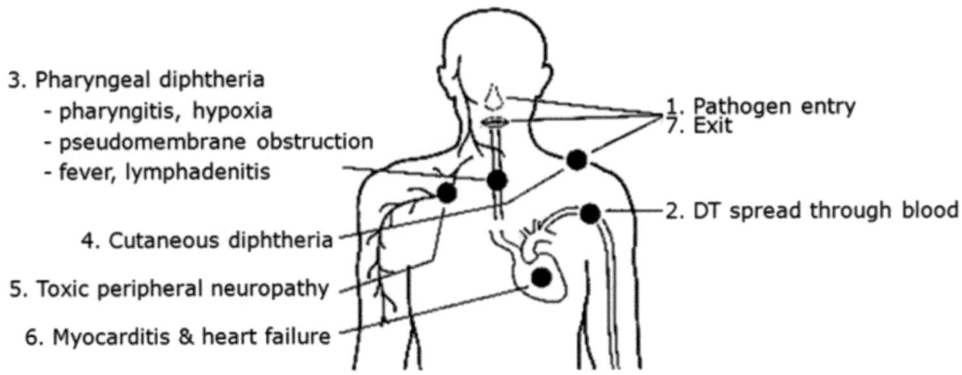

Fig. 2. Pathogenesis of the diphtheria disease. The illustration summarizes clinical manifestations of both pharyngeal and cutaneous diphtheria as well as the spread of the disease which involves blood-borne diphtheria toxin (DT) rather than distribution and dissemination of the pathogen *C. diphtheriae*. Systemic complications are indicated by the occurrence of toxic peripheral neurotrophy and toxic myocarditis eventually causing congestive heart failure. The scheme represents a modified version inspired by a comprehensive diphtheria review (Murphy, 1996)

Diphtheria pathogenesis is largely determined by the capacity of virulent *C. diphtheriae* biotypes (see below) to produce the deadly DT and to colonize and multiply in skin lesions or nasopharyngeal cavities. Since both determinants are encoded by the bacterium carrying a lysogenic beta prophage (Freeman, 1951; Bishai & Murphy, 1988), virulence results from the combined effects of the bacterial and phage genomes (Fig. 3). Even though avirulent *C. diphtheriae* strains seldom associate with the disease, it has been documented that non-toxigenic strains may acquire virulence following lysogenic conversion *in situ* (see below). Although it is clear that events other than production and secretion of DT promote host tissue colonization, detailed knowledge about *C. diphtheriae* factors involved in virulence is scarce. Putative roles in the colonization process have been discussed for a sialic acid splitting neuraminidase from the pathogen and for a corynebacterial cell surface component known as cord factor, i.e. 6,6'-di-O-mycoloyl-α, α-D-trehalose (reviewed by Murphy, 1996). The emergence of continuously changing lysotypes in the pathogen's population is likely due to their ability to compete more efficiently in segments of the nasopharyngeal ecologic niche. Thus, a given lysotype may persist for a while only to be replaced during later stages in the infection by another one that is more adapted to its niche.

Diphtheria is a contagious disease; although toxigenic strains have been isolated from horses, the pathogen *C. diphtheriae* is usually spread by direct physical contact among humans, namely by droplets or through inhaling aerosols of infected individuals. In addition, *in situ* conversion of avirulent strains to pathogenic ones may involve lateral gene transfer following bacterial lysis and release of the DT encoding phage gene (Freeman, 1951; Holmes & Barksdale, 1969). In regions of active immunization programs, isolated focal outbreaks can be associated with carriers who returned from visits to regions still endemic for diphtheria. In the US, Europe and elsewhere, diphtheria was a disease typical of children before mass immunization with diphtheria toxoid. Today, virulent biotypes of *C. diphtheriae* are rarely isolated and clinical diphtheria has largely been eradicated from industrialized nations through global vaccination schemes. Due to effective Diphtheria–Pertussis–Tetanus (DPT) vaccines, the number of diphtheria cases among school-aged children in the US has significantly dropped from 52 in 1980-2000 to 3 in 2000-2007 (Atkinson et al., 2007). For adults, however, vaccine boosts, are strongly advocated since immunity wears off with age and 30-60% of adults are estimated to be at risk, in particular, persons travelling to countries in which diphtheria has not been fully eradicated but poses a constant endemic health-threat. In the 1980s and 1994, public health breakdown in Sweden and Russia caused epidemic clinical diphtheria (Rappuoli et al., 1988) with officials recording more than 80,000 cases including 2,000 deaths. Focal outbreaks reported thereafter were almost certainly associated with diphtheria carriers who returned from Russia to Europe and the US.

4. Host defence, diagnosis and control

Recognition that systemic organ damage associated with diphtheria is due to the action of the lethal DT rather than dissemination of blood-borne pathogens led to the development of a highly successful toxoid vaccine in which inactivated DT that remains antigenic is able to raise an immune response. The toxoid is prepared by incubating DT with formaldehyde at 37° C under alkaline conditions. Although immunization with the toxoid has made diphtheria a rare disease, diphtheria outbreaks do still occur in non-immunized and immune-compromised groups. Control of diphtheria, therefore, depends upon adequate immunization with antigenically intact yet inactivated diphtheria toxoid. Immunization against diphtheria should begin in the second month of life with a series of three primary doses spaced 4 to 8 weeks apart, followed by a fourth dose approximately 1 year after the last primary inoculation. Diphtheria toxoid is widely used as a component in the DPT vaccine (see above). Epidemiologic surveys have shown that immunization against diphtheria is approximately 97% effective. Although mass immunization against diphtheria is practiced in the United States and Europe and there is an adequate immunization rate in children, a large proportion of the adult population may have antibody titers that are below the protective level. The adult population should be reimmunized with diphtheria toxoid every 10 years (see above). Indeed, booster immunization with diphtheria-tetanus toxoids should be administered to persons traveling to regions with high rates of endemic diphtheria (Central and South America, Africa, Asia, Russia and Eastern Europe). In recent years, the use of highly purified toxoid preparations for immunization has minimized the occasional severe hypersensitivity reaction.

Although antibiotics (e.g. penicillin and erythromycin) are used as part of the treatment of patients who present with diphtheria, prompt passive immunization with diphtherial antitoxin is most effective in reducing the fatality rate. The long half-life of specific antitoxin in the circulation is an important factor in ensuring effective neutralization of diphtheria toxin; however, to be effective, the antitoxin must react with the toxin before it becomes internalized into the cell. Protection and immunity towards diphtheria involves an antibody response to DT following clinical disease or a formaldehyde-inactivated diphtheria toxoid following immunization. Immunization with diphtheria toxoid is extraordinarily effective. Diphtheria patients must be promptly treated with antitoxin to neutralize circulating DT.

Clinical diagnosis of diphtheria requires bacteriologic laboratory confirmation of toxigenic *C. diphtheriae* in throat or lesion cultures. For primary isolation, a variety of media may be used including Löffler, Müller-Miller tellurite or Tinsdale tellurite agars. Sterile cotton-tipped applicators are used to swab the pharyngeal tonsils or their beds. Calcium alginate swabs may be inserted through both nares to collect nasopharyngeal samples for culture. Since diphtheritic lesions are often covered with a pseudomembrane (see above) the surface of the lesion may have to be carefully exposed before swabbing with the applicator. In addition to the determination of biotype and lysotype of *C. diphtheriae* isolates, it is possible to use molecular biology techniques in the study of diphtheria outbreaks and pathogen identification. The latter may involve restriction endonuclease digestion patterns of *C. diphtheriae* chromosomal DNA as well as the use of the cloned DT gene (*tox*; see below) or specific corynebacterial insertion sequences as genetic probes (von Hunolstein et al., 2003).

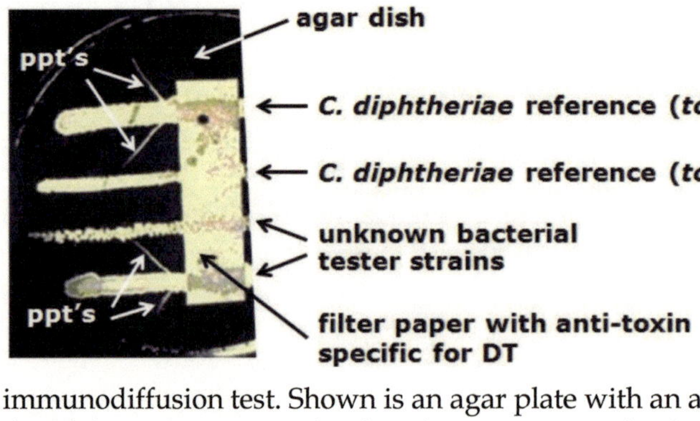

Fig. 3. The Elek immunodiffusion test. Shown is an agar plate with an antitoxin soaked filter that is inoculated with known toxigenic (*tox*$^+$) and non-toxigenic (*tox*$^-$) isolates of *C. diphtheriae* and unknown bacterial tester strains. The thin white lines (arrows) represent anti-toxin/DT precipitates ("ppt's") indicating bacterial DT production. Permission to show Rahul Gladwin's blog data (http://www.rahulgladwin.com/noteblog/bacteriology/what-is-an-eleks-test.php) is acknowledged.

For many years, the Schick test has been established to assess immunity to diphtheria toxin, although today it has been replaced in many regions by serologic tests for specific antibodies to diphtheria toxin. In the Schick test, 0.0124 microgram of diphtheria toxoid in 0.2 millilitre is injected intradermally at a control site and a small amount of diphtheria toxin (ca. 0.8 nanogram in 0.2 millilitre) is injected intradermally into the forearm (test site). Usually, after 48 and 96 hours respecitively, readings are taken with non-specific skin reactions generally peaking by 48 hours. After 96 hours, an erythematous reaction with some possible necrosis at the test site indicates non-sufficient antitoxic immunity for neutralization of DT to occur (≤ 0.03 IU/millilitre). Inflammation at either test or control sites after 48 hours is indicative for a hypersensitivity reaction to the antigen preparation. In many instances, DT is only partially purified prior to inactivation with formaldehyde (see above) and as a result, preparations of toxoid may contain other corynebacterial products, which may elicit a (false positive) hypersensitivity reaction in some individuals.

Following initial isolation, *C. diphtheriae* may be identified as *mitis*, *intermedius*, or *gravis* biotype (see below) on the basis of physiological parameters including carbohydrate fermentation profiles and hemolysis on sheep blood agar plates. The toxigenicity of *C. diphtheriae* strains is determined by a variety of *in vitro* and *in vivo* tests. The most common *in vitro* assay for toxigenicity is the Elek immunodiffusion test (Fig. 3), which is based on the double diffusion of DT and antitoxin in an agar medium. A sterile, antitoxin-saturated filter paper strip is embedded in the culture medium and *C. diphtheriae* isolates are streak-inoculated at a 90° angle to the filter paper. The production of DT can be readily detected within 18 to 48 hours by the formation of a toxin-antitoxin precipitating band in the agar. Alternatively, many eukaryotic cell lines (e.g. African green monkey kidney or Chinese hamster ovary) are sensitive to DT, enabling *in vitro* tissue culture tests to be used for detection of toxin and DT-dependent ADP ribosylation of the cellular target protein, eukaryotic translation elongation factor 2 (EF2, see below). Several highly sensitive *in vivo* tests for DT have also been described (e.g. guinea pig challenge test, rabbit skin test). Clinical diagnosis depends upon culture-proven toxigenic *C. diphtheriae* infection of the skin, nose, or throat combined with clinical signs of nasopharyngeal diphtheria, i.e. dysphagia, sore throat, bloody nasal discharge, formation of pseudomembranes etc.

5. The diphtheria pathogen *Corynebacterium diphtheriae*

5.1 *C. diphtheriae* and diphtheria toxin (DT) production

Diphtheria is caused by *Corynebacterium diphtheriae*, in particular its pathovarieties or biotypes *gravis*, *intermedius* and *mitis* (reviewed by Murphy, 1996). The bacterial cells are Gram-positive, club-shaped, non-motile and non-capsulated (Fig. 1). Cultures grown in tissue or *in vitro* often contain typical cell wall spots that may affect the Gram reaction and are composed of characteristic polymetaphosphate inclusions; these are stainable with methylene-blue and appear as purple granules (Fig. 1). Although the three biotypes differ in colony morphology, growth performance and virulence, they all share the ability to secrete the lethal protein: diphtheria toxin (DT). Intriguingly, DT is specified for by *tox*, a gene carried on one of a family of related corynebacteriophages integrated into the host chromosome of *C. diphtheriae* (Fig. 4) (for review, see Bishai & Murphy 1988). That DT is encoded by the prophage gene was demonstrated when non-pathogenic strains of *C. diphtheriae* became lysogenically converted upon infection with a bacterial virus known as beta phage (Freeman, 1957; Holmes & Barksdale, 1969). Moreover, mutant phages gave rise to nontoxic material that cross-reacted with diphtheria antitoxins, albeit being significantly shorter than full-length DT (Uchida et al., 1971).

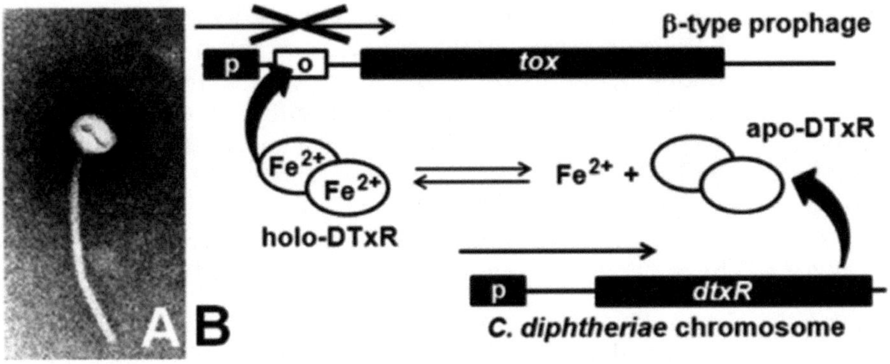

Fig. 4. Phage origin of *tox,* the structural gene encoding diphtheria toxin (DT), and model for *tox* gene regulation in the bacterial host *C. diphtheriae*. (A) Electron micrograph of the beta corynebacteriophage (for review, see Calendar, 1988) which carries the DT gene *tox* and upon infection and genomic integration converts non-toxigenic strains of *C. diphtheriae* into virulent ones. (B) Model of regulated *tox* gene expression by the repressor DTxR. Regulation of the phage *tox* gene depends on DTxR, a Fe^{2+}-binding and iron-responsive repressor dimer that is encoded by the *dtxR* gene on the *C. diphtheriae* genome (Tao, et al., 1994). This is why expression of the *tox* gene depends on the physiological state of the microbial host: under low iron conditions, Fe^{2+} ions dissociate from DTxR and liberate the *tox* gene operator from occupation by DTxR. This leads to *tox* gene derepression and DT can be expressed and secreted into the culture medium. In the presence of iron and upon binding Fe^{2+} ions, the holo-form of DTxR is recruited to the operator region upstream of *tox* and thereby prevents transcription of the DT gene by RNA polymerase to occur (D'Aquino et al., 2005). Upon depletion of Fe^{2+} from the medium, the holo-repressor complex (holo-DTxR) dissociates into its inactive apo-form (apo-DTxR) and the *tox* gene is relieved from transcriptional repression. The authors acknowledge permission by Professor Kenneth Todar, University of Wisconsin, USA, to reproduce a modified version of the electron micrograph (Todar, 2004) representing corynebacteriophage beta.

For optimal growth, some *C. diphtheriae* pathogens require thiamine or biotin and cultivation of most biotypes of *C. diphtheriae* depend on supplementation with nicotinic and pantothenic acids. In addition to being restricted to lysogenic bacteria, expression of the DT gene *tox* is controlled by an iron-responsive host repressor termed DTxR (Fig. 4) (Tao, et al., 1994). Thus, even though the *tox* gene is of viral origin, its regulation at the level of transcriptional repression/activation is coupled to the iron metabolism of the bacterial host (Tao, et al., 1994; D'Aquino et al., 2005). Therefore, optimal DT production is preferably achieved under conditions of low iron levels using culture medium that has been thoroughly deferrated. As for a physiological role of DT, the *tox* gene itself is not essential for the phage cycle and both synthesis and release of DT are not coupled to phage-induced lysis of *C. diphtheriae* cells. Also, it remains to be seen whether the lethal protein, which may account for ~5% of total protein expression in *C. diphtheriae*, benefits the bacterial life style in one way or another.

Nonetheless, by killing epithelial cells from infected pharyngeal niches, DT may contribute to colonization and virulence of the bacterial pathogen.

As early as 1887, Löffler described avirulent cells of *C. diphtheriae* from healthy individuals that were indistinguishable from virulent ones isolated from patients. It is now known that avirulent strains can be converted to virulent ones following infection with *tox* carrying corynebacteriophages *in vitro* and *in situ*. To this end, genetic drift of DT including horizontal gene transfer has not been described so that DT production appears to be confined to the three biotypes of *C. diphtheriae*. In addition to *C. diphtheriae*, other species of the genus *Corynebacterium* may occasionally cause infection of the nasopharnyx and the skin. These include *C. ulcerans, C. pseudotuberculosis, C. pseudodiphtheriticum* and *C. xerosis* with the latter two being capable of producing pyrazinamidase, an intriguing enzyme which converts pyrazinamide (also used in prodrug treatment of *Mycobacterium tuberculosis*) to pyrazinoic acid (McClatchy et al., 1981). In veterinary medicine, *C. renale* and *C. kutscheri* are important pathogens which cause respectively, pyelonephritis in cattle and latent infections in mice.

5.2 DT, an A/B prototype toxin with ADP-ribosyltransferase activity

In sensitive species of humans, monkeys or rabbits, DT is extremely potent with as little as 100 nanograms of DT per kilogram of body weight being lethal. Protein structural analysis has revealed that DT, which is a 535 amino acid residue protein, is organized into individual protein domains with three distinct pathological functions: an N-terminal catalytic ADP-ribosyltransferase domain (i), a receptor binding domain for docking onto target cells (ii) and a transmembrane domain for subcellular delivery of the catalytic domain (iii) (Fig. 5) (Collier & Kandel, 1971; Gill & Pappenheimer, 1971; Gill & Dinius, 1971). Similar to the plant toxin ricin or *Pseudomonas* exotoxin A (ETA), DT is a prototype member of the classical A/B family of toxins (Lord & Roberts, 2005; Sandvig et al., 2005). In their secreted exo-forms, they mature by partial proteolysis into the N-terminal and C-terminal fragments A and B, respectively, which are held together by a disulfide bridge. While fragment B carries the receptor binding domain and the transmembrane motif (see above), segment A harbours the catalytic domain of DT.

Cell intoxication by DT is a multi-step process (Fig. 6) and involves (1) DT docking onto the cell surface receptor, (2) DT uptake and internalization by receptor-mediated endocytosis, (3) acidification of the endocytic vesicle by an ATP-driven proton pump, (4) uncoupling of fragment A from the A/B toxin and (5) delivery of the cytotoxic domain from the lumen of the endocytic vesicle into the cytosol (reviewed by Collier, 2001 and Ratts & Murphy, 2005). Next, by virtue of its catalytic activity, fragment A of DT targets the eukaryotic translation elongation factor 2 (EF2) for NAD^+-dependent ADP-ribosylation (Fig. 6) (Collier & Cole, 1969; Pappenheimer, 1977). The resulting post-translational modification of EF2 by DT inhibits the essential elongation function of EF2 during *de novo* protein synthesis and eventually, leads to cell death (Fig. 6) (Van Ness et al., 1980; Sitikov et al., 1984). DT is an extremely potent agent and it has been demonstrated that subcellular import of a single molecule of its ADP-ribosylating domain toxin is sufficient for cell death induction. Studies on archaeal and eukaryal cells, which can both be killed by DT, demonstrate that the ADP-ribosylation reaction of DT is conserved and requires an exotic and highly modified histidine residue (Kimata & Kohno, 1994) in the EF2 target protein which is also known as diphthamide (Fig. 7). Intriguingly, the EF2 analogues from the bacterial pathogens undergo no such diphthamide modification, which explains why *C. diphtheriae* cells are auto-immune and protected against their own ADP-ribosylase killer toxin (reviewed by Collier, 2001 and Ratts & Murphy, 2005).

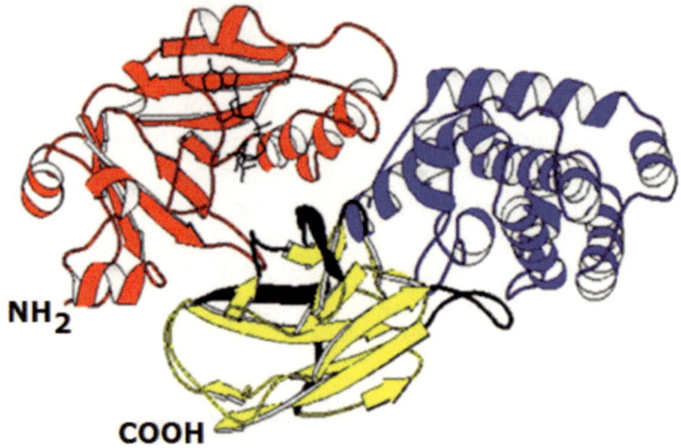

Fig. 5. MolScript-based ribbon diagram highlighting the modular domain organization of the DT monomer. The amino and carboxyl termini of full length DT are indicated (NH_2 and COOH, respectively). The domain in red represents the N-terminal ADP-ribosyltransferase catalytic centre which accounts for cytotoxic ADP-ribosylation and inactivation of the DT target protein EF2; the yellow motif illustrates the C-terminal binding domain important for cell surface attachment and receptor-mediated endocytosis of DT; the protein domain in blue is the transmembrane motif responsible for endosome insertion and subsequent subcellular release of the cytotoxic ADP-ribosylase domain. Permission by Professor Kenneth Todar, University of Wisconsin, USA, to reproduce a modified version of the illustration (Todar, 2004) is gratefully acknowledged.

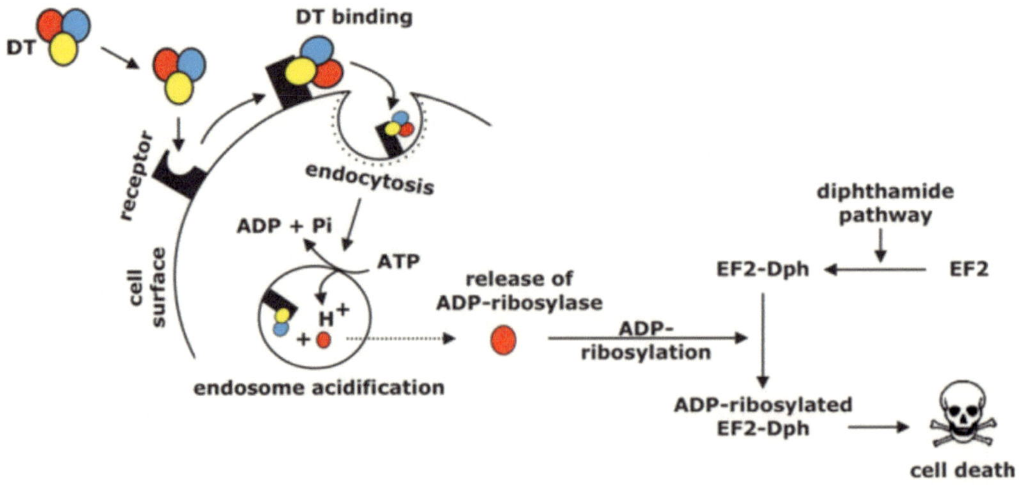

Fig. 6. Schematic diagram of eukaryotic target cell intoxication by DT. The toxin (with domain colour coding as introduced in Fig. 5) binds to its cell surface receptor by virtue of

its receptor binding (yellow) domain and is internalized by receptor-mediated endocytosis using clathrin-coated endosomes. Upon endosome acidification by a proton pump ATPase (pH ~5.1) located in the membrane of endocytic vesicles, the catalytic ADP-ribosylase domain (red) of DT becomes uncoupled from the receptor binding (yellow) and transmembrane (blue) domains. The catalytic domain is delivered to the cytosol and targets diphthamide-modified EF2 for ADP-ribosylation. This results in EF2 inactivation, inhibition of protein synthesis and eventually, death of the target cell. Scheme depiction has been inspired by previous DT reviews (for details see, Murphy, 1996; Collier, 2001; Todar 2004; Ratts & Murphy, 2005).

6. Diphthamide modification of eukaryotic translation elongation factor 2 (EF2)

6.1 Posttranslational biosynthesis of diphthamide on EF2

Diphthamide synthesis on EF2 operates through a complex pathway, which has been conserved among lower and higher eukaryotes (Chen et al., 1985; Moehring et al., 1984; Liu et al., 2004). In the budding yeast *Saccharomyces cerevisiae,* diphthamide biosynthesis requires at least five genes, *DPH1-DPH5* (Liu et al., 2004), two mammalian homologues of which (*DPH1/OVCA1* & *DPH3/KTI11*) are intriguingly involved in embryonic development and cell proliferation in rodents and humans (Fichtner & Schaffrath, 2002; Chen & Behringer, 2004; Fichtner et al., 2003; Liu & Leppla, 2003; Nobukuni et al., 2005; Liu et al., 2006). Though complex in nature, the diphthamide pathway has been shown to be molecularly dissectable. In *S. cerevisiae,* genetic screens selecting for resistance towards DT led to the isolation of diphthamide mutants that corresponded to five individual complementation groups (*dph1-dph5*) (Chen et al., 1985).

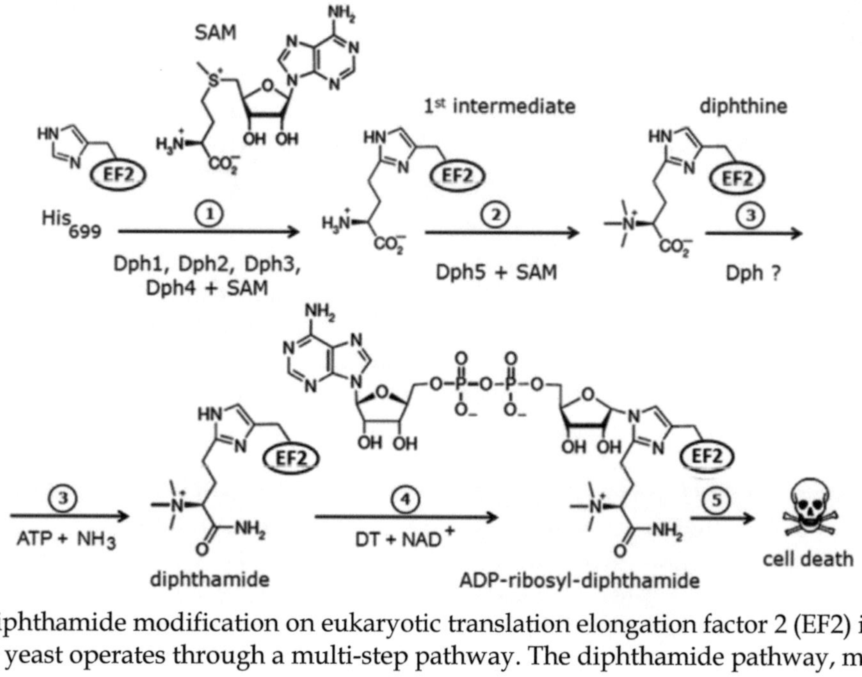

Fig. 7. Diphthamide modification on eukaryotic translation elongation factor 2 (EF2) in budding yeast operates through a multi-step pathway. The diphthamide pathway, modified

after Zhang et al. (2010), involves known and elusive (?) steps with the intermediates 2-(3-carboxyl-3-aminopropyl)-histidine and diphthine being generated. Abbreviations used: S-adenosylmethionine (SAM); adenosine triphosphate (ATP); nicotinamide adenine dinucleotide (NAD^+). The pathway culminates in diphthamide-driven ADP-ribosylation of EF2 (ADP-ribosyl-diphthamide) by DT and other bacterial ADP-ribosylase toxins, including *Pseudomonas* exotoxin A or *Vibrio cholerae* cholix toxin (Zhang et al., 2008; Jørgensen et al., 2008) all of which induce cell death.

Diphthamide biosynthesis involves stepwise modifications starting with the transfer of the 3-amino-3-carboxypropyl (ACP) group from S-adenosylmethionine (SAM) to the C-2 position of the imidazole ring in the target histidine residue (EF2 His_{600} from the archaeon *Pyrococcus horikoshii;* EF2 His_{699} from budding yeast; EF2 His_{715} in mammals) (Fig. 7). In yeast, this step depends on the diphthamide factors Dph1, Dph2, and Dph3 which all interact with each other (Fichtner et al., 2003; Liu et al., 2004; Bär et al., 2008) as well as Dph4, a J-protein (Webb et al., 2008) potentially chaperoning the Dph1-Dph3 complex. Eventually, Dph1-Dph4 action generates the first intermediate of the diphthamide modification pathway: 2-[3-carboxyl-3-aminopropyl]-histidine (Fig. 7) (Zhang et al., 2010). Next, the ammonium group of the intermediate undergoes trimethylation yielding the second intermediate diphthine (Fig. 7). This step is at least in part catalyzed by the protein methyltransferase Dph5 and requires three molecules of the methyl donor SAM (Fig. 7) (Chen & Bodley, 1988; Mattheakis et al., 1992). Finally, the carboxyl group of diphthine undergoes amidation (Fig. 7) in a process that is potentially catalyzed rather than spontaneous or non-enzymatic and likely to involve an as of yet unassigned ATP-dependent amidase (Fig. 7) (Liu et al., 2004). Once fully modified, the N-1 position of the diphthamide-imidazole ring (Fig. 7) is the site for NAD^+-dependent ADP-ribosylation by DT. Intriguingly, other microbial ADP ribosylase toxins including *Pseudomonas* exotoxin A [ETA] (Zhang et al., 2008) and *Vibrio cholera* cholix toxin (Jørgensen et al., 2008) are known to target the dipththamide residue of EF2 in a highly similar, if not identical, manner. Eventually, ADP-ribosyl-diphthamide, the resulting terminal modification, irreversibly inactivates the translation elongation function of EF2 (Fig. 7) (Sitikov et al., 1984).

As for the elusive and terminal amidation step, no DT resistant yeast mutants have been identified to date, probably because diphthine is a substrate (though poor) for ADP-ribosylating toxins. Provided terminal amidation was an enzymatically catalysed process rather than a spontaneous one (see above), amidase-deficient mutants may still display DT sensitivity, which is why the amidase in question may have repeatedly escaped identification in the above screens for DT resistance. It will be interesting to see whether this also holds true for screens involving EF2 inhibitors or antagonists that are not related to DT but share with DT a common requirement for diphthamide modification of EF2. This is of particular interest in the light of recent evidence that *dph1, dph2, dph3, dph4* and *dph5* deletion mutants from yeast not only are protected against DT (Fig. 8) but are also all resistant to growth inhibition by sordarin (Fig. 8) (Bär et al., 2008; Botet et al., 2008). The latter is an ascomycetous glycoside (Hauser & Sigg, 1971) whose antifungal activity obviously depends on diphthamide, but that operates by selectively blocking the EF2-ribosome complex rather than inhibiting EF2 by ADP-ribosylation (Dominguez et al., 1999).

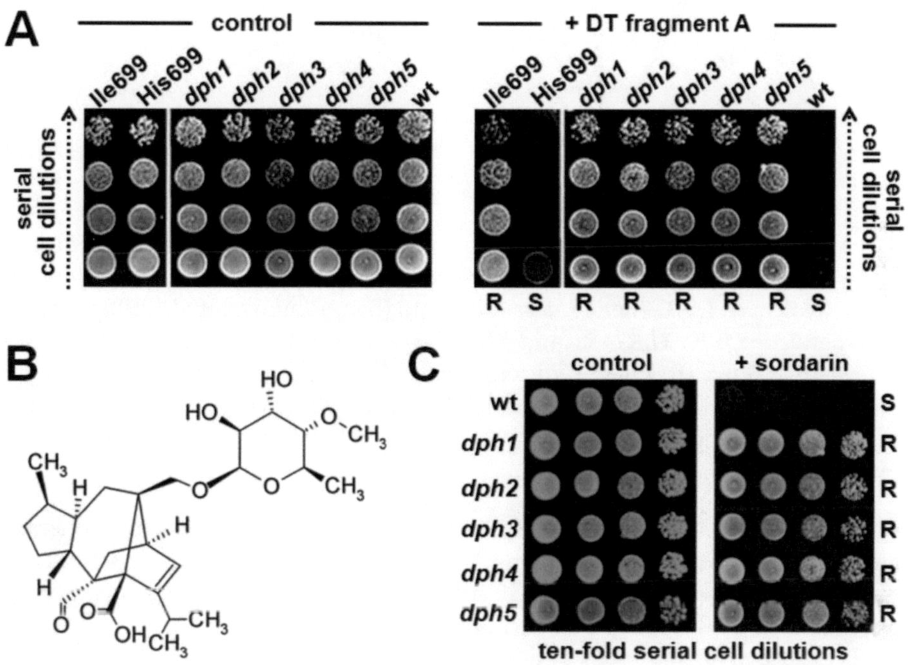

Fig. 8. Diphthamide modification is essentially required for growth inhibition of yeast cells by DT and by the antifungal sordarin. (A) DT resistance due to defects in diphthamide synthesis on EF2. Yeast cells with an EF2 diphthamide target residue substitution (His699Ile) (Kimata & Kohno, 1994) and diphthamide mutants (*dph1, dph2, dph3, dph4* and *dph5*) (Chen et al., 1985) resist (R) against conditional expression of the lethal DT fragment A while wild-type cells (wt; His699) remain sensitive (S) to the ADP-ribosylase and are killed (right panel). Empty vector control (left panel) shows the growth control in the absence of DT. (B) Chemical formula of sordarin, an EF2-specific antifungal and ribosome inhibitor. (C) Like DT, sordarin action requires diphthamide synthesis on EF2. Wild-type (wt) parental strain W303 and its diphthamide mutants (*dph1-dph5*) were cultivated in the absence (control) or presence of the antifungal (+ sordarin). A resistant (R) cell response is distinguished from sensitivity (S).

A

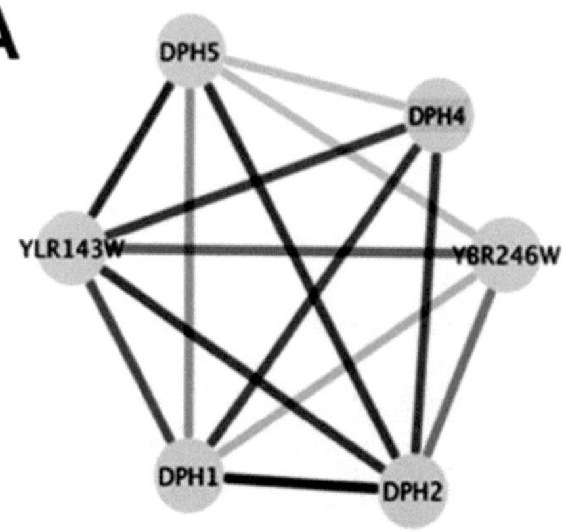

B

Gene	correlation score*
DPH2	0.314
DPH4	0.248
YLR143w	0.234
DPH5	0.182
YBR246w	0.158

* profiles correlated to *dph1* traits

Fig. 9. Based on synthetic genetic array (SGA) analysis, yeast Open Reading Frames (ORFs) *YLR143w* and *YBR246w* represent loci that are potentially related to the *DPH* genes and the diphthamide pathway. (A) Genetic interaction data (Baryshnikova et al., 2010) indicating relatedness between ORFs *YLR143w* and *YBR246w* and diphthamide synthesis genes *DPH1*, *DPH2*, *DPH4* and *DPH5*. (B) Phenotypic clustering (Carette et al., 2009) and phenotypic scores, in relation to dipthamide mutant *dph1*, between *YBR246w* and *DPH5* genes as well as *YLR143w* and *DPH4* suggest both ORFs to be related to *DPH1* and to the diphthamide modification pathway.

In an effort to further analyze the relationships among individual components of the diphthamide pathway, we found that the Dph1, Dph2 and Dph3 proteins form a protein complex whose assembly is crucial for diphthamide formation and consequently for ADP-ribosylation of EF2 by DT (Fig. 10). Strikingly, the *DPH3* gene from budding yeast was shown to be allelic with the locus Killer Toxin Insensitive 11 (*KTI11*) (Butler et al., 1994). *KTI11* was shown to be required for the *Kluyveromyces lactis* tRNAse toxin zymocin to kill other yeast species including *S. cerevisiae* (Fichtner & Schaffrath, 2002). In particular, the Kti11/Dph3 gene product was shown to be involved in a tRNA modification pathway that is essential for the tRNase activity of zymocin to cleave target tRNAs and cause yeast cell death by way of tRNA depletion (Huang et a., 2005; Lu et al., 2006; Jablonowski & Schaffrath, 2007; Jablonowski et al., 2006; Kheir et al., 2011). In addition to interacting with Dph1, Dph2 and EF2 (Fichtner et al., 2003; Bär et al., 2008), Dph3/Kti11 was furthermore shown to communicate with other proteins (Kti13: Zabel et al., 2008) or protein complexes (Rvs161•Rvs167; Elongator complex: Fichtner et al., 2003; Krogan et al., 2006) suggesting multiple roles for Kti11/Dph3 in processes not necessarily limited to the diphthamide modification pathway. In support of such versatility, DelGIP1 (the human homologue of yeast Kti11/Dph3) interacts with deafness locus-associated guanine nucleotide exchange factor (DelGEF) and the DelGIP1•DelGEF protein complex affects exocyst-dependent secretion of proteoglycans (Sjölinder et al., 2002, 2004). Also, our group was able to show that conditional phenotypes and stress-inducible growth defects of a yeast mutant with a single *KTI11/DPH3* gene deletion were more severe and pronounced in relation to rather mild defects of yeast mutants lacking *DPH1* or *DPH2* gene function (Bär et al., 2008), supporting its role in a wider range of cellular functions in yeast. Atomic absorption spectroscopy has recently shown that the Kti11/Dph3 protein folds into a closed compact and globular protein structure with its C-terminal alpha-helix protruding outward (Sun et al., 2005). Moreover, the protein co-ordinates a zinc ion via a $Zn(Cys)_4$ binding module that is highly conserved among Kti11/Dph3 homologues from plants, animals and humans (Proudfood et al., 2008). Presumably, it is this motif that is engaged in the putative electron-carrier activity recently proposed for Kti11/Dph3 by Proudfood et al. (2008). In line with this notion, both single and multiple Cys substitutions of the four critical residues in the potential $Zn(Cys)_4$ binding module cause inactivation of the Kti11/Dph3 variants and traits including resistance to growth inhibition by DT, sordarin and zymocin that are identical to the phenotypes of null-mutants lacking *KTI11/DPH3* gene function (Fichtner & Schaffrath, 2002; Bär et al., 2008).

Strikingly, the multi-step pathway for diphthamide formation and EF2 modification (Fig. 7) has been conserved from lower to higher eukaryotes. Among the five budding yeast diphthamide genes (*DPH1*, *DPH2*, *DPH3*, *DPH4* and *DPH5*) (Fig. 7), there are two mammalian homologues (*DPH1/OVCA1* and *DPH3/KTI11*) that are required for cell proliferation, tumourigenesis and neuronal development in mice and human cells. As a result, defects in *DPH3/KTI11* are associated with neurodegeneration in mice (Liu et al., 2006) and mutations in *OVCA1/DPH1* have identified a tumour suppressor role for this diphthamide-related gene product in the context of ovarian cancer (Chen & Behringer, 2004). In an effort to further study diphthamide function and the interrelation between components of the diphthamide pathway, we found by co-immune precipitation and tandem affinity purification protocols that the Dph1, Dph2 and Dph3 factors form a protein complex, assembly of which is crucial for EF2 ADP-riboslyation by DT (Fichtner et al., 2003; Bär et al., 2008). Moreover, we and others discovered that the Dph1-Dph5 proteins are all required for the cytotoxic activity of sordarin (Bär et al., 2008; Botet et al., 2008), another EF2-related antifungal and translation inhibitor (Justice et al., 1998).

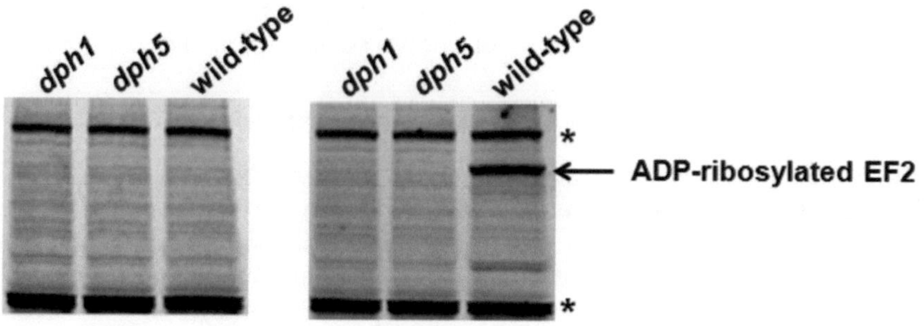

Fig. 10. Yeast diphthamide modification mutants evade ADP-ribosylation of EF2 by DT. Shown are EF2 ADP ribosylation assays on total protein extracts from the indicated yeast strain backgrounds in the absence (left panel) and presence (right panel) of recombinant DT. When using biotin-labeled NAD^+ as donor for the *in vitro* ADP ribosylation assay, wild-type strains display EF2 ADP-ribosylation acceptor activity (indicated by the arrow) whereas diphthamide mutans *dph1* and *dph5* fail to do so. The asterisks denote unspecific signals in proteins irrespective of DT treatment and/or strain backgrounds tested.

In a search for new diphthamide-related factors, two novel and uncharacterized open reading frames (ORFs), YBR246w and YLR143w, have been identified recently as new potential components for diphthamide biosynthesis using genetic screens in human and yeast cells (Botet et al., 2008; Carette et al., 2009). Based on synthetic genetic interaction data deposited at the genetic interaction database (GID; University of Toronto, Canada) (Baryshnikova et al., 2010) and the significance of the phenotypic correlation scores, both budding yeast ORFs are predicted to have EF2-related functions (Fig. 9). In addition, possible effector roles of YBR246w and YLR143w for EF2 specific antifungals including sordarin are becoming evident: when deleted, these new loci not only affect the communication between Dph5 and EF2 but also phenocopy traits (including sordarin resistance) that are typical of *dph1*, *dph2*, *dph3*, *dph4* and *dph5* mutants from yeast (Bär et al., 2008; Botet et al., 2008; Carette et al., 2009). Although being aware that the sordarin phenotype may also be ascribable to defects in EF2-unrelated genes that are required for binding and/or import of the deadly antifungal (Botet et al., 2008), we consider these ORFs to be candidate diphthamide biosynthesis genes. In support of this notion, preliminary data based on *in vitro* EF2 modification assays demonstrate that inactivation of YBR246w and YLR143w eliminates the ADP-ribosylation acceptor activity of EF2 in the presence of DT. Since this is a trait that is specific to the *bona fide* diphthamide synthesis defect of *dph1*, *dph2*, *dph3*, *dph4* and *dph5* mutants (Liu & Leppla, 2003; Liu et al., 2004) (Fig. 10), YBR246w or YLR184w deletion may cause a diphthamide defect, too, which abolishes DT-dependent ADP-ribosylation of EF2.

To sum up, diphthamide incorporation of EF2 is not only pathologically relevant for ADP-ribosylation by DT but also crucial for toxicity of the antifungal sordarin. Physiologically, the dipthamide pathway appears to be important for mRNA translation as well as proper cell proliferation and neural development in eukaryal cells. Surprisingly, our data imply that formation of diphthamide is genetically more complex than originally anticipated (Chen et al., 1985; Liu et al., 2004) and that the pathway may comprise more gene products than the five Dph1-Dph5 members known to date (Carette et al., 2009). For future work, it will be significant to define the roles of new diphthamide candidates and how they may relate to or communicate with the other known pathway members.

6.2 Biological significance for diphthamide modification of EF2

Diphthamide on EF2 is the target for bacterial ADP-ribosylase toxins (DT; ETA; cholix) and also affects toxicity of sordarin and ricin, a ribosome inhibiting protein toxin from plants (Gupta et al. 2008). Although this emphasizes its varied pathological relevance, the physiological significance of diphthamide remains enigmatic and elusive. Nonetheless, the evolutionary conservation of the diphthamide pathway among eukaryotes strongly suggests that diphthamide will be important in processes including mRNA translation. In support of this notion, evidence from research groups including our own has shown that diphthamide defects increase translational frame-shifting (Ortiz et al., 2006; Bär et al., 2008). Moreover, homologues of diphthamide synthesis genes (*DPH1/OVCA1* and *DPH3/KTI11*) affect the proliferation and development of mammalian cells, which is why inactivation of *DPH3/KTI11* is associated with tRNA modification defects and neurodegeneration and mutations in *DPH1/OVCA1* revealed a tumour suppressor role for this diphthamide synthesis gene in ovarian cancer (Chen & Behringer, 2004; Nobukuni et al., 2005; Huang et al., 2005; Liu et al., 2006; Kim et al., 2010).

Whether or not this implies structural or regulatory roles for diphthamide in mRNA translation remains to be seen. The latter, however, is intriguing with the emergence of a cellular ADP-ribosyltransferase that resembles the diphthamide-dependent ADP-ribosylation reaction by DT (Lee & Iglewski, 1984; Jäger et al., 2011). As a result, diphthamide may be envisioned to be used as an on/off switch for endogenous ADP-ribosylation of EF2 and control of mRNA translation and protein synthesis. Irrespective of unclear physiological functions, recent genetic data imply that the diphthamide pathway is more complex than originally anticipated and likely to comprise further components, in addition to Dph1-Dph5 (Carette et al., 2009). For future research, it will be therefore crucial to define the identity of new diphthamide synthesis candidates and provide insights into how they communicate with known members of the pathway.

7. Engineering DT chimera for use in cell-specific proliferation control

Protein engineering is a new and rapidly developing area within the field of molecular biology; it brings together recombinant DNA methodologies and solid phase DNA synthesis in the design and construction of chimeric genes whose products have unique properties. Through a combination of protein engineering and DT structure-function studies, it has been possible to genetically substitute the native DT receptor-binding domain B (Figs. 5 and 6) with a variety of polypeptide hormones and cytokines (e.g. α-melanocyte-stimulating hormone [α-MSH], interleukin [IL] 2, IL-4, IL-6, IL-7, epidermal growth factor, etc) (Foss, 2001; Kreitman, 2006, 2009). The resulting fusion toxins or chimera combine the receptor-binding specificity of the cytokine with the catalytic ADP-ribosylase domain of DT. In each instance, the chimeric proteins have unique properties and selectively attack only those target cells that bear the appropriate target cell receptor on the cell surface. One of these engineered fusion toxins, DAB389IL-2 (ONTAK) (Le Maistre et al., 1992), has been evaluated in clinical trials for the treatment of human lymphomas, in which cells with high affinity IL-2 receptors play a major role in pathogenesis. Administration of ONTAK has been shown to be well tolerated, safe and to induce durable remission from disease in the absence of undesired side effects. Moreover, ONTAK and its predecessor, DAB486IL-2 (Le Maistre et al., 1992) have demonstrated activity in a variety of diseases, including cutaneous T cell lymphoma (CTCL), psoriasis, rheumatoid arthritis and HIV infection. Hence, DT based fusion toxins are important biological agents for the treatment of certain tumours or disorders in which specific cell surface receptors can be selectively targeted (Hesketh et al., 1993; Van der Spek et al., 1994; Foss, 2001; Kreitman, 2006, 2009) and it is likely that such DT chimera will be providing further and important new biological tools for selected cell targeting and DT-dependent inactivation of protein biosynthesis, a fundamental biological process with key roles for cell cycling and cancer formation (White-Gilbertson et al., 2009).

8. Conclusion

Diphtheria represents one of the best studied bacterial diseases of humans with its etiology, mode of transmission, pathogenic mechanism and molecular basis of DT structure and function being clearly established. Consequently, highly effective methods for treatment and prevention of diphtheria have been developed and many contributions to the fields of medical microbiology, immunology and molecular biology as well as to our understanding of host-bacterial interactions and pathogenesis have been made possible by studying diphtheria and DT. Diphtheria is caused by *C. diphtheriae*, pathovar. *gravis*, *intermedius* and *mitis*, three biotypes that differ in virulence and growth performance but share the ability to secrete the lethal ADP ribosylase toxin DT, the protein product of a lysogenic phage gene. The DT gene *tox* is under control of an iron-responsive repressor (DtxR) so that DT production is limited under conditions of low iron levels and to lysogenic bacteria only. DT is a typical A/B toxin containing two fragments that are proteolytically processed from a single precursor and held together by a disulfide bridge. The A fragment is catalytically active and the B fragment promotes receptor-mediated endocytosis of DT. Upon import, the A subunit is cleaved-off from the B fragment and gets released into the cytoplasm. Here, DT unfolds its toxicity and ADP-ribosylates eukaryotic translation elongation factor 2 (EF2). ADP-ribosylation of EF2 by DT is irreversible, eventually inhibiting mRNA translation and protein synthesis and inducing the death of the target cell. Studies from archaeal and eukaryal target cells demonstrate that the ADP-ribosylase activity of DT requires diphthamide, a highly modified histidine residue in EF2. Intriguingly, the EF2 analogues from *Corynebacteria* lack diphthamide, which explains why the DT producers are immune to their own toxin.

Strikingly, diphthamide formation on EF2 operates through a multi-step pathway that is conserved among archaea and eukaryotes. In the yeast *S. cerevisiae*, it comprises at least five different genes, *DPH1-DPH5*, of which two mammalian homologues (*DPH1/OVCA1* & *DPH3/KTI11*) are required for cell proliferation, tumourigenesis and neuronal development. As a result, defects in *DPH3/KTI11* are associated with neurodegeneration and mutations in *OVCA1/DPH1* have identified a tumour suppressor role for the diphthamide-related product in ovarian cancer. In an effort to further study the diphthamide pathway, we found that the Dph1, Dph2 and Dph3 factors form a protein complex, assembly of which is crucial for EF2 ADP-riboslyation by DT. Moreover, all five Dph1-Dph5 proteins are required for the cytotoxic activity of sordarin, another EF2-related inhibitor. In a search for novel diphthamide-related genes from yeast by use of synthetic genetic array (SGA) analysis and the genetic interaction database (GID), we identified two open reading frames (ORFs: YBR246W; YLR143w) previously implicated in antifungal activity of DT and sordarin. In line with predicted EF2 roles, deletion mutants lacking YBR246W or YLR184w are resistant towards doses of sordarin that are lethal to wild-type yeast cells. Moreover, EF2 modification assays in the presence of DT demonstrate that protein extracts from the deletion strains lack ADP-ribosylation acceptor activity of EF2. This suggests that YBR246W or YLR184w inactivation may have caused a diphthamide biosynthetic defect, which abrogates DT-dependent ADP-ribosylation of EF2. In sum, diphthamide incorporation of EF2 is not only relevant for ADP-ribosylation by DT but also crucial for toxicity of the antifungal sordarin. Physiologically, the dipthamide pathway appears to be important for mRNA translation as well as proper cell proliferation and neural development in eukaryal cells. Surprisingly, our data imply that formation of diphthamide is genetically more complex than originally anticipated and that the pathway may comprise more than the five Dph1-Dph5 gene products known to date.

Finally, the study of diphtheria toxin structure/function relationships has clearly shown DT toxin to be a three-domain protein with individual roles for receptor binding, endocytosis and catalysis (i.e. NAD^+-dependent ADP-ribosylation). Through protein engineering, a rapidly developing area within the field of molecular biology that brings together recombinant DNA methodologies and solid phase DNA synthesis, the design of diphtheria fusion toxin genes has been feasible whose products have unique properties. Thus, it has been possible to genetically substitute the native diphtheria toxin receptor-binding domain with a variety of polypeptide hormones and cytokines so that the resulting fusion toxins combine the receptor-binding specificity of the cytokine with the ADP ribosylase activity of DT. The fusion toxins can selectively intoxicate only those cells which bear the appropriate targeted receptor. It is likely that such DT-based fusion toxins will be important new biological agents for the treatment of tumours/disorders in which specific cell surface receptors may need to be targeted.

9. Acknowledgment

Support to SL by the US National Institute of Allergy and Infectious Diseases Intramural Programme and by the Biotechnology and Biological Sciences Research Council (BBSRC) to MJRS (BB/F0191629/1) and RS (BB/F019106/1) is gratefully acknowledged. SU has been awarded an *OVCA1* PhD studentship through the HOPE Foundation for Cancer Research, UK, and receives support from the Department of Genetics, University of Leicester, UK. RS greatfully acknowledges support from the Feodor Lynen Fellowship (3.1-3. FLF-DEU/1037031) Alumnus Programme of the Alexander von Humboldt Foundation, Bonn, Germany.

10. References

Atkinson, W., Hamborsky, J., McIntyre, L., & Wolfe, S. (eds.) (2007). *Diphtheria*. In: Epidemiology and Prevention of Vaccine-Preventable Diseases (The Pink Book) (10 ed.). Washington DC: Public Health Foundation. pp. 59–70.

Baryshnikova, A., Costanzo, M., Dixon, S., Vizeacoumar, F.J., Myers, C.L., Andrews, B., & Boone, C. (2010). Synthetic genetic array (SGA) analysis in *Saccharomyces cerevisiae* and *Schizosaccharomyces pombe*. *Methods in Enzymology* 470: 145-179.

Bär, C., Zabel. R., Liu, S., Stark, M.J., & Schaffrath, R. (2008). A versatile partner of eukaryotic protein complexes that is involved in multiple biological processes: Kti11/Dph3. *Mol Microbiol* 69: 1221-1233.

Bishai, W.R., & Murphy, J.R. (1988). Bacteriophage gene products that cause human disease. In Calendar, R. (ed.): *The Bacteriophages*. Plenum, New York.

Botet, J., Rodríguez-Mateos, M., Ballesta, J.P., Revuelta, J.L., & Remacha, M. (2008). A chemical genomic screen in *Saccharomyces cerevisiae* reveals a role for diphthamidation of translation elongation factor 2 in inhibition of protein synthesis by sordarin. *Antimicrobial Agents and Chemotherapy* 52: 1623-1629.

Broudy, T.B., Pancholi, V., & Fischetti, V.A. (2001). Induction of lysogenic bacteriophage and phage-associated toxin from group a streptococci during coculture with human pharyngeal cells. *Infection and Immunity* 69: 1440-1443.

Butler, A.R., White, J.H., Folawiyo, Y., Edlin, A., Gardiner, D., & Stark, M.J. (1994). Two *Saccharomyces cerevisiae* genes which control sensitivity to G1 arrest induced by *Kluyveromyces lactis* toxin. *Molecular and Cellular Biology* 14: 6306-6316.

Calendar, R. (1988). *The Bacteriophages*, Plenum, New York.

Carette, J.E., Guimaraes, C.P., Varadarajan, M., Park, A.S., Wuethrich, I., Godarova, A., Kotecki, M., Cochran, B.H., Spooner, E., Ploegh, H.L., & Brummelkamp, T.R. (2009). Haploid genetic screens in human cells identify host factors used by pathogens. *Science* 326: 1231-1235.

Chen, C.M., & Behringer, R.R. (2004). Ovca1 regulates cell proliferation, embryonic development, and tumorigenesis. *Genes and Development* 18: 320-332.

Chen, J.Y., Bodley, J.W. (1988). Biosynthesis of diphthamide in *Saccharomyces cerevisiae.* Partial purification and characterization of a specific S-adenosylmethionine:elongation factor 2 methyltransferase. *Journal of Biological Chemistry* 263: 11692-11696.

Chen, J.Y., Bodley, J.W., & Livingston, D.M. (1985). Diphtheria toxin-resistant mutants of *Saccharomyces cerevisiae. Molecular and Cellular Biology* 5: 3357-3360.

Collier, R.J. (2001). Understanding the mode of action of diphtheria toxin: a perspective on progress during the 20th century. *Toxicon* 39: 1793–1803.

Collier, R.J., & Cole, H.A. (1969). Diphtheria toxin subunit active in vitro. *Science* 164: 1179-1181.

Collier, R.J., & Kandel, J. (1971). Structure and activity of diphtheria toxin. I. Thiol-dependent dissociation of a fraction of toxin into enzymically active and inactive fragments. *Journal of Biological Chemistry* 246: 1496-1503.

D'Aquino, J.A., Tetenbaum-Novatt, J., White, A., Berkovitch, F., & Ringe, D. (2005). Mechanism of metal ion activation of the diphtheria toxin repressor DtxR. *Proceedings of the National Academy of Sciences of the United States of America* 102: 18408-18413.

Dominguez, J.M., Gomez-Lorenzo, M.G., & Martin, J.J. (1999). Sordarin inhibits fungal protein synthesis by blocking translocation differently to fusidic acid. *Journal of Biological Chemistry* 274: 22423-22427.

Faruque, S.M., & Nair, G.B. (2002). Molecular ecology of toxigenic *Vibrio cholerae. Microbiology and Immunology* 46: 59–66.

Fichtner, L., & Schaffrath, R. (2002). *KTI11* and *KTI13, Saccharomyces cerevisiae* genes controlling sensitivity to G1 arrest induced by *Kluyveromyces* lactis zymocin. *Molecular Microbiology* 44: 865-875.

Fichtner, L., Jablonowski, D., Schierhorn, A., Kitamoto, H.K., Stark, M.J., & Schaffrath, R. (2003). Elongator's toxin-target (TOT) function is nuclear localization sequence dependent and suppressed by post-translational modification. *Molecular Microbiology* 49: 1297-1307.

Foss, F.M. (2001). Interleukin-2 fusion toxin: targeted therapy for cutaneous T cell lymphoma. *Annals of the New York Academy of Sciences* 941: 166-176.

Freeman, V.J. (1951). Studies on the virulence of bacteriophage-infected strains of *Corynebacterium diphtheriae. Journal of Bacteriology* 61: 675–688.

Gill, D.M., & Dinius, L.L. (1971). Observations on the structure of diphtheria toxin. *Journal of Biological Chemistry* 246: 1485-1491.

Gill, D.M., & Pappenheimer, A.M. (1971). Structure-activity relationships in diphtheria toxin. *Journal of Biological Chemistry* 246: 1492-1495.

Gunge, N. (1983). Yeast DNA plasmids. *Annual Reviews of Microbiology* 37: 253-276.

Gupta, P.K., Liu, S., Batavia, M.P., & Leppla, S.H. (2008). The diphthamide modification on elongation factor-2 renders mammalian cells resistant to ricin. *Cellular Microbiology* 10: 1687-1694.

Hauser, D., & Sigg, H,P. (1971). Isolierung und Abbau von Sordarin. *Helvetica Chimica Acta* 54: 1178-1190.

Havaldar, P.V., Sankpal, M.N., & Doddannavar, R.P. (2000). Diphtheritic myocarditis: clinical and laboratory parameters of prognosis and fatal outcome. *Annals of Tropical Paediatrics* 20: 209–215.

Hesketh, P., Caguioa, P., Koh, H., Dewey, H., Facada, A., McCaffrey, R., Parker, K., Nylen, P., Woodworth, T. (1993). Clinical activity of a cytotoxic fusion protein in the treatment of cutaneous T cell lymphoma. *Journal of Clinical Oncology* 11: 1682-1690.

Holmes, R. K., & Barksdale, L. (1969). Genetic analysis of tox+ and tox- bacteriophages of *Corynebacterium diphtheriae*. *Journal of Virology* 3: 586-598.

Huang, B., Johansson, M.J., & Byström, A.S. (2005). An early step in wobble uridine tRNA modification requires the Elongator complex. *RNA* 11: 424-436.

Huang, A., De Grandis, S., Friesen, J., Karmali, M., Petric, M., Congi, R., & Brunton, J.L. (1986). Cloning and expression of the genes specifying Shiga-like toxin production in *Escherichia coli* H19. *Journal of Bacteriology* 166: 375-379.

Jablonowski, D., & Schaffrath, R. (2007). Zymocin, a composite chitinase and tRNase killer toxin from yeast. *Biochemical Society Transactions* 35: 1533-1537.

Jablonowski, D., Zink, S., Mehlgarten, C., Daum, G., & Schaffrath, R. (2007). $tRNA^{Glu}$ wobble uridine methylation by Trm9 identifies Elongator's key role for zymocin-induced cell death in yeast. *Molecular Microbiology* 59: 677-688.

Jäger, D., Werdan, K., & Müller-Werdan, U. (2011). Endogenous ADP-ribosylation of elongation factor-2 by interleukin-1β. *Molecular and Cellular Biochemistry* 348: 125-128.

Johnson, L.P., Tomai, M.A., & Schlievert, P.M. (1986). Bacteriophage involvement in group A streptococcal pyrogenic exotoxin A production. *Journal of Bacteriology* 166: 623-627.

Jørgensen, R., Purdy, A.E., Fieldhouse, R.J., Kimber, M.S., Bartlett, D.H. & Merrill, A.R. (2008). Cholix toxin, a novel ADP-ribosylating factor from *Vibrio cholerae*. *Journal of Biological Chemistry* 283: 10671-10678.

Justice, M.C., Hsu, M.J., Tse, B., Ku, T., Balkovec, J., Schmatz, D., & Nielsen, J. (1998). Elongation factor 2 as a novel target for selective inhibition of fungal protein synthesis. *Journal of Biological Chemistry* 273: 3148-3151.

Kaufmann, G. (2000). Anticodon nucleases. *Trends in Biochemical Sciences* 25: 70-74.

Kheir, E., Bär, C., Jablonowski, D., & Schaffrath, R. (2011). Cell growth control by tRNase ribotoxins from bacteria and yeast. In: Mendez-Vilas A., ed., *Science and Technology against Microbial Pathogens. Research, Development and Evaluation*, World Scientific Publishing Ltd; pp. 398-402.

Kim, S., Johnson, W., Chen, C., Sewell, A.K., Byström, A.S., & Han, M. (2010) Allele-specific suppressors of lin-1(R175Opal) identify functions of MOC-3 and DPH-3 in tRNA modification complexes in *Caenorhabditis elegans*. *Genetics* 185: 1235-1247.

Kimata, Y., & Kohno, K. (1994). Elongation factor 2 mutants deficient in diphthamide formation show temperature-sensitive cell growth. *Journal of Biological Chemistry* 269: 13497-13501.

Kreitman, R.J. (2006). Immunotoxins for targeted cancer therapy. *Journal of the American Association of Pharmaceutical Scientists* 8: E532-551.

Kreitman, R.J. (2009). Recombinant immunotoxins containing truncated bacterial toxins for the treatment of hematologic malignancies. *BioDrugs* 23: 1-13.

Krogan, N.J., Cagney, G., Yu, H., Zhong, G., Guo, X., Ignatchenko, A., Li, J., Pu, S., Datta, N., Tikuisis, A.P., Punna, T., Peregrín-Alvarez, J.M., Shales, M., Zhang, X., Davey, M., Robinson, M.D., Paccanaro, A., Bray, J.E., Sheung, A., Beattie, B., Richards, D.P., Canadien, V., Lalev, A., Mena, F., Wong, P., Starostine, A., Canete, M.M., Vlasblom, J., Wu, S., Orsi, C., Collins, S.R., Chandran, S., Haw, R., Rilstone, J.J., Gandi, K., Thompson, N.J., Musso, G., St Onge, P., Ghanny, S., Lam, M.H., Butland, G., Altaf-Ul, A.M., Kanaya, S., Shilatifard, A., O'Shea, E., Weissman, J.S., Ingles, C.J., Hughes,

T.R., Parkinson, J., Gerstein, M., Wodak, S.J., Emili, A., & Greenblatt, J.F. (2006). Global landscape of protein complexes in the yeast *Saccharomyces cerevisiae*. *Nature* 440: 637-643.

Lee, H., & Iglewski, W.J. (1984). Cellular ADP-ribosyltransferase with the same mechanism of action as diphtheria toxin and Pseudomonas toxin A. *Proceedings of the National Academy of Sciences of the United States of America* 81: 2703-2707.

Leis, S., Spindler, J., Reiter, J., Breinig, F., & Schmitt, M.J. (2005). *S. cerevisiae*K28 toxin - a secreted virus toxin of the A/B family of protein toxins. In: Schmitt, M.J., Schaffrath, R. (eds.) *Topics in Current Genetics, Microbial Protein Toxins*, vol. 11, Springer-Verlag, Berlin, Heidelberg, New York, pp. 111-132.

Le Maistre, C.F., Craig, F.E., Meneghetti, C., McMullin, B., Parker, K., Reuben, J., Boldt, D.H., Rosenblum, M., & Woodworth, T. (1992). Phase I trial of a 90-minute infusion of the fusion toxin DAB486 IL-2 in hematological cancers. *Cancer Research* 53: 3930-3934.

Liu, S., & Leppla, S.H. (2003). Retroviral insertional mutagenesis identifies a small protein required for synthesis of diphthamide, the target of bacterial ADP-ribosylating toxins. *Molecular Cell* 12: 603-613.

Liu, S., Milne, G.T., Kuremsky, J.G., Fink, G.R., & Leppla, S.H. (2004). Identification of the proteins required for biosynthesis of diphthamide, the target of bacterial ADP-ribosylating toxins on translation elongation factor 2. *Molecular and Cellular Biology* 24: 9487-9497.

Liu, S., Wiggins, J.F., Sreenath, T., Kulkarni, A.B., Ward, J.M., & Leppla, S.H. (2006). Dph3, a small protein required for diphthamide biosynthesis, is essential in mouse development. *Molecular and Cellular Biology* 26: 3835-3841.

Lord, J.L, & Roberts, L.M. (2005). Ricin: structure, synthesis and mode of action. In: Schmitt MJ, Schaffrath R, eds. *Topics in Current Genetics, Microbial Protein Toxins*, vol. 11, Springer-Verlag, Berlin, Heidelberg, New York; pp. 215-233.

Lu, J., Huang, B., Esberg, A., Johansson, M.J., & Byström, A.S. (2006). The *Kluyveromyces lactis* gamma-toxin targets tRNA anticodons. *RNA* 11: 1648-1654.

Mattheakis, L.C., Shen, W.H., & Collier, R.J. (1992). *DPH5*, a methyltransferase gene required for diphthamide biosynthesis in *Saccharomyces cerevisiae*. *Molecular and Cellular Biology* 12: 4026-4037.

McClatchy, J.K., Tsang, A.Y., & Cernich, M.S. (1981). Use of pyrazinamidase activity on Mycobacterium tuberculosis as a rapid method for determination of pyrazinamide susceptibility. *Antimicrobial Agents and Chemotherapy* 20: 556–557.

Meinhardt, F., Schaffrath, R., & Larsen, M. (1997). Microbial linear plasmids. *Applied Microbiology and Biotechnology* 47: 329-336.

Moehring, T.J., Danley, D.E., Moehring, J.M. (1984) *In vitro* biosynthesis of diphthamide, studied with mutant Chinese hamster ovary cells resistant to diphtheria toxin. *Molecular and Cellular Biology* 4: 642-650.

Murphy, J.R. (1996). *Corynebacterium diphtheriae*. In: Baron S, ed. *Medical Microbiology*, 4th edition, Chapter 32, The University of Texas Medical Branch at Galveston, 1996. Available at: http://www.ncbi.nlm.nih.gov/books/NBK7971/

Newland, J.W., Strockbine, N.A., Miller, S.F., O'Brien, A.D., & Holmes, R.K. (1985). Cloning of Shiga-like toxin structural genes from a toxin converting phage of *Escherichia coli*. *Science* 230: 179-181.

Nobukuni, Y., Kohno, K., & Miyagawa, K. (2005). Gene trap mutagenesis-based forward genetic approach reveals that the tumor suppressor *OVCA1* is a component of the biosynthetic pathway of diphthamide on elongation factor 2. *Journal of Biological Chemistry* 280: 10572-10577.

Ortiz, P.A., Ulloque, R., Kihara, G.K., Zheng, H., & Kinzy, T.G. (2006). Translation elongation factor 2 anticodon mimicry domain mutants affect fidelity and diphtheria toxin resistance. *Journal of Biological Chemistry* 281: 32639–32648.

Pappenheimer, A.M. (1977). Diphtheria toxin. *Annual Review of Biochemistry* 46: 69-94.

Pappenheimer, A.M., (1984). Diphtheria. In Germanier, R. (ed.) *Bacterial Vaccines*. Academic Press, San Diego.

Proudfoot, M., Sanders, S.A., Singer, A., Zhang, R., Brown, G., Binkowski, A., Xu, L., Lukin, J.A., Murzin, A.G., Joachimiak, A., Arrowsmith, C.H., Edwards, A.M., Savchenko, A.V., & Yakunin AF. (2008). Biochemical and structural characterization of a novel family of cystathionine beta-synthase domain proteins fused to a Zn ribbon-like domain. *Journal of Molecular Biology* 375: 301-315.

Rappuoli, R., Perugini, M., & Falsen, E. (1988). Molecular epidemiology of the 1984–1986 outbreak of diphtheria in Sweden. *New England Journal of Medicine* 318: 12-14.

Ratts, R., & Murphy, J.R. (2005). Diphtheria toxin, diphtheria-related fusion protein toxins and the molecular mechanism of their action against eukaryotic cells. In: Schmitt MJ, Schaffrath R, eds. *Topics in Current Genetics, Microbial Protein Toxins*, vol. 11, Springer-Verlag, Berlin, Heidelberg, New York; pp. 1-20.

Roux, E., & Yersin, A. (1888) Contribution al'etude de la diphtheriae. *Annales de l'Institut Pasteur* 2: 629-661.

Sandvig, K., Wälchli, S., & Lauvrak, S.U. (2005). Shiga toixns and their mechnaisms of cell entry. In: Schmitt MJ, Schaffrath R, eds. *Topics in Current Genetics, Microbial Protein Toxins*, vol. 11, Springer-Verlag, Berlin, Heidelberg, New York; pp. 35-53.

Schaffrath, R., & Meinhardt, F. (2005) *Kluyveromyces lactis* zymocin and other plasmid-encoded yeast killer toxins. In: Schmitt, M.J., Schaffrath, R. (eds.) *Topics in Current Genetics, Microbial Protein Toxins*, vol. 11, Springer-Verlag, Berlin, Heidelberg, New York, pp. 133-155.

Schaffrath, R., Meinhardt, F., Meacock, P.A. (1999). Molecular manipulation of *Kluyveromyceslactis* linear DNA plasmids: Gene targeting and plasmid shuffles. *FEMS Microbiology Letters* 178: 201-210.

Schmitt, M.J., & Schaffrath, R. (2005) *Microbial Protein Toxins, Topics in Current Genetics*, vol. 11, Springer-Verlag, Berlin, Heidelberg, New York.

Sitikov, A.S., Davydova, E.K., Bezlepkina, T.A., Ovchinnikov, L.P., & Spirin, A.S. (1984). Eukaryotic elongation factor 2 loses its non-specific affinity for RNA and leaves polyribosomes as a result of ADP-ribosylation. *FEBS Letters* 176: 406-410.

Sjölinder, M., Uhlmann, J., & Ponstingl, H. (2002). DelGEF, a homologue of the Ran guanine nucleotide exchange factor RanGEF, binds to the exocyst component Sec5 and modulates secretion. *FEBS Letters* 532: 211-215.

Sjölinder, M., Uhlmann, J., & Ponstingl, H. (2004). Characterisation of an evolutionary conserved protein interacting with the putative guanine nucleotide exchange factor DelGEF and modulating secretion. *Experimental Cell Research* 294: 68-76.

Solders, G, Nennesmo, I., & Persson, A. (1989). Diphtheritic neuropathy, an analysis based on muscle and nerve biopsy and repeated neurophysiological and autonomic function tests. *Journal of Neurology, Neurosurgery and Psychiatry* 52: 876–880.

Sugisaki, Y., Gunge, N., Sakaguchi, K., Yamasaki, M., & Tamura, G. (1985). Transfer of DNA killer plasmids from *Kluyveromyces lactis* to *Kluyveromyces fragilis* and *Candida pseudotropicalis*. *Journal of Bacteriology* 164: 1373-1375.

Sun, J., Zhang, J., Wu, F., Xu, C., Li, S., Zhao, W., Wu, Z., Wu, J., Zhou, C.Z., & Shi, Y. (2005). Solution structure of Kti11p from *Saccharomyces cerevisiae* reveals a novel zinc-binding module. *Biochemistry* 44: 8801-8809.

Tao, X., Schiering, N., Zeng, H.Y., Ringe, D., & Murphy, J.R. (1994). Iron, DtxR, and the regulation of diphtheria toxin expression. *Molecular Microbiology* 14:191-197.

Todar, K. (2004). Web Review of Todar's Online Textbook of Bacteriology. *The Good, the Bad, and the Deadly*. Chapter Diptheria (*Corynebacterium diphtheriae*).

Tokunaga, M., Kawamura, A., Kitada, K., Hishinuma, F. (1990). Secretion of killer toxin encoded on the linear DNA plasmid pGKL1 from *Saccharomyces cerevisiae*. *Journal of Biological Chemistry* 265: 17274-17280.

Uchida, T., Gill, D.M., & Pappenheimer, A.M. (1971). Mutation in the structural gene for diphtheria toxin carried by temperate phage. *Nature - New Biology* 233: 8-11.

Uthman, S., Kheir, E., Bär, C., Jablonowski, D., & Schaffrath, R. (2011). Growth inhibition strategies based on antimicrobial microbes/toxins. In: *Science against Microbial Pathogens: Communicating Current Research and Technological Advances*, Mendez-Vilas A., ed., Formatex, Badajoz, Spain, in press.

Van der Spek, J., Cosenza, L., Woodworth, T., Nichols JC, Murphy J.R. (1994). Diphtheria toxin-related cytokine fusion proteins: elongation factor 2 as a target for the treatment of neoplastic disease. *Molecular and Cellular Biochemistry* 138: 151-156.

Van Ness, B.G., Howard, J.B., & Bodley, J.W. (1980). ADP-ribosylation of elongation factor 2 by diphtheria toxin. NMR spectra and proposed structures of ribosyl-diphthamide and its hydrolysis products *Journal of Biological Chemistry* 255: 10710-10716.

von Hunolstein, C., Alfarone, G., Scopetti, F., Pataracchia, M., La Valle, R., Franchi, F., Pacciani, L., Manera, A., Giammanco, A., Farinelli, S., Engler, K, De Zoysa, A., & Efstratiou, A. (2003). Molecular epidemiology and characteristics of Corynebacterium diphtheriae and Corynebacterium ulcerans strains isolated in Italy during the 1990s. *Journal of Medical Microbiology* 52: 181-188.

Waldor, M.K., & Mekalanos, J.J. (1996). Lysogenic conversion by a filamentous phage encoding cholera toxin. *Science* 272: 1910–1914.

Webb, T.R., Cross, S.H., McKie, L., Edgar, R., Vizor, L., Harrison, J., Peters, J., & Jackson, I.J. (2008). Diphthamide modification of eEF2 requires a J-domain protein and is essential for normal development. *Journal of Cell Science* 121: 3140-3145.

White-Gilbertson, S., Kurtz, D.T., & Voelkel-Johnson, C. (2009). The role of protein synthesis in cell cycling and cancer. *Molecular Oncology* 3: 402-408.

Willshaw, G.A., Smith, H.R., Scotland, S.M., & Rowe, B. (1985). Cloning of genes determining the production of vero cytotoxin by *Escherichia coli*. *Journal of General Microbiology* 131: 3047-3053.

Zabel, R., Bär, C., Mehlgarten, C., & Schaffrath, R. (2008). Yeast alpha-tubulin suppressor Ats1/Kti13 relates to the Elongator complex and interacts with Elongator partner protein Kti11. *Molecular Microbiology* 69: 175-187.

Zhang, Y., Liu, S., Lajoie, G., & Merrill A.R. (2008). The role of the diphthamide-containing loop within eukaryotic elongation factor 2 in ADP-ribosylation by *Pseudomonas aeruginosa* exotoxin A. *Biochemical Journal* 413: 163-174.

Zhang, Y., Zhu, X., Torelli, A.T., Lee, M., Dzikovski, B., Koralewski, R.M., Wang, E., Freed, J., Krebs, C., Ealick, S.E., & Lin, H. (2010). Diphthamide biosynthesis requires an organic radical generated by an iron-sulphur enzyme. *Nature* 465: 891-896.

18

Diphtheria Toxin and Cytosolic Translocation Factors

Ryan C. Ratts[1] and John R. Murphy[2]
[1]*Dartmouth Medical School*
[2]*Boston University School of Medicine*
USA

1. Introduction

Diphtheria Toxin (DT) was the first investigated bacterial protein toxin. As one of the most extensively studied bacterial protein toxins, it has served as a model system for the analysis of other protein toxins (Pappenheimer, 1977). As reviewed by Pappenheimer, Loeffler identified *Corynebacterium diphtheriae* as the causative agent of diphtheria in 1884, and the toxin was first described in the culture medium of *C. diphtheriae* by Roux and Yersin in 1888. The gene for DT is encoded by a family of closely related corynebacteriophages (Uchida et al., 1971; Greenfield et al., 1983), and is expressed only under conditions of iron deprivation (Pappenheimer, 1977). Regulation of DT expression is under control of the iron-activated diphtheria toxin repressor, DTxR, which is encoded in the *C. diphtheriae* genome and inhibits transcription of DT in the presence of iron and other transition metal ions (Love and Murphy, 2000).

DT is translated with a 25 amino acid signal peptide and is co-translationally secreted as a single 535 amino acid residue polypeptide chain with a molecular weight of 58 kDa (Smith, 1980; Kaczorek et al., 1983). Biochemical analysis of DT demonstrated that proteolytic 'nicking' of the toxin *in vitro* results in two fragments, A and B, which remain covalently attached by an inter-chain disulfide bond (Gill and Pappenheimer, 1971). Fragment A contains the enzymatic activity (Collier and Kandel, 1971), whereas Fragment B mediates binding to cell surface receptors and facilitates the cytosolic entry of fragment A (Drazin et al., 1971). X-ray crystallographic analysis, at a resolution of 2.5 Å, demonstrated that DT is composed of three structural domains: the amino terminal catalytic (C) domain corresponds to fragment A (21 kDa), and the transmembrane (T) and carboxy terminal receptor binding (R) domains comprise fragment B (37 kDa) (Figure 1) (Choe et al., 1992). A disulfide bond between Cys186 and Cys201 subtends a 14 amino acid protease sensitive loop and connects fragment A with fragment B (Gill and Pappenheimer, 1971). Furin mediated cleavage within this loop and retention of the disulfide bond have been shown to be pre-requisites for intoxication of eukaryotic cells (Ariansen et al., 1993; Tsuneoka et al., 1993).

Once delivered into cytosol, the C-domain catalyzes the NAD+-dependent ADP-ribosylation of elongation factor 2 (EF-2). EF-2 is a soluble translocase involved in protein synthesis, and is the only known substrate for the DT C domain in eukaryotic cells (Pappenheimer, 1977). Transfer of the ADP-ribosyl moiety of NAD^+ to a modified histidine residue in EF-2 (diphthamide) results in the irreversible arrest of chain elongation during protein synthesis (Collier and Cole, 1969), leading to cell death by apoptosis.

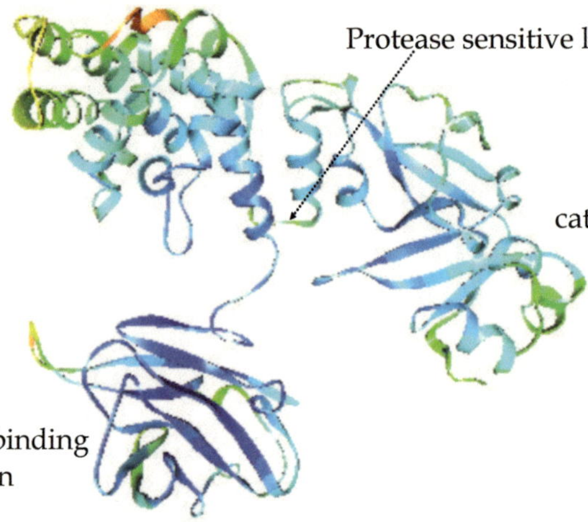

Fig. 1. X-Ray Crystallographic Structure of Diphtheria Toxin. PDB 1 MDT. Modified from Choe et al., 1992.

2. Receptor binding

Intoxication by DT involves an ordered sequence of events in which each structural domain of the toxin plays a precise and essential role and begins with toxin binding to cells expressing the heparin binding epidermal growth factor-like precursor (Figure 2) (Naglich et al., 1992). The sensitivity of targeted cells to intoxication by DT is roughly related to the number of receptors present on the cell surface, and is also enhanced by the diphtheria toxin receptor associated protein 27, DTRAP 27, which is the primate homologue of human CD9 (Mitamura et al., 1992). Human CD9 antigen, which is associated with the DT receptor but not DT itself, enhances sensitivity to DT through an unknown mechanism (Brown et al, 1993; Iwamoto et al., 1994),. In contrast to other AB toxins - such as abrin, ricin, and cholera - neither gangliosides nor galactosides have any effect on DT binding and intoxication (Pappenheimer, 1977).

In 1896, Paul Ehrlic coined the phrase "Zauberkugeln", or "magic bullet," for specifically targeting cells causing disease. This dream was realized almost a hundred years later by Murphy et al. (1986) with the design and synthesis of DT based fusion protein toxins that were targeted toward specific eukaryotic cell receptors. Substitution of the native R domain with a surrogate ligand results in the formation of a fusion protein toxin construct that targets cells expressing the appropriate cell surface receptor. The first genetically engineered fusion protein toxin, $DAB_{486}MSH$, consisted of DT fragment A and a portion of fragment B fused to α-melanocyte stimulating hormone (α-MSH) (Murphy et al., 1986). While this fusion protein toxin construct was prone to degradation, human interleukin 2 (IL-2) was selected as the next surrogate receptor binding domain and DAB_{486}IL-2 was next constructed (Williams et al., 1987). DAB_{486}IL-2 proved resistant to degradation, was

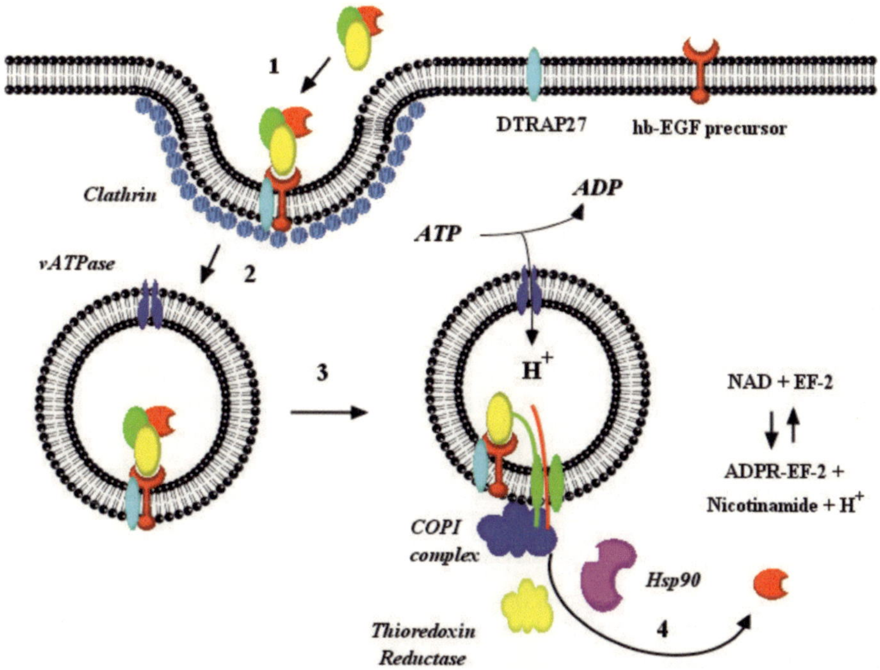

Fig. 2. Schematic Overiew of DT Intoxication. (1) DT binds to its cell surface receptor (2) Internalization of clathrin coated pits into early endosomal vesicles (3) Acidification of the endosomal lumen induces DT T domain insertion and pore formation (4) Translocation and cytosolic release of the DT C domain is facilitated by COPI complex, Thioredoxin Reductase and Hsp90. Refolded DT C domain catalyzes the ADP-ribosylation of EF-2. Diphtheria toxin: yellow = receptor binding (R) domain; green = transmembrane (T) domain; red = catalytic (C) domain. Reproduced from Murphy (2011).

remarkably potent (IC_{50} of 1 x 10^{-11} M), and was specifically targeted to cells only expressing high affinity IL-2 receptors (Bacha et al., 1980; Williams et al., 1990). Subsequent in-frame deletion analysis of the carboxy terminal residues in the DT portion of DAB_{486}IL-2 demonstrated that incorporation of a smaller portion of the diphtheria toxin fragment B, DAB_{389}IL-2, resulted in a chimeric toxin that was 10-fold more cytotoxic (Williams et al., 1990).

In the case of DAB_{389}IL-2, only the high affinity and intermediate affinity IL-2 receptor - toxin complexes are internalized (Waters et al., 1990). The specific expression of the high affinity IL-2 receptor on only activated and proliferating T-cells made DAB_{389}IL-2 a potential therapeutic agent for the treatment of both T-cell mediated malignancies and autoimmune diseases (Ratts and vanderSpek, 2002). In 1999, DAB_{389}IL-2 (ONTAK®) was the first fusion protein toxin construct approved by the U.S. Food and Drug Administration for clinical use in humans, and is currently used for the treatment of CD25 positive refractory cutaneous T cell lymphoma (Ratts and vanderSpek,2002). In designing fusion protein constructs, only those surrogate ligands that trigger clathrin dependent endocytosis, analogous to the mechanism of entry of endogenous DT, are functional. There are currently more than 20 different fusion protein toxins under clinical development. Since DAB_{389}IL-2 binds with greater affinity to its receptor compared to native DT, this fusion protein toxin has proven to be an effective and novel probe for studying internalization of the C-domain by target cells.

3. Endocytosis

Receptor bound DT is concentrated in clathrin coated pits and internalized into clathrin coated vesicles (CCVs), which are then converted into early endosomes (Moya et al. 1985). Assembly of the clathrin coat is inhibited by depletion of intercellular potassium, and cells are protected against DT under such conditions (Moya et al., 1985; Sandvig et al., 1985). Sequestration of the coated pit from the plasma membrane requires additional proteins, including the GTPase dynamin (Simpson et al., 1998). Simpson et al. (1998) demonstrated that over expression of dominant negative dynamin blocks clathrin dependent endocytosis and protects cells against DT. Successful detachment of the coated pit results in CCVs which are subsequently released into the cytoplasm. After entering the cytoplasm, the CCVs are uncoated in an ATPase dependent manner and the subsequent homotypic fusion of uncoated vesicles results in the formation of early endosomes (Luzio et al., 2001). The clathrin triskelon is replaced with a new set of protein components on the vesicle membrane that includes Arf-1, COPI complex, Rab-5, early endosomal antigen (EEA1), and vesicular (v)-ATPase. Although the precise mechanism is unclear, the dynamic docking and release of these factors activates the process of membrane fusion through the formation of a fusion pore and activation of v-ATPase (Luzio et al, 2001).

The characteristic feature of endosomes is acidification of the lumen by v-ATPase. Acidification promotes protein sorting by dissociating ligand-receptor complexes and allowing some receptors to be recycled back to the plasma membrane. Acidification is also required for the formation of endosomal carrier vesicles (ECVs), which carry ligands and non-dissociated ligand-receptor complexes from early to late endosomes. Bafilomycin A1, a specific inhibitor of v-ATPase, blocks acidification and prevents the formation of ECVs, resulting in the accumulation of early endosomes (Bowman, et al.,1988). The formation of ECVs requires the binding of both β'COP (Sec 27) and ADP-ribosylation factor 1 (ARF1) to the cytoplasmic surface of the endosomal membrane, and binding of both factors is dependent upon a low pH within the endosomal lumen (Aniento et al., 1996). Inward invaginations of the endosomal membrane also occurs during ECV formation, resulting in the production of multi-vesicular bodies (Futter et al., 1996).

Several studies have confirmed the early endosomal compartment as the site fragment A translocation. Merion et al. (1983) showed that endosomes isolated from DT resistant mutants of chinese hamster ovary (CHO)-K1 cells were defective in acidification. In contrast, lysosomes isolated from the same mutants were not defective in acidification, suggesting that the endosomal compartment was the site of fragment A translocation (Merion et al., 1983). Umata et al. (1990) demonstrated that Bafilomycin A1, which prevents acidification of the endosomal lumen, protected cells against DT intoxication.

Cell fractionation experiments provided the best evidence that DT translocation occurs from early endosomes (Papini et al., 1993a; Papini et al. 1993b; Lemichez et al., 1997). While the DT C domain is most efficiently translocated from early endosomes, the majority of the toxin is actually sorted into ECVs and late endosomes where translocation of the C domain into the cytosol is marginal (Lemichez et al., 1997). Toxin trapped within ECVs and late endosomes is ultimately targeted for lysosomes and degraded. Lemichez et al. (1997) provided two possible explanations for why toxin failed to translocate from ECVs or late endosomes: First, there might be cytosolic factors specific to early endosomes required for translocation. Second, translocation events might actually be occurring in the ECVs, but such events within the multi-vesicular body would result in the vectorial transfer of the DT C domain into the lumen of another intra-vaculolar vesicle rather than the cytosol.

4. Role for acidification

Ammonium salts (e.g., NH_4Cl), glutamine and other amines, and choloroquine were the first compounds found to inhibit the cytosolic entry of the DT (Kim et al., 1965; Sandvig et al., 1980). Although these compounds had no effect upon neither enzymatic activity nor receptor binding, these reagents did protect sensitive cells against DT intoxication. Choloroquine and ammonium salts are ionophores, and they raise the luminal pH of endosomes and lysosomes. These results led to the hypothesis that passage of DT through a low pH compartment was a required step for intoxication. Umata et al. (1990) confirmed this hypothesis by demonstrating that acidification of the endosomal lumen by membrane associated vesicular (v)-ATPase was a required step in DT intoxication.

In contrast to the endosomal route, low pH (5.5) exposure of toxin bound to the surface of cells results in decreased protein synthesis even in the presence of choloroquine and ammonium ions (Sandvig et al., 1980). This same study demonstrated that the entry of pre-nicked diphtheria toxin through the cell membrane in the low pH environment was time and temperature dependent. Using the same system, Sandvig and Olsnses (1981) also demonstrated that the cytosolic entry of the DT C domain could be blocked by the metabolic inhibitors 2-deoxyglucose and sodium azide, implying that a cellular ATPase was required for the membrane translocation of the DT C domain (Sandvig et al., 1981).

Pronase protection assays were used to examine which portions of DT inserted into the plasma membrane when toxin bound cells were exposed to low pH (Moskaug et al., 1991). Moskaug et al. (1991) found a translocated fragment A (20 kD) in the cytosol and a plasma membrane associated 25 kDa peptide derived from fragment B. Furthermore, an inwardly directed proton gradient was required for the translocation of fragment A, but not for membrane insertion of fragment B (Sandvig et al., 1988). Analogously, it has also been shown that translocation of fragment A requires a lower pH as compared to the membrane insertion of fragment B (Falnes et al., 1992).

5. Pore formation

Exposure of DT transmembrane (T) domain to artificial lipid bilayers at low pH results in spontaneous membrane insertion and the formation of voltage dependent and cation selective channels (Boquet et al., 1976; Donovan et al., 1981). Kagan et al. (1981) observed a channel diameter of approximately 18-22 Å, which is theoretically large enough to accommodate the passage of a fully denatured fragment A. The crystal structure of DT shows that the T domain is composed of nine α-helices (TH1-9) and their connecting loops, and that the helices are arranged in three layers (Figure 1, Choe et al., 1992). The first three helices (TH1-3) comprise the first layer and are amphipathic in nature. Helices TH5, 6, and 7 compose a second hydrophobic layer. The third, central core layer is composed of the hydrophobic helices TH8 and 9, connected by transmembrane loop 5 (TL5).

Insertion of this third α-helical layer (Th8-9) is required for pore formation, which is then stabilized by the second α-helical layer (TH5, 6, and 7). Assays used to measure the formation and conductance of membrane pores, such as patch clamp experiments, molecular marker exclusion studies, and pH sensitive dyes have been used in conjunction with diphtheria toxin mutants to demonstrate the importance of specific residues in pore formation and support this model of helix insertion (Figure 3). Upon acidifcation of the endosomal lumen, residues Glu 349 and Asp 352 located at the tip of loop (TL5) connecting TH8 and TH9 are protonated, and the third helical layer spontaneously inserts into the membrane and forms a cation selective channel (O'Keefe et al., 1992; Mindell et al., 1994). Deletion or disruption of these helices by introducing proline residues ablates channel formation and results in non-cytotoxic mutants (vanderSpek et al., 1994a; Hu et al., 1998), suggesting that the full length helices arranged in a specific conformation is required for channel formation. While helices TH8 and 9 alone can create pores (Silverman et al., 1994), pore formation by TH8 and 9 alone is not sufficient for effective delivery of the C domain (vanderSpek et al., 1994a).

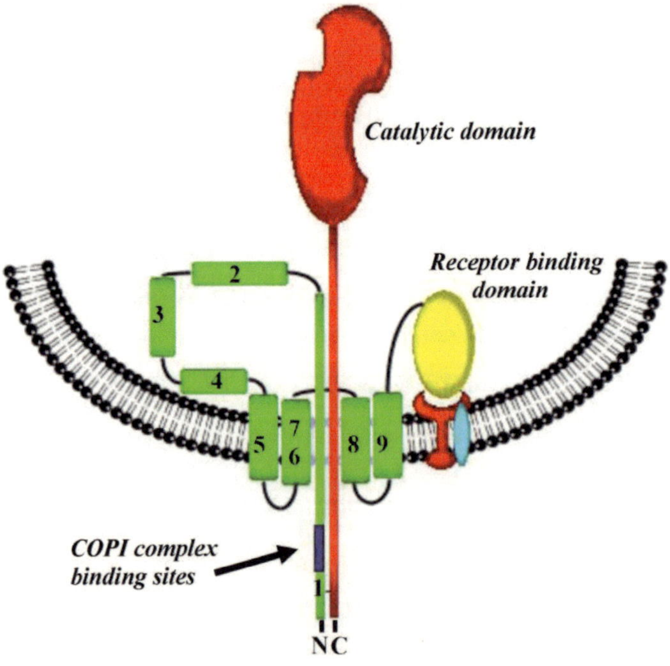

Fig. 3. Schematic of DT transmembrane (T) domain membrane insertion and pore formation. Following furin mediated nicking at Arg194 and denaturation of the catalytic (C) domain, the *N*-terminal portion of the T domain with the disulfide bond linked *C*-terminal end of the C domain is threaded into the pore. Emergence of one or more of the KXKXX motifs in first alpha helix (TH1) of the T domain on the cytosolic side of the vesicle membrane allows for binding of the COPI complex required for translocation of the catalytic domain. Reproduced from Murphy (2011).

The role that the Pro 345 residue, located at the end of TH8, plays in channel formation remains unclear. Mutation of Pro 345 to either a Glu residue, an α-helix former, or to a Gln residue, an α-helix breaker, resulted in a marked decrease in DT toxicity (Johnson et al., 1993). The *cis-trans* isomerization of proline by membrane associated peptidylprolyl *cis-trans* isomerases (PPIases), or cyclophilins, is important in the gating mechanisms of other cation selective channels, and a role for PPIases in DT channel formation or translocation of the DT C domain have been proposed (Johnson et al., 1993).

Following membrane insertion of the third helical layer, the second helical layer is subsequently inserted next and is thought to stabilize the channel formed by helices TH8 and 9 (Cabiaux et al., 1993; Cabiaux et al. 1994). Insertion of proline residues into the second helical layer of DAB_{389}IL-2 resulted in non-cytotoxic mutants with abnormal channel formation (Hu et al., 1998). Although this layer is not required for channel formation, it appears that the second helical layer is required for the formation of productive channels capable of supporting C domain translocation across the early endosomal membrane.

Deletion of the first three helices of DAB_{389}IL-2 resulted in a non-cytotoxic mutant that still formed characteristic channels and retained enzymatic activity (vanderSpek et al., 1993). The amino terminal residues of TH1 are translocated across the membrane and presented to the cytosol (Madshus et al., 1994a). Replacement of the charged residues in TH1 with uncharged residues strongly inhibits translocation of TH1 (Madshus et al., 1994a, vanderSpek et al., 1994b). The insertion of proline residues into the first helical layer also resulted in non-cytotoxic mutants that formed characteristic channels and retained enzymatic activity (Hu et al., 1998).

Taken together, these results suggested that the first helical layer facilitates the orientation and insertion of the C domain through the nascent channel formed by the T domain. Assuming that the disulfide bond connecting fragments A and fragment B remains intact, translocation of amino terminal residues of TH1 across the endosomal membrane would be anticipated to effectively thread the carboxy terminal residues of the C domain through the nascent channel and present them to the cytosol (vanderSpek et al., 1994b), and this work implied possible interactions with an unidentified translocation apparatus. These early findings were prescient of the recent identification of the T1 motif in TH1 by Ratts et al (2005) and role of the di-lysine motif KXKXX in recruiting components COPI complex required for toxin entry that is discussed below (Trujillo et al., 2010).

6. Unfolding of the catalytic domain

Unfolding of the DT C domain occurs *in vitro* in acidic conditions similar to those found inside the lumen of the endosome, and unfolding is required for delivery. Given the limited size of the pore, unfolding of the DT C domain was postulated as a pre-requisite for translocation (Donovan et al., 1981; Kagan et al., 1981). The necessity for complete denaturation of the DT C domain prior to translocation was then indirectly demonstrated by (Wiedlocha et al., 1992) and by (Falnes et al., 1994). Wiedlocha et al. (1992) fused acidic fibroblast growth factor (aFGF) to the amino terminus of fragment A. This aFGF-DT fusion protein construct was cytotoxic, confirming the observation that polypeptides fused to fragment A are delivered into the cytosol of targeted cells (Stenmark et al., 1991). In the presence of heparin, however, aFGF retains a rigid tertiary structure and the aFGF-DT fusion protein was no longer cytotoxic, implying that unfolding is a requirement for delivery through the nascent channel formed by the T domain. Falsnes et al. (1994) also created a double cysteine mutant which formed a disulfide bond within fragment A. With the disulfide bond intact, unfolding of fragment A does not occur. This mutant retained ADP-ribosyltransferase activity, but it was not cytotoxic. Taken together, these studies indicated that the cytosolic delivery of the C domain occurs in at least a partially unfolded state and that once delivered into the cytosol, the C domain must be refolded into an active conformation.

7. Reduction of the interchain disulfide bond

The C domain is separated from the T and R domains by a protease sensitive loop that is sub-tended by the disulfide bond between residues Cys 186 and Cys 201. Upon binding and internalization of the toxin-receptor complex, this loop is nicked by the enzyme furin (Tsuneoka et al., 1993). Retention of the interchain disulfide bond following nicking is a pre-requisite for intoxication (Falsnes et al., 1992), and it presumably mediates threading the DT C domain through the channel formed by the T domain. The pivotal role of reducing the inter-chain disulfide bond is underscored by the observation that reduction and release of the C domain appears to be the rate limiting step for the entire intoxication process (Papini et al., 1993b).

The precise location where reduction of the DT inter-chain dilsulfide bond occurs remains somewhat controversial. Moskaug et al. (1987) showed that only membrane permeate sulfhydryl blockers were able to prevent the release of the C-domain into cytosol. Papini et al. (1993b) reported that reduction of the DT interchain disulfide bond occurs after the low pH induced membrane insertion of the T domain within the early endosome. Since unreduced DT C domain and membrane inserted DT fragment B are both targeted for proteolytic degradation (Madshus et al. 1994b), these results suggested that reduction of the interchain disulfide bond occurs during or post-translocation. In contrast, Ryser et al. (1991) found that membrane impermeate sulfhydryl blockers prevented DT intoxication, and proposed that reduction occurs prior to translocation, presumably on the cell surface or within the endosomal lumen. *In vitro* studies have shown that thioredoxin 1 (Trx-1) (12 kDa) reduces the DT inter-chain disulfide bond under acidic conditions (Moskaug et al., 1987). This result is consistent with observations that exposure of the DT interchain disulfide bond on the protein surface occurs upon denaturation (Blewitt et al., 1985). Trx-1 is predominately cytosolic, but a shorter form (10 kDa) is actively secreted by a non-classical ER-Golgi independent pathway and is present on the luminal side of the endosomal membrane (Rosen et al., 1995). It is not known whether or not Trx-1 interacts directly with DT *in vivo.*

8. Model for autonomous delivery

Initial studies of T domain insertion and pore formation in artificial lipid bilayers in the presence of a pH gradient led to the hypothesis of autonomous delivery of the C domain, and Deleers et al (1983) first suggested that a pH gradient was required to facilitate C-domain delivery. Shiver and Donovan (1987), using asolectin vesicles, demonstrated that diphtheria toxin could deliver its own C-domain across the artificial bilayer in a pH dependent fashion, independent of added proteins or factors. These studies demonstrated a requirement for a pH gradient, in which the endocytic vesicle luminal pH is optimally between 4.7 and 5.5 and the cytosolic pH is at or near 7.4. The topography of DT inserted into both cell plasma membranes and artificial bilayers has been studied using protease digestion and analyzing the enzymatic cleavage products (Moskaug et al, 1991, Cabiaux et al, 1994). Although insertion of transmembrane helices 8 and 9 is a common finding of these studies, discrepancies arise in interpreting cleavage products that include the C-domain and whether or not they represent translocation intermediates (Madhus, 1994). Taken together, the apparent ability of DT to transfer its C-domain across synthetic lipid bilayers, in the absence of other proteins, led to a model of autonomous C-domain delivery.

The model of autonomous C-domain delivery was advanced by Oh et al. (1999) using planar lipid membranes and DT labeled with an *N*-terminal histidine tag (6× His). Since addition of Ni2+ to the *trans* compartment prevented the rapid closure of pores, these investigators concluded that the N- terminal end of the C-domain containing the His tag was translocated from the *cis* to the *trans* side of the lipid bilayer upon channel formation by the T-domain. These investigators also used biotin to label cysteine site-directed mutants at either position 58 or 148. The addition of streptavidin to the *trans* side of the planar lipid membrane also interfered with the channel closure. Again, these results suggested that Cys_{58} and Cys_{148} were on the *trans* side of the membrane following channel formation.

Also using artificial lipid bilayers, Ren et al. (1999) demonstrated that in a low pH environment, the presence of proteins in a partly unfolded molten globule-like conformation (e.g. unfolded C-domain) were able to convert the T domain from a shallow membrane inserted form to a fully *trans*- membrane inserted form. Hammond et al (2002) confirmed that the DT T-domain has chaperonin-like properties, but also observed that the T domain had a significantly greater affinity for other molten globule-like polypeptides compared to its own C-domain. The chaperonin-like property of membrane inserted T domain towards unfolded substrates under acidic conditions has been confirmed (Hayashibara *et al*, 2005; Chassaing *et al.*, 2011).

In the autonomous translocation model, delivery of the C-domain is thought to be achieved through the chaperonin-like activity of the T-domain. Although these studies clearly demonstrate ability for DT to utilize a pH gradient, in conjunction with a relatively high membrane potential, to mediate autonomous translocation *in vitro*, it is not at all clear that these conditions occur *in vivo*. Many proteins are imbedded in the endosomal membrane and decorate both the luminal and cytosolic face of endocytic vesicles, and the impact these proteins may have on toxin delivery across the endosomal membrane are not included in artificial membrane bilayer systems. Since protease digestion patterns of DT inserted into planar lipid bilayers differ from those of DT inserted into the plasma membrane (Moskaug et al., 1991; Cabiaux et al., 1994), it seems likely that interaction(s) between the toxin and proteins associated with the endosomal membrane influence the orientation and/or stoichiometry of T-domain membrane insertion and translocation of the C-domain.

9. Model for facilitated delivery

A role for cellular factors in facilitating DT membrane translocation was first suggested by Sandvig and Olsnses (1981) with their observation that the successful delivery of toxin artificially inserted into the plasma membrane under acidic conditions required the function of a cellular ATPase. This hypothesis was expanded by Kaneda et al (1984), who established hybrid cell lines resistant to DT and demonstrated that the resistance of these cell lines appeared to be independent of receptor binding, receptor trafficking, and susceptibility of EF2 to ADP-ribosylation. They concluded that the resistance of these hybrid lines was due to cellular factors required for toxin entry.

The rationale for cellular factors facilitating the delivery of the DT C-domain across the endosomal membrane is congruent with other known and similar mechanisms of protein translocation across membranes within eukaryotic cells such as mitochondrial import, ER synthesis, and the retrograde translocation of toxins from the ER. During mitochondrial import, an electrochemical membrane potential is initially required for insertion of the proteins synthesized in the cytosol into the translocation complex and its subsequent transfer to the translocation complex present on the mitochondrial inner membrane (Bauer et al., 2000). The inward movement of the protein, however, requires unfolding and its translocation into the mitochondrial matrix is mediated by an ATP dependent import motor consisting of at least three components, including mitochondrial heat shock protein 70 (Hsp 70) (Bauer et al., 2000). The translocation of newly synthesized proteins into the ER occurs co-translationally through channels formed by the Sec 61 translocon complex (Tsai et al., 2002). Bip, an ER luminal resident homologue of Hsp 70, functions analogously to mitochondrial Hsp 70 in mediating protein translocation into the ER lumen (Baker et al., 1996). In contrast, the ERAD pathway involves the retro-translocation of misfolded proteins, as well as several toxins (*e.g.* cholera, pseudomonas exotoxin A, ricin), from the ER lumen into the cytosol through the same Sec 61 channel (Tsai et al., 2002). In ERAD, as reviewed by Tsai et al (2002), misfolded luminal proteins are recognized and unfolded by chaperones prior to retro-translocation through the Sec 61 channel. Cellular factors that are conserved from yeast to humans, are then required for the extraction of from the ER membrane and their subsequent release into the cytosol. In all of these systems, translocation is facilitated by the sequential binding and refolding of denatured proteins by chaperonins as they emerge through the membrane.

Lemichez et al (1997) provided the first direct evidence supporting the hypothesis that delivery of the C-domain across the endosomal membrane requires both ATP and cytosolic factors. This pivotal study demonstrated that DT translocation occurs from within early endosomes, and that Bafilomycin A1 resulted in the accumulation of DT within the lumen of arrested early endosomes. These investigators established an *in vitro* translocation assay system using purified early endosomes pre-loaded with DT from cells treated with bafilomycin A1. The *in vitro* translocation of the C-domain across the endosomal membrane required the addition of both ATP and cytosolic factors. Lemichez et al (1997) also observed that DT co-localizes with β′COP in tubular structures, and that antibodies to β′COP inhibited the *in vitro* translocation of the DT C domain across the endosomal membrane.

10. Defining the DT Cytosolic Translocation Factor (CTF) complex

Using the *in vitro* translocation assay developed by Lemichez *et al.* (1997) as a purification assay, Ratts *et al.* (2003) confirmed and extended the observations that cytosolic translocation factors (CTFs) are essential for the translocation and release of the DT C-domain from the lumen of early endosomes pre-loaded with the fusion protein toxin DAB_{389}IL-2. Control endosomes loaded with horse radish peroxidase and a pH sensitive dye

(OG514) demonstrated that endosomal lysis did not occur and that the cytosolic factors were not required for endosomal acidification, respectively, under assay conditions. Protein complexes mediating toxin translocation were then partially purified from both human and yeast cytosolic extracts, and individual proteins were identified using mass spectrometry sequencing. The potential role of individual proteins as putative CTFs were then examined using specific inhibitors and/or neutralizing antibodies. Ratts et al (2003) showed that both heat shock protein 90 (Hsp 90) and thioredoxin reductase 1 (TrR-1), and their yeast homologues Hsp 82 and TrR, respectively, are components of the CTF complex required for DT entry. Importantly, CTF activity was limited to the translocation step and neither factor inhibited the enzymatic ADP-ribosylation of EF2 by the DT C-domain. Finally, a physiologic role for Hsp 90 and TrR-1 was confirmed using specific inhibitors in cytotoxicity assays to protect cells against toxin. Although Hsp 90, TrR-1, β-COP have all been confirmed as CTFs for the entry of diphtheria toxin, these factors alone are not sufficient for translocation (Ratts et al., 2003; Ratts et al 2005). The additional required components of the CTF remain to be identified. The *in vitro* translocation assay utilized by Lemichez et al (1997) and Ratts et al (2003) cannot distinguish between direct translocation of the DT C domain across the endosomal membrane and the release of the DT C domain from the cytosolic surface of the endosomal membrane. In either scenario, the assay system does accurately assess the physiological delivery of C-domain from lumen of early endosomes into the cytosol and the *in vitro* translocation assay has rapidly become the gold standard for studying toxin translocation across the endosomal membrane.

Protein complexes of similar composition to the diphtheria toxin CTF complex have been described in the protein-trapping proteomic analysis of yeast by Ho et al. (2002). Cyclophilin (Cpr6) trapped complexes from yeast contain Hsp 82, TrR-1 and Sec 27 (β-COP) (Ho et al, 2002). There are two considerations for interpreting the data obtained from protein-trapping proteomic analysis: First, the protein complexes are most likely of heterologous nature. Second, only the proteins that were readily detectable are included. Cyclophilin is functionally active in Hsp 90 chaperonin complexes, and a role for cyclophilin as a putative CTF will be discussed below. Surprisingly, EF-2 is present in several yeast complexes containing the diphtheria toxin CTFs (Ho et al., 2002), and Hsp 90 has previously been shown to directly interact with elongation factor-2 kinase (Palmquist et al., 1994). Recently, Bektas et al. (2011) provided evidence that EF-2 itself may augment the *in vitro* translocation of the DT C domain across endosomal membranes in the presence of actin filaments .

10.1 Hsp 90 functions as a CTF

Hsp 90 is ubiquitously expressed and comprises the core of several multi-molecular chaperonin complexes that are highly conserved in eukaryotes (Schulte et al., 1998). These complexes also contain additional chaperones, co-chaperones, and adapter proteins. Interaction of these proteins with Hsp 90 is mediated through a tetracopeptide repeat acceptor site (TPR domain) found in Hsp 90, and the formation of discrete subcomplexes with distinct co-chaperones mediates Hsp 90 substrate recognition (Caplan, 1999). Although Hsp 90 does not usually directly bind nor refold nascent polypeptides, it is known to refold a growing list of proteins including membrane associated protein kinases (Bijlmakers et al., 2000). In addition to its refolding activity, Hsp 90 complexes are also known to regulate the trafficking of membrane associated proteins through interactions with cytoskeletal motors (Pratt et al., 1999).

Ratts et al (2003) established a functional role for human Hsp 90, and the yeast homologue Hsp 82, as a component of the CTF complex by immunoprecipitation and the use of specific inhibitors in both the *in vitro* translocation assay and cytotoxicity assays. Using the Hsp 90 specific inhibitors geldanamycin and radicicol, Ratts et al (2003) demonstrated that Hsp 90 ATPase activity is capable of refolding *in vitro* denatured DT C domain into a biologically active conformation. Geldanamycin binds to the Hsp 90 active site, blocks the binding of ATP, and consequently inhibits substrate dissociation from the Hsp 90 refolding complex (Grenert et al., 1997). Radicicol, different in structure from geldanamycin, binds to a different location within the ATP binding pocket of Hsp 90 but also blocks the binding of ATP, and consequently inhibits substrate dissociation from the Hsp 90 refolding complex (Schulte et al., 1998).

Surprisingly, neither the addition of geldanamycin nor radicicol alone inhibited the *in vitro* translocation of the DT C-domain (Ratts et al., 2003). There are several reports demonstrating the synergistic inhibitory effects of geldanamycin and radicicol on Hsp 90, and inhibition is thought to result from either the disruption of substrate binding or the interaction with co-chaperonins (Schulte et al., 1998). When both inhibitors were used together, the *in vitro* translocation of the DT C-domain was inhibited (Ratts et al., 2003). The synergistic inhibition of C domain translocation was specific to Hsp 90, and protected cells against toxin. These results indicated that refolding of the denatured C-domain into an active conformation and translocation of the C domain across the early endosomal membrane were mutually exclusive events, and that redundant mechanisms exist for refolding any unfolded DT C domain following translocation. Dmochewitz et al (2011) confirmed and extended the observations made by Ratts et al (2003) using the anthrax pore to deliver the DT C domain across endosomal membranes *in vitro*. In this system, the *in vitro* translocation of the DT C domain across endosomal membranes was dependent on Hsp 90 ATPase activity. This study also demonstrated that the *in vitro* translocation of the DT C domain through the anthrax pore required the activity of cyclophilin, a known Hsp-90 co-chaperone. Dmochewitz et al. (2011) also provided the first evidence for interaction between the DT C domain and Hsp 90, either directly or in the presence of an adaptor protein.

Hsp 90 mediates the entry of other bacterial toxins from the lumen of endosomes including the *C. botulinum* C2 toxins (Haug et al., 2003), iota toxin (Haug et al., 2004), and *C. perfingens* toxin (Haug et al. 2004). Like diphtheria toxin, passage through a low pH compartment and unfolding of the *C. botulinum* C2 toxin catalytic domain are pre-requisites for entry (Barth et al., 2011). In the case of the *C. botulinum* C2 toxins, Haug et al (2003) clearly demonstrated that Hsp 90 ATPase activity was not acting as an allosteric regulator of v-ATPase, and ruled out the possibility that Hsp 90 inhibition resulted in the enhanced proteosomal degradation of toxin. In addition to bacterial protein toxins, Hsp 90 has also been show to to mediate the endosomal membrane translocation of the HIV viral TAT protein (Vendeville et al, 2004), the endogenous protein fibroblast growth factor (Wesche, et al. 2006). Hsp 90 mediated translocation is not limited to the endosomal membrane, and Hsp 90 function is also required cytosolic entry of cholera toxin, another ADP-ribosylating toxin, from the ER via the ERAD pathway (Taylor et al, 2010).

Subtle differences between these toxins and their interaction with CTFs may reveal insight into the precise molecular role of Hsp 90 within the CTF complex. All of the bacterial protein toxins requiring Hsp 90 for cytosolic entry that have been identified to date are ADP-ribosyltransferases, and Barth (2011) has hypothesized that there is some conserved component of the ADP-ribosyltransferase domain that mediates interaction with Hsp 90, either directly or indirectly through an adaptor protein or co-chaperone.

10.2 TrR-1 functions as a CTF

TrR-1 is an ubiquitously expressed homodimeric NADPH-dependent flavin adenine dinucleotide containing reductase, and is the only protein known to date to reduce thioredoxin (Trx-1) (Mustacich et al., 2000). Trx-1 reduces *in vitro* the DT inter-chain disulfide bond under acidic conditions (Moskaug et al., 1987), and reduced Trx-1 has also been shown to bind a variety of misfolded cytosolic proteins and directly facilitate refolding (Hawkins et al., 1991). Ratts et al (2003) established a functional role for TrR-1 and the yeast homologue as a component of the CTF complex by both immunoprecipitation, affinity depletion, and the use of the TrR-1 specific inhibitor *cis*-13-retinoic acid in both *in vitro* translocation assays and cytotoxicity assays. Under reducing conditions, TrR-1 was an essential component of the CTF complex indicating that it is structurally present or directly interacting with other CTFs that are required for DT C domain translocation, and this role is independent of its enzymatic activity. Ratts et al. (2003) demonstrated that TrR-1 function *in vitro* is required for translocation and/or release of the C-domain from early endosome under non-reducing conditions.

TrR-1 may be important for the entry of other bacterial protein toxins. TrR-1 reduces *in vitro* the inter-chain disulfide bond in both the botulinum neurotoxins and tetanus neurotoxins (Kistner et al., 1992; Kistner et al., 1993). These toxins are organized in a similar fashion to DT, and their mechanism across endosomal membranes parallels that of DT (Montecucco et al., 1996). An *in vivo* role for TrR-1 in mediating the entry of these neurotoxins, however, has not been shown. A role for TrR-1 in the intoxication of ricin has recently been reported by Bellisola et al. (2004), who showed that Trx and PDI mediated *in vitro* reduction of the ricin inter-chain disulfide bond depends upon TrR-1 activity under non-reducing conditions. When cytosolic extracts were depleted of TrR-1, effective reduction of ricin into two fragments still occurred, but protein(s) or protein fragment(s) of 15 kDa were associated with the ricin catalytic domain. Bellisola et al. (2004) hypothesized that this factor(s) associated with the ricin catalytic domain were chaperones required for toxin entry.

10.3 Cyclophilin may function as a CTF

Cyclophilin is a peptidylprolyl *cis-trans* isomerase and co-chaperone of Hsp 90, and mammalian cyclophilin - Hsp 90 complexes are conserved in yeast (Dolinski et al., 1998). A potential role for proyl isomerases in DT T domain membrane insertion and channel formation has been proposed (See Pore Formation above). Cyclophilin does facilitate the cytosolic entry of the *C. botulinum* C2 toxin, *C. perfingens* toxin, and the *C difficile* actin-ADP ribosylating CDT toxin (Kaiser et al., 2011). Dmochewitz et al (2011) demonstrated that *in vitro* translocation of the DT C domain across endosomal membranes using the anthrax pore was inhibited by cyclosporin, a specific inhibitor of cyclophilin. It has not yet been demonstrated, however, if translocation of the DT C domain using the DT T domain requires cyclophilin. Cyclophilin has not yet been identified in the purified diphtheria CTF complex, but cyclophilin trapped complexes from yeast do contain the other known CTFs required for diphtheria toxin entry. Although additional analysis is required to confirm that cyclophilin plays a role in the diphtheria toxin CTF complex, cyclophilin does play a role in the entry of other toxins.

11. Identification of the T1 motif

Since a highly conserved CTF complex is required for DT entry, we reasoned that a sequence specific binding site mediating interaction between toxin and the CTF complex exists. Given the common route of entry of diphtheria toxin, the anthrax lethal and edema factors, and the botulinum neurotoxins across endosomal membranes, we performed *in silico* sequence analysis of these toxins. Initial analysis was limited to portions of the DT C domain (residues 140-193) and T domain (residues 194-272) which were hypothesized to be the first portions of the toxin threaded through the nascent pore and presented to cytosol, using position-specific-iterated (PSI)-BLAST (Basic Local Alignment Search Tool) analysis (Karlin and Altschul, 1990). This initial analysis elucidated a 12 amino acid motif corresponding to DT residues 212-223 in transmembrane helix 1, and was therefore named the T1 motif (Figure 4) (Ratts dissertation 2004). Next, *in silico* analysis of the entire primary amino acid sequence of DT that employed PSI-BLAST, Clustal W Alignment (Thompson et al, 1994), and MEME (Multiple Expectation maximization for Motif Elucidation) (Bailey et al, 1994) using overlapping 12 amino acid sequences from DT to probe the data base revealed a conserved 10 amino acid motif corresponding to the same region within diphtheria toxin, anthrax lethal factor, anthrax edema factor and botulinum neurotoxins serotype A, C, and D (Figure 4) (Ratts et al., 2005). Although these two methods essentially defined the same motif, the two algorithm derived consensus sequences contain subtle differences highlighting the import of functional analysis to confirm any physiological relevance such motifs may have in mediating protein-protein interactions.

Anthrax			p-value
Edema Factor	50-65	EKNKTEKEKFKDSINN	2.4 x 10-7
	404-420	KLDHLRIEELKENGII	1.8 x 10-6
Lethal Factor	27- 42	ERNKTQEEHLKEIMKH	5.5 x 10-8
Botulinum neurotoxin			
Serotype A	719-734	AKVNTQIDLIRKKMKE	5.4 x 10-6
	828-843	GTLIGQVDRLKDKVNN	2.1 x 10-7
Serotype C1	755-770	ENIKSQVENLKNSLDV	2.4 x 10-9
Serotype D	751-766	ENIKSQVENLKNSLDV	2.4 x 10-9
Diphtheria toxin			
	212-227	DKTKTKIESLKEHGPI	9.0 x 10-8
MEME Consensus		TQIENLKEKGX	
Blast Consensus		EKXKTXXEXLKE	

```
DT    198-SSLSCINLDWDVIRDKTKTKIESLKEHGPIKNKMSESPNKTVSEEKAKQYLEE-250
LF     10-KEKEKNKDENKRDEERNKTQEEHLKEIMKHIVKIEKGEEAVKKEAAEKLLEKV-65
```

Fig. 4. BLAST and MEME analysis of anthrax edema and lethal factor (LF), botulinum neurotoxins, and diphtheria toxin (DT). P-values are for toxins compared to MEME consensus sequence. Longer sequence for LF and DT are shown indicating the flanking di-lysine motifs as underlined and described in the text.

For each toxin, the T1 motif is positioned on the surface of the protein within an amphipathic alpha helix that is located in a region of the toxin consistent with potential function in the translocation process. For diphtheria, the T1 motif is present within the first amphipathic helix of the DT T domain - TH1 – which is responsible for threading the DT C domain into the nascent pore formed by the remainder of the T domain. Deletion of TH1, proline disruption of TH1, or change in the charge distribution within this region all result in the loss of toxicity (vanderSpek et al., 1993; vanderSpek et al., 1994b). Furthermore, these mutations had no effect upon receptor binding, channel conductance in artificial lipid bilayers, nor the ADP-ribosyltransferase activity of the C domain.

The proposed 'entry' motif is also consistent with the known mechanism of entry for anthrax lethal factor. Anthrax toxin is a binary complex assembled from three distinct protein chains: protective antigen (PA), lethal factor (LF), and edema factor (EF) (for review see Mourez et al., 2002). Protective antigen (PA83) binds to a universal cell surface receptor and a 20 kDa fragment is removed by furin digestion (Molloy et al., 1992). The remaining 63 kDa fragment (PA63) remains on the cell surface and spontaneously oligomerizes into a heptamer. The heptameric complex is then capable of binding either LF or EF (Pimental et al., 2004). The overall route of entry closely follows that of diphtheria. PA bound with either LF or EF, is internalized into an endosomal compartment, where acidification induces a conformational change in PA, driving membrane insertion and formation of a cation selective channel (Abrami et al 2003; Blaustein et al., 1989). Wesche et al. (1998) showed that the acid-induced translocation of LF, like diphtheria, must undergo complete unfolding for passage through the channel formed by PA, and is then refolded into an active conformation in the cytosol (Wesche et al., 1998). In contrast, EF remains associated with the vesicle compartment (Guidi-Rontani et al., 2000). In the case of anthrax LF, the putative entry motif is located between amino acid residues 27 - 39 in the mature protein, a region N-terminal to the PA binding domain. Analysis of anthrax LF N-terminal deletion mutagenesis (Arora and Leppla, 1993) demonstrated that the deletion of amino acids 1 - 40 in lethal factor results in a complete loss of toxicity for macrophages. More recently, Lacy et al. (2002) confirmed these results, and also showed that deletion of the N-terminal 27 amino acids had no effect. Although results by Lacy et al. (2002) suggested that the deletion of amino acid residues 1-40 may abrogate LF binding to PA, it is clear that the region is required for toxicity.

12. β COP Functions as a CTF

To demonstrate that the T1 motif mediates physiologically relevant interaction with CTFs, Ratts et al. (2005) engineered toxin resistant cells by transfecting a mini-gene encoding the T1 motif (amino acids 210-229 of DT). Cells expressing the T1 peptide were resistant to both $DAB_{389}IL-2$ and wild type DT, but were not protected against pseudomonas exotoxin A which enters cells through the ER and once delivered to the cytosol inhibits protein synthesis via an identical NAD+ dependent ribosylation of EF2. These results suggested that the T1 motif was not interfering with receptor binding, receptor trafficking, nor inhibiting the ability of toxin to ADP-ribosylate EF-2. Ratts et al (2005) then showed that knockdown of the T1 motif mini-gene using siRNA restored sensitivity to toxin, and we reasoned the T1 peptide was inhibiting an essential protein-protein interaction with CTFs.

In order to confirm such an interaction, a fusion protein was constructed between GST and DT amino residues 140-271 (Ratts et al., 2005). Because other regions outside the T1 motif might also be important in the entry process we used a longer segment of DT, corresponding to regions of T domain and C domain that are first threaded through the pore and presented to the cytosol. While the T1 motif alone might be sufficient in blocking protein-protein interactions, additional regions of the toxin may be required for actually binding CTFs. In pull down experiments, Ratts et al (2005) affinity purified several proteins that specifically bound to DT140-271, and identified them by mass spectrometry sequencing. One of these identified proteins was β-COP. Using labeled [35S]-β-COP that was synthesized *in vitro* using a rabbit reticulocyte transcription and translation reaction mixture, we found that GST-DT140-271 specifically bound β-COP and that bind was inhibited by synthetic T1-motif peptide. Confirming and extending Lemichez et al. (1997), there results suggested direct interaction between toxin and β-COP via the T1 motif.

A role for the DT T1 Motif in mediating the cytosolic entry of anthrax lethal factor (LF) was demonstrated by Tamayo et al. (2008) using an *in vitro* translocation assay consisting of early endosomes pre-loaded with anthrax protective antigen (PA) and the anthrax LFn-DTa fusion protein construct. The LFn-DTa is a fusion protein consisting of the LF binding domain for PA and the C domain of diphtheria. Tamayo et al. (2008) clearly demonstrated that the anthrax LFn-DTa fusion protein construct was translocated across the endosomal membrane in an ATP and cytosol dependent fashion, and this observation was confirmed by Dmochewitz et al (2011). Tamayo et al. (2008) also demonstrated using GST-LFn pull downs that the T1 motif in anthrax lethal factor directly binds β-COP, as well as zeta (ζ)-COP, and that a synthetic peptide containing the DT T1 motif blocked this interaction.

13. Lysines adjacent to the T1 motif region bind COPI

COPI is a heptameric structure that is composed of α-, β-, β'-, γ-, ε-, δ-, δ-subunits, and this complex functions to facilitate endosomal vesicular trafficking, the retrograde transport of vesicles between Golgi compartments, and between the Golgi apparatus and the endoplasmic reticulum (Serafini et al, 1991; Waters et al., 1991; Whitney et al., 1995). As previously mentioned, both β'COP (Sec 27) and ADP-ribosylation factor 1 (ARF1) bind to the cytoplasmic surface of the endosomal membrane to promote ECV formation, and the binding of both factors is dependent upon a low endosomal lumen pH (Aniento et al., 1996). COPI complexes have also been shown to be recruited to the cytosolic surface of vesicle membranes *en bloc* by Arf-GTP (Donaldson et al, 1992; Palmer et al., 1993). The recognition of di-lysine motifs (KXKXX, KKXX) by coatomer in the cytoplasmic tails of cargo proteins is well established (Cosson et al., 1994; Eugster et al., 2004). Interactions between COPI and the p23/24 adaptor is also mediated by a di-lysine motif, and is thought stabilize coatomer binding to the membrane surface (Harter et al., 1998).

Trujillo et al (2010) hypothesized that the multiple di-lysine motifs adjacent to the T1 motif in DT are the specific amino acid residues that interact with coatomer. This hypothesis was then confirmed by site-directed mutagenesis of the specific lysine residues K213, K215, K217, and K222 demonstrating that at least three of the four lysine residues in the region of the T1 motif are required for both COPI binding and for the cytotoxic activity of DAB389IL-2 (Trujillo et al., 2010). Using a similar *in vitro* COPI precipitation assay as described by Hudson and Draper (1997), Trujillo et al (2010) demonstrated that synthetic peptides of the DT T domain transmembrane helix 1 would cross-link and induce precipitation of COPI complexes *in vitro*. Synthetic peptides containing lysine to alanine mutations at either the N-terminal or C-terminal end of the peptide, or all five positions failed to precipitate COPI *in vitro.* The addition of monoamine 1,3-cyclohexanebis (methylamine), CBM, to the reaction mixture also blocked peptide binding to COPI complex. Trujillo et al. (2010) also demonstrated that DT directly interacts with only the β-COP and γ_1-COP components.

These observations suggested that the ε-amino moieties of the lysine residues immediately adjacent to the T1 motif specifically bind to COPI, and Trujillo et al (2010) reasoned that this region within DT was functioning as a mimetic of the cytoplasmic tail regions of either the cargo or p23/24 adaptor proteins that are normally recognized by COPI. This theory was validated by domain swapping the 13 amino acid COPI binding sequence from the cytoplasmic tail region of the p23 adaptor protein with native T1 motif and adjacent upstream lysine residues in $DAB_{389}IL-2$. The COPI domain swap fusion toxin mutant $DAB_{(212p23)389}IL-2$ retained full cytotoxic potency relative to the wild type-fusion protein toxin (Trujillo et al., 2010). Regardless of sequence, a major role for the DT transmembrane helix 1 is COPI complex binding and this interaction is essential for toxin entry.

14. A new model for translocation

The autonomous model for entry explains the initial steps in toxin translocation across the endosomal membrane, while the completion of translocation and release of the DT C domain into cytosol requires cytosolic factors. Acidification within the endosomal lumen promotes unfolding of the C domain and membrane insertion of the T domain in a mutually augmented process. It is not known if any host cell proteins help facilitate unfolding. The chaperonin-like qualities of the T domain then appear to thread the C-terminal end of the C domain, connected by its disulfide bond to the *N*-terminal end of the T domain, into the nascent pore. Presentation of the di-lysine motifs (KXKXX) in the N-terminal end of the T domain to the cytosolic side of the endosomal membrane then allows for targeting of the toxin by the COPI complex. Coatomer recognition of the toxin as cargo or a p23 mimetic essentially designates the N-terminal end of the T domain for "retrieval" into endogenous membrane sorting pathways. The effect of coatomer is to normally retrieve, or pull, membrane bound proteins into carrier vesicles. The effect of retrieving, or pulling, the mobile region of the N-terminal T domain actually results in the "retrieval" of the disulfide linked C domain through the pore and facilitating its complete translocation.

During this translocation process, Hsp 90 and TrR-1 perform critical steps that are required for toxin entry. Coatomer binding is a dynamic process consisting of many factors, and whether or not Hsp 90 and TrR-1 directly interact with the toxin or are rather involved in regulating or stabilizing coatomer remains to be elucidated. It is interesting that coatomer stabilization and release from the membrane is regulated by an endogenous ADP-ribosylation factor, and that the role of Hsp 90 in mediating toxin entry appears to be limited to toxins whose catalytic domains, like diphtheria, are ADP-ribosyltransferases. Likewise, the potential role for cyclophilin within the CTF complex also needs clarification.

Potential models for Hsp 90 function in the CTF complex include (but are not limited to): power stoke, regulation of other CTFs, Brownian ratchet, or architectural adaptor. The power stroke model implies that the Hsp 90 ATPase functions as a motor that directly drives the translocation, and is unlikely to apply to diphtheria entry since Ratts et al. (2003) demonstrated that translocation of the DT C domain across the endosomal membrane did not require processive cycles of Hsp 90 ATPase function. Dmochewitz (et al. 2011) has demonstrated interaction between the C domain and Hsp 90, implying that Hsp 90's role is direct rather than indirect, i.e. regulatory, within the CTF complex. In the Brownian ratchet model, Hsp 90 would bind to progressive nascent regions of translocating C domain, preventing retrograde translocation back into the endosome. In other words, Hsp 90 binding and stabilization of exposed hydrophobic residues in the DT C domain as they emerge from the endosome effectively facilitates translocation. The Brownian ratchet model would be consistent with the observed synergistic inhibition by geldanamycin and radical - only when both inhibitors are used concomitantly, the emerging diphtheria toxin residues are no longer recognized by Hsp 90 and translocation is inhibited. Alternatively, Hsp 90 may function merely as an architectural adaptor, i.e. scaffold, within the CTF complex mediating a purely structural interaction between the toxin C domain and other CTFs.

Whether or not TrR-1 directly reduces the DT inter-chain disulfide bond *in vivo* remains unknown. It is possible that TrR-1 first reduces another reductase, which then directly reduces the DT inter-chain disulfide bond. Potential candidates include (Trx-1), presumably present on the endosomal membrane. Thioredoxin peroxidases, such as the alkyl hydroperoxide reductase-1 (Ahp1) identified in the yeast partially purified CTF complex; or a hitherto unidentified reductase, such as the novel protein YOR011C identified in the yeast partially purified CTF complex that bears homology to known NADPH oxidoreductases (Ratts et al. 2003). Conversely, another reductase might first reduces the DT inter-chain disulfide bond, and TrR-1 then subsequently mediates the release of the DT C domain by reducing the newly formed intermediate disulfide bond. A third possibility is that TrR-1 plays no role in reduction of the DT inter-chain disulfide bond during intoxication. Rather, TrR-1 may be responsible for the reduction of a key component of the CTF machinery required for translocation. For example, the reactivity of the free cysteines in Hsp 90 have been implicated in mediating chaperonin activity (Nardai et al., 2000).

As we learn more about toxin entry, our models will continue to need refinement. In the case of anthrax lethal factor, for example, Tamayo et al. (2011) recently reported that the chaperone Grp78 is required for intoxication and it unfolds the LF catalytic domain within the endosomal lumen. This finding appears to contradict long held beliefs that unfolding of the anthrax LF catalytic domain naturally occurs solely under acidic conditions *in vitro* and that the pore formed by protective antigen has chaperonin-like properties that facilitates autonomous delivery - both of which parallel and are analogous to models of diphtheria toxin entry. The report by Tamayo et al. (2011) reiterates the importance of studying toxin entry in biologically relevant systems containing the heterogeneous population of proteins naturally encountered by the toxin during intoxication. While the chaperones facilitating translocation of anthrax LF and DT have so far been found on opposite sides of the endosomal membrane, the entry of both toxins requires COPI binding in the cytosol. The identification of any other additional CTFs will further refine our models of toxin entry.

15. Conclusion

Diphtheria was the first investigated bacterial protein toxin, and more than a century later remains a paradigm for toxin entry. While there is no longer any question that cytosolic translocation factors (CTFs) facilitate the entry of diphtheria toxin, much work remains. The remaining components of the CTF complex required for the cytosolic entry of diphtheria toxin need to be identified, and the precise role each cellular factor performs during translocation requires definition. Current methods for the purification of CTF complexes remain limited, and novel techniques that are more cost effective and readily available are desperately needed.

It is now apparent that a divergent group of toxins have convergently evolved to exploit similar mechanisms of entry to that of diphtheria toxin, and comparing and contrasting the differences in the CTF complexes for each toxin will serve as a valuable probe into the endogenous functions of coatomer assembly, cyclophilin and Hsp 90 function, thioredoxin redox pathways, and any other yet unidentified factors. Defining the precise molecular interaction between toxins and the CTF complex will allow for the design of novel therapeutics targeted towards virulence factors. Indeed, geldanamycin has already been shown to protect rat ileal gut from cholera toxin (Taylor et al., 2010) and clinical trials will likely soon follow. In light of the apparent evolutionary pressures, it is tempting to hypothesize that the CTF complex described for diphtheria toxin entry endogenously participates in discrete inter-intracellular signaling mechanisms that are highly conserved in eukaryotes.

16. Acknowledgements

Ryan Ratts is supported by a Hitchcock Foundation Pilot Research Grant. John Murphy is supported by Public Health Service grant AI-021628 and by grant AI-057159 from the New England Regional Center of Excellence in Emerging Infectious Diseases and Biodefense.

17. References

Abrami, L, Liu, S, Cosson, P., Leppla, S.H., and van der Goot, F.G. Anthrax toxin triggers endocytosis of its receptor via a lipid raft-mediated clathrin-dependent process. *J Cell Biol* 2003 160: 321-328.

Aniento, F, Emans, S, Griffiths, G, & Gruenberg, J. An endosomal bCOP is involved in the pH-dependent formation of transport vesicles destined for late endosomes. *J Cell Biol*, 1993; 133: 29-41.

Ariansen, S, Afanasiev, BN, Moskaug, JO, Stenmark, H, Madhaus, IH, & Olsnes, S. Membrane translocation of diphtheria toxin A-fragment: role of carboxy-terminal region. *Biochemistry*, 1993; 32: 83-90.

Arora, N. and Leppla, S.H. Residues 1-254 of anthrax lethal factor are sufficient to cause cellular uptake of fused polypeptides. *J Biol chem.* 268: 3334-41

Bacha, P, Waters, C, Williams, J, Murphy, JR, & Strom, TB. Interleukin-2 targeted cytotoxicity: Selective action of a diphtheria toxin-related interleukin-2 fusion protein. *J Exp Med*, 1988; 167: 612-622.

Bailey, T.L.; Elkan, C. Fitting a mixture model by expectation maximization to discover motifs in biopolymers. *Proc. Int. Conf. Intell. Syst. Mol. Biol.* 1994, 2, 28–36.

Baker, A, Kaplan CP, & Pool, MR. Protein targeting and translocation, a comparative review. *Biol Rev Camb Philos Soc* 1996, 71(4):637-702.

Bauer, M. F., S. Hofmann, W. Neupert and M. Brunner. Protein translocation into mitochondria: the role of TIM complexes. *Trends Cell Biol* 2000, 10(1): 25-31.

Barth, H. Exploring the role of host cell chaperones/PPIases during cellular up-take of bacterial ADP-ribosylating toxins as basis for novel pharmacological strategies to protect mammalian cells against these virulence foactors. *Naunyn. Schmiedebergs Arch. Pharmacol.* 2011, *383*, 237–245.

Bektaş M, Hacıosmanoğlu E, Ozerman B, Varol B, Nurten R, Bermek E. On diphtheria toxin fragment A release into the cytosol-Cytochalasin D effect and involvement of actin filaments and eukaryotic elongation factor 2. Int J Biochem Cell Biol. 2011 Jun 12.

Bellisola, G., G. Fracasso, R. Ippoliti, G. Menestrina, A. Rosen, S. Solda, S. Udali, R. Tomazzolli, G. Tridente and M. Colombatti. Reductive activation of ricin and ricin A-chain immunotoxins by protein disulfide isomerase and thioredoxin reductase. Biochem Pharmacol 2004, 67(9): 1721-31.

Bijlmakers, M. J. and M. Marsh. Hsp90 is essential for the synthesis and subsequent membrane association, but not the maintenance, of the Src-kinase p56(lck). Mol Biol Cell 2000, 11(5): 1585-95.

Blaustein, RO, Koehler, TM, Collier, RJ, & Finkelstein, A. Anthrax toxin: channel forming activity of PA in planar phospholipid bilayers. *Proc Natl Acad Sci, USA*, 1989; 86: 2209-2213.

Blewitt, M. G., L. A. Chung and E. London. Effect of pH on the conformation of diphtheria toxin and its implications for membrane penetration. Biochemistry 1985, 24(20): 5458-64.

Bowman, E.J.; Siebers, A.; Altendorf, K. Bafilomycins: A class of inhibitors of membrane ATPases from microorganisms, animal cells, and plant cells. *Proc. Natl. Acad. Sci. USA* 1988, *85*, 7972–7976.

Boquet, P, Silverman MS, Pappenheimer, AM, Jr, & Vernon WB. Binding of Triton X-100 to diphtheria toxin, cross reacting material 45, and their fragments. *Proc Natl Acad Sci, USA*, 1976; 73: 4449-4453.

Brown, JG, Almond, BD, Naglich, JG, & Eidels L. Hypersensitivity to DT by mouse cells expressing both DT receptor and CD9 antigen. *Proc Natl Acad Sci, USA*, 1993; 90: 8184-8188.

Cabiaux, V.; Quertenmont, P.; Conrath, K.; Brasseur, R.; Capiau, C.; Ruysschaert, J.M. Topology of diphtheria toxin B fragment inserted in lipid vesicles. *Mol. Microbiol.* 1994, *11*, 43–50.

Caplan, A. J. Hsp90's secrets unfold: new insights from structural and functional studies. *Trends Cell Biol* 1999, 9(7): 262-8.

Chassaing, A, Prichard, S. Araye-Guet, A, Barbier, J, Forge V., & Gillet D. Solution and membrane-bound chaperone activity of DT T domain towards the C domain. *FEBS* 2011, Epub Feb 18.

Choe et al., S Choe, M J Bennett, G Fujii, P M Curmi, K A Kantardjieff, R J Collier and D Eisenberg The crystal structure of diphtheria toxin. *Nature* 1992 357(6375): 216-22.

Collier, R. J. and H. A. Cole. Diphtheria toxin subunit active in vitro. *Science* 1969 164 (884): 1179-81.

Collier, R.J.; Kandel, J. Structure and activity of diphtheria toxin. I. Thiol-dependent dissociation of a fraction of toxin into enzymically active and inactive fragments. *J. Biol. Chem.* 1971, *246*, 1496–1503.

Cosson, P.; Letourneur, F. Coatomer interaction with di-lysine endoplasmic retention motifs. *Science* 1994, *263*, 1629–1631.

Deleers, M.; Beugnier, N.; Falgmagne, P.; Cabiaux, V.; Ruysschaert, J.M. Localization in diphtheria toxin fragemnt B of a region that induces pore formation in planar lipid bilayers at low pH. *FEBS Lett.* 1983, *160*, 82–86.

Dmochewitz L, Lillich M, Kaiser E, Jennings LD, Lang AE, Buchner J, Fischer G, Aktories K, Collier RJ, Barth H Role of CypA and Hsp90 in membrane translocation mediated by anthrax protective antigen. *Cell Microbiol.* 2010 Oct 14

Donaldson, J.G.; Cassel, D.; Kahn, R.A.; Klausner, R.D. ADP-ribosylation factor, a small GTP-binding protein, is required for binding of coatomer protein beta-COP to membranes. *Proc. Natl. Acad. Sci. USA* 1992, *89*, 6408–6412.

Dolinski, K. J., M. E. Cardenas and J. Heitman (1998). CNS1 encodes an essential p60/Sti1 homolog in Saccharomyces cerevisiae that suppresses cyclophilin 40 mutations and interacts with Hsp90. Mol Cell Biol 1998, 18(12): 7344-52.

Donovan, Jj, Simon, MI, Draper RK, & Montal, M. Diphtheria toxin forms transmembrane channels in planar lipid bilayers. *Proc Natl Acad Sci, USA*, 1981; *78:* 172-176.

Drazin, R, Kandel, J, & Collier, RJ. Structure and activity of DT II. Attack by trypsin at a specific site within the intact molecule. *J Biol Chem*, 1971; 246: 1504-1510.

Duprez, V, Smoljanovic, M, Lieb, M, & Dautry-Varsat, A. Trafficking of interleukin 2 and transferring in endosomal fraction of T cells. J cell Sci, 1994; 107: 1289-1295.

Eugster, A.; Frigerio, G.; Dale, M.; Duden, R. The alpha- and beta'-COP WD40 domains mediate cargo-selective interactions with distinct di-lysine motifs. *Mol. Biol. Cell* 2004, *15*, 1011–1023.

Falnes, PO, Madshus, IH, Sandvig, K, & Olsnes, S. Replacement of negative by positive charges in the presumed membrane-inserted part of diphtheria toxin B fragment. Effect on membrane translocation and on formation of cation channels. *J Biol Chem*, 1992; 267: 12284-12290.

Falnes, P. O., S. Choe, I. H. Madshus, B. A. Wilson and S. Olsnes Inhibition of membrane translocation of diphtheria toxin A-fragment by internal disulfide bridges *J Biol Chem* 1994 269(11): 8402-7.

Futter, C. E., A. Pearse, L. J. Hewlett and C. R. Hopkins. Multivesicular endosomes containing internalized EGF-EGF receptor complexes mature and then fuse directly with lysosomes. J Cell Biol 1996. 132(6): 1011-23.

Gill, DM, & Pappenheimer, AM, Jr. Structure activity relationships in diphtheria toxin. *J Biol Chem*, 1971; 246: 1485-1491.

Greenfield L, Bjorn MJ, Horn G, Fong D, Buck GA, Collier RJ, & Kaplan D. Nucleotide sequence of the structural gene for diphtheria toxin carried by corynebacteriophage *Proc Natl Acad Sci, USA*, 1983; 80: 6853-6857.

Grenert, J. P., W. P. Sullivan, P. Fadden, T. A. Haystead, J. Clark, E. Mimnaugh, H. Krutzsch, H. J. Ochel, T. W. Schulte, E. Sausville, et al.. The amino-terminal domain of heat shock protein 90 (hsp90) that binds geldanamycin is an ATP/ADP switch domain that regulates hsp90 conformation. J Biol Chem 1997, 272: 23843-50.

Guidi-Rontani, C, Weber-Levy, M, Mock, M, & Cabiaux, V. Translocation of Bacillus anthracis lethal and oedema factors across endosome membranes. *Cell Microbiol*, 2000; 2: 259-264.

Hammond, K., G. A. Caputo and E. London Interaction of the membrane-inserted diphtheria toxin T domain with peptides and its possible implications for chaperone-like T domain behavior. Biochemistry 2002, 41: 3243-53.

Haug G, Aktories K, Barth H. The host cell chaperone Hsp90 is necessary for cytotoxic action of the binary iota-like toxins. *Infect Immun.* 2004 May;72(5):3066-8

Haug G, Leemhuis J, Tiemann D, Meyer DK, Aktories K, Barth H The host cell chaperone Hsp90 is essential for translocation of the binary Clostridium botulinum C2 toxin into the cytosol. *J Biol Chem.* 2003 Aug 22;278(34):32266-74.

Hawkins, H. C., E. C. Blackburn and R. B. Freedman (1991a). Comparison of the activities of protein disulphide-isomerase and thioredoxin in catalysing disulphide isomerization in a protein substrate. Biochem J 1991, 275: 349-53.

Hayashibara, M.; London, E. Topography of diphtheria toxin A chain inserted into lipid vesicles. *Biochemistry* 2005, *44*, 2183–2196.

Harter, C.; Weiland, F.T. A single binding site for dilysine retrieval motifs and p23 with the gamma subunit of coatomer. *Proc. Natl. Acad. Sci. USA* 1998, *95*, 11649–11654.

Hudson, R.T.; Draper, R.K. Interaction of coatomer with aminoglycoside antibiotics: evidence that coatomer has at least two dilysine binding sites. *Mol. Biol. Cell* 1997, *8*, 1901–1910.

Ho, Y., A. Gruhler, A. Heilbut, G. D. Bader, L. Moore, S. L. Adams, A. Millar, P. Taylor, K. Bennett, K. Boutilier, et al. Systematic identification of protein complexes in Saccharomyces cerevisiae by mass spectrometry. *Nature* 2002 415(6868): 180-3.

Hu, H-Y, Hunth PD, Murphy, JR, & vanderSpek, JC. The effects of helix breaking mutations in the diphtheria toxin transmembrane domain helix layers of the fusion toxin DAB_{389}IL-2. *Protein engn*, 1998; 11: 101-107.

Iwamoto, R.; Higashiyama, S.; Mitamura, T.; Taniguchi, N.; Klagsbrun, M.; Mekada, E. Heparin-binding EGF-like growth factor, which acts as the DT receptor, forms a complex with membrane protein DRAP27/CD9, which up-regulates functional receptors and DT sensitivity. *EMBO J.* 1994, *13*, 2322–2330.

Johnson, V. G., P. J. Nicholls, W. H. Habig and R. J. Youle. The role of proline 345 in diphtheria toxin translocation. *J Biol Chem* 1993, 268(5): 3514-9.

Kaczorek M, Delpeyroux F, Chenciner N, Streek RE, Murphy JR, Boquet P, & Tiollais P. Nucleotide sequence and expression of the diphtheria *tox*228 gene in *Escherichia coli. Science*, 1983; Science, 221: 855-858.

Kagan, BL, Finkelstein, A, & Colombini, M. Diphtheria toxin fragment forms large pores in phospholipids bilayer membranes. *Proc Natl Acad Sci, USA*, 1981; 78: 4950-4954.

Kaiser, E., Kroll, C., Ernst, K., Schwan, C, Popoff, M, Fischer, G, Buchner, J, Aktories, K, Barth, H. Membrane translocation of binary ADP-ribosylating toxins from C. difficile and C. perfingines is facilitated by cyclophilin and Hsp 90. Infect Immun, 2011 Epub Jul 18.

Kaneda, Y., Uchida, T., Mekada, E.; Nakanishi, M.; Okada, Y. Entry of diphtheria toxin into cells: possible existence of cellular factor(s) for entry of diphtheria toxin into cells was studied in somatic cell hybrids and hybrid toxins. *J. Cell Biol.* 1984, *98*, 466–472.

Karlin, S and Altschul, SF. Methods for assessing the statistical significance of molecular sequence features by using general scoring themes. *Proc Natl Acad Sci USA* 1990, 87(6)2264-8.

Kim, K.; Groman, N.B. *In vitro* inhibition of diphtheria toxin action by ammonium salts and amines. *J. Bacteriol.* 1965, *90*, 1552–1556.

Kistner, A. and E. Habermann. Reductive cleavage of tetanus toxin and botulinum neurotoxin A by the thioredoxin system from brain. Evidence for two redox isomers of tetanus toxin. *Naunyn Schmiedebergs Arch Pharmacol* 1992, 345(2): 227-34.

Kistner, A., D. Sanders and E. Habermann. Disulfide formation in reduced tetanus toxin by thioredoxin: the pharmacological role of interchain covalent and noncovalent bonds. *Toxicon* 1993, 31(11): 1423-34.

Lacy, D. B. and R. J. Collier, Structure and function of anthrax toxin. *Curr Top Microbiol Immunol* 2002, 271: 61-85.

Lemichez, E, Bomsel, M, Devilliers, G, vanderSpek, J, Murphy, JR, Lukianov, EV, Olsnes, S, & Boquet, P. Membrane translocation of diphtheria toxin fragment A exploits early to late endosome trafficking machinery. *Molec Microbiol*, 1997; 23: 445-457.

Love, J.F. and Murphy, J.R. Design and development of a novel genetic probe for the analysis of repressor-operator interactions. *J Microbiol Methods* 2002, 51(1):63-72.

Luzio, J. P., B. M. Mullock, P. R. Pryor, M. R. Lindsay, D. E. James and R. C. Piper, Relationship between endosomes and lysosomes. *Biochem Soc Trans 2001*, 29: 476-80.

Madshus, I.H. The *N*-terminal alpha-helix of fragment B of diphtheria toxin promotes translocation of fragment A into the cytoplasm of eukaryotic cells. *J. Biol. Chem.* 1994, *269*, 17723–17729.

Madshus, I.H.; Wiedlocha, A.; Sandvig, K. Intermediates in translocation of diphtheria toxin across the plasma membrane. *J. Biol. Chem.* 1994, *269*, 4648–4652.

Merion, M., P. Schlesinger, R. M. Brooks, J. M. Moehring, T. J. Moehring and W. S. Sly. Defective acidification of endosomes in Chinese hamster ovary cell mutants "cross-resistant" to toxins and viruses. *Proc Natl Acad Sci U S A* 1983, 80(17): 5315-9.

Mindell, J.A.; Silverman, J.A.; Collier, R.J.; Finkelstein, A. Structure function relationships in diphtheria toxin channels: II. A residue responsible for the channel's dependence on *trans* pH. *J. Memb. Biol.* 1994, *137*, 29–44.

Mitamura, T, Iwamoto, R, Umata, T, Yomo, T, Urabe, M, Tsuneoka, M, & Mekada, E. The 27-kD DT receptor-associated protein (DTRAP27) from Vero cells is the monkey homolog of human CD9 antigen: expression of DRAP27 elevates the number of DT receptors on toxin sensitive cells. J Cell Biol, 1992; 118: 1389-1399.

Molloy, SS, Bresnahan, PA, Leppla, SH, Klimpel, KR, & Thomas, G. Human furin is a calcium-dependent serine endoprotease that recognizes the sequence Arg-X-X-Arg and efficiently cleaves anthrax toxin protective antigen. *J Biol Chem*, 1992; 267: 16396-16402.

Montecucco, C., E. Papini and G. Schiavo. Bacterial protein toxins and cell vesicle trafficking. *Experientia* 1996, 52(12): 1026-32.

Moskaug, J. O., K. Sandvig and S. Olsnes. Cell-mediated reduction of the interfragment disulfide in nicked DT. A new system to study toxin entry at low pH." *J Biol Chem* 1987, 262(21): 10339-45.

Moskaug, JO, Stenmark, H, & Olsnes, S. Insertion of diphtheria toxin B-fragment into the plasma membrane at low pH. Characterization and topology of inserted regions. *J Biol Chem*, 1991; 266: 2652-2659.

Mourez, M, Lacy, DB, Cunningham, K, Legmann, R, Sellman, BR, Mogridge, J, & Collier RJ. 2001: a year of major advances in anthrax toxin research. *Trends in Microbiology*, 2002; 10: 287-293.

Moya, M.; Dautry-Varsat, A.; Goud, B.; Louvard, D.; Boquet, P. Inhibition of coated pit formation in Hep2 cells blocks the cytotoxicity of diphtheria toxin but not that of ricin toxin. *J. Cell Biol.* 1985, *101*, 548–559.

Murphy, JR. Mechanism of DT C domain delivery to eukaryotic cell cytosol and the cellular factors that directly participate in the process. *Toxins*, 2011, 3(3):294-308.

Murphy, J.R.; Bishai, W.; Borowski, M.; Miyanohara, A.; Boyd, J.; Nagle, S. Genetic construction, expression, and melanoma-selective cytotoxicity of a diphtheria toxin-related alpha-melanocyte-stimulating hormone fusion protein. *Proc. Natl. Acad. Sci. USA* 1986, *83*, 8258–8262.

Mustacich, D. and G. Powis. Thioredoxin reductase. *Biochem J* 2000, 346 Pt 1: 1-8.

Naglich, JG, Matherall, JE, Russell, DW, & Eidels L. Expression cloning of a diphtheria toxin receptor: identity with a heparin-binding EGF-like growth factor precursor. *Cell,* 1992; 69: 1051-1061.

Nardai, G., B. Sass, J. Eber, G. Orosz and P. Csermely. Reactive cysteines of the 90-kDa heat shock protein, Hsp90. *Arch Biochem Biophys* 2000, 384(1): 59-67.

Oh, JO, Senzel, L, Collier, RJ, & Finkelstein, A. Translocation of the catalytic domain of diphtheria toxin across planar phospholipids bilayers by its own T-domain. Proc *Natl Acad Sci, USA,* 1999; 96: 8467-8470.

O'Keefe, DO, Cabiaux, V, Choe, S, Eisenberg, D, & Collier, RJ. pH-dependent insertion of proteins into membranes: B-chain mutation of diphtheria toxin that inhibits membrane translocation, Glu-349-Lys. *Proc Natl Acad Sci, USA,* 1992; 89: 6202-6206.

Palmer, D.J.; Helms, J.B.; Beckers, C.J.; Orci, L.; Rothman, J.E. Binding of coatomer to Golgi membranes requires ADP-ribosylation factor. *J. Biol. Chem.* 1993, *268,* 12083–12089.

Palmquist, K., B. Riis, A. Nilsson and O. Nygard.. Interaction of the calcium and calmodulin regulated eEF-2 kinase with heat shock protein 90. *FEBS Lett* 1994, 349(2): 239-42.

Papini, E., R. Rappuoli, M. Murgia and C. Montecucco. Cell penetration of diphtheria toxin. Reduction of the interchain disulfide bridge is the rate-limiting step of translocation in the cytosol. *J Biol Chem* 1993, 268(3): 1567-74.

Pappenheimer, AM, Jr. Diphtheria toxin. *Annu. Rev. Biochem.,* 1977; 46: 69-94.

Pimental, R.A., Christensen, K.A., Krantz, B.A., and Collier, R.J. (2004) Anthrax toxin complexes: heptameric protective antigen can bind lethal factor and edema factor simultaneously. *Biochem Biophys Res Commun* 322: 258-262

Pratt, W. B., A. M. Silverstein and M. D. Galigniana. A model for the cytoplasmic trafficking of signalling proteins involving the hsp90-binding immunophilins and p50cdc37. *Cell Signal* 1999, 11(12): 839-51.

Ratts, R. Purification, Identification and Characterization of the DT CTF complex. PhD Thesis. Copyright 2004. Boston University

Ratts R, Trujillo C, Bharti A, vanderSpek J, Harrison R, Murphy JR A conserved motif in transmembrane helix 1 of DT mediates catalytic domain delivery to the cytosol. Proc Natl Acad Sci U S A. 2005 Oct 25;102(43):15635-40. Epub 2005 Oct 17.

Ratts, R and vanderSpek, JC. DT: structure function and its clinical applications. In, *Chimeric Toxins.* H. Lorberboum-Galski and P. Lazarovici (Eds). Taylor and Francis, London 2002, 14-36

Ratts, R, Zeng, H, Berg EA, Blue, C, McComb, ME, Costello, CE, vanderSpek, JC, & Murphy, R. The cytosolic entry of diphtheria toxin catalytic domain requires a host cell cytosolic translocation factor complex. *J Cell Biol,* 2003 Mar 31;160(7):1139-50

Ren, J, Kachel, K, Kim, H, Malenbaum, S, Collier, RJ, & London, E. Interaction of diphtheria toxin T domain with molten globule-like proteins and its implicatios for translocation. *Science,* 1999; 248: 955-957.

Rosen, A., P. Lundman, M. Carlsson, K. Bhavani, B. R. Srinivasa, G. Kjellstrom, K. Nilsson and A. Holmgren. A CD4+ T cell line-secreted factor, growth promoting for normal and leukemic B cells, identified as thioredoxin. *Int Immunol* 1995, 7(4): 625-33.

Ryser, H-J, Mandel, R, & Ghani, F. Cell surface sulfhydryls are required for the cytotoxicity of DT but not ricin toxin in Chinese hamster ovary cells. *J Biol Chem,* 1991; 266: 18439-18442.

Sandvig, K. and S. Olsnes. Diphtheria toxin entry into cells is facilitated by low pH. *J Cell Biol* 1980, 87(3 Pt 1): 828-32.

Sandvig, K. and S. Olsnes. Rapid entry of nicked diphtheria toxin into cells at low pH. Characterization of the entry process and effects of low pH on the toxin molecule. *J Biol Chem* 1981, 256(17): 9068-76.

Sandvig, K. and S. Olsnes. Diphtheria toxin-induced channels in Vero cells selective for monovalent cations. *J Biol Chem* 1988, 263(25): 12352-9.

Sandvig, K., A. Sundan and S. Olsnes. Effect of potassium depletion of cells on their sensitivity to diphtheria toxin and pseudomonas toxin. *J Cell Physiol* 1985, 124(1): 54-60.

Serafini, T.; Stenbeck, G.; Brecht, A.; Lottspiech, F.; Orci, L.; Rothman, J.E.; Wieland, F.T. A coat subunit of Golgi-derived nonclathrin—coated vesicles with homology to the clathrin-coated vesicle protein beta-adaptin. *Nature* 1991, *349*, 215–220.

Schulte, T. W., S. Akinaga, S. Soga, W. Sullivan, B. Stensgard, D. Toft and L. M. Neckers. Antibiotic radicicol binds to the N-terminal domain of Hsp90 and shares important biologic activities with geldanamycin. *Cell Stress Chaperones* 1998, 3(2): 100-8.

Shiver, J.W.; Donovan, J.J. Interactions of diphtheria toxin with lipid vesicles: Determinants of ion channel formation. *Biochim. Biophys. Acta* 1987, *903*, 48–55.

Silverman, J.A.; Mindell, J.A.; Collier, R.J.; Finkelstein, A. Structure-function relationships in diphtheria toxin channels: I. Determining a minimal channel-forming domain. *J. Membr. Biol.* 1994, *137*, 17–28.

Simpson, J.C.; Smith, D.C.; Roberts, L.M.; Lord, J.M. Expression of mutant dynamin protects cells against diphtheria toxin but not against ricin. *Exp. Cell Res.* 1998, *239*, 293–300.

Smith, WP, Tai, PC, Murphy, JR, & Davis BD. A precursor in the cotranslational secretion of diphtheria toxin. *J Bacteriol*, 1980; 141: 184-189.

Stenmark, H., S. Olsnes and I. H. Madshus. Elimination of the disulphide bridge in fragment B of diphtheria toxin: effect on membrane insertion, channel formation, and ATP binding. *Mol Microbiol* 1991, 5(3): 595-606.

Tamayo AG, Bharti A, Trujillo C, Harrison R, Murphy JR. COPI coatomer complex proteins facilitate the translocation of anthrax lethal factor across vesicular membranes in vitro. *Proc Natl Acad Sci* U S A. 2008 Apr 1;105(13):5254-9.

Tamayo AG., Slater, L, Taylor-Parker, J, Bharti, A., Harrison, R., Hung, D, Murphy, JR. GRP78(BiP) facilitates the cytosolic delivery of anthrax lethal factor (LF) in vivo and functions as an unfoldase in vitro. Mol Microbiol 2011, 81(5): 1390-401.

Taylor M, Navarro-Garcia F, Huerta J, Burress H, Massey S, Ireton K, Teter K. Hsp90 is required for transfer of the cholera toxin A1 subunit from the endoplasmic reticulum to the cytosol. *J Biol Chem.* 2010 Oct 8;285(41):31261-7. Epub 2010 Jul 28.

Thompson, J.D.; Higgins, D.G.; Gibson, T.J. CLUSTAL W: Improving the sensitivity of progressive multiple sequence alignment through sequence weighting, position-specific gap penalties, weight matrix choice. *Nucleic Acids Res.* 1994, *22*, 4673–4680.

Trujillo C, Taylor-Parker J, Harrison R, Murphy JR Essential lysine residues within transmembrane helix 1 of diphtheria toxin facilitate COPI binding and catalytic domain entry. *Mol Microbiol.* 2010 May;76(4):1010-9. Epub 2010 Apr 14.

Tsai, B., Y. Ye and T. A. Rapoport. Retro-translocation of proteins from the endoplasmic reticulum into the cytosol. *Nat Rev Mol Cell Biol* 2002, 3(4): 246-55.

Tsuneoka, M, Nakayama, K, Hatsuzawa, K, Komada, M, Kitamura, N, & Mekada E. Evidence for the involvement of furin in cleavage and activation of diphtheria toxin. *J Biol Chem*, 1993; 268: 26461-26465.

Uchida, T, Gill, DM, & Pappenheimer, AM, Jr. Mutation in the structural gene for diphtheria toxin carried by temperate phage . *Nature*, 1971; 233: 8-11.

Umata, T.; Moriyama, Y.; Futai, M.; Mekada, E. The cytotoxic action of diphtheria toxin and its degradation in intact Vero cells are inhibited by bafilomycin A1, a specific inhibitor of vacuolar-type H(+)-ATPase. *J. Biol. Chem.* 1990, *265*, 21940–21945.

Waters, CA, Schimke, P, Snider, CE, Itoh, K, Smith, KA, Nichols, JC, Strom, TB, & Murphy, JR. Interleukin-2 receptor targeted cytotoxicity: Receptor requirements for entry of IL-2-toxin into cells. *Eur J Immunol*, 1990; 20: 785-791.

Waters, M.G.; Serafini, T.; Rothman, J.E. Coatomer a cytosolic protein complex containing subunits of non-clathrin-coated Golgi transport vesicles. *Nature* 1991, *349*, 248–251.

Wesche, J, Malecki, J, Wiedlocha A, Skjerpen, CS and Olsnes, S. FGF-1 and FGF-2 require the cytosolic chaperone Hsp 90 for translocation into the cytosol and nucleus. *J Cell Sci* 2006, 119:4332-41

Wesche, J, Elliott, JL, Falnes, PO, Olsnes, S, Z& Collier, RJ. Characterization of membrane translocation by anthrax protective antigen. *Biochemistry*, 1998; 37: 15737-15746.

Whitney, J.A.; Gomez, M.; Sheff, D.; Kries, T.E.; Mellman, I. Cytoplasmic coat proteins involved in endosome function. *Cell* 1995, *83*, 703–713.

Wiedlocha, A., I. H. Madshus, H. Mach, C. R. Middaugh and S. Olsnes. Tight folding of acidic fibroblast growth factor prevents its translocation to the cytosol with diphtheria toxin as vector. 1992 *Embo J* 11(13): 4835-42.

Williams, D, Parker, K, Bishai, W, Borowski, M, Genbauffe, F, Strom, TB, & Murphy, JR. DT receptor binding domain substitution with IL-2: genetic construction and properties of the DT-related IL-2 fusion protein. *Protein Engn*, 1987; 1: 493-498.

Williams, DP, Snider, CE, Strom TB, & Murphy JR. Structure function analysis of IL-2-toxin (DAB_{486}IL-2): Fragment B sequences required for the delivery of fragment A to the cytosol of target cells. *J Biol Chem*, 1990; 265: 11885-11889.

VanderSpek, C, Cassidy, D, Genbauffe, F, Huynh, PD, & Murphy, JR. An intact transmembrane helix 9 is essential for the efficient delivery of the diphtheria toxin catalytic domain to the cytosol of target cells. *J Biol Chem*, 1994; 269: 21455-21459.

VanderSpek, C, Howland, K, Friedman, T, & Murphy, JR. Maintenance of the hydrophobic face of the diphtheria toxin amphipathic transmembrane helix 1 is essential for the efficient delivery of the catalytic domain to the cytosol of target cells. *Protein Engn*, 1994; 7: 985-989.

vanderSpek JC, Mindel J, Finkelstein A, & Murphy JR. Structure function analysis of the transmembrane domain of the interleukin-2 receptor targeted fusion toxin DAB_{389}IL-2: The amphipathic helical region of the transmembrane is essential for the efficient delivery of the catalytic domain to the cytosol of target cells. *J Biol Chem*, 1993; 90: 8524-8528.

Vendeville A, Rayne F, Bonhoure A, Bettache N, Montcourrier P, Beaumelle B.HIV-1 Tat enters T cells using coated pits before translocating from acidified endosomes and elicitinbiological responses. *Mol Biol Cell.* 2004 May;15(5):2347-60

19

Pattern Recognition Receptors and Infectious Diseases

Ardi Liaunardy Jopeace[1], Chris B. Howard[1], Ben L. Murton[1],
Alexander D. Edwards[2] and Tom P. Monie[1]
[1]*Department of Biochemistry, University of Cambridge and*
[2]*School of Pharmacy, University of Reading*
United Kingdom

1. Introduction

1.1 The innate immune system

Our bodies are under constant attack from pathogens. Despite this continual bombardment, under normal circumstances we remain healthy for most of our lives. This protection against infectious and harmful agents is provided by our immune system. The immune system can be broken into two elements: adaptive immunity and innate immunity. Adaptive immunity is a specific response targeted against particular pathogens through, for example, cytotoxic T cells and antibody production. The adaptive immune system has the potential to raise a defence against any invading pathogen. However, this is a relatively slow and energy expensive process. Innate immunity in contrast provides a non-specific response against any pathogen via a variety of components and processes. These include: barrier functions, complement, natural killer (NK) cells, antimicrobial peptides, mucosal secretions, pattern recognition receptors (PRRs) and the commensal micro-organisms. Innate immunity is responsible for clearing the majority of pathogen exposures that would result in infection before the adaptive system is even involved. This chapter will focus upon the role of one particular arm of the innate immune response to infectious diseases – Pattern Recognition Receptors. It will broadly address the mechanisms by which PRRs recognise the pathogens, the effects this has and the types if response it has. It will also bring in examples of evasion strategies used by pathogens to avoid detection and touch on the impact of polymorphisms in the receptors. Finally we will discuss the role of PRRs in a key defence against infectious diseases, vaccination.

1.2 Targets for innate immune recognition by PRRs

PRRs are protein molecules encoded in the genome and not subject to rearrangement or variation during the lifetime of an individual. PRRs function as molecular sensors of infection and are predominantly found on critical immune cells such as macrophages and dendritic cells (DC). However, other cell types likely to come into contact with pathogens, for example epithelial cells, also express subsets of these receptors. Given the absence of functional rearrangement how do PRRs recognise pathogens from diverse families possessing such diverse biology and patterns of infection?

Firstly, the innate immune system is designed to recognise biological components that are common to many pathogens. These are known as pathogen-associated molecular patterns (PAMPs). This means, for example, that a receptor is able to respond to all bacteria that have common components in their cell walls rather than a specific protein that is found on only one type of micro-organism (Table 1).

Secondly, there are a number of families of receptors, and many receptors in each family (Section 2, Table 1). This limited diversity allows the innate immune system to respond, not only to different PAMPs, but also PAMPs found in either the extracellular space or an intracellular environment. By having multiple sites for detection of diverse targets, it is unlikely that any given pathogen will be able to evade all of the levels of detection.

Thirdly, and most importantly, the receptors are able to mount a coordinated response to pathogen infection because of extensive cross-talk and communication between the different signalling pathways. This again minimises the possibility of a pathogen being able to evade the innate immune response. Overall, the innate immune response is primarily designed to induce inflammation at the site of infection, recruit inflammatory cells and mediators and begin to potentiate the adaptive immune system. The coordinated nature of the innate response ensures that any response initiated is robust enough to meet the threat.

Stimulatory Pathogen Associated Molecular Pattern (PAMP)	Pattern Recognition Receptor (PRR)	Signalling Adapter Protein	Transcriptional or Cellular Pathway Activated
Toll-like receptors (TLRs)			
Bacterial cell wall components	TLR2 homo/heterodimers	MyD88	NFκB / AP1
LPS	TLR4 (plasma membrane)	MyD88	NFκB / AP1
LPS	TLR4 (endosome)	TRIF	IRF3 / NFκB / AP1
Flagellin	TLR5	MyD88	NFκB / AP1
dsRNA	TLR3	TRIF	IRF3 / NFκB / AP1
ssRNA	TLR7	MyD88	IRF7 / NFκB
Nod-like receptors (NLRs)			
iE-DAP	NOD1	RIP2	NFκB
MDP	NOD2	RIP2/CARD9	NFκB / AP1
e.g. Pore-forming toxins, nucleic acid	NLRP3	ASC	Caspase-1 activation
Retinoic acid-inducible gene I-like receptors (RLRs)			
dsRNA	RIG-I	MAVS	IRF3 / AP1 / NFκB
C-type lectin receptors (CLRs)			
β-glucans	Dectin-1	Syk	NFκB

Table 1. Pattern Recognition Receptor (PRR) Activation and Outputs. The activation and signalling of PRRs is a complex, multi-factorial process. Activatory ligands (blue column) are recognised by specific PRRs (pink column). This leads to the recruitment of adaptor signalling proteins (lilac column) and the activation of intracellular signalling cascades. The net result is the up-regulation of transcriptional activators or specific cellular processing events (green column).

1.3 Innate immune signalling overview

PRR activation and signalling is a complex multifactorial process that results in remarkably similar outcomes (Figure 1). For example: upregulation of NFκB (Nuclear Factor kappa B) and IRF (interferon (IFN) regulatory factor) family transcription factors; stimulation of the stress kinase pathways (e.g. mitogen-activated protein kinases (MAPK)); and activation of caspase-1 (Figure 1). Ultimately this results in up-regulation of pro-inflammatory cytokines, chemokines and anti-viral proteins. PRRs are activated by PAMPs. Endogenous molecules, such as ATP and heat shock proteins, can also act as ligands for some PRRs. These endogenous ligands are collectively known as damage associated molecular patterns (DAMPs). PRR activation results in conformational changes in the proteins, activates intracellular signalling pathways to amplify the signal and initiates the innate response (Figure 1). Assembly of the downstream signalling complex is reliant on the involvement of specific adapter proteins to recruit signalling components and act as molecular scaffolds for complex assembly. PRRs use specific adaptors and different adaptor proteins result in the activation of different signalling pathways (see Section 2; Table 1).

1.4 Physiological outcomes of innate immune activation

The targets of the transcription factors produced as a result of PRR stimulation are pro-inflammatory effectors, the most important of which are tumour necrosis factor (TNF), interleukin (IL)-1 and IL-6. The pro-inflammatory signals modify the permeability of the vasculature around a site of infection to increase recruitment of specialised immune cells, such as monocytes and macrophages. This leads to the classic signs of infection; redness, heat, swelling and pain. At a cellular level these effectors can regulate cellular death in localised areas of infection, but also coordinate events in the whole body through the activation of the acute-phase response. The production of anti-viral type I IFNs induces apoptosis in infected cells, thereby removing the virus from the system, but also triggers resistance to viral infection in neighbouring cells and so helps restrict the spread of infection.

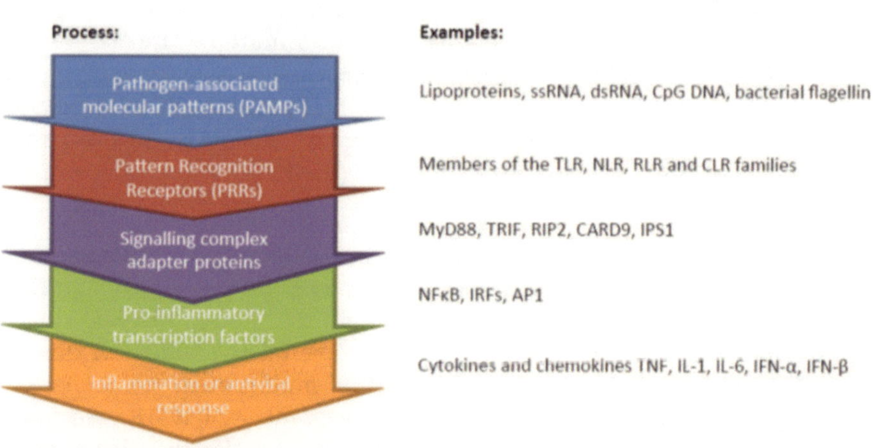

Fig. 1. Overview of innate immune signalling pathways and components. Activation begins with recognition of a stimulatory ligand, such as a pathogen-associated molecular pattern and results in an inflammatory or antiviral response from the cell.

The cellular and molecular changes associated with PRR activation are both complex and subtle. They create a response that can be shaped to deal with the specific nature of the infection. In macrophages many genes that modify their direct involvement in fighting infection and help repair damaged tissues are activated in response to PRR stimulation. Other cells, including monocytes, neutrophils, T-cells and B-cells can also be recruited to either directly help with the immune response or aid in the activation of the adaptive immune system.

2. Pattern recognition receptor families

PRRs are classified into four main families: Toll-like receptors (TLRs); Nucleotide binding leucine rich repeat (NLR) containing receptors, also known as NOD-like receptors; Retinoic acid-inducible gene I (RIG-I)-like receptors; and the C-type lectin receptors. The following sections provide brief details on the general signalling strategy of each of these families as well as specific examples of stimulatory ligands and physiological responses.

2.1 Toll-like receptors (TLRs)

TLRs are type 1 membrane proteins. They were the first components discovered in what we now regard as the innate immune system. TLRs use leucine-rich repeats (LRRs) to detect and bind ligand (Monie et al., 2009). LRRs have a conserved structural backbone which provides a scaffold on which variation can be built (Figure 2). Hence, LRRs from different receptors recognise a diverse range of PAMPs. In humans, TLR1, 2, 4, 5, 6 and 10 project their LRRs into the extracellular space, whereas TLR3, 7, 8 and 9 are compartmentalised to sample the contents of the endosomes.

TLRs signal in dimeric complexes after ligand binding (Figures 2 and 3). In general these are homodimeric complexes except for TLR2 which forms a heterodimer with TLR1 or TLR6. It has also been reported that TLR4 is capable of forming a signalling complex with TLR6. However, in this instance the receptor is involved in sterile inflammation and, in conjunction with CD36 responds to endogenous danger signals rather than PAMPs (Stewart et al., 2009). It is conceivable that following activation multiple dimeric TLR receptors cluster together in specific regions of the cellular membrane in order to augment signalling. Extracellular TLRs generally recognise components found on the outer surfaces of pathogens, such as lipoproteins and flagellin. Endosomal TLRs meanwhile recognise nucleic acids such as CpG-DNA, double-stranded RNA (dsRNA) and single stranded RNA (ssRNA).

The cytoplasmic Toll/IL-1 receptor (TIR) domain (Figure 2) mediates downstream signalling through adaptor recruitment. Based upon adaptor usage TLR signalling can be divided into two categories; those that signal through the protein myeloid differentiation factor 88 (MyD88) and those that don't. MyD88 is recruited to the TIR domains of an activated TLR and results in the formation of a multiprotein complex termed the myddosome (Figure 3). The myddosome contains a number of IL-1R-associated kinases (IRAKs) which direct signalling down specific pathways. Firstly, degradation of the inhibitory protein IκB (inhibitor of kappa B) releases the transcription factor NFκB; and secondly, the MAP (mitogen activated protein) kinase pathway activates the c-fos/jun transcription factor. These signals combine to drive expression of pro-inflammatory cytokines from NFκB and AP1 responsive genes respectively. The endosomal TLRs use the same pathway to activate NFκB and members of the IRF-family of transcription factors that activate expression of type I interferons needed to combat viral infection.

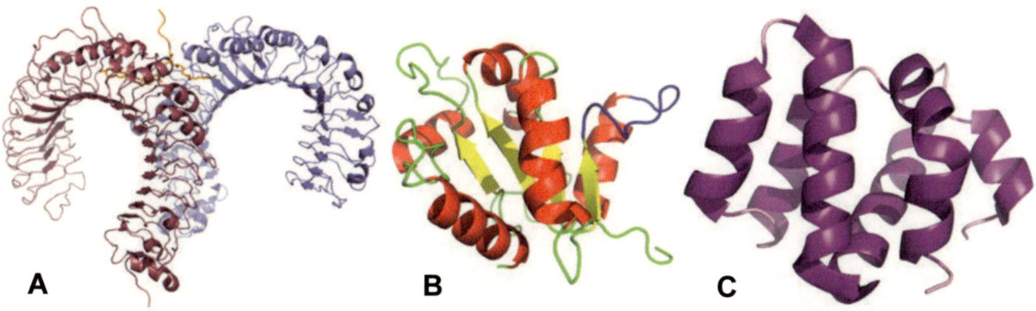

Fig. 2. Selected secondary structures of functional domains from PRRs. (A) Leucine rich repeat (LRR) containing ectodomains of TLR1 (blue) and TLR2 (purple). The synthetic ligand PAM3CYK4 (orange) stimulates heterodimerisation and formation of a signalling competent complex. (B) Toll/IL-1 receptor (TIR) domain of TLR2. The central beta-sheet core (yellow) is surrounded by five alpha helices. The BB loop, between the second beta-sheet and second alpha helix, is coloured blue. The BB loop is a key region of the TIR domain for downstream signalling activation and adaptor recruitment. (C) The caspase activation and recruitment domain (CARD) of the NLR family member NOD1. The CARD domain is a six-helix bundle involved in protein-protein interactions.

The MyD88-independent pathways use the adapter TIR-related adaptor protein inducing IFNβ (TRIF) in combination usually with the adaptor protein TRAM (TRIF-related adaptor molecule). This pathway is used to drive expression of IFN-β either in response to dsRNA detection by TLR3, or TLR4 signalling from the endosome rather than the plasma membrane. There is however significant cross-talk between the pathways. Adaptor proteins have recently been shown to be important in the susceptibility to infectious disease. This is exemplified by the adaptor Mal (MyD88-adaptor like), which is involved in recruitment of MyD88 to the TIR domain of TLR2 and TLR4. In this instance heterozygotic carriage of a single nucleotide polymorphism that results in the amino acid change serine to leucine at residue one-hundred-and-eighty in the TIR domain appears to be protective against the development of sepsis, invasive pneumococcal disease, bacteremia, malaria and tuberculosis (Ferwerda et al., 2009a; Khor et al., 2007)

2.2 Nucleotide binding leucine rich repeat containing receptors (NLRs)

The NLRs are a large family of cytoplasmic PRRs, of which there are at least 23 members. They share a characteristic domain organisation comprising of an N-terminal protein interaction domain, a central nucleotide binding region and C-terminal leucine-rich repeats (Figure 2). Currently the precise method of receptor activation by all the different ligands remains to be elucidated for the NLR family. There are two main groups in the NLR family based on the nature of their N-terminal domain. These are the NLRC sub-family who possess caspase activation and recruitment domain (CARDs) (Figure 2), and the Pyrin domain containing NLRP sub-family.

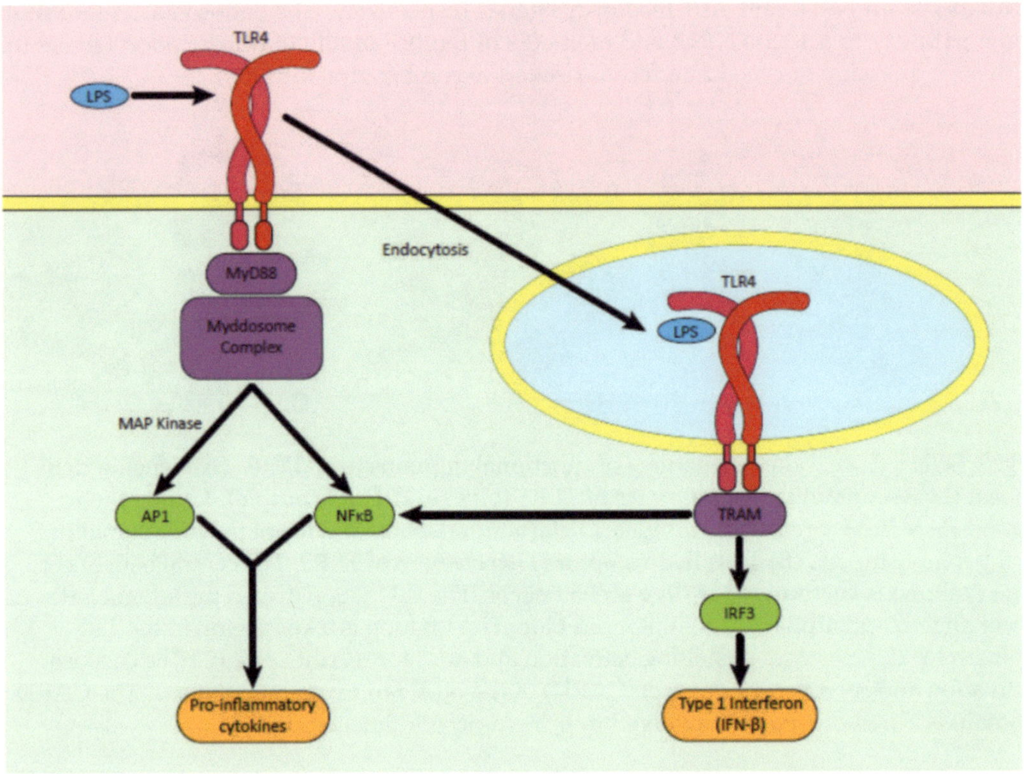

Fig. 3. Simplified schematic of TLR signalling exemplified by TLR4. Ligands are coloured blue, receptors are red, adaptor proteins purple, pro-inflammatory transcription factors green, and cellular outputs orange.

NLR signalling pathways can be broadly split into two: 1) upregulation of NFκB and activation of pro-inflammatory genes; 2) Inflammasome formation, caspase-1 activation and secretion of IL-1β and IL-18 (Figure 4). The first pathway is utilised by the prototypical NLRC family members NOD1 and NOD2. These receptors bind to PAMPs derived from bacterial peptidoglycan (Table 1). The activated NLRs signal through the adapter Receptor Interacting Protein 2 (RIP2) to drive the release of NFκB into the nucleus by the same processes employed by TLRs. In a further demonstration of PRR cross-talk, Nod2 also activates the MAP kinase pathway using a different adapter, CARD9, to upregulate pro-inflammatory gene expression from AP1 dependent promoters. The inflammasome forming NLRs consist, to date, of NLRP1, NLRP3 and NLRC4. The NLRP family members recruit the protein ASC (apoptosis-associated speck-like protein containing a CARD) through homotyoic Pyrin:Pyrin interactions. ASC also possesses a CARD domain which recruits pro-caspase 1 to the inflammasome complex. Self-cleavage of pro-caspase 1 releases active caspase-1 which subsequently cleaves pro-IL-1β and pro-IL-18 into their mature forms for secretion from the cell. Both IL-1β and IL-18 are proinflammatory and they play crucial roles in host defence against pathogens. IL-1β is responsible for the generation of systemic and local immune responses by causing fever, activating lymphocytes and recruiting them along with neutrophils to the site of infection. IL-18 lacks the pyrogenic nature of IL-1β but is involved in induction of IFN-γ production by T-cells and NK cells to drive T-helper cell type 1 (Th1) responses during adaptive immunity development. The NLRC4 inflammasome can activate caspase-1 in an ASC-dependent and -independent manner. Pro-IL-1β and pro-IL-18 are both expressed in an NFκB dependent manner. Hence their cellular levels are increased by TLR and NLR activation. The inflammasome can then be activated in response to a diverse selection of ligands, increasing the levels of IL-1β and IL-18 and amplifying the initial response to many PAMPs.

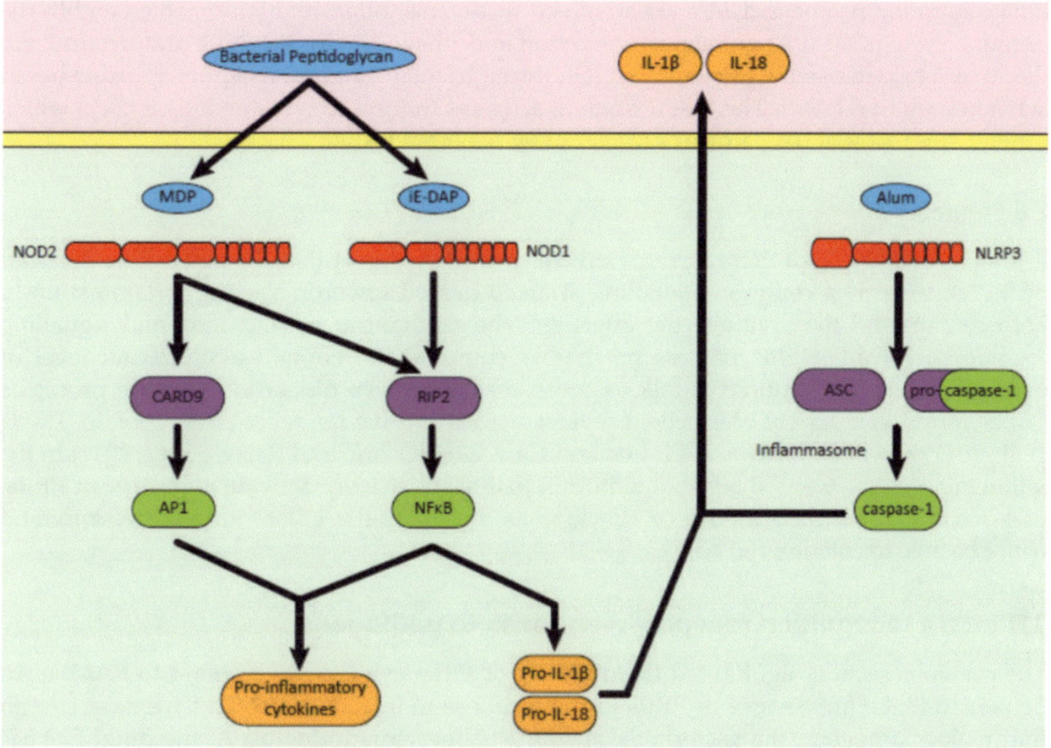

Fig. 4. Simplified representation of NLR family member signalling. Ligands are coloured blue, receptors are red, adaptor proteins purple, pro-inflammatory transcription factors green, and cellular outputs orange. Caspase-1 activation ultimately results in cell death through the process of pyroptosis.

2.3 Retinoic acid-inducible gene I-like receptors (RLRs)

RLRs are a small family of PRRs that detect intracellular RNA. RLRs use CARDs to interact with downstream signalling components. Activation results in expression of type I IFNs and other pro-inflammatory cytokines. In conjunction with endosomal TLRs the RLRs provide a robust antiviral response. RIG-I recognises short uncapped dsRNA or ssRNA, whereas melanoma differentiation-associated 5 (MDA5) detects longer dsRNA such as poly (I:C). Both proteins signal by forming CARD:CARD interactions with MAVS (mitochondrial antiviral signalling protein; also known as IFN-β-promoter stimulator 1 (IPS-1)) which is localised on the exterior membrane of the mitochondria. This activates the IRF transcription factors, but again leads to co-stimulation of the MAP kinase pathway as seen in the signalling of the other PRRs. The RLRs are also involved in sensing and triggering a response to cytoplasmic DNAs which can be transcribed by RNA polymerase III into dsRNA.

2.4 C-type lectin receptors (CLRs)

CLRs are characterised by the presence of a C-type lectin domain. Over 1000 proteins in the human genome could be described as CLRs, however, only a few specifically modulate the innate immune response. CLRs are involved in diverse, often regulatory, roles within the immune system, such as antigen presentation and phagocytosis. Dectin-1 and dectin-2 are the best characterised CLRs and signal through their immunoreceptor tyrosine-based activation motif (ITAM). The ITAM domain activates the spleen tyrosine kinase (Syk) which upregulates many of the pathways triggered by the other PRRs.

2.5 Summary

It is clear that although there is much diversity in the range of PAMPs that can be detected by PRRs, there is a common signalling strategy geared towards causing inflammation to both contain and then remove the infection. The mechanism of activation and signalling cascades involved in this process are highly complex and contain a significant level of overlap, redundancy and cross-talk. A more comprehensive discussion of these processes can be found in a variety of excellent review articles and the references they contain (Davis et al., 2011; Kawai and Akira, 2011; Loo and Gale, 2011; Osorio and Reis e Sousa, 2011).In the following sections we will see that although pathogens usually activate a number of PRRs, they have adapted their modes of attack so as to bypass the innate immune system, and hence be able to colonise the body.

3. Pattern recognition receptor responses to pathogens

The previous section highlighted the diversity of PRRs available to respond to PAMPs. To demonstrate the importance of PRRs in the response to infectious diseases we have chosen four major pathogens; the bacteria *Salmonella spp.*, the virus Influenza A, the fungi *Candida albicans*, and the parasite *Schistosoma mansoni*. Here we describe the importance of PRRs in the recognition of these pathogens and induction of an innate immune response against them. As will become apparent the innate immune system has evolved so that multiple PRRs recognise different PAMPs from the same pathogen.

Pathogens, like higher organisms, also undergo evolutionary pressure to survive. In essence this can be viewed as a host-pathogen arms race. Successful pathogens are able to evade, limit, or manipulate detection by PRRs, and in some cases, utilise PRR signalling pathways for their own benefit. Pathogen survival can be augmented in a number of ways. These include targeting the recognition receptor, the signalling transduction event, and the key effector proteins of the innate immune system (Hajishengallis and Lambris, 2011). The innate immune system is a common target for immune evasion strategies for two primary reasons. Firstly, it is the initial host defence encountered by the pathogens upon infection. Secondly, the innate immune system is essential for the development of adaptive immunity. Consequently, by exploiting the innate immune system, pathogens can undermine the whole immune response of the host. Many different mechanisms are employed by pathogens to subvert immune signalling. These include: the use of immunomodulatory proteins; receptor antagonists; the induction of immunosuppression; activation of host immune inhibitory receptors; reduced expression, or alteration, of the PAMP; and manipulation of PRR crosstalk. In short successful pathogens are able to survive for longer in, and colonise, the host through maintenance of a careful balance between innate immune activation and suppression. In addition to identifying the key PRR-pathogen interactions we will provide examples highlighting the ability of these organisms to survive in the host and evade the innate immune response.

3.1 PRRs and Salmonella

3.1.1 *Salmonella* is a Gram-negative bacterium that causes food-borne diseases

Salmonella is a Gram-negative (Figure 5), rod-shaped, flagellated, bacterium which invades, and replicates and survives within, immune cells such as macrophages (Coburn et al., 2007). There are over 2500 serotypes of *Salmonella enterica*. *S. enterica typhi* and *S. enterica typhimurium* cause typhoid fever and enterocolitis respectively in humans. These diseases affect millions of people globally causing around 600,000 deaths annually, mostly in infants and immunocompromised patients.

Salmonella is transmitted via the faeco-oral route following ingestion of contaminated food, water or animal products, or close contact with an infected individual. Infection predominantly occurs in the epithelial lining of the intestine with intestinal epithelial cells (IECs) and macrophages being key cells for both bacterial uptake and immunity. IECs act not only as physical barriers to infection, but also contribute to the innate immune response following PRR activation. Bacterial uptake by macrophages (and dendritic cells) results in stimulation of a wide range of PRRs and can also serve as a route to systemic infection. The pathophysiology of *Salmonella* infections is strongly connected to the strong inflammatory response from the host. Interaction between host PRRs and *Salmonella* virulence factors influence the pathology, morbidity, and mortality at different stages of infection.

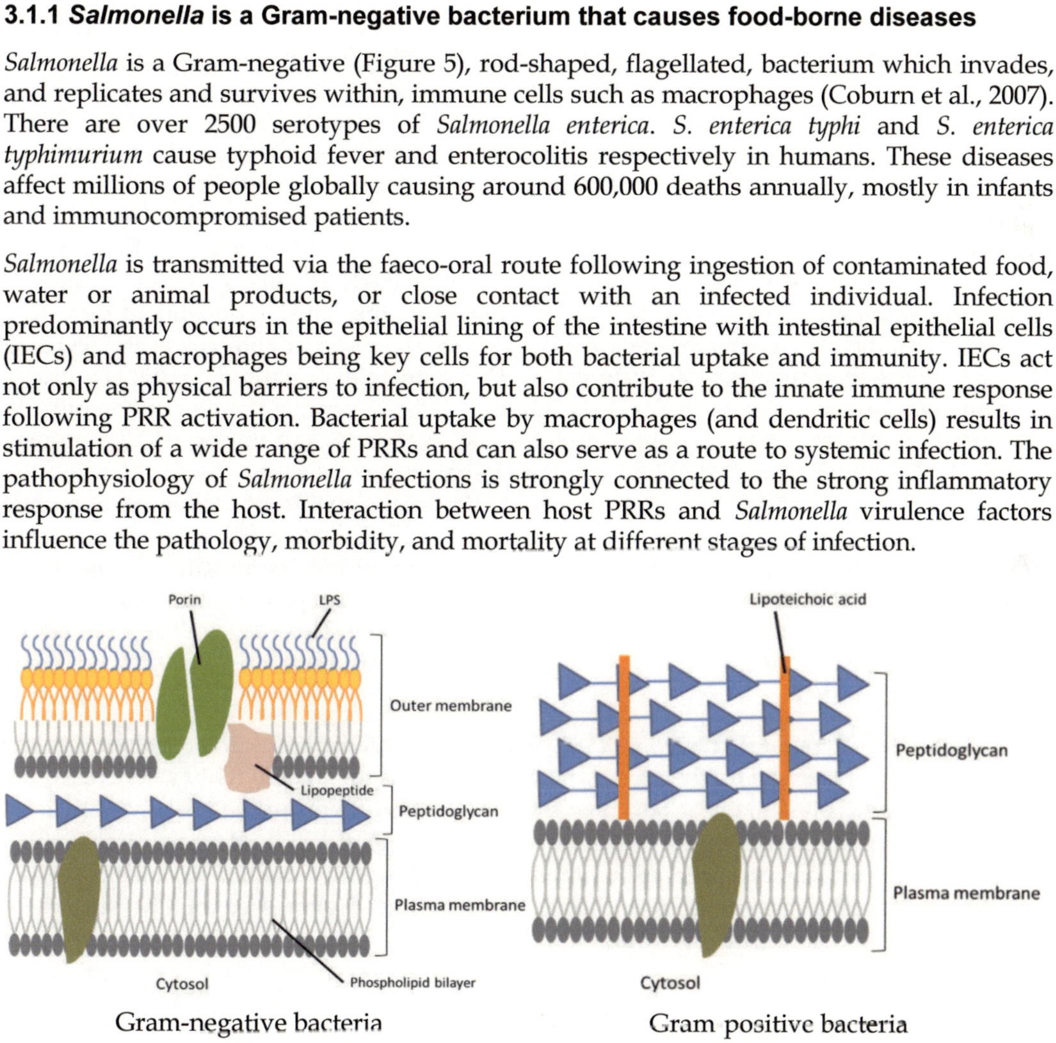

Fig. 5. Schematic of the cell wall structure of Gram-negative (left-hand image) and Gram-positive (right-hand image) bacteria highlighting the key components of each type of bacterial wall. Salmonella is a rod-shaped Gram-negative bacterium. Two key PAMPs associated with Salmonella are LPS and lipopeptide which activate TLR4 and TLR2 respectively. In addition, the surface of Salmonella possesses flagella, another potent immunostimulatory molecule.

3.1.2 *Salmonella* PAMPs and PRR activation

Salmonella is recognised by a wide range of PRRs: TLR1, 2, 4, 5, 6, and 9; NLRC4; NLRP3; NOD1 and NOD2 (Hold et. al., 2011). Of these the key PRRs are TLR2, TLR4, TLR5 and NLRC4. Cell culture studies and mouse models have identified several *Salmonella* PAMPs responsible for PRR activation. Of particular importance are LPS, lipoproteins and flagellin (Figure 5). Flagellin provides an interesting example of a ligand that is able to activate two distinct receptors (TLR5 and NLRC4) leading to distinct immune responses (Franchi et al., 2006; Hayashi et al., 2001).

LPS and lipoproteins lead to classical activation of TLR4 and TLR2 signalling pathways respectively (Section 2.1). The importance of TLR2 signalling is influenced by the severity of infection, playing a key role at high multiplicities of infection. In contrast, the role of TLR4 appears essential at all levels of Salmonella infection (Spiller et al., 2008; Talbot et al., 2009). TLR4 activation by LPS requires several co-receptors such as: myeloid-differentiation 2 (MD2), cluster of differentiation 14 (CD14), and LPS-binding protein (LBP). The TLR4 signalling pathway is different from all other TLRs as its activation results in two separate signalling cascades: MyD88-dependent and MyD88-independent pathways which result in NF-κB activation and IFN-β and NFκB activation respectively (Figure 3). This activation is regulated temporally and spatially as it is been suggested that MyD88-dependent signalling occurs first on the plasma membrane, following which the receptor complex is endocytosed after which it will sequentially activate the MyD88-independent pathway. This is a classic example of the use of subcellular localisation of the receptor signalling complex to determine use of downstream adaptor proteins and the specifics of the signalling pathway activated. The importance of TLR4 in the response to *Salmonella* is highlighted by observations that mice possessing defects in TLR4 are incapable of mounting a normal immune response to *Salmonella typhimurium* infection (Talbot et al., 2009). It appears that the relative importance of different TLR and adaptor proteins in combating *Salmonella* is dependent upon the bacterial load. For example, the adaptor protein Mal only appears important at low multiplicities of infection (Kenny et al., 2009). This may well be a deliberate ploy on the part of the host to manage the severity of the response at a level which reflects the severity of infection.

TLR5 recognises monomeric flagellin. TLR5 is expressed on the basolateral surface, not the apical surface, of polarised epithelial cells so only responds to flagellin that has breached the epithelial barrier. This is likely to be a host strategy to stop inappropriate immune activation by flagellated commensal bacteria in the lumen (Gewirtz et al., 2001; Hayashi et al., 2001) . Once the bacterium has breached the epithelial barrier flagellin can then be detected by the baso-laterally located receptor. In addition, TLR5 is found expressed on the surface of immune cells such as macrophages and DCs.

The mechanism of flagellin recognition by TLR5 is interesting as only monomeric flagellin is recognised. This is because the TLR5 binding site is buried in the functional flagellar filament. This is one of the bacterium's ways of evading the host immune system. A single filamentous flagella consists of 11 protofilaments, each of which contains four globular domains (D0-D3) (Figure 6). The recognition site for TLR5 is contained in the N-terminal D1 domain. This region is essential for motility and is consequently highly conserved (Smith et al., 2003). Mutations within D1 have been shown to abolish recognition by TLR5, bacterial motility, and to disrupt protofilament assembly. In particular differences in amino acids 89-

96 have been implicated in the ability of some species of bacteria to evade immune detection by TLR5 (Andersen-Nissen et al., 2005).

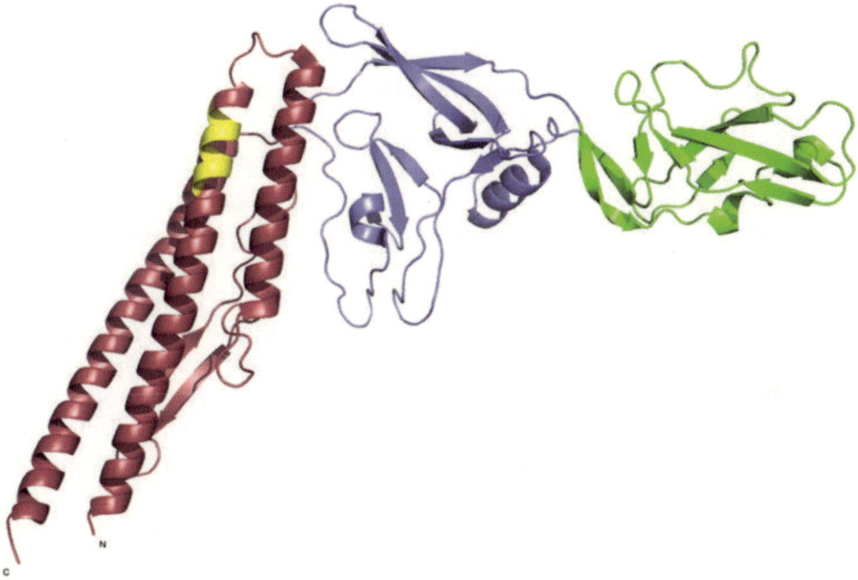

Fig. 6. Crystal structure of FliC flagellin from *S. typhimurium* (pdb entry 1io1). Domain colouring is: D1 - light purple; D2 - blue; D3 - green; the yellow region in D1 corresponds to amino acids 89-96.

Prior to detection by TLR5, flagella has to be depolymerised into its monomeric form. Direct contact between the bacterium and the host cell triggers the *de novo* synthesis and secretion of monomeric flagellin into the host cell via T3SS (Subramanian and Qadri, 2006). This process is triggered by the bacterium sensing lysophospholipids produced by the host cells upon infection and is important for initial inflammatory and innate immune responses by IECs. Following activation TLR5 forms a homodimer and initiates MyD88-dependent signalling cascades (Figure 3) as part of the innate immune response. One effect of this is to recruit neutrophils and macrophages to the site of infection.

Once *Salmonella* has breached the epithelia it can be phagocytosed by macrophages. The bacterium can reside and replicate inside a Salmonella-containing vesicle. Fragments of flagellin enter into the cytoplasm, probably via a type III secretion system, from where it stimulates the NLR family receptor NLRC4 (Franchi et al., 2006). NLRC4 is also activated by the protein PrgJ, a component of the type III secretion system expressed by the *Salmonella* pathogenicity island (SPI)-1 (Miao et al., 2010). The mechanisms of NLRC4 activation by bacteria such as Salmonella are complex and seem to follow some form of temporal cascade. The net effect is that activation of NLRC4 leads to inflammasome formation, caspase-1 activation and secretion of IL-1β and IL-18. In addition, caspase-1 activation via NLRC4 can trigger macrophage death through pyroptosis. Pyroptosis is a caspase-1 dependent, programmed cell death event that has features of both apoptosis and necrosis. The process of pyroptosis results in the release of pro-inflammatory cellular contents and also serves to limit intracellular bacterial replication (Roy and Zamboni, 2006) (Figure 4).

3.1.3 Modulation of the innate immune response by *Salmonella*

Salmonella is capable of infecting, surviving, and multiplying within macrophages. This requires multiple virulence proteins which are predominantly encoded on the SPI-2 pathogenicity island. These factors enable the bacterium to resist the oxidative burst and maturation of phagosomes and lysosomes. In fact the bacterium modifies these endocytic vacuoles and generates an environment conducive to bacterial replication - the salmonella containing vacuole (SCV) (Figure 7).

In addition to acting as a trigger of NLRC4 signalling (Section 3.1.2) the T3SS allows proteins to be injected into the cell cytoplasm that modulate cellular function. A major role of these proteins is to alter cytoskeletal function and permit bacterial entry. In addition, *Salmonella* also secretes an immunomodulatory protein SipB. The precise role and mechanism of action of SipB is unknown. However, the protein is capable of interacting with caspase-1 and consequently altering the signalling pathways involved in caspase-1 activation and downstream functionality (Hersh et al., 1999). Other bacteria also produce proteins that modulate immune signalling. For example, it has recently been shown that *Escherichia coli* and *Brucella melitensis* produce TIR domain containing virulence factors that inhibit TLR signalling by directly blocking MyD88 adaptor protein function through a homotypic TIR-TIR interaction (Cirl et al., 2008).

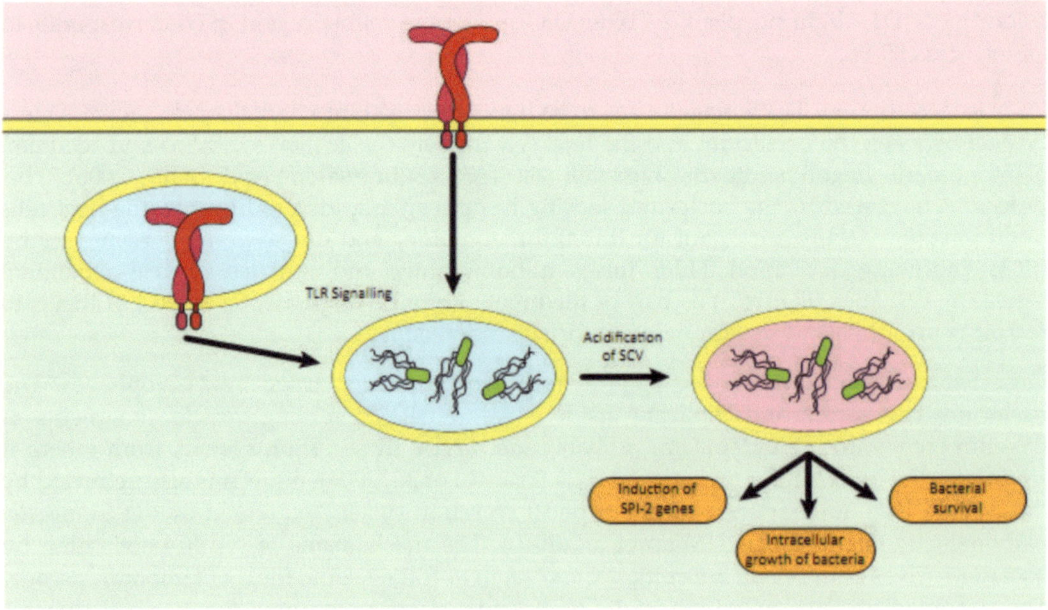

Fig. 7. Formation of a *Salmonella* containing vacuole (SCV) promotes *Salmonella* survival and virulence inside host macrophages. SCV formation appears to be dependent on functional TLR signalling and requires acidification to activate expression of the *Salmonella* pro-survival genes.

3.1.4 Altering PAMP properties as a way to evade immune detection

Salmonella flagellin is a readily available and common target recognised by both extracellular, TLR5, and intracellular, NLRC4, PRRs. Although many PAMPs cannot be altered and changed in order to evade the immune response this is not the case for flagellin. *Salmonella* has been found to downregulate flagellin expression once it is inside macrophages, although how quickly this happens is unclear. A loss of flagellin expression will obviously reduce the potential for immune stimulation, but it has yet to be determined whether this occurs in a timeframe that will influence PRR activation. As TLR5 recognises monomeric flagellin mechanisms that increase flagellum stability and reduce the release of monomeric subunits will also reduce immune activation.

Some other flagellated bacteria have adopted a mechanism in which they express flagellin lacking the proinflammatory regions found in Salmonella FliC (Section 3.1.2). The classic example is *Helicobacter Pylori*. *H.pylori* express the flagellin proteins FlaA and FlaB. These subunits retain the ability to assemble motile flagella, but lack the TLR5 stimulatory regions. This was elegantly demonstrated by experiments in which the comparable sequence from *H.pylori* flagellin was substituted into *Salmonella* FliC. The mutant flagellin lost the ability to activate TLR5.

3.2 PRRs and viral PAMPs

Viruses are more abundant than bacteria; they are also very diverse genetically and evolve rapidly. Viruses are obligate parasites and can only survive and replicate inside host cells. They have different virulence components and simpler structural features in comparison to bacteria. The requirement on the host cell for replication makes viral nucleic acids the key viral PAMPs. Consequently, only a subset of PRRs can detect them. These include: NLRP3; NOD2; TLR3, 7, 8, and 9; and the RIG-I like receptors (Kanneganti, 2010; Perry et al., 2005) (Table 2).

PAMP	PRR	Adapter	Cytokines
Toll-like receptors (TLRs)			
dsRNA	TLR3	TRIF	IFN-β/ pro-inflammatory
G/U rich ssRNA	TLR7	MyD88	IFN-α/ pro-inflammatory
G/U rich ssRNA	TLR8	MyD88	IFN-α
unmethylated CpG DNA motifs	TLR9	MyD88	IFN-α
Nod-like receptors (NLRs)			
ssRNA	NOD2	MAVS	Type I IFNs
Viral RNA	NLRP3	ASC	IL-1β/IL-18
Retinoic acid-inducible gene I-like receptors (RLRs)			
5′ triphosphate ssRNA	RIG-I	MAVS/ASC/CARD9	Type-I IFNs/ IL-1β

Table 2. Natural viral PAMPs are recognised by PRRs and stimulate cytokine production. Viral nucleic acids generally differ from host nucleic acids through the presence of specific motifs and also their subcellular localisation. Viral nucleic acid (blue column) is recognised by specific PRRs (pink column) and this leads to receptor activation. The activated receptor recruits specific adaptor proteins and initiates signalling cascades. The net result of this is the secretion of cytokines.

The host response to viral infection results in the production of anti-viral agents such as type I IFNs that interfere with viral replication and survival inside host cells, and pro-inflammatory cytokines such as IL-1β and IL-18. Type I IFNs are the key players in innate immune response against viral infection. We will expand the discussion on role of PRRs in viral infection by considering the example of influenza virus.

3.2.1 Recognition of influenza by TLRs

Influenza is a negative-sense ssRNA virus that causes pulmonary inflammation and chronic lung diseases. The symptoms vary from fever and inflammation to death, depending on the strain of the virus and the host response. Influenza enters host cells by endocytosis following recognition of sialic acid residues by the viral haemagglutinin protein. This is followed by pH-dependent fusion of the viral and endosomal membranes allowing release of the viral core into the cytosol. The exact sequence of events that subsequently leads to recognition of influenza by PRRs is still largely unknown. Influenza PAMPs can be recognised by a variety of PRRs (Figure 8 and Table 2). However, the majority of immunopathology appears to result from TLR7, NLRP3 and RIG-I activation (Ichinohe, 2010). Plasmacytoid dendritic cells (pDCs) are the major cell-type responsible for mounting an immune response to influenza through the secretion of high amounts of type I IFNs and proinflammatory cytokines (Perry et al., 2005). Macrophages, nasal airway epithelial cells and monocytes have also been found to respond to influenza. Secreted type I IFNs interact with IFN receptors causing expression of type I IFN-stimulated genes with antiviral properties. For example, increased expression of RIG-I like receptors and proteins involved in the inhibition of viral transcription and trafficking. Type I IFNs also influence the development of adaptive immunity such as increasing expression of costimulatory molecules on macrophages and DCs, aiding maturation of DCs, and the activation of T and NK cells.

pDCs are professional antigen presenting cells. Following endocytic uptake of virus particles the virus is degraded and can contact endosomal PRRs. The presence of ssRNA in the endosome activates TLR7 (Lund et al., 2004) which signals in a MyD88-dependent manner to activate IRF3 and IRF7 transcription factors for the expression of type I IFNs. ssRNA recognition by TLR7 appears to require endosomal acidification before the receptor can form a homodimer and initiate the signalling pathways. TLR7 and MyD88 are both required for the type I IFN response to influenza ssRNA in pDCs. Studies have shown that mice deficient in either TLR7 or MyD88 are unable to respond to influenza virus (Diebold et al., 2004; Lund et al., 2004). TLR7 is also expressed in other cell types such as macrophages and conventional DCs, however TLR7 activation in these cell types only result in expression of proinflammatory cytokines. This difference is due to different signalling adaptor proteins present in these different cell types. Human naïve B cells and effector memory $CD4^{+}$ T cells also express and signal through TLR7 activation (Wang et al., 2006).

The TLR7 response to influenza ssRNA is independent of viral replication. In contrast, there is evidence that dsRNA can induce type I IFN production via a TLR7- and MyD88-independent pathway that requires viral replication (Guillot et al., 2005). Even though influenza is a ssRNA virus, dsRNA molecules are synthesised during the replicative stage of the virus. Certainly TLR3 recognises endosomal dsRNA from influenza virus (Guillot et al., 2005). The downstream signalling proceeds not through MyD88, but the adaptor TRIF to activate IRF3 and late-phase NF-κB. The importance of dsRNA recognition in influenza infection is supported by the observation that the influenza protein NS1, which sequesters viral dsRNA, inhibits type I IFN induction upon viral infection (Lu et al., 1995).

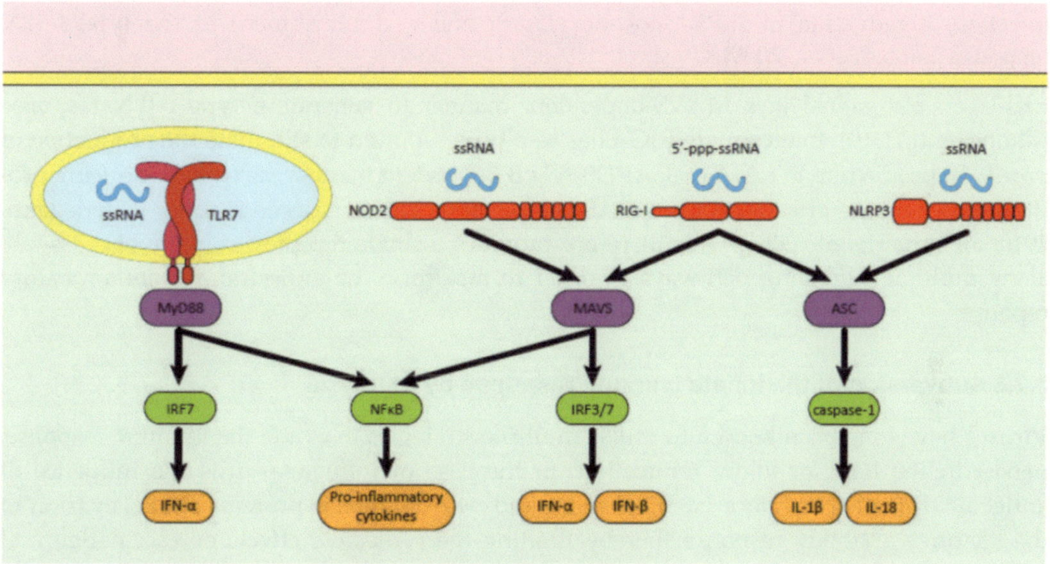

Fig. 8. Cytoplasmic and endosomal PRRs that recognise PAMPs from ssRNA virus such as influenza. Different PRRs can activate different pathways, and some pathways are shared by several PRRs.

3.2.2 Recognition of influenza by NLR and RLRs

Influenza can be recognised by the NLRP3 inflammasome, RIG-I and potentially NOD2 (Kanneganti, 2010). Activation of these signalling pathways results in the activation of caspase-1, IL-1β and IL-18; the production of inflammatory cytokines; and the secretion of type I IFNs via MAVS engagement. Each of these receptors is located in the cytoplasm and hence responds to the presence of RNA, 5'-phosphate ssRNA, or ssRNA within the cytoplasm. This contrasts to TLR7 which responds to ssRNA in the endosomal compartment. In the case of NLRP3 it is unknown whether viral RNA is a directly activating ligand for the receptor. Indeed it is more likely in this instance that the presence of viral RNA in the cytoplasm leads to a homeostatic disruption that in turn activates NLRP3, stimulates inflammasome formation, and initiates a protective innate immune response.

NOD2 and NLRP3 elicit different immune responses to viral RNA (Fig. 6). NLRP3 stimulation leads to activation of caspase 1 and subsequent processing of the pro forms of IL-1β and IL-18 via inflammasome formation. Both IL-1β and IL-18 are important in the clearance of influenza infection as mice which lack the IL-1 receptor and consequently can't respond to these cytokines show impaired viral clearance and increased mortality (Schmitz et al., 2005). Unlike NLRP3, NOD2 does not form an inflammasome. The primary role of NOD2 seems to be the detection of the bacterial peptidoglycan fragment muramyl dipeptide and signalling through NF-κB regulated pathways. However, more recently NOD2 has been reported to respond to viral ssRNA (Sabbah et al., 2009). Viral ssRNA results in activation of an alternative MAVS-dependent NOD2 signalling cascade in which NOD2 relocalises to the mitochondria and ultimately activates IRF3. This leads to the induction of an antiviral type I IFN response. A loss of NOD2 led to an increase in the susceptibility of mice to influenza infection, a reduction in IRF3 phosphorylation and a diminishment of the type I IFN response (Sabbah et al., 2009).

RIG-I can also signal in a MAVS-dependent manner to generate a type I IFN response (Kanneganti, 2010). Interestingly RIG-I has also been reported to stimulate the production of pro-IL-1β production in a MAVS-CARD9-NFkB dependent manner; as well as inducing pro-IL-1β processing and secretion in an ASC-dependent inflammasome manner (Kanneganti, 2010; Pichlmair et al., 2006). This therefore provides a single receptor example of cross-talk along multiple signalling pathways in order to maximise the anti-viral and inflammatory reponse.

3.2.3 Subversion of the innate immune response by influenza

Viruses have long been known to utilise multiple strategies to evade the immune response, persist in the host, or allow reinfection. In the case of influenza virus the influence of antigenic drift in the surface haemaglutinin and neurominidase proteins allows evasion of the adaptive antibody response thereby limiting the protective effects of vaccination and facilitating influenza epidemics. Antigenic shift is a more extreme, and less common, evasion strategy in which viruses from different species undergo recombination to create a new potentially pandemic viral strain. Commonly recombination occurs between human and avian viral strains.

Influenza virus also employs various strategies to disrupt the innate immune response; either by interfering with PRR mediated detection of viral components, or through modulation of signalling cascades. The viral non-structural protein (NS)1 is a good example of a protein that targets a specific signalling pathways to avoid detection. NS1 has the potential to inhibit the activation of caspase 1 and the production of type I IFNs. Interestingly there does appear to be strain-dependent variation in activity of NS1 in this respect. The N-terminal region of NS1 appears to be important for the inhibition of inflammasome-dependent immune responses; specifically through inhibition of caspase-1 activation, and hence IL-1β and IL-18 production (Kanneganti, 2010). NS1 has also been reported to inhibit RIG-I-MAVS-dependent antiviral signalling (Bowie and Unterholzner, 2008). Pichlmair and colleagues, reported that NS1 binds directly to RIG-I and inhibits its activation, thereby reducing type I IFN production (Pichlmair et al., 2006). However, the exact molecular mechanism of how NS1 inhibits RIG-I signalling is not clear. This interaction may directly antagonise RIG-I function, or it could involve other proteins that are required for proper signalling. For example, NS1 also sequesters dsRNA so that they cannot be detected by dsRNA-recognising PRRs such as TLR3 and PKR. More recently, Gack and co-workers showed that NS1 inhibits RIG-I signalling by inhibiting activation of ubiquitin ligase tripartite motif (TRIM)25; a crucial component of the RIG-I signalling cascade required for activation of RIG-I through ubiquitination within the CARD domain (Gack et al., 2007).

3.3 PRRs and *Candida albicans*

3.3.1 *Candida albicans*

The yeast *Candida albicans* is a common human commensal that colonises mucocutaneous surfaces of the oral cavity, gastrointestinal tract and vagina. *Candida albicans* is often a benign member of the mucosal flora. However, under specific host conditions, such as a change in immune status or commensal species, *Candida albicans* can proliferate in a saprophytic state and become an opportunistic pathogen. This usually results in mucosal diseases, but on occasion the infection may become systemic and life-threatening. A specific example is nosocomial candidiasis in hospital patients with a compromised immune system. *Candida albicans* can differentiate in yeast, pseudohyphal and hyphal forms. The hyphal form is often linked to disease as it facilitates infection of epithelial cells and tissue damage. In addition to hyphae *Candida* species enhance their pathogenicity through biofilm formation and secretion of proteases and toxins. The balance between the commensal and pathogenic state is what makes *Candida albicans* a useful study case for looking at the interplay between host PRRs and PAMPs, and the dynamics that lead to protection/tolerance or infection.

3.3.2 Induction of an immune response by *Candida albicans*

It is hypothesised that the initial interaction between the host immune cell and specific *C.albicans* PAMPs is critical for deciding whether the immune response is protective or invasive. Studies suggest that a prolonged anti-inflammatory response against *C. albicans*, including increased production of IL-10, IL-4 and differentiation of regulatory/suppressive T cell subsets facilitates invasion and the initial development of disease. In the absence of IL-10 there is a switch to a protective response by the innate immune system. This includes stimulation of inflammatory cytokines such as IL-12, TNFα, and IL-6; and progression towards a Th17 response leading to IL-17 and IL-22 production to clear the infection. Further evidence for the role of IL-10 as a modulator of yeast infection is suggested by animal models. IL-10 deficient mice are protected against the toxic effects of *C.albicans* infection and show a decline in inflammatory markers associated with yeast infections. In contrast, inclusion of IL-4 and IL-10 in a gastrointestinal model of yeast infection facilitates invasion rather than protection.

Interaction studies between host immune cells and *Candida albicans* have identified various PRRs that recognise yeast derived PAMPs, and facilitate protective responses via the pro-inflammatory pathway. Most yeast and fungal PAMPs have been identified in the cell wall, a complex matrix consisting of glucans, mannans, mannoproteins and glycolipids. Several receptors including TLR4 and the C-type lectins Dectin-2, Mincle and the macrophage mannose receptor bind to mannans of *Candida* species. Dectin-1, lactosylceramide complement receptor-3 and scavenger receptors recognise β-glucans of *Candida.*

3.3.3 TLR sensing of *Candida albicans*

TLRs are involved in the immune response against *C. albicans* as well as other fungal agents, particularly TLR2 and to a lesser extent TLR4. Both pathogenic and commensal forms of *C. albicans* are involved in TLR-dependent signalling, in addition to other commensal yeasts such as *Saccromyces cerevisiae.* TLR2 recognises phospholipomannan components of the fungal cell wall. TLR4 is activated by α-mannans on *C. albicans* and initiates the production of IL-12 by host immune cells and a subsequent protective Th1 response. TLR4 polymorphisms Asp299Gly/Thr399Ile are associated with an increased susceptibility to *C. albicans* infection in the bloodstream, with an increase in IL-10 levels being the contributing factor (Van der Graaf et al., 2006). In addition to a pro-inflammatory response, TLR2 activation may also lead to the production of IL-10 and generation of T regulatory cells and a non-protective Th2 response. This is supported by data on TLR2 KO mice which are more resistant to *Candida* infection. The TLR2 polymorphism R753G gives rise to patients with enhanced *Candida* sepsis, suggesting that TLR2 is an important PRR for regulation of *Candida* infections (Woehrle et al., 2008). Indeed, TLR2 signalling complexes may modulate the Th1/Th2 (IL-10) balance in response to fungi by switching between pro- and anti-inflammatory responses. TLR signalling occurs in crosstalk with the carbohydrate specific PRRs, the C-type and S-type lectins, to regulate *C. albicans* infection.

3.3.4 CLR recognition of *Candida albicans*

CLRs such as Dectin-1, Dectin-2, Mincle, DC-SIGN (SIGNR1, mouse homolog) and mannose receptor (MR) are key PRRs in the immune response against fungi. The interaction of CLRs with PAMPs is mediated via carbohydrate recognition domains (CRD), which facilitate internalisation, degradation and antigenic presentation. CLRs signal via the Syk pathway to initiate an inflammatory response using an ITAM motif in their cytoplasmic tail. Some CLRs such as Dectin-2, lack an ITAM motif and instead utilise adaptor molecules such as the Fc receptor γ chain and the DNAX-activating protein (DAP12) which have an ITAM motif for signalling.

Dectin-1, which is expressed in neutrophils, macrophages and DCs, is a specific receptor for β-1,3 glucans, located in the cell walls of fungi, such as *Saccharomyces cerevisiae* (zymosan) and *Candida albicans.* Dectin-1 signalling pathways are not completely understood. It is proposed that Dectin-1 mediated responses may require crosstalk with TLRs, NLRs, tetraspanins and the DC-SIGN receptor. Dectin-1 binds and internalises β-glucans, and mediates its own signalling pathway which includes the production of reactive oxygen species (ROS) also termed an oxidative burst, activation of NFκβ and secretion of proinflammatory cytokines. Following ligand recognition via the CRD, Dectin-1 is phosphorylated by the tyrosine kinase Src, which recruits Syk to the ITAM motif to activate MAPKs and NFAT. This Syk interaction also mediates formation of the CARD9-Bcl10-Malt1 complex, which stimulates NFκβ and the secretion of proinflammatory cytokines. This ultimately leads to a Th17 T cell response. Th17 cells are particularly important for anti-microbial immunity at the epithelial and mucosal barriers and produce cytokines such as IL-17 and IL-22 which stimulate anti-microbial proteins. A lack of Th17 cells leaves the host susceptible to invasion by opportunistic pathogens such as *C.albicans*.

A recent study suggests that Malt-1 activation of the NFκβ subunit C-Rel is important for induction of Th17 enhancing cytokines IL1β and IL23. It was also evident that Dectin-1 activates all components of the NFκβ complex, whereas Dectin-2 specifically activates C-Rel (Gringhuis et al., 2011). Recent studies suggest that Dectin-1 NFκβ activation is induced by zymosan, whereas hyphal forms of *C.albicans* activate NFκβ via Dectin-2. Hyphae stimulation in *C.albicans* also facilitates association of CARD-9 with Bcl10, in a Dectin-2 specific manner (Bi et al., 2010). This is a good example of how different PRRs of the host have distinguished between pathogenic (hyphae producing) and commensal forms of *Candida albicans.*

The ability of Dectin-1 to activate Th17 responses assists in the prevention of fungal infection. Loss of Dectin-1 in KO mice and Dectin-1 polymorphisms in humans makes the host more susceptible to infection (Ferwerda et al., 2009b). In *C.albicans* infection, β-glucans may also stimulate Th17 and regulatory T cell responses via a Dectin-1/TLR2 crosstalk, in addition to the Dectin-1 specific pro-inflammatory cytokine response (Gantner et al., 2003; LeibundGut-Landmann et al., 2007). This Dectin-1/TLR2 response also involves the production of prostaglandin E2, which upregulates Th17 dependent cytokines IL-6 and IL-23 (Smeekens et al., 2010). Dectin-1 also synergises with TLR2 and TLR4 for the production of TNFα and there is evidence to suggest that Dectin-1 and TLR2/6 pathways crosstalk to enhance responses by each receptor. Furthermore, Dectin-1 activation also upregulates pro-IL-1β for subsequent activation by the NLRP3 inflammasome (Cheng et al., 2011).

Dectin-1 also associates with Galectin-3, an S-type lectin that binds to β-1,2 mannosides present in the cell wall of *Candida albicans,* an interaction that is required for proinflammatory responses in fungi. The Dectin1-Galectin-3 complex modulates TNFα levels, whereby a decrease in galectin-3 corresponds to a decrease in TNFα. Mutant *C.albicans* expressing more β-glucan on the cell wall surface had reduced galectin-3 binding and a reduction in the protective pro-inflammatory response. Hence, association between Galectin-3 and Dectin-1 can modulate the proinflammatory response to help distinguish between pathogenic and nonpathogenic fungi (Esteban et al., 2011).

Dectin-2 recognises several fungal species including *C.albicans* and interacts with PAMPs of high mannose content, specifically α-linked mannans and zymosan. Dectin-2 also activates NFκβ and a Th17 response via the Syk-CARD9 pathway, as well as MAPKs via a CARD9 independent pathway. However unlike Dectin-1, it couples to Syk indirectly utilising the ITAM motif of the Fc receptor. A recent study has suggested that it is Dectin-2, rather than Dectin-1, that is more involved in the Th17 response to *C.albicans* and their hyphae, with IL-1β and IL-23 induction being Dectin-2 dependent. DCs from Dectin-2 KO mice show a limited cytokine response to α-mannans (Saijo et al., 2010).

Macrophage inducible C-type lectin (Mincle) binds to yeast cell wall components, specifically α-linked mannans, and like Dectin-2 also uses the Fc receptor to signal in a Syk-CARD9 dependent matter. Mincle has also been linked to TLR2 responses. DC-SIGN and its mouse homolog (SIGNR1) recognises complex mannoside structures on the surface of yeast facilitating internalisation. SIGNR1 specifically binds zymosan as well as live and heat killed *C.albicans.* SIGNR1 has also been reported to modulate TLR4 dependent signalling and to itself induce a proinflammatory response against *C.albicans* (Takahara et al., 2011). SIGNR1 may also interact with Dectin-1 to enhance Syk dependent pathways.

There is recent evidence to suggest that the interaction of *candida albicans* with glucan (Dectin-1) and mannan (Dectin-2) specific receptors, works in combination with the adaptor protein MyD88 to activate phospholipase A_2 and the production of eicosanoids, which are important modulators of inflammation (Suram et al., 2010).

3.4 PRRs and *Schistosoma mansoni*

3.4.1 Schistosoma infection and immunity

The parasitic worm Schistosoma represents the fourth most prevalent helminth infection worldwide affecting 200 million people. In schistosomiasis, the human parasitic disease caused by helminths, the parasite takes on various forms during its lifecycle, which presents a variety of PAMPs to the host and contribute to the developing host immune response. The lifecycle of *S.mansoni* in mammalian hosts begins when the larval stage (cercariae) is released from an intermediate host (snail; genus *Biomphalaria)* and then infects host cells, where it transforms into adult worms. Hosts infected with these parasites accumulate hundreds of intravascular worms which secrete various antigenic molecules into the blood which continuously trigger the host inflammatory response and facilitate prolonged colonisation. During *S.mansoni* infection, the adult worms can survive for many years, where they evade the host immune response, by establishing a balance between host activation and immune suppression. The adult worms also produce hundreds of eggs daily over a life period of 5 to 30 years. A Th2 anti-inflammatory response is triggered by the presence of eggs as well as soluble antigens secreted by the eggs, whereas a Th1 inflammatory specific response is more likely when adult worms interact with host immune cells.

3.4.2 Recognition of *Schistosoma mansoni* by PRRs

Schistosoma mansoni produces various glycoconjugates (glycoproteins and glycolipids) that interact with PRRs of the innate immune system and potentially modulate the function of host immune cells (Figure 9). The mouse model of schistosomiasis identified that Schistosoma glycoconjugates containing Lacto-N-fucopentaose III (LNFPIII) induce a Th2 response in collaboration with TLR4. Also the schistosomal tegument has been reported to activate inflammatory responses in DCs via a TLR4/MyD88 pathway. Schistosomiasis is also associated with high levels of endotoxemia and elevated levels of high mobility group 1 (HMGB1) protein, which is a ligand for TLR2, TLR4 and the RAGE receptor.

Lysophosphatidylserine (Lyso-PS) and dsRNA from the eggs of *S.mansoni* also activate TLR2 and TLR3 inflammation pathways respectively. Soluble schistosomal egg antigens (SEA) inhibit TNFα and IL-6 secretion originating from TLR signalling pathways. This TLR suppression occurs at the same time as NLRP3 activation and IL-1β production (Ritter et al., 2010). SEA binds to the Dectin-2/FcRγ complex and signals via the Syk pathway to induce ROS and potassium efflux, known effectors of the inflammasome NLRP3. *S.mansoni* infection of mice without inflammasome components ASC and NLRP3 failed to induce an inflammatory response indicated by the lowered IL-1β levels and the downregulation of T cell responses.

CLRs also recognise glycans associated with schistosomes using one or more CRD (Figure 9). The CLRs DC-SIGN, macrophage galactose type lectin (MGL) and MR on human DCs, bind specific glycans on the SEA of *S.mansoni*. This binding facilitates internalisation of the SEA and promotion of a Th2 response. DC-SIGN can also bind to the larval form of *S.mansoni* via glycolipids. Human DCs primed with adult worm glycolipids switch towards a Th1 immune response and induce an inflammatory cytokine cascade. DC-SIGN binds to fucose components of the glycolipid of the worm and helps activate TLR4 signalling and inflammation (van Stijn et al., 2010). It is proposed that DC-SIGN recruits glycolipids and then presents them to TLR4, via a TLR4-DC-SIGN complex in lipid rafts.

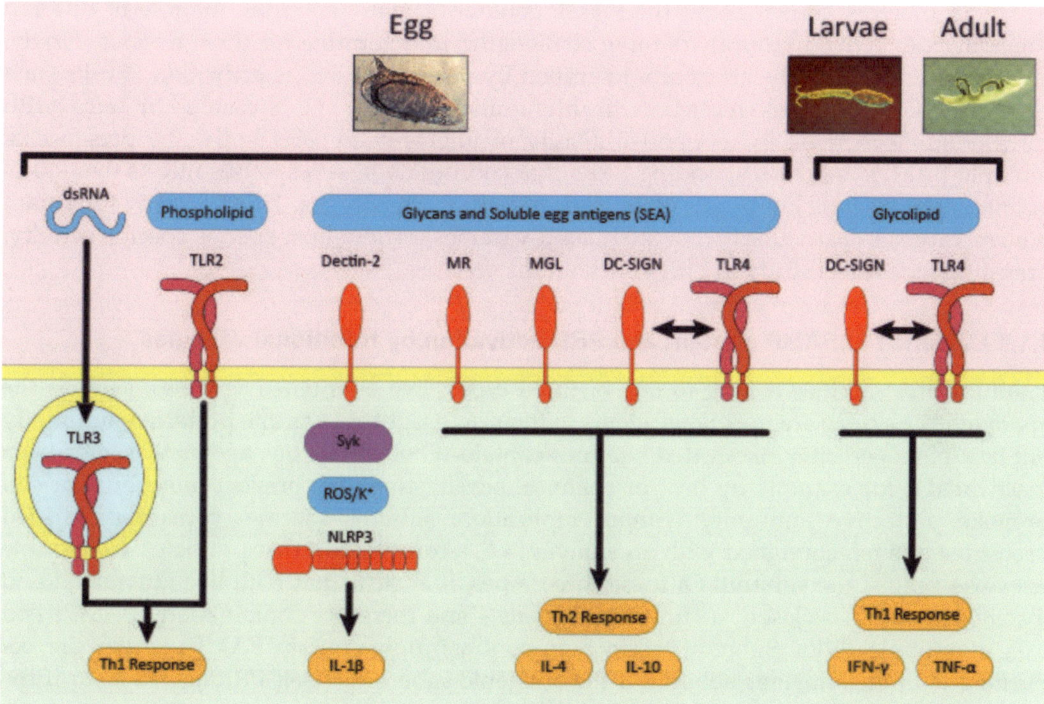

Fig. 9. PRRs involved in the immune response against schistosomal PAMPs at different stages of the schistosomes lifecycle. The activation of a Th1 (inflammatory) and a Th2 (humoral) response demonstrates the ability of the parasite to regulate infection. Pictures of schistosoma egg, larvae and adult reproduced with the permission of David Dunne.

4. The role of PRRs in immunisation against infectious disease

Immunisation is a crucial and highly successful defence against many infectious diseases including: measles, tetanus, diphtheria, rubella, polio and tuberculosis. Over recent years it has become apparent that PRRs play a major and crucial role in the processes of immune priming and polarization. These new findings have been applied to vaccine research in two major areas: firstly to determine the molecular mechanism of action of known vaccines and adjuvants; and secondly new adjuvant components have been developed that target specific PRRs in a quest towards rationally designed 'customised' vaccines.

4.1 The role of PRRs in current vaccines

PRRs are important for the priming of adaptive immune responses (Section 3.3). It is not surprising that many current vaccines also function, at least in part, by activating PRRs. Studies with knock-out mice have shown that PRRs are critical for the optimal function of several known vaccines. However, PRRs are not necessary for all vaccines to induce protective immune responses, and several vaccines instead trigger alternative pro-inflammatory pathways that appear to primarily recognize tissue or cellular injury rather than PAMPs.

Although much is known about the PAMP content of many vaccines, the role of PRRs in triggering protective immunity is more challenging to determine for three reasons. Firstly, individual PAMPs can be efficiently identified by measuring innate activation of cells such as DC *in vitro* whereas induction of immunity can only be measured *in vivo* with corresponding increase in cost and difficulty of interpretation. Secondly, the presence of multiple PAMPs and corresponding PRRs that coordinate host responses means that study of immunity in single knockouts often leads to partial phenotypes. Thirdly, many important human vaccines- particularly live attenuated vaccines - show host-species specific activity, preventing the direct study in PRR knockout mice.

4.1.1 Evidence of PAMP content and PRR activation by traditional vaccines

Traditionally, vaccines belong to one of three types: live attenuated vaccines, such as the eponymous *vaccinia,* are infectious agents in their own right, and prime protective immunity but lack pathogenicity; inactivated vaccines contain whole infectious agents that have been inactivated - for example by heat or chemical sterilization - to prevent infection, but still provoke protective immunity without replication; subunit vaccines contain a purified protective antigen combined with an adjuvant i.e. a formulation that promotes an immune response against the subunit. Of these three types, it is clear that both live attenuated and inactivated vaccines closely resemble pathogens - and therefore contain many PAMPs and trigger multiple PRRs. Subunit vaccines, in contrast, only contain PAMPs if they are co-purified with the antigenic subunit, if the antigenic subunit is itself PRR agonistic, or if the adjuvant activates PRRs (see 4.1.2, 4.1.3 and 4.1.4).

4.1.2 PRR activation by live attenuated vaccines

Our oldest vaccines are live attenuated pathogens. Yet they are also the most poorly understood due to the complex interplay between parasite and host. Live attenuated vaccines contain a plethora of PAMPs. For example, live attenuated bacterial vaccines such as *Mycobacterium tuberculosis* BCG and live oral Typhoid Fever vaccine are rich in well known PAMPs such as bacterial DNA, lipopolysaccharides and lipopeptides. Two major challenges in characterizing PRR triggering by live attenuated viral vaccines are the fact that PAMP content and location changes during the infectious cycle (e.g. production of different types of nucleic acids, viral entry into host cells); and the presence of PRR inhibitors can obscure signaling.

Vaccinia is one of the best studied live attenuated vaccines. The importance of PRRs in vaccinia virus sensing became clear very early on with the discovery that its genome encodes inhibitors of IL-1 and TLR signaling (Bowie et al., 2000). Host responses to vaccinia are complex. Pathways act separately and synergistically, and there are diverse responses from different cell types. Studies of viral-induced cytokine production from cells from knockout mice have started to unpick this complexity and demonstrated that vaccinia can trigger multiple PRR including TLR2/TLR6, (Delaloye et al., 2009; Zhu et al., 2007), the RLR MDA-5 (Delaloye et al., 2009), and TLR8 (Martinez et al., 2010). The inflammasome component NALP3 is also required for maximal cytokine responses (Delaloye et al., 2009).

Although the rich PAMP content of live attenuated vaccines has been characterised, understanding fully how PRR triggering induces protective adaptive immunity still remains a challenge. For example, MyD88-/- mice show reduced protection from experimental tuberculosis after vaccination with BCG (Fremond et al., 2004). And studies of the mouse Typhoid model *Salmonella* typhimurium suggest that TLRs and MyD88 are required in a range of cell types for optimal function of oral live attenuated bacterial vaccines (Dougan et al., 2011). Likewise, although the precise PRR requirement for protective immunity to vaccinia cannot be determined due to the lack of appropriate (or safe) models, TLR2 and MyD88 knockout mice do show partial reduction in MVA-specific T cell responses and CD8+ T cell IFNγ secretion (Zhu et al., 2007).

4.1.3 PRR activation by inactivated vaccines

Inactivated vaccines are generally simpler to study because they have a fixed content, do not undergo metabolic changes, and in general do not subvert host signaling. Furthermore, a great deal is known about the PAMP content of inactivated organisms since killed microbes have been of great use for decades as a source of 'natural' PAMPs in the identification and study of PRRs.

Recently, a major pathway for viral nucleic acid recognition - viral ssRNA triggering TLR7 - was initially identified by study of IFNα production by pDC in response to heat-inactivated influenza virus (Diebold et al., 2004) (Section 3.2.1). Indeed, in the absence of TLR7 whole inactivated influenza virus vaccine loses immunogenicity (Geeraedts et al., 2008). This study highlighted in particular the importance of TLR7 in driving a particular class of immune response - specifically Th1 immunity - reinforcing the notion that PRR triggering controls immune response polarization as well as magnitude. In contrast, split virus or subunit vaccines, which are less potent but considered safer, showed little TLR7 dependence presumably as a result of loss of the packaged viral ssRNA that potently stimulates TLR7 during production (Geeraedts et al., 2008). Of course these studies into the PRR requirements of vaccines have been performed in mouse models and to date the importance of PRR signaling for protective immunity in humans has yet to be determined, and may show different patterns.

Evidence for the need for TLR signaling for the activity of inactivated bacterial vaccines comes from the whole cell Pertussis vaccine. Although this vaccine contains a wide range of bacterial PAMPs, TLR4 and TRIF but not TLR2 knockout mice showed reduced immunity. This suggests that LPS is more critical than lipopeptides for induction of adaptive responses in this instance (Fransen et al., 2010).

4.1.4 PRR triggering by subunit vaccines

At first sight, subunit vaccines should not contain PAMPs because the critical microbial 'subunit' should be an antigen, i.e. target for adaptive - not innate - immune responses. But although simpler and purer than whole inactivated vaccines, many current human subunit vaccines still contain microbe-derived PAMPs either co-purified with the antigen or in some cases the antigenic subunit is itself a PRR agonist. Thus, meningitis vaccines based on purified outer membrane vesicle preparations of Neisseria meningitides contain both LPS and TLR2-stimulatory lipopeptides, and require TLR4 and TRIF signaling for optimal immune priming (Fransen et al., 2010). As well as PAMPs co-purified with antigenic subunits, many non-protein protective antigens such as polysaccharides or lipoproteins can directly trigger PRR. For example, the outer-surface lipoprotein (OspA) subunit of Borrelia burgdorferi activates TLR2 and has been used as an effective human vaccine against Lyme disease. This particular antigenic PAMP not only shows reduced immunogenicity in TLR2 knockout mice, but human hyporesponsiveness to the vaccine is associated with low TLR1 expression (Alexopoulou et al., 2002).

4.1.5 PAMP-free triggering of PRRs by adjuvants

The sections above have introduced the importance of TLRs in the development of immunity following vaccination. It is now becoming apparent that other PRRs, and stimulation of alternative proinflammatory pathways, can be important for vaccine functionality. There is evidence that some vaccine adjuvants can induce long-lasting and protective immune responses independently of TLR-based signalling pathways (Gavin et al., 2006; Nemazee et al., 2006). Furthermore, the majority of recently developed human adjuvant formulations, such as emulsions (Reed et al., 2009), do not obviously contain microbial components and are therefore unlikely to contain PAMPs. The NLRP3 inflammasome has been shown to be activated by the common adjuvant alum, however it is currently debatable as to whether this activation is required for the adjuvant activity of alum (De Gregorio et al., 2009; Franchi and Nunez, 2008; Li et al., 2008; McKee et al., 2009). Several other PAMP-free adjuvant formulations, including oil emulsions, saponins and microparticles made from biodegradeable polymer poly(lactic-co-glycolic acid) also trigger NALP3-dependent immune activation (Williams et al., 2010). In addition, the Syk/CARD9 pathway is activated by the potent adjuvant additive, trehalose 6,6-dibehenate, a synthetic mimic of a mycobacterial cell wall component (Werninghaus et al., 2009).

4.2 Implications of PRR research findings for the development of new vaccines

There is still a large demand for better vaccines in order to reduce costs, improve potency and efficacy, to tackle diseases which currently lack a vaccine (e.g. Human Immunodeficiency Virus) and to respond quickly to new challenges from infectious diseases (e.g. pandemic influenza). Understanding how PRRs contribute to protective immunity and how this can be modulated are key if vaccines are to improve.

One area of particular importance to vaccine development is the need to rationally design new adjuvants with greater potency than current ones such as alum (Mbow et al., 2010; Reed et al., 2009; Leroux-Roels, 2010). Selective triggering of different PRRs and DC subsets are thought to be major points of control of immune polarization (Iwasaki and Medzhitov, 2004; Kapsenberg, 2003). It follows therefore that not only are new adjuvants needed, but these must be engineered to stimulate the correct PRR on the optimal cell type. The most clinically relevant illustration of the benefits of adding PRR agonists to increase adjuvant activity is GSK's adjuvant AS 04, which incorporates the TLR4 agonist monophosphoryl lipid A (MPLA) to alum (Didierlaurent et al., 2009). The human papilloma virus virus-like particle vaccine Cervarix is formulated with AS 04, which may account for its apparent increased potency compared to Gardasil, a similar VLP vaccine that uses alum without MPLA (Einstein et al., 2009). Interestingly MPLA appears to preferentially activate TLR4 signalling through the TRIF:TRAM pathway and not Mal:MYD88 (Mata-Haro et al., 2007).

Without doubt the role of synthetic PRR-specific agonists as additives to vaccine adjuvants will become a developing and increasingly important field of research. Of course given the potent immunostimulatory properties of PRR agonists care will have to be taken to avoid potentially damaging, or fatal, systemic effects.

4.2.1 TLR agonists in adjuvants

As well as the benefits of adding MPLA to alum, a wide range of TLR agonists have been shown to promote immunity when added to antigens. These include TLR2-stimulatory lipopeptides such as MALP-2, the TLR5 agonist flagellin, TLR9-stimulatory CpG oligos, small molecule TLR7/8 agonists such as imidazoquinolines, the TLR3 agonist polyI:C and various modified RNA and DNA oligos that can act on TLR3,7 and/or 9. TLR triggering, such as by CpG oligos or imidazoquinolines, frequently promotes Th1 responses (Schnare et al., 2001), but there are a number of exceptions, including Th2 induction by lipopeptides and flagellin that trigger TLR2 and TLR5 respectively (Didierlaurent et al., 2004; Redecke et al., 2004). It has become clear that for maximal potency and benefits the TLR agonist requires linking in some way with the target antigen. For example, agonists have been covalently coupled to proteins; synthesized directly in combination with the TLR agonist; or antigen and PRR agonists can be immobilised together on a particulate scaffold. The importance of linking PRR agonists with antigen was demonstrated in a recent study where peptides were co-encapsulated with a TLR9 agonist using the biodegradeable polymer PLGA; only when antigen and CpG oligonucleotides were present in the same PLGA microsphere was an effective cytotoxic T cell response achieved (Schlosser et al., 2008).

4.2.2 Combinatorial PRR triggering

Just as most microbes contain a number of different PAMPs and trigger several PRR, there is a need to combine PRR triggers in adjuvants for synergistic effects, and to closely mimic pathogens. The best studied example of synergistic PRR signaling comes from the activation of TLR2 combined with signaling through the CLEC dectin-1 (Gantner et al., 2003; Underhill, 2007). PRR signaling also synergises with other proinflammatory pathways. Major examples include the interplay between T cell feedback signals through CD40 expressed on PRR-stimulated DC (Schulz et al., 2000), and the requirement of NALP3 for maximal response to various PRR including vaccinia (Delaloye et al., 2009).

5. Conclusions

Without doubt PRRs have a crucial role to play in the detection of, and response to, infectious diseases. The repertoire and versatility of the host in detecting PAMPS and associated danger signals is outstanding and continually expanding. In fact this is only matched by the steps taken by pathogens to circumvent these defence strategies. As research progresses in this field it is becoming increasingly apparent that although the outputs of PRR activation are broadly similar - i.e. pro-inflammatory cytokine induction, caspase-1 processing and IFN induction - the mechanisms by which this takes place are actually remarkably subtle. There is significant crosstalk between TLR, NLR, CLR and RLR signalling pathways. In addition, there is clear redundancy in function between different receptors that helps to ensure appropriate recognition of, and response to, pathogens. The complexity of the signalling crosstalk is only likely to increase as our understanding of these systems improves.

Another key area in which PRR recognition of infectious diseases is becoming increasingly important is the development of adaptive immunity. The innate response seems to play a vital role in directing the nature of the adaptive response, particularly in relation to driving development of particular T-cell subsets. This is a rapidly developing area and the search for rational vaccine design makes it critical to infectious disease research. The study of the cellular and molecular biology of PRRs has provided a strong theoretical and experimental foundation for the rational design of vaccine adjuvants. This new understanding must be harnessed to provide a complete toolkit for custom adjuvant design. However, in common with other biomedical disciplines, clinical uptake typically lags behind scientific discovery and we wait to see how best this knowledge can be transferred to provide clinical benefit.

6. Acknowledgements

The work in our group is funded by The Wellcome Trust (TPM; WT0805090MA) and the Biotechnology and Biological Sciences Research Council (TPM; RG52820). We thank David Dunne for the images of *Schistosoma* eggs, larvae and adult worms used in Figure 9.

7. References

Alexopoulou, L., Thomas, V., Schnare, M., Lobet, Y., Anguita, J., Schoen, R.T., Medzhitov, R., Fikrig, E., and Flavell, R.A. (2002). Hyporesponsiveness to vaccination with Borrelia burgdorferi OspA in humans and in TLR1- and TLR2-deficient mice. Nat Med *8*, 878-884.

Andersen-Nissen, E., Smith, K.D., Strobe, K.L., Barrett, S.L., Cookson, B.T., Logan, S.M., and Aderem, A. (2005). Evasion of Toll-like receptor 5 by flagellated bacteria. Proc Natl Acad Sci U S A *102*, 9247-9252.

Bi, L., Gojestani, S., Wu, W., Hsu, Y.M., Zhu, J., Ariizumi, K., and Lin, X. (2010). CARD9 mediates dectin-2-induced IkappaBalpha kinase ubiquitination leading to activation of NF-kappaB in response to stimulation by the hyphal form of Candida albicans. J Biol Chem *285*, 25969-25977.

Bowie, A., Kiss-Toth, E., Symons, J.A., Smith, G.L., Dower, S.K., and O'Neill, L.A. (2000). A46R and A52R from vaccinia virus are antagonists of host IL-1 and toll-like receptor signaling. Proc Natl Acad Sci U S A *97*, 10162-10167.

Bowie, A.G., and Unterholzner, L. (2008). Viral evasion and subversion of pattern-recognition receptor signalling. Nat Rev Immunol *8*, 911-922.

Cheng, S.C., van de Veerdonk, F.L., Lenardon, M., Stoffels, M., Plantinga, T., Smeekens, S., Rizzetto, L., Mukaremera, L., Preechasuth, K., Cavalieri, D., *et al.* (2011). The dectin-1/inflammasome pathway is responsible for the induction of protective T-helper 17 responses that discriminate between yeasts and hyphae of Candida albicans. J Leukoc Biol *90*, 357-366.

Cirl, C., Wieser, A., Yadav, M., Duerr, S., Schubert, S., Fischer, H., Stappert, D., Wantia, N., Rodriguez, N., Wagner, H., *et al.* (2008). Subversion of Toll-like receptor signaling by a unique family of bacterial Toll/interleukin-1 receptor domain-containing proteins. Nat Med *14*, 399-406.

Coburn, B., Grassl, G.A., and Finlay, B.B. (2007). Salmonella, the host and disease: a brief review. Immunol Cell Biol *85*, 112-118.

Davis, B.K., Wen, H., and Ting, J.P. (2011). The inflammasome NLRs in immunity, inflammation, and associated diseases. Annu Rev Immunol *29*, 707-735.

De Gregorio, E., D'Oro, U., and Wack, A. (2009). Immunology of TLR-independent vaccine adjuvants. Curr Opin Immunol *21*, 339-345.

Delaloye, J., Roger, T., Steiner-Tardivel, Q.G., Le Roy, D., Knaup Reymond, M., Akira, S., Petrilli, V., Gomez, C.E., Perdiguero, B., Tschopp, J., *et al.* (2009). Innate immune sensing of modified vaccinia virus Ankara (MVA) is mediated by TLR2-TLR6, MDA-5 and the NALP3 inflammasome. PLoS Pathog *5*, e1000480.

Didierlaurent, A., Ferrero, I., Otten, L.A., Dubois, B., Reinhardt, M., Carlsen, H., Blomhoff, R., Akira, S., Kraehenbuhl, J.P., and Sirard, J.C. (2004). Flagellin promotes myeloid differentiation factor 88-dependent development of Th2-type response. J Immunol *172*, 6922-6930.

Didierlaurent, A.M., Morel, S., Lockman, L., Giannini, S.L., Bisteau, M., Carlsen, H., Kielland, A., Vosters, O., Vanderheyde, N., Schiavetti, F., *et al.* (2009). AS04, an aluminum salt- and TLR4 agonist-based adjuvant system, induces a transient localized innate immune response leading to enhanced adaptive immunity. J Immunol *183*, 6186-6197.

Diebold, S.S., Kaisho, T., Hemmi, H., Akira, S., and Reis e Sousa, C. (2004). Innate antiviral responses by means of TLR7-mediated recognition of single-stranded RNA. Science *303*, 1529-1531.

Dougan, G., John, V., Palmer, S., and Mastroeni, P. (2011). Immunity to salmonellosis. Immunol Rev *240*, 196-210.

Einstein, M.H., Baron, M., Levin, M.J., Chatterjee, A., Edwards, R.P., Zepp, F., Carletti, I., Dessy, F.J., Trofa, A.F., Schuind, A., *et al.* (2009). Comparison of the immunogenicity and safety of Cervarix and Gardasil human papillomavirus (HPV) cervical cancer vaccines in healthy women aged 18-45 years. Hum Vaccin *5*, 705-719.

Esteban, A., Popp, M.W., Vyas, V.K., Strijbis, K., Ploegh, H.L., and Fink, G.R. (2011). Fungal recognition is mediated by the association of dectin-1 and galectin-3 in macrophages. Proceedings of the National Academy of Sciences *108*, 14270-14275.

Ferwerda, B., Alonso, S., Banahan, K., McCall, M.B., Giamarellos-Bourboulis, E.J., Ramakers, B.P., Mouktaroudi, M., Fain, P.R., Izagirre, N., Syafruddin, D., *et al.* (2009a). Functional and genetic evidence that the Mal/TIRAP allele variant 180L has been selected by providing protection against septic shock. Proc Natl Acad Sci U S A *106*, 10272-10277.

Ferwerda, B., Ferwerda, G., Plantinga, T.S., Willment, J.A., van Spriel, A.B., Venselaar, H., Elbers, C.C., Johnson, M.D., Cambi, A., Huysamen, C., *et al.* (2009b). Human dectin-1 deficiency and mucocutaneous fungal infections. N Engl J Med *361*, 1760-1767.

Franchi, L., Amer, A., Body-Malapel, M., Kanneganti, T.D., Ozoren, N., Jagirdar, R., Inohara, N., Vandenabeele, P., Bertin, J., Coyle, A., *et al.* (2006). Cytosolic flagellin requires Ipaf for activation of caspase-1 and interleukin 1beta in salmonella-infected macrophages. Nat Immunol *7*, 576-582.

Franchi, L., and Nunez, G. (2008). The Nlrp3 inflammasome is critical for aluminium hydroxide-mediated IL-1beta secretion but dispensable for adjuvant activity. Eur J Immunol *38*, 2085-2089.

Fransen, F., Stenger, R.M., Poelen, M.C., van Dijken, H.H., Kuipers, B., Boog, C.J., van Putten, J.P., van Els, C.A., and van der Ley, P. (2010). Differential effect of TLR2 and TLR4 on the immune response after immunization with a vaccine against Neisseria meningitidis or Bordetella pertussis. PLoS One *5*, e15692.

Fremond, C.M., Yeremeev, V., Nicolle, D.M., Jacobs, M., Quesniaux, V.F., and Ryffel, B. (2004). Fatal Mycobacterium tuberculosis infection despite adaptive immune response in the absence of MyD88. J Clin Invest *114*, 1790-1799.

Gack, M.U., Shin, Y.C., Joo, C.H., Urano, T., Liang, C., Sun, L., Takeuchi, O., Akira, S., Chen, Z., Inoue, S., *et al.* (2007). TRIM25 RING-finger E3 ubiquitin ligase is essential for RIG-I-mediated antiviral activity. Nature *446*, 916-920.

Gantner, B.N., Simmons, R.M., Canavera, S.J., Akira, S., and Underhill, D.M. (2003). Collaborative induction of inflammatory responses by dectin-1 and Toll-like receptor 2. J Exp Med *197*, 1107-1117.

Gavin, A.L., Hoebe, K., Duong, B., Ota, T., Martin, C., Beutler, B., and Nemazee, D. (2006). Adjuvant-enhanced antibody responses in the absence of toll-like receptor signaling. Science *314*, 1936-1938.

Geeraedts, F., Goutagny, N., Hornung, V., Severa, M., de Haan, A., Pool, J., Wilschut, J., Fitzgerald, K.A., and Huckriede, A. (2008). Superior immunogenicity of inactivated whole virus H5N1 influenza vaccine is primarily controlled by Toll-like receptor signalling. PLoS Pathog *4*, e1000138.

Gewirtz, A.T., Navas, T.A., Lyons, S., Godowski, P.J., and Madara, J.L. (2001). Cutting edge: bacterial flagellin activates basolaterally expressed TLR5 to induce epithelial proinflammatory gene expression. J Immunol *167*, 1882-1885.

Gringhuis, S.I., Wevers, B.A., Kaptein, T.M., van Capel, T.M., Theelen, B., Boekhout, T., de Jong, E.C., and Geijtenbeek, T.B. (2011). Selective C-Rel activation via Malt1 controls anti-fungal T(H)-17 immunity by dectin-1 and dectin-2. PLoS Pathog *7*, e1001259.

Guillot, L., Le Goffic, R., Bloch, S., Escriou, N., Akira, S., Chignard, M., and Si-Tahar, M. (2005). Involvement of toll-like receptor 3 in the immune response of lung epithelial cells to double-stranded RNA and influenza A virus. J Biol Chem *280*, 5571-5580.

Hajishengallis, G., and Lambris, J.D. (2011). Microbial manipulation of receptor crosstalk in innate immunity. Nat Rev Immunol *11*, 187-200.

Hayashi, F., Smith, K.D., Ozinsky, A., Hawn, T.R., Yi, E.C., Goodlett, D.R., Eng, J.K., Akira, S., Underhill, D.M., and Aderem, A. (2001). The innate immune response to bacterial flagellin is mediated by Toll-like receptor 5. Nature *410*, 1099-1103.

Hersh, D., Monack, D.M., Smith, M.R., Ghori, N., Falkow, S., and Zychlinsky, A. (1999). The Salmonella invasin SipB induces macrophage apoptosis by binding to caspase-1. Proc Natl Acad Sci U S A *96*, 2396-2401.

Ichinohe, T. (2010). Respective roles of TLR, RIG-I and NLRP3 in influenza virus infection and immunity: impact on vaccine design. Expert Rev Vaccines *9*, 1315-1324.

Iwasaki, A., and Medzhitov, R. (2004). Toll-like receptor control of the adaptive immune responses. Nat Immunol *5*, 987-995.

Kanneganti, T.-D. (2010). Central roles of NLRs and inflammasomes in viral infection. Nat Rev Immunol *10*, 688-698.

Kapsenberg, M.L. (2003). Dendritic-cell control of pathogen-driven T-cell polarization. Nat Rev Immunol *3*, 984-993.

Kawai, T., and Akira, S. (2011). Toll-like receptors and their crosstalk with other innate receptors in infection and immunity. Immunity *34*, 637-650.

Kenny, E.F., Talbot, S., Gong, M., Golenbock, D.T., Bryant, C.E., and O'Neill, L.A.J. (2009). MyD88 Adaptor-Like Is Not Essential for TLR2 Signaling and Inhibits Signaling by TLR3. J Immunol *183*, 3642-3651.

Khor, C.C., Chapman, S.J., Vannberg, F.O., Dunne, A., Murphy, C., Ling, E.Y., Frodsham, A.J., Walley, A.J., Kyrieleis, O., Khan, A., *et al.* (2007). A Mal functional variant is associated with protection against invasive pneumococcal disease, bacteremia, malaria and tuberculosis. Nat Genet *39*, 523-528.

LeibundGut-Landmann, S., Gross, O., Robinson, M.J., Osorio, F., Slack, E.C., Tsoni, S.V., Schweighoffer, E., Tybulewicz, V., Brown, G.D., Ruland, J., *et al.* (2007). Syk- and CARD9-dependent coupling of innate immunity to the induction of T helper cells that produce interleukin 17. Nat Immunol *8*, 630-638.

Leroux-Roels, G. (2010). Unmet needs in modern vaccinology: adjuvants to improve the immune response. Vaccine *28 Suppl 3*, C25-36.

Li, H., Willingham, S.B., Ting, J.P., and Re, F. (2008). Cutting edge: inflammasome activation by alum and alum's adjuvant effect are mediated by NLRP3. J Immunol *181*, 17-21.

Loo, Y.M., and Gale, M., Jr. (2011). Immune signaling by RIG-I-like receptors. Immunity *34*, 680-692.

Lu, Y., Wambach, M., Katze, M.G., and Krug, R.M. (1995). Binding of the influenza virus NS1 protein to double-stranded RNA inhibits the activation of the protein kinase that phosphorylates the elF-2 translation initiation factor. Virology *214*, 222-228.

Lund, J.M., Alexopoulou, L., Sato, A., Karow, M., Adams, N.C., Gale, N.W., Iwasaki, A., and Flavell, R.A. (2004). Recognition of single-stranded RNA viruses by Toll-like receptor 7. Proc Natl Acad Sci U S A *101*, 5598-5603.

Martinez, J., Huang, X., and Yang, Y. (2010). Toll-like receptor 8-mediated activation of murine plasmacytoid dendritic cells by vaccinia viral DNA. Proc Natl Acad Sci U S A *107*, 6442-6447.

Mata-Haro, V., Cekic, C., Martin, M., Chilton, P.M., Casella, C.R., and Mitchell, T.C. (2007). The vaccine adjuvant monophosphoryl lipid A as a TRIF-biased agonist of TLR4. Science *316*, 1628-1632.

Mbow, M.L., De Gregorio, E., Valiante, N.M., and Rappuoli, R. (2010). New adjuvants for human vaccines. Curr Opin Immunol *22*, 411-416.

McKee, A.S., Munks, M.W., MacLeod, M.K., Fleenor, C.J., Van Rooijen, N., Kappler, J.W., and Marrack, P. (2009). Alum induces innate immune responses through macrophage and mast cell sensors, but these sensors are not required for alum to act as an adjuvant for specific immunity. J Immunol *183*, 4403-4414.

Miao, E.A., Mao, D.P., Yudkovsky, N., Bonneau, R., Lorang, C.G., Warren, S.E., Leaf, I.A., and Aderem, A. (2010). Innate immune detection of the type III secretion apparatus through the NLRC4 inflammasome. Proceedings of the National Academy of Sciences *107*, 3076-3080.

Monie, T.P., Bryant, C.E., and Gay, N.J. (2009). Activating immunity: lessons from the TLRs and NLRs. Trends Biochem Sci *34*, 553-561.

Nemazee, D., Gavin, A., Hoebe, K., and Beutler, B. (2006). Immunology: Toll-like receptors and antibody responses. Nature *441*, E4; discussion E4.

Osorio, F., and Reis e Sousa, C. (2011). Myeloid C-type lectin receptors in pathogen recognition and host defense. Immunity *34*, 651-664.

Perry, A.K., Chen, G., Zheng, D., Tang, H., and Cheng, G. (2005). The host type I interferon response to viral and bacterial infections. Cell Res *15*, 407-422.

Pichlmair, A., Schulz, O., Tan, C.P., Naslund, T.I., Liljestrom, P., Weber, F., and Reis e Sousa, C. (2006). RIG-I-mediated antiviral responses to single-stranded RNA bearing 5'-phosphates. Science *314*, 997-1001.

Redecke, V., Häcker, H., Datta, S.K., Fermin, A., Pitha, P.M., Broide, D.H., and Raz, E. (2004). Cutting Edge: Activation of Toll-Like Receptor 2 Induces a Th2 Immune Response and Promotes Experimental Asthma. The Journal of Immunology *172*, 2739-2743.

Reed, S.G., Bertholet, S., Coler, R.N., and Friede, M. (2009). New horizons in adjuvants for vaccine development. Trends Immunol *30*, 23-32.

Ritter, M., Gross, O., Kays, S., Ruland, J., Nimmerjahn, F., Saijo, S., Tschopp, J., Layland, L.E., and Prazeres da Costa, C. (2010). Schistosoma mansoni triggers Dectin-2, which activates the Nlrp3 inflammasome and alters adaptive immune responses. Proc Natl Acad Sci U S A *107*, 20459-20464.

Roy, C.R., and Zamboni, D.S. (2006). Cytosolic detection of flagellin: a deadly twist. Nat Immunol *7*, 549-551.

Sabbah, A., Chang, T.H., Harnack, R., Frohlich, V., Tominaga, K., Dube, P.H., Xiang, Y., and Bose, S. (2009). Activation of innate immune antiviral responses by Nod2. Nat Immunol *10*, 1073-1080.

Saijo, S., Ikeda, S., Yamabe, K., Kakuta, S., Ishigame, H., Akitsu, A., Fujikado, N., Kusaka, T., Kubo, S., Chung, S.H., *et al.* (2010). Dectin-2 recognition of alpha-mannans and induction of Th17 cell differentiation is essential for host defense against Candida albicans. Immunity *32*, 681-691.

Schlosser, E., Mueller, M., Fischer, S., Basta, S., Busch, D.H., Gander, B., and Groettrup, M. (2008). TLR ligands and antigen need to be coencapsulated into the same biodegradable microsphere for the generation of potent cytotoxic T lymphocyte responses. Vaccine *26*, 1626-1637.

Schmitz, N., Kurrer, M., Bachmann, M.F., and Kopf, M. (2005). Interleukin-1 is responsible for acute lung immunopathology but increases survival of respiratory influenza virus infection. J Virol *79*, 6441-6448.

Schnare, M., Barton, G.M., Holt, A.C., Takeda, K., Akira, S., and Medzhitov, R. (2001). Toll-like receptors control activation of adaptive immune responses. Nat Immunol *2*, 947-950.

Schulz, O., Edwards, A.D., Schito, M., Aliberti, J., Manickasingham, S., Sher, A., and Reis e Sousa, C. (2000). CD40 triggering of heterodimeric IL-12 p70 production by dendritic cells in vivo requires a microbial priming signal. Immunity *13*, 453-462.

Smeekens, S.P., van de Veerdonk, F.L., van der Meer, J.W., Kullberg, B.J., Joosten, L.A., and Netea, M.G. (2010). The Candida Th17 response is dependent on mannan- and beta-glucan-induced prostaglandin E2. Int Immunol *22*, 889-895.

Smith, K.D., Andersen-Nissen, E., Hayashi, F., Strobe, K., Bergman, M.A., Barrett, S.L., Cookson, B.T., and Aderem, A. (2003). Toll-like receptor 5 recognizes a conserved site on flagellin required for protofilament formation and bacterial motility. Nat Immunol *4*, 1247-1253.

Spiller, S., Elson, G., Ferstl, R., Dreher, S., Mueller, T., Freudenberg, M., Daubeuf, B., Wagner, H., and Kirschning, C.J. (2008). TLR4-induced IFN-gamma production increases TLR2 sensitivity and drives Gram-negative sepsis in mice. J Exp Med *205*, 1747-1754.

Stewart, C.R., Stuart, L.M., Wilkinson, K., van Gils, J.M., Deng, J., Halle, A., Rayner, K.J., Boyer, L., Zhong, R., Frazier, W.A., *et al.* (2009). CD36 ligands promote sterile inflammation through assembly of a Toll-like receptor 4 and 6 heterodimer. Nat Immunol *11*, 155-161.

Subramanian, N., and Qadri, A. (2006). Lysophospholipid sensing triggers secretion of flagellin from pathogenic salmonella. Nat Immunol *7*, 583-589.

Suram, S., Gangelhoff, T.A., Taylor, P.R., Rosas, M., Brown, G.D., Bonventre, J.V., Akira, S., Uematsu, S., Williams, D.L., Murphy, R.C., *et al.* (2010). Pathways regulating cytosolic phospholipase A2 activation and eicosanoid production in macrophages by Candida albicans. J Biol Chem *285*, 30676-30685.

Takahara, K., Tokieda, S., Nagaoka, K., Takeda, T., Kimura, Y., and Inaba, K. (2011). C-type lectin SIGNR1 enhances cellular oxidative burst response against C. albicans in cooperation with Dectin-1. Eur J Immunol *41*, 1435-1444.

Talbot, S., Tötemeyer, S., Yamamoto, M., Akira, S., Hughes, K., Gray, D., Barr, T., Mastroeni, P., Maskell, D.J., and Bryant, C.E. (2009). Toll-like receptor 4 signalling through MyD88 is essential to control <i>Salmonella enterica</i> serovar Typhimurium infection, but not for the initiation of bacterial clearance. Immunology *128*, 472-483.

Underhill, D.M. (2007). Collaboration between the innate immune receptors dectin-1, TLRs, and Nods. Immunol Rev *219*, 75-87.

Van der Graaf, C.A., Netea, M.G., Morre, S.A., Den Heijer, M., Verweij, P.E., Van der Meer, J.W., and Kullberg, B.J. (2006). Toll-like receptor 4 Asp299Gly/Thr399Ile polymorphisms are a risk factor for Candida bloodstream infection. Eur Cytokine Netw *17*, 29-34.

van Stijn, C.M., Meyer, S., van den Broek, M., Bruijns, S.C., van Kooyk, Y., Geyer, R., and van Die, I. (2010). Schistosoma mansoni worm glycolipids induce an inflammatory phenotype in human dendritic cells by cooperation of TLR4 and DC-SIGN. Mol Immunol *47*, 1544-1552.

Wang, J.P., Liu, P., Latz, E., Golenbock, D.T., Finberg, R.W., and Libraty, D.H. (2006). Flavivirus activation of plasmacytoid dendritic cells delineates key elements of TLR7 signaling beyond endosomal recognition. J Immunol *177*, 7114-7121.

Werninghaus, K., Babiak, A., Gross, O., Holscher, C., Dietrich, H., Agger, E.M., Mages, J., Mocsai, A., Schoenen, H., Finger, K., *et al.* (2009). Adjuvanticity of a synthetic cord factor analogue for subunit Mycobacterium tuberculosis vaccination requires FcRgamma-Syk-Card9-dependent innate immune activation. J Exp Med *206*, 89-97.

Williams, A., Flavell, R.A., and Eisenbarth, S.C. (2010). The role of NOD-like Receptors in shaping adaptive immunity. Curr Opin Immunol *22*, 34-40.

Woehrle, T., Du, W., Goetz, A., Hsu, H.Y., Joos, T.O., Weiss, M., Bauer, U., Brueckner, U.B., and Marion Schneider, E. (2008). Pathogen specific cytokine release reveals an effect of TLR2 Arg753Gln during Candida sepsis in humans. Cytokine *41*, 322-329.

Zhu, J., Martinez, J., Huang, X., and Yang, Y. (2007). Innate immunity against vaccinia virus is mediated by TLR2 and requires TLR-independent production of IFN-beta. Blood *109*, 619-625.

20

Stem Cells in Infectious Diseases

Ramesh Chandra Rai, Debapriya Bhattacharya and Gobardhan Das
Immunology Group, International Centre for Genetic Engineering and Biotechnology, New Delhi, India

1. Introduction

Stem cells are unspecialized cells found in embryos (blastocyst stage) and in various tissues of adults. They divide mitotically to self renew and can differentiate into different types of cells in appropriate conditions for specific functions. They serve as cell reservoirs for purpose of repair of damaged tissues of the body. Recent research suggests that stem cells especially mesenchymal stem cells have immuno-modulatory characteristics. Due to this property many trials are being conducted with transplantation of MSCs in treating diseases which arise from immunological abuses. These cells have capacity of specific homing and thus can repair infection induced injuries of various organs of body. Evidences suggest that mesenchymal stem cells could on the other hand be a potential target for treatment of tuberculosis.

Even after more than a century of its discovery in 1882 by Robert Koch, *Mycobacterium tuberculosis* (*M. tb*) continues to be one of the leading causes of mortality and morbidity in humans among infectious diseases. One third of global population is latently infected with *M. tb* (World Health Organisation November 2010), and is a cause of around two million deaths each year. The majority of infected individuals remain asymptomatic until there is any perturbation of host immune responses. Currently available vaccine, Bacillus Calmette-Guérin (BCG) is effective only in disseminated TB in young children. On the contrary, its efficacy dramatically varies in adult pulmonary TB depending on ethnicity and geographical locations. Current therapy of TB is very effective and is adopted by internationally recognized Directly Observed Treatment Short course (DOTS) programme. However, this regimen of therapy consists of multiple antibiotics for an extended period of time, and thus incorporates the risk of developing drug resistance. In fact, non-compliance is the central cause for generation of multiple and extensively drug resistant (MDR and XDR) forms of TB (Peter A. Otto *et al.*, 2008). Therefore, there is an urgent need for alternative therapeutic targets and newer strategies for treatment of *Mycobacterium tuberculosis* infections.

Considerable efforts have been made to uncover the strategy used by the harbouring tubercular bacilli to induce persistent/latent infection. Only recently, it has been clearly demonstrated that mesenchymal stem cells (MSCs) play a "Janus" like activity and establish a dynamic equilibrium. MSCs position themselves in between harbouring bacilli and host protective T cells. Therefore, MSCs could be a potential therapeutic target for treatment of latent tuberculosis (Raghuvanshi S. *et al.*, 2010). They are recruited at the site of infection and do not allow *M. tb* to spread but at the same time suppress host immune response mounted against the pathogen, thus preventing complete elimination of pathogen from the host (Raghuvanshi S. *et al.*, 2010). These results shed a light on possible new ways for treating tuberculosis, which has been a major killer of humans for centuries.

2. Stem cells and various diseases

Due to self renewal and multi-lineage differentiation capabilities, transplantation of stem cells has emerged as a very promising way of treatment of many diseases. Stem cell therapy of different diseases involves the local delivery of stem cells to injured/ infected site or their systemic transfusion. Owing the ability to differentiate into various lineages, stem cells hold therapeutic potential for treatment of many non-infectious and infectious diseases.

2.1 Non-infectious diseases

Mesenchymal stem cells can manipulate host immune responses; they have been used for treating/preventing many diseases which arise because of irregularities of immune system or host responses. Also the infused stem cells are able to differentiate to a particular type of cell after reaching the site in response to local signals. Although this notion have not yet been demonstrated very well. Many reports suggest their use in case of cardiovascular, lung fibrosis, neural and orthopaedic diseases (Barry FP and Murphy JM, 2004; Ortiz LA. *et al.*, 2003).

In a study by Teng, YD. *et al.*, 2002, have shown improvement in injured spinal cord by transplanting neural stem cell in adult rat. These approaches can also be extended to treat the conditions of stroke and other neurodegenerative diseases (Barry FP. and Murphy JM, 2004). Recently Lin H. *et al.*, 2011, reported positive therapeutic use of MSCs in different liver diseases and inherited metabolic disorders. They have shown that cytokines produced from MSCs can attenuate inflammatory injury to the liver and prevent apoptosis of liver cells. Also MSCs helped in regaining the proliferation and function of hepatocytes.

2.1.1 Auto-immune diseases

When immune system of human body recognises its own component as non-self, it starts immune response against it. This leads to auto-immune diseases such as inflammatory bowel disease, arthritis etc. In inflammatory bowel disease which includes ulcerative colitis and Crohn's disease, the intestine become inflamed (Melgar S and Shanahan F, 2010; Siegmund B and Zeitz M, 2011). This is due to immune reaction of person's body towards its own intestinal tissues. In case of arthritis especially in rheumatoid arthritis, there is inflammation of joints due to overt immune responses. This leads to damage of joints which is due to inflammation of joint lining tissues. So, objective of treatments will be suppression of immune responses.

2.1.2 Graft Versus Host Diseases (GVHD)

It is a situation when host immune system rejects transplanted organ or part of it as a non-self. Infiltration of MSCs can suppress host immune response and thus can prevent GVHD

(Le Blanc K, *et al.*, 2004; Tse WT, 2003). Prolonged survival of skin graft was observed when MSCs were used (Bartholomew A, *et al.*, 2002). So it can reverse the process of rejection and GVHD when used in transplantation (Bobis S., *et al.*, 2006; Le Blank K and Ringden O., 2005). GVHD was not observed in case of patients with metachromatic leukodystrophy and Hurler's syndrome after MSCs were infused (Koc, O. N. *et al.*, 2002).

In such situations immuno-suppressive effect of MSCs can help in preventing these diseases.

2.2 Infectious diseases

There is growing understanding among scientific community that many of infectious diseases may be cured or controlled using stem cells. Stem cell therapy can also be used in general to fight infections e.g. sepsis, a life threatening condition which arises from spread of an infection throughout the body and body's response to it. Report from Mei SH. *et al.*, 2010; suggest that sepsis could be treated successfully by transplanting mesenchymal stem cells to the patient.

2.2.1 Stem cell therapy for treatment of HIV infection

Stem cell therapy for treatment of HIV is under intensive investigation in recent times. Scientists are trying to reconstitute HIV-resistant lymphoid and myeloid system in experimental mice model to combat HIV infections (Holt, N. *et al.*, 2010; Steven G Deeks and Joseph M McCune, 2010). Holt, N. *et al.* 2010, engineered human hematopoietic cells to disrupt the CCR5 receptors which are utilized by viruses for their entry. When these engineered cells are transplanted to mice, they confer resistance towards the HIV infections. When CCR5 disrupted stem cells transplanted in a HIV patient, patient remained free of virus for 20 months even in absence of antiretroviral therapies (Hütter G *et al.*, 2009).

In a similar kind of approach Kitchen SG. *et al.*, 2009, demonstrated that hematopoietic stem cells could be engineered to target HIV infected cells. They generated CD8+ cytotoxic T cell lymphocytes which express transgenic-human anti-HIV T cell receptor. After cloning and transplantation to mice model, these cells were able to kill cells which were infected with HIV and were displaying its antigens.

2.2.2 Stem cell therapy for treatment of malaria

Malaria, which is characterized by invasion of erythrocytes by *Plasmodium*, leads to extreme perturbation of hematopoiesis. Severe destruction of red blood cells causes anaemia, thus posing pressure on bone marrow to meet the requirement of myeloid cells. Scientists from National Institute for Medical Research, UK, have identified an atypical progenitor cells from malaria infected mice which can give rise to a lineage of cells capable of fighting this disease (Belyaev, NN, 2010). Transplantation of these cells into mice with severe malaria helped mice recover from the disease. Other reports also supports stem cell therapy for malaria treatment (Saei, AA. and Ahmadian, S., 2009). Stem cells can also be engineered to produce erythrocytes with modified hemoglobin as its variants are associated with protection from malaria.

Approaches may differ but stem cells are in focus for treatment of many diseases. The current reports from our lab suggest that tuberculosis could be prevented possibly by targeting mesenchymal stem cells.

3. Tuberculosis and its treatment options

Mycobacterium tuberculosis infects humans through aerial route and thus lungs are the primary organ for its infection. Subsequently infection spreads to other organs of body such as spleen and lymph nodes. Recruitment of macrophages and lymphocytes at the site of infection leads to formation of granuloma which is small area of inflammation due to tissue injury or infection and a hallmark of tuberculosis. Many other diseases are also associated with the formation of granulomas such as sarcoidosis, histoplasmosis, syphilis, Crohn's disease etc. Granulomas are formed when immune cells contains a foreign substance after recognition which could not get cleared by body's immune system. They are characterized by presence of macrophages and infectious agent besides other cells and body matrix such as lymphocytes, neutrophils, eosinophils, fibroblasts and collagen.

In case of tuberculosis granulomas are formed at the site of infection where *Mycobacterium tuberculosis* remains as a latent infection. Infection to the macrophages of lungs leads to secretion of several of chemokines which attracts lymphocytes and neutrophils. These cells are able to contain pathogen inside granuloma, thus preventing the spread of bacterium to other parts of body and further inflammation. In other words granulomas are hiding place of bacteria in the infected organs. Final outcome of these interactions and whether it will lead to disease condition or not depends on the strength of host immune response.

Host immune response blocks spread of infection and prevents disease condition but it is not able to completely remove *M. tb* from body. Its persistent infection in a person converts into diseased condition when there is suppression of immunity such as in case of AIIDS. As HIV infection compromises immunity, the person will become highly susceptible to active tuberculosis as latent infection turns into active form (Goletti D, *et al.*, 1996). Co-existence of both TB and HIV fuel each other worsening the patient's condition. Immunosuppression in HIV patients occur as a result of decrease in number of $CD4^+$ T cells and leads to progression of TB. One report suggests that the chances of getting TB increases from 4% to 49% when there is decrease in $CD4^+$ T cells from 200 cells/μl to 100 cells/μl (Jones BE *et al.*, 1993). On the other hand *Mycobacterium tuberculosis* infection facilitates replication of HIV. This is done by cytokines such as TNF-α and IL-6 secreted from *M. tb* infected macrophages (Havlir DV and Barnes PF 1999; Nakata K, *et al.*, 1997). These cytokines creates a microenvironment which are inductive to HIV replication (Goletti D, *et al.* 1996). Thus, both HIV and *M. tb* can shorten the lifespan of patients by working together.

4. Bacillus Calmette–Gue´rin (BCG) and its efficacy

Bacillus Calmette–Gue´rin (BCG) vaccine is prepared from attenuated strain of *Mycobacterium bovis*. This strain has become avirulent due to continuous passages in artificial medium for a long time but still remained antigenic, being used as vaccine to prevent tuberculosis. But its effectiveness is not 100% and does not last longer (Colditz GA *et al.*, 1994). At the maximum it can provide protection up to 15 years depending on many factors including geographical conditions. Directly Observed Treatment, Short Course (DOTS) is a world health organisation (WHO) recommended treatment for tuberculosis. It was launched in India in 1997 as a revised national tuberculosis control programme. Before launching the programme, it was tested from 1993-1996. The key components of this programme are as follows-

i. Political commitment to control TB;
ii. Case detection by sputum smear microscopy examination among symptomatic patients;
iii. Patients are given anti- TB drugs under the direct observation of the health care provider/community DOT provider;
iv. Regular, uninterrupted supply of anti-TB drugs; and
v. Systematic recording and reporting system that allows assessment of treatment results of each and every patient and of whole TB control programme.

Treatment of tuberculosis involves- isoniazid, rifampicin, ethambutol, pyrazinamide daily for two months, followed by four months of isoniazid and rifampicin given three times a week. Sometimes one or the other drugs are omitted during treatment depending on the patient's condition. Later in 2006; WHO launched stop TB programme as a multi-dimensional approach to fight this disease at international level and better management of treatment strategies.

5. Mesenchymal stem cells (MSCs) and its role in *M. tb* infection

Discovered by A. J. Friedenstein in 1968 (Friedenstein, AJ. *et al.*,1974) MSCs are a subset of non-haematopoietic pleuripotent cells found in adult bone marrow and are capable of differentiating into adipocytes, fibroblasts and even myoblasts (Ren G. *et al.*, 2010). The mesenchymal stem cell name to these cells was given by Caplan. They have very high capacity to proliferate *in vitro* and don't loose proliferation capacity for a long time (Sundin, M. *et al.*, 2006). After their discovery and growing understanding of their role in the modulation of host immune response, they have been thought to be an important tool for regenerative medicine and immunotherapy. Although there are no exclusive markers for MSCs, they are characterized by their ability to differentiate into different kinds of cells mentioned above and by the combined surface expressions of $CD29^{+}CD44^{+}Sca\text{-}1^{+}CD45^{-}CD11b^{-}CD11c^{-}Gr\text{-}1^{-}F4/80^{-}MHC\text{-}II^{-}MHC\text{-}I^{low}$ (Ren G. *et al.*, 2008 and 2010).

MSCs are immuno-suppressive in nature and they exert their effect only when they are stimulated. Unstimulated MSCs are not capable of performing this effect (Yufang Shi *et al.*, 2010). MSCs have been shown to prevent rejection of allogenic skin grafts (Xu G, *et al.* 2007), graft versus host diseases (K. Le Blanc and O. Ringden, 2006), and therefore are helpful in treating auto-immune disorders. They are able to alter function of T cells, B cells, dendritic cells (DCs) and natural killer (NK) cells (Ren G. *et al.*, 2010). This is done by cytokines secreted by MSCs and through direct cell-cell contact. MSCs produce number of cytokines, signalling molecules and growth factors which can suppress inflammatory response and may also lead to trophic effects (Caplan AI and Dennis JE. 2006; Lin H. *et al.*, 2011). Their regulatory effect on immune system, such as anti-proliferative (Bartholomew A, *et al.*, 2002; Di Nicola M *et al.*, 2002; Le Blank K *et al.*, 2003; Sudres M, *et al.*, 2006) and anti-inflammatory roles makes them an important candidate for therapy of many inflammatory diseases (Newman RE *et al.*, 2009).

Mesenchymal stem cells have ability to create a microenvironment which helps in engraftment. The expressions of major histocompatibility I (MHC I) molecules are less on these cells and they lack human leukocyte antigen (HLA) class II and costimulatory molecules such as CD40, CD80 and CD86 (Krampera, M. *et al.*, 2003). Low level expression of MSC I can still activate T cells but they become anergic as there is no secondary signals or co-stimulation (Javazon EH. *et al.*, 2004; Wong RS. 2011). Also low level expression of MHC I prevent these cells from being destroyed by natural killer cells (Moretta A. *et al.*, 2001). They generally do not express MHC II molecules on their surface (Le Blank K. *et al.*, 2003) but could be immunogenic in certain circumstances (Le Blank K. *et al.*, 2003; Stagg J. *et al.*, 2006). The above characteristics help them to be less immunogenic (Herrero C. and Perez-Simon, J. A. 2010) and also have ability of interaction with components of both innate and adaptive immune system. Suppression of T and B cell proliferation and their activation makes them useful for treatment of different infectious and non-infectious diseases such as tuberculosis, graft versus host disease and various auto-immune diseases (Sundin, M. *et al.*, 2006). These cells have ability to migrate specifically to the site of injury. This has been shown in many of diseases involving injury of tissues and cartilages.

5.1 Effector molecules of mesenchymal stem cells

The molecular players which perform immunosuppression are mainly nitric oxide (NO), indoleamine 2,3-dioxygenase (IDO) and prostaglandin E2 (PGE2) (Ren G. *et al.*, 2008). Three nitric oxide synthases catalyse the synthesis of NO, which by interacting with many receptors and enzymes plays critical role in immune-suppression. It affects the phenotype of T cells and impairs its proliferation and function affecting TCR mediated signalling (Hoffman, RA. *et al.*, 2002). MSCs has been shown to express many chemokine receptors such as CCR1, CCR4, CCR5 and CCR10, thus in response to many of the cytokines, they move to desired destination (Von Luttichau *et al.*, 2005).

5.2 Host immune response

Both innate and adaptive immunity plays role against *Mycobacterium tuberculosis* infection. Host immune response against *Mycobacterium tuberculosis* is Th1 rather than Th2 mediated as IFN-γ knock out mice fails to mount immune response against its infection (Schroder K *et al.*, 2004). Of note, IFN-γ plays suppressive role for Th2 cell differentiation. *M. tb* evades host protective immune responses by modulating various immune mechanisms that includes down regulations of Major Histocompatibility Complex (MHCs), co-stimulatory molecules, and up-regulating production of immune suppressive cytokines viz. TGF-β and IL-10, and prostaglandins. Each of these targets is extensively studied for therapeutic interventions. However, it has been mostly unsuccessful. It is now evident that MSCs confine harbouring bacteria and segregate host protective responses. Cell mediated immunity is required for protection from *M. tb*. But *M. tb* has evolved mechanisms to evade the host immune response and remains as persistent infection inside the granuloma.

5.3 Balance between immune response and disease outcome

After *M. tb* infection, macrophage and lymphocytes are mobilized to the site of infection, resulting in formation of granuloma. Thus cells of innate and adaptive immune system of body surround the pathogen. Recognition of pathogen associated molecular patterns leads to activation of T cells which secrete IFN-γ. Since *M. tb* is an intracellular pathogen, effector T cells plays crucial role in host immunity against this pathogen. To evade the host defence mechanism, pathogen recruits MSCs at the periphery of granuloma (Raghuvanshi S. *et al.*,

2010). Reports from various groups suggest that MSC interferes with antigen presenting cell functionality, block the differentiation of B cells. They also suppress natural killer cell and T cell responses. Both naïve and memory T cell responses were inhibited by MSCs. The suppression is due to cell cycle arrest at G0/G1 stage of T cells (Glennie S. *et al.*, 2005). They induce Th2 cells to produce interleukin-4 (IL-4) and also inhibit the production of interferon-γ thus creating an anti-inflammatory state. MSCs also arrest B cells at G0/G1 stage of their cell cycle besides suppressing their differentiation (Corcione, A. *et al.*, 2006; Tabera, S. *et al.*, 2008) and inhibit immunoglobulin production (Herrero, C. and Perez Simon J. A. 2010). MSCs also hinder functional differentiation of dendritic cells (Jiang XX., *et al.*, 2005; Ramasamy R., *et al.*, 2007). Besides above mentioned roles there is conflicting reports regarding immune-suppression effect of MSCs in murine models *in vivo* (Muriel Sudres *et al.*, 2006).

Pro-inflammatory cytokines induces MSCs to secrete several cytokines/ chemokines (IL-10, TGF-β, IDO and PGE2) and nitric oxide (NO). Together they perform immuno-suppression (Ren G. *at al.*, 2008) and also induce regulatory T cells which prevent killing of *M. tb* by cytotoxic T cells (Scott-Browne JP *et al.*, 2007). NO inhibits T cell proliferation, production of cytokines, and induce tolerance (Niedbala, W. *et al.*, 2006; Ren G. *et al.*, 2008). NO diffuses rapidly to the vicinity but its active concentration drops very fast as it is highly unstable (Ren G. *et al.*, 2008). It is effective only up to a distance of 100 micrometer (J.R. Lancaster Jr., 1997). To perform immunosuppressive activity, T cells must be held in close proximity to the MSCs. This is done by MSC surface molecules such as intercellular adhesion molecule-1 (ICAM1) and vascular cell adhesion molecule-1 (VCAM1), which are shown to interact with T cells and hold them close to the mesenchymal stem cells (Ren G. *et al.*, 2010 and 2011). Thus besides soluble factors secreted from MSCs, cell surface molecules on MSCs also play crucial role in immune suppression against *Mycobacterium tuberculosis* (Xu G, *et al.* 2007; Shi Y. *et al.*, 2010).

In mice after infection by *Mycobacterium tuberculosis*, MSCs exclusively infiltrate to infected organs such as lungs and spleen (Raghuvanshi S. *et al.*, 2010). They have not been found to the uninfected organs of the infected person. This report suggests that immune suppression by MSC is local and confines to the infection site only. Although MSCs recruited at the site of infection contains pathogen inside granulomas, it also prevents killing of *Mycobacterium tuberculosis* by suppressing the host immunity. These cells intercept immune cells from the pathogen by being there physically and helping to establish equilibrium between host and the pathogen (Figure 1). In other words, *M. tb* rely on MSCs to establish long lasting infection which should be intervened to achieve objective of treating tuberculosis.

6. Issues in therapy with stem cells

Therapy with stem cells have shown hope for treatment of those diseases which otherwise seems to be untreatable. But this approach also has its own risks. Utilization of MSCs for therapeutic use is like a double edged sword putting patient at the danger of cancer. The anti-proliferative effects of these cells are often associated with anti-apoptotic effect also, which may leads to tumour progression, metastasis and drug resistance. So even with vast therapeutic potential of stem cells in various non-infectious and infectious diseases, there

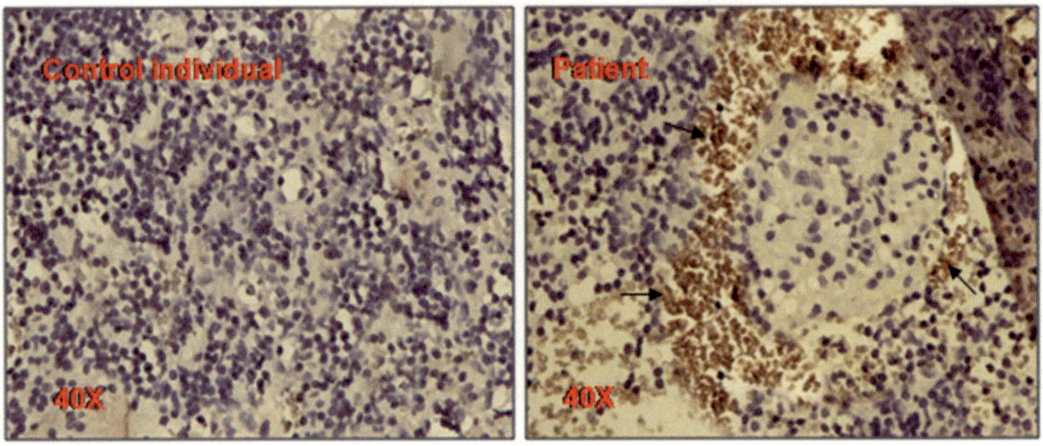

Fig. 1. Immunohistochemical staining for the presence of MSCs (arrows) in granuloma-containing lymph node of patients with tuberculosis. Adapted from Raghuvanshi S. *et al.*, PNAS, 2010.

are some issues which have to be addressed before its actual implementation. Some of them are as follows-

i. Reach of the administered stem cell to its desired destination such as injured tissue and infected/affected organ. Also the effect of endogenous population of the stem cells should be considered.
ii. Proper understanding of the host immune response against the administered stem cell.
iii. Dose of the transplanted stem cells. Also being animal product for administration into patients, long term safety issues has to be understood.
iv. Risk to the patient with secondary infections in case of immune suppression of the host by stem cells. Immuno-compromised condition of the patient may lead to infection of fungus, bacteria and viruses. This should be considered while going for stem cell infiltration and should be tested clinically (Sundin, M. *et al.*, 2006).
v. Although anti-tumor response of MSCs has been observed, they can also suppress anti-tumor immune response. MSCs can be potentially tumorogenic by direct transformation. So, use of MSCs for therapy of patients with high risk to cancer should be avoided.

Since allogenic MSCs are little immunogenic, the other choice should be administration of autologous MSCs. Clinical applications of autologous MSCs of bone marrow has been successfully shown in case of MDR tuberculosis (Erokhin VV., *et al.*, 2008). They have shown that systemic transplantation of the autologous MSCs stopped the bacterial discharge and lung tissue cavities were resolved in tuberculosis patients infected with resistant forms of *Mycobacterium tuberculosis*. Contrary to the role of MSCs in various diseases which have been discussed earlier, where transplantation of these cells is required for treatments of various diseases, report from our lab suggest them as a target for treatment of tuberculosis.

7. Conclusion and future perspectives

Use of stem cells for treatment of many diseases is the area of intensive research these days with many clinical trials undergoing. Mesenchymal stem cells are the main cell type being used due to their longevity and less ethical issues. Still there are many concerns as discussed including their immunogenicity. Suppression of immune system is the other major concern which poses serious threat of other infections to the patients. Studies from our lab using mouse model of tuberculosis suggest role of mesenchymal stem cells in this disease. Besides currently available strategies for treatment of tuberculosis, the probable new target such as MSCs holds promise in the current scenario of MDR and XDR tuberculosis. Targeting MSCs will also wouldn't lead to generation of any new resistance in pathogen as one does not need to target them directly rather manipulate the host immune response. In the coming future we may be able to use MSCs as an immuno-therapeutic target for the treatment of tuberculosis.

8. Acknowledgements

Authors would like to thank Wellcome-DBT India Alliance; Department of Biotechnology, Government of India and Council of Scientific and Industrial Research, Government of India for financial support.

9. References

Barry FP. and Murphy JM, Mesenchymal stem cells: clinical applications and biological characterization. Int J Biochem Cell Biol. 2004, 36 (4): 568-84.

Bartholomew A, Sturgeon C, Siatskas M, Ferrer K, McIntosh K, Patil S, Hardy W, Devine S, Ucker D, Deans R, Moseley A, Hoffman R, Mesenchymal stem cells suppress lymphocyte proliferation in vitro and prolong skin graft survival in vivo. Exp Hematol. 2002, 30 (1): 42-8.

Belyaev NN, Brown DE, Diaz AI, Rae A, Jarra W, Thompson J, Langhorne J, Potocnik AJ, Induction of an IL7-R(+)c-Kit(hi) myelolymphoid progenitor critically dependent on IFN-gamma signaling during acute malaria. Nat Immunol. 2010; 11(6): 477-85.

Bobis S, Jarocha D, Majka M; Mesenchymal stem cells: characteristics and clinical applications. Folia Histochem Cytobiol. 2006; 44(4): 215-30.

Caplan AI, and Dennis JE. Mesenchymal stem cells as trophic mediators. J Cell Biochem. 2006; 98(5): 1076-84.

Colditz GA, Brewer TF, Berkey CS (1994). "Efficacy of BCG Vaccine in the Prevention of Tuberculosis". J Am Med Assoc 271 (9): 698–702.

Corcione A, Benvenuto F, Ferretti E, Giunti D, Cappiello V, Cazzanti F, Risso M, Gualandi F, Mancardi GL, Pistoia V, Uccelli A., Human mesenchymal stem cells modulate B-cell functions. Blood, 2006, 1; 107 (1): 367-72.

Di Nicola M, Carlo-Stella C, Magni M, Milanesi M, Longoni PD, Matteucci P, Grisanti S, Gianni AM., Human bone marrow stromal cells suppress T-lymphocyte proliferation induced by cellular or nonspecific mitogenic stimuli, Blood. 2002; 99(10): 3838-43.

Erokhin VV, Vasil'eva IA, Konopliannikov AG, Chukanov VI, Tsyb AF, Bagdasarian TR, Danilenko AA, Lepekhina LA, Kal'sina SSh, Semenkova IV, Agaeva EV. Systemic transplantation of autologous mesenchymal stem cells of the bone marrow in the treatment of patients with multidrug-resistant pulmonary tuberculosis. Probl Tuberk Bolezn Legk. 2008; (10): 3-6.

Friedenstein AJ, Chailakhyan RK, Latsinik NV, Panasyuk AF, Keiliss-Borok IV. Stromal cells responsible for transferring the microenvironment of the hemopoietic tissues. Cloning in vitro and retransplantation in vivo, Transplantation. 1974; 17 (4): 331-40.

Glennie S, Soeiro I, Dyson PJ, Lam EW, Dazzi F, Bone marrow mesenchymal stem cells induce division arrest anergy of activated T cells, Blood. 2005; 105(7):2821-7.

Goletti D, Weissman D, Jackson RW, et al. Effect of *Mycobacterium tuberculosis* on HIV replication: role of immune activation. J Immunol. 1996; 157: 1271-1278.

Havlir DV, Barnes PF. Tuberculosis in patients with human immunodeficiency virus infection. N Engl J Med. 1999; 340: 367-373.

Herrero C, Pérez-Simón JA, Immunomodulatory effect of mesenchymal stem cells., Braz J Med Biol Res. 2010; 43(5): 425-30.

Hütter G, Nowak D, Mossner M, Ganepola S, Müssig A, Allers K, Schneider T, Hofmann J, Kücherer C, Blau O, Blau IW, Hofmann WK, Thiel E, Long-term control of HIV by CCR5 Delta32/Delta32 stem-cell transplantation. N Engl J Med. 2009; 360(7): 692-8.

Hoffman RA, Mahidhara RS, Wolf-Johnston AS, Lu L, Thomson AW, Simmons RL. Differential modulation of CD4 and CD8 T-cell proliferation by induction of nitric oxide synthesis in antigen presenting cells, Transplantation. 2002; 74(6): 836-45.

Holt N, Wang J, Kim K, Friedman G, Wang X, Taupin V, Crooks G. M., Kohn DB, Gregory PD, Holmes MC and Cannon PM. Human hematopoietic stem/ progenitor cells modified by zink-finger nucleases targeted to CCR5 control HIV-1 in vivo. Nature Biotechnol. 2010; 28 (8): 839-47.

Javazon EH, Beggs KJ, Flake AW. Mesenchymal stem cells: paradoxes of passaging. Exp Hematol. 2004; 32(5): 414-25.

Jiang XX, Zhang Y, Liu B, Zhang SX, Wu Y, Yu XD, Mao N., Human mesenchymal stem cells inhibit differentiation and function of monocyte-derived dendritic cells, Blood. 2005; 105(10): 4120-6.

Jones BE, Young SM, Antoniskis D, Davidson PT, Kramer F, Barnes PF, Relationship of the manifestations of tuberculosis to CD4 cell counts in patients with human immunodeficiency virus infection. Am Rev Respir Dis. 1993;148(5):1292-7.

Le Blanc K, Rasmusson I, Sundberg B, Götherström C, Hassan M, Uzunel M, Ringdén O. Treatment of severe acute graft-versus-host disease with third party haploidentical mesenchymal stem cells. Lancet. 2004; 363(9419):1439-41.

Le Blanc K and Ringdén O, Immunobiology of human mesenchymal stem cells and future use in hematopoietic stem cell transplantation, Biol Blood Marrow Transplant. 2005; 11(5): 321-34.

Le Blanc K and Ringden O., Mesenchymal stem cells: Properties and role in clinical bone marrow transplantation, Curr. Opin. Immunol. (2006), 18, pp. 586–591.

Le Blanc K, Tammik C, Rosendahl K, Zetterberg E, Ringdén O., HLA expression and immunologic properties of differentiated and undifferentiated mesenchymal stem cells, Exp Hematol. 2003; 31(10): 890-6.

Le Blanc K, Tammik L, Sundberg B, Haynesworth SE, Ringdén O., Mesenchymal stem cells inhibit and stimulate mixed lymphocyte cultures and mitogenic responses independently of the major histocompatibility complex., Scand J Immunol. 2003; 57(1): 11-20.

Kitchen SG, Bennett M, Galić Z, Kim J, Xu Q, Young A, Lieberman A, Joseph A, Goldstein H, Ng H, Yang O, Zack JA. Engineering antigen-specific T cells from genetically modified human hematopoietic stem cells in immunodeficient mice. PLoS One. 2009; 4(12)

Koç ON, Day J, Nieder M, Gerson SL, Lazarus HM, Krivit W. Allogeneic mesenchymal stem cell infusion for treatment of metachromatic leukodystrophy (MLD) and Hurler syndrome (MPS-IH), Bone Marrow Transplant. 2002; 30(4): 215-22.

Krampera M, Glennie S, Dyson J, Scott D, Laylor R, Simpson E, Dazzi F, Bone marrow mesenchymal stem cells inhibit the response of naive and memory antigen-specific T cells to their cognate peptide, Blood. 2003; 101(9): 3722-9.

Lancaster J.R. Jr., A tutorial on the diffusibility and reactivity of free nitric oxide. Nitric Oxide 1 (1997), pp. 18–30.

Lazebnik LB, Konopliannikov AG, Kniazev OV, Parfenov AI, Tsaregorodtseva TM, Ruchkina IN, Khomeriki SG, Rogozina VA, Konopliannikova OA. Use of allogeneic mesenchymal stem cells in the treatment of intestinal inflammatory diseases. Ter Arkh. 2010; 82(2): 38-43.

Lazebnik LB, Konopliannikov AG, Parfenov AI, Kniazev OV, Parfenov AI, Ruchkina IN, Khomeriki SG, Rogozina VA, Konopliannikova OA, Tsaregorodtseva TM. Application of allogeneic mesenchymal stem cells in complex patients treatment with ulcerative colitis. Eksp Klin Gastroenterol. 2009; (5): 4-12.

Lin H, Xu R, Zhang Z, Chen L, Shi M, Wang FS, Implications of the immunoregulatory functions of mesenchymal stem cells in the treatment of human liver diseases. Cell Mol Immunol. 2011, 8(1): 19-22.

Mei SH, Haitsma JJ, Dos Santos CC, Deng Y, Lai PF, Slutsky AS, Liles WC, Stewart DJ. Mesenchymal Stem Cells Reduce Inflammation while Enhancing Bacterial Clearance and Improving Survival in Sepsis. Am J Respir Crit Care Med. 2010 Oct 15; 182(8): 1047-57.

Melgar S and Shanahan F, Inflammatory bowel disease- from mechanisms to treatment strategies. Autoimmunity. 2010; 43(7): 463-77.

Moretta A, Bottino C, Vitale M, Pende D, Cantoni C, Mingari MC, Biassoni R, Moretta L. Activating receptors and coreceptors involved in human natural killer cell-mediated cytolysis. Annu Rev Immunol. 2001; 19: 197-223.

Nakata K, Rom WN, Honda Y, et al. *Mycobacterium tuberculosis* enhances human immunodeficiency virus-1 replication in the lung. Am J Respir Crit Care Med. 1997; 155: 996-1003.

Newman RE, Yoo D, LeRoux MA, Danilkovitch-Miagkova A. Treatment of inflammatory diseases with mesenchymal stem cells. Inflamm Allergy Drug Targets. 2009; 8(2):110-23.

Niedbala W., B. Cai and F.Y. Liew, Role of nitric oxide in the regulation of T cell functions, Ann. Rheum. *Dis.* 65 (Suppl 3) (2006), pp. iii37–iii40.

Ortiz LA, Gambelli F, McBride C, Gaupp D, Baddoo M, Kaminski N, Phinney DG. Mesenchymal stem cell engraftment in lung is enhanced in response to bleomycin exposure and ameliorates its fibrotic effects. Proc Natl Acad Sci U S A. 2003; 100(14): 8407-11.

Peter A. Otto, A. Agid, Suzan and Mushtaha, MDR-TB is in town; and might be tugging along XDR-TB. SSMJ Vol 2 Issue 3 (www.southernsudanmedicaljournal.com).

Raghuvanshi S, Sharma P, Singh S, Van Kaer L, Das G. Mycobacterium tuberculosis evades host immunity by recruiting mesenchymal stem cells. Proc Natl Acad Sci U S A. 2010, 107(50): 21653-8.

Ramasamy R, Fazekasova H, Lam EW, Soeiro I, Lombardi G, Dazzi F. Mesenchymal stem cells inhibit dendritic cell differentiation and function by preventing entry into the cell cycle, Transplantation. 2007; 83(1): 71-6.

Ren G, Zhang L, Zhao X, Xu G, Zhang Y, Roberts AI, Zhao RC, Shi Y. Mesenchymal stem cell-mediated immunosuppression occurs via concerted action of chemokines and nitric oxide. Cell Stem Cell. 2008, 7; 2(2): 141-50.

Ren G, Zhao X, Zhang L, Zhang J, L'Huillier A, Ling W, Roberts AI, Le AD, Shi S, Shao C, Shi Y. Inflammatory cytokine-induced intercellular adhesion molecule-1 and vascular cell adhesion molecule-1 in mesenchymal stem cells are critical for immunosuppression. J Immunol. 2010; 184(5): 2321-8.

Saei, A. A. and Ahmadian, S. Stem cell engineering might be protective against severe malaria Bioscience Hypotheses Volume 2, Issue 1, 2009, Pages 48-49.

Schroder K, Hertzog PJ, Ravasi T, Hume DA. Interferon-gamma: an overview of signals, mechanisms and functions". J. Leukoc. Biol. 2004, 75(2): 163–89.

Scott-Browne JP, Shafiani S, Tucker-Heard G, Ishida-Tsubota K, Fontenot JD, Rudensky AY, Bevan MJ, Urdahl KB. Expansion and function of Foxp3-expressing T regulatory cells during tuberculosis. J Exp Med. 2007;204(9): 2159-69.

Shi Y, Hu G, Su J, Li W, Chen Q, Shou P, Xu C, Chen X, Huang Y, Zhu Z, Huang X, Han X, Xie N, Ren G. Mesenchymal stem cells: a new strategy for immunosuppression and tissue repair. Cell Res. 2010; 20(5): 510-8.

Siegmund B and Zeitz M, Innate and adaptive immunity in inflammatory bowel disease. World J Gastroenterol. 2011; 17(27): 3178-83.

Stagg J, Pommey S, Eliopoulos N, Galipeau J, Interferon-gamma-stimulated marrow stromal cells: a new type of nonhematopoietic antigen-presenting cell, Blood. 2006; 107(6): 2570-7.

Steven G Deeks and Joseph M McCune, Can HIV be cured with stem cell therapy? Nature Biotechnology, 2010, 28, 807–810.

Sundin M, Orvell C, Rasmusson I, Sundberg B, Ringdén O, Le Blanc K, Mesenchymal stem cells are susceptible to human herpesviruses, but viral DNA cannot be detected in the healthy seropositive individual, Bone Marrow Transplant. 2006; 37(11): 1051-9.

Sudres M, Norol F, Trenado A, Grégoire S, Charlotte F, Levacher B, Lataillade JJ, Bourin P, Holy X, Vernant JP, Klatzmann D, Cohen JL. Bone marrow mesenchymal stem cells suppress lymphocyte proliferation in vitro but fail to prevent graft-versus-host disease in mice. J Immunol. 2006; 176(12): 7761-7.

Tabera S, Pérez-Simón JA, Díez-Campelo M, Sánchez-Abarca LI, Blanco B, López A, Benito A, Ocio E, Sánchez-Guijo FM, Cañizo C, San Miguel JF, The effect of mesenchymal stem cells on the viability, proliferation and differentiation of B-lymphocytes, Haematologica. 2008; 93(9):1301-9.

Teng YD, Lavik EB, Qu X, Park KI, Ourednik J, Zurakowski D, Langer R, Snyder EY; Functional recovery following traumatic spinal cord injury mediated by a unique polymer scaffold seeded with neural stem cells; Proc Natl Acad Sci U S A. 2002; 99(5): 3024-9.

Tse WT, Pendleton JD, Beyer WM, Egalka MC, Guinan EC., Suppression of allogeneic T-cell proliferation by human marrow stromal cells: implications in transplantation, Transplantation. 2003, 75(3): 389-97.

Xu G, Zhang L, Ren G, Yuan Z, Zhang Y, Zhao RC, Shi Y. Immunosuppressive properties of cloned bone marrow mesenchymal stem cells. Cell Res. 2007; 17(3): 240-8.

Von Lüttichau I, Notohamiprodjo M, Wechselberger A, Peters C, Henger A, Seliger C, Djafarzadeh R, Huss R, Nelson PJ. Human adult CD34- progenitor cells functionally express the chemokine receptors CCR1, CCR4, CCR7, CXCR5, and CCR10 but not CXCR4, Stem Cells Dev. 2005; 14(3): 329-36.

Wong RS, Mesenchymal stem cells: angels or demons? J Biomed Biotechnol. 2011; 2011: 459510.

21

The Importance of Haem vs Non-Haem Iron in the Survival and Pathogenesis of *Brucella abortus*

Marta A. Almirón[1], Nidia E. Lucero[2] and Norberto A. Sanjuan[3]
[1]Universidad Nacional de San Martín/Instituto de Investigaciones Biotecnológicas
[2]Instituto Nacional de Enfermedades Infecciosas-ANLIS "Dr. C. G. Malbrán", Departamento de Bacteriología,
[3]Universidad de Buenos Aires/ Facultad de Medicina/ Departamento de Microbiología
Argentina

1. Introduction

The genus *Brucella* belongs to the alpha-group of proteobacteria, along with plant pathogens as *Agrobacterium* and symbionts as *Rhizobium* and *Bradyrhizobium*. Several *Brucella* species, highly related at the genetic level, have been identified as the etiological agents of brucellosis. Each one has shown a preferred host although they can infect other animals. Animal brucellosis is usually endemic in developing countries and its main impact is economic. Human brucellosis is difficult to diagnose because symptoms are extremely variable. Few live vaccines are available for animals only, not for humans. The main problems with this pathogen are the lack of virulence factors commonly identified in other bacteria and the ability to establish a niche inside eukaryotic cells, where they replicate and survive evading the immune response and the action of other antibacterial molecules.

In general, the pathogenic mechanisms used by bacteria have been related to iron because this essential cellular nutrient is scarce and not easily available for bacteria either in body fluids or inside eukaryotic cells. Thus, the iron deficient environment that bacteria encounter during infection induces genes which products are needed to support effective survival and thus they became part of virulence factors. Most of them are related to the acquisition of ionic iron or iron-containing molecules (Schaible & Kaufmann, 2004).

In the case of *Brucella*, much effort has been put into the study of this organism under iron limitation. The first reports about the nutritional preferences showed an absolute requirement for iron (Gerhardt, 1958). Further studies, mainly on *Brucella abortus* (the causative agent of brucellosis in cattle) have shown that *Brucella* produce two catecholic compounds, 2,3-dyhidroxybenzoic acid (2,3-DHBA) and brucebactin, as siderophores under iron limitation (Gonzalez Carrero et al., 2002; Lopez-Goñi et al., 1992). However, experimental evidence on mutants unable to synthesize those molecules failed to demonstrate that their production is critical for bacterial replication inside macrophages (Bellaire et al., 1999; Jain et al., 2011). In addition, a mutant in the main iron-response regulator gene, with deficient synthesis of siderophores and increased intracellular haem content, showed a better replication pattern inside professional phagocytes than wild type (Martinez et al., 2006). On the other hand, a *B.*

abortus mutant that can not ensemble iron into protoporphyrin IX to produce its own haem was unable to survive inside professional phagocytes (Almiron et al., 2001). Another *B. abortus* mutant that can not internalize haem from the medium showed significant attenuation in cultured murine macrophages (Paulley et al., 2007). None of these two mutants could establish a wild-type pattern of infection in the mice model. Therefore, taking into consideration all these results, it seems that under iron limitation, as one of the stress conditions that probably *Brucella* face during infection, the acquisition or biosynthesis of haem renders more benefits to survive than the acquisition of iron. In agreement with this, we found that a mutation in the main iron-reservoir protein of *B. abortus* did not affect its replication inside professional phagocytes (Almiron & Ugalde, 2010).

For a long time, a link has been established between the preference of *Brucella* to use erythritol as a carbon and energy source and the pathogenesis of this organism, based on experimental data (Smith et al., 1962). This molecule is present at high concentrations in placental trophoblast, the preferred niche for *Brucella*. One of the plausible explanations to this link is the bacterial necessity for iron to catabolized erythritol. Without interfering with this theory, it is apparent that placenta is a membranous-vascular organ that receives nutrients from the mother´s blood providing in this way a high content of haem. Additionally, haem is known to be the main iron source inside eukaryotic cells.

2. Involvement of iron in the replication of *B. abortus*

B. abortus, like most pathogenic bacteria, presents an absolute requirement for the micronutrient iron to support growth (Gerardt, 1958). Bacteria utilize iron as a cofactor or as a prosthetic group for essential enzymes that participates in many biological processes, such as metabolism, respiration, oxygen transport, and gene regulation. Iron is one of the most abundant elements in nature but its bioavailability is reduced under physiological conditions. The oxidised Fe^{3+} ferric form is predominant in the environment under aerobic atmospheres with very low solubility at neutral pH (10^{-18} M), and even lower (10^{-36}M) in solution due to its tendency to hydrolyze and form polymers (Andrews et al., 2003). In animals, iron is bound to proteins in order to keep the metal soluble and to avoid toxic reactions due to its redox potential. Intracellularly, iron is chelated by a porphyrin ring giving rise to haem. However, the chelated metal iron can undergo reversible oxidative changes and thus haem is mainly associated to proteins. In this way, free iron is practically unavailable for bacteria in the host.

B. abortus is able to acquire iron in different ways. Directly, through the synthesis and secretion of two catecholic siderophores, 2,3-DHBA and the more complex compound derived from this known as brucebactin. Both of them are synthesized by the enzymes encoded in the *dhbCEBA* operon in response to iron limitation (Gonzalez Carrero et al., 2002; Lopez-Goñi et al., 1992). The indirect way is by the incorporation of haemin as an iron source (Almirón et al., 2001; Paulley et al., 2007).

B. abortus stores iron mainly in a bacterioferritin. This molecule represents a ferritin that contains haem. In *Brucella*, the bacterioferritin is a homopolymer that accumulates approximately 70% of the intracellular iron (Almirón & Ugalde, 2010). Another protein considered as a miniferritin, Dps, is expressed in *Brucella* and could be contributing with iron storage in this pathogen during the stationary phase of growth (Almiron et al., 1992;

Lamontagne et al., 2009). According to the phenotype of a *B. abortus bfr* mutant it was suggested that this microorganism senses the Bfr-bound iron available for metabolism, by an unknown mechanism, and thus regulates iron homeostasis independently of the external iron concentration (Almiron & Ugalde, 2010).

2.1 Extracellular survival

The acquisition of iron from the environment is a process tightly regulated by bacteria in order to keep iron homeostasis. An excess of free intracellular iron can be devastating for bacterial survival. The iron-uptake system by siderophores, low-molecular chelators with high-affinity towards ferric iron, means the production of the compounds plus the proteins needed for transportation and reception of ferric-siderophores complexes. The transport is usually mediated by the energy-transducing TonB-ExbB-ExbD system in Gram-negative bacteria (Andrews et al., 2003).

In this regard, the TonB system, an ABC transporter, and a putative GTPase were shown to be involved in iron acquisition of *B. melitensis*. The *exbB*, *dstC* and *dugA* genes are needed for the assimilation of DHBA and /or ferric citrate (Danese et al., 2004). Is it probably that they have the same effect in *B. abortus*.

2.1.1 The complex regulation of siderophore biosynthesis

The *B. abortus dhbCEBA* operon is repressed during growth under iron-sufficient conditions while it is highly induced under iron limitation (Lopez-Goñi et al., 1992). The transcriptional regulators acting on the promoter region of the *dhbCEBA* operon are Irr and DhbR. The iron-response regulator, Irr, is a member of the Fur family, and DhbR of the AraC family. Both proteins have demonstrated to interact with the DNA *in vitro* by the electrophoretic mobility shift assay (Anderson et al., 2008; Martinez et al., 2006). The *B. abortus irr* gene is constitutively transcribed regardless of the external iron concentration, but no protein could be detected under iron-sufficient conditions (Martinez et al., 2005). The transcription of *dhbR* is iron repressible and seems to be under the transcriptional control of Irr. A putative binding site for Irr was found between the -35 and -10 regions related to the transcriptional start of the *dhbR* gene (Anderson et al., 2008). The induction of *dhbC* transcription by Irr and DhbR has been correlated with the reduced production of siderophores in the culture media of the *irr* and *dhbR* mutants, respectively, and in comparison with the wild type. In both studies, the transcription was analyzed by constructing *dhbC*-lacZ fusions. To study the Irr regulation, the fusion was carried out to the *B. abortus* chromosome causing a mutation in the gene that enabled the strain to produce siderophores. In this case, a two-fold induction was observed in the wild type in comparison with the *irr* mutant (Martinez et al., 2006). In the other work, the authors assayed the β-galactosidase activity of a plasmid-borne lacZ fusion expressed in different genetic backgrounds. Interestingly, they found equivalent reduction in the enzyme activity expressed either in *B. abortus dhbR* or in *B. abortus dhbC* mutants. In this way, the authors corroborated that DhbR needs siderophores as a coinducer to repress transcription. This mode of action was described for other AraC-like regulators (Anderson et al., 2008). If DhbR acts in this way, the cause of the remaining levels of the enzyme activity detected in the *B. abortus irr dhbC* mutant under iron limitation should be investigated.

Neither Irr nor DhbR are involved in the transcriptional repression of the *dhbCEBA* operon. In order to have an accurate control of iron metabolism, the Irr protein is unstable under iron-sufficient conditions. The *Brucella* genome encodes two *irr* paralogues as other members of the alpha-proteobacteria group (Martinez et al., 2005). It has not been studied yet if the *B. abortus irr* ortologue is expressed and plays a role in iron-dependent regulation.

Other regulators that could be involved in iron homeostasis have been described by genomic sequence analysis, like RirA (Johnston et al., 2007; Rodionov et al., 2006). But, the lack of experimental results limits our understanding of this subject in *Brucella*.

Beyond this, the fact that more than two regulators modulate the transcription of the genes involved in the biosynthesis of both siderophores is an indication of the importance of the non-haem iron acquisition in the survival of *Brucella* under iron limitation. The idea that siderophores contribute to the virulence of several pathogens -such as *Escherichia coli* and *Vibrio cholerae*- is based on the capacity they give to the bacteria to acquire an essential nutrient under iron limitation. However, this role has not been well defined in *Brucella* yet, as we will discuss below.

2.1.2 Could erythritol be related to siderophore production due to its osmotic property?

The attenuation of a *B. abortus dhbC* mutant in pregnant cattle settled the bases for the relationship between iron acquisition and erythritol catabolism (Bellaire et al., 2003a). Bellaire and colleagues found that the production of siderophores was stimulated by the presence of erythritol in the media, and this effect was also observed at transcriptional level. The wild-type *B. abortus* harboring a plasmid-borne *dhbC-lacZ* fusion showed an increment in the β-galactosidase levels when grown in the presence of erythritol than that observed when this polyalcohol was not added. In order to explain this observation, they hypothesized that wild-type *B. abortus* experience an increased demand for iron in order to catabolize erythritol, since one of the enzymes involved in this metabolic pathway needs iron as a cofactor.

Interestingly, we found that if instead of the minimal media MG (usually employed to test siderophore production in *B. abortus* strains) we used the minimal media MM, no siderophores detection was possible after bacterial growth although iron was not present. The composition of this defined media is: $(NH_4)_2SO_4$ 2 g, KH_2PO_4 7 g, glucose 4 g, casaminoacids 10 g, $MnCl_2$ 100 μg, $MgSO_4$ 100 mg, biotin 2 μg, nicotinic acid 0.4 mg, piridoxal 0.4 mg, thiamin 0.4 mg and pantoteic acid 0.4 mg per liter; pH 7. A comparative look at the composition of both media led us to find a remarkable difference related to NaCl and glycerol, present in 7.5 g/l (128mM) and 37.5 g/l respectively in MG media. Thus, we decided to supplement MM with NaCl and glycerol and test for catechole production.

The results presented in Table 1 indicate that the *B. abortus* siderophore production was induced by increasing amounts of NaCl or glycerol. Moreover, both osmolytes act in a synergistic mode when added together to the MM media. An increment in siderophore production was also obtained when manitol was added to MM, suggesting that the phenotype was not restricted to ionic osmolytes. To test if this induction was exerted at transcriptional level, the β-galactosidase of the *B. abortus* chromosomal *dhbC-lacZ* fusion was

Medium	MM	MM	MM	MM	MM	MG
NaCl (g/l)	-	5	10	-	10	-
Glicerol (g/l)	-	-	-	37,5	37,5	-
[SD]/OD_{600}	1.9	13.0	34.4	21.3	122.6	51.4

Table 1. Effects of NaCl and glycerol on *B. abortus* siderophore production. *B. abortus* siderophore secretion expressed as nmol/ml related to cell density from the wild-type 2308 strain grown in MG or MM media supplemented with NaCl and glycerol at the indicated concentrations. Data are from one experiment made in duplicates and representative of more than four independent experiments.

measured in MM media supplemented with different amounts of NaCl. The results, as shown in Table 2, demonstrate that osmolality plays a role in *dhbC* transcription and consequently in siderophore secretion.

mM NaCl in MM	0	50	100	200
β-galactosidase (Miller units)	21.8	23.2	93.3	439.1

Table 2. Effects of NaCl on the *B. abortus dhbC* transcription. β-Galactosidase activity from *B. abortus dhbC-lacZ* grown in MM supplemented with NaCl at the indicated concentrations. Data are representative of at least three independent experiments.

Even though *Bacillus subtilis* is a Gram-positive bacterium, it produces a similar catechol molecule, 2,3-dihydroxybenzoate, that is finally modified to render the siderophore bacillibactin with stronger chelation capacity than the precursor. The enzymes that participate in their biosynthetic pathway are encoded in the *dhbACEBF* operon. It was reported that high salinity causes iron limitation in *B. subtilis* and triggers the derepression of iron-controlled genes present in the operon mentioned before (Hoffmann et al., 2002). Iron limitation as well as high salinity led to the accumulation of comparable amounts of siderophores in the bacterial culture. This phenotype as well as the growth deficiency observed under high salinity could be reduced by an excess of iron. In this microorganism, the ferric uptake regulator Fur is repressing the genes when sufficient iron is present (Hoffmann et al., 2002). In this relation, it should be noted that erythritol is an osmolyte and curiously, it has been shown that the growth of the *B. abortus dhbC* mutant in iron-limited media supplemented with erythritol is enhanced by the addition of iron (Bellaire et al., 2003a).

Similarly, a *B. abortus entF* mutant presented a growth deficiency under iron limitation in comparison with wild type, which was reverted by the addition of iron (Jain et al., 2011). The product of *entF* is involved in the production of brucebactin (Gonzalez Carrero et al., 2002). It was shown that the *B. abortus entF* mutant was not able to increase the number of viable cells when incubated under iron limitation. Interestingly, the mutant culture had not lost viability before a period of 192 h of incubation as an indication that the internal-iron content was enough to support metabolism in the experimental conditions used. Instead, a decrease in the number of viable cells was observed when the medium was supplemented with erythritol, but this phenotype was reverted by the addition of iron salts. These data indicate, besides the role that the product of *entF* could have in the erythritol metabolism as suggested, the relationship between siderophore production and erythritol. Is it possible that *Brucella* needs to acquire iron in order to survive under osmotic pressure?

No data about the growth phenotype of iron-depleted cells in media containing erythritol has been reported. This information may be important if it is considered that the host imposes iron limitation as a defense mechanism against microbial infection (Schaible & Kaufmann, 2004). Under this circumstance, it is likely to find iron-depleted bacteria from host's samples. A similar situation could be considered if the bacterial samples came from environment. Taking into account that *Brucella* modulates iron-dependent gene regulation according to their iron content and independently of the external iron concentration, it should be appropriate to test the survival efficiency of iron-depleted *brucella* in media that contain erythritol, such as the modified Brucella selective medium that has been developed to be used for diagnostic purposes (Her et al., 2010).

2.1.3 Fur regulation

Bfr is a homopolymeric hemoprotein that functions as the main iron-reservoir of *Brucella*. As other members of the alpha-proteobacteria group, the *Brucella* iron-dependent regulation responds to the internal iron concentration (Almirón & Ugalde, 2010). Hence, a mutation in the *B. abortus bfr* induces siderophore biosynthesis and secretion earlier than in the wild-type strain under iron limitation (Almirón & Ugalde, 2010). It has been described that the promoter region of the *dhbCEBA* operon is subjected to the regulation of Irr and DhbR proteins under iron limitation. Both were able to bind the promoter region *in vitro*. The same region has also two putative Fur boxes. Fur is the main iron-dependent regulator in many bacteria. It usually represses genes when bound to iron. Therefore, if iron is not available there should be a derepression of fur-regulated genes. In order to understand whether Fur participates in the *dhbCEBA* regulation we constructed mutants by inserting a kanamicin-resistant cassette in the amplified *fur* gene and then, by carring this mutation to the chromosome of the wild-type *B. abortus* 2308 and the isogenic *bfr* or *dhbC-lacZ* mutants by homologous recombination as described previously (Martinez, 2004). As shown in Figure 1, we determined the β-galactosidase activity of the chromosomal *dhbC*-lacZ fusion in the background of the parental and *fur* mutant strains. We included the *bfr dhbC* mutant strain for comparative purpose (Almirón & Ugalde, 2010).

The experiments were done when cells were grown in MG or iron-supplemented MG. Although the absence of Fur did not produce the same effect on the *dhbC* transcription, the small induction observed among cultures at $OD_{600} \leq 1$ led us to look more precisely at siderophore production in the wild-type, *bfr* and *fur* isogenic mutants.

It is interesting to note that when the cells have the possibility to acquire external iron by means of siderophores, the results can be different. While the wild type did not sense internal iron limitation during the first hours of incubation in MG, the consequence of Fur absence is equivalent to the internal-iron deficiency produced by the mutation in *bfr*, in terms of siderophore secretion (Figure 2A). In contrast, in the presence of external iron the *bfr* mutant represses the biosynthesis as wild type, while *fur* did not (Figure 2B). To determine if the repression observed in *bfr* mutant was due to Fur, a *B. abortus bfr fur* double mutant was constructed. The results suggest that Fur is regulating siderophore production

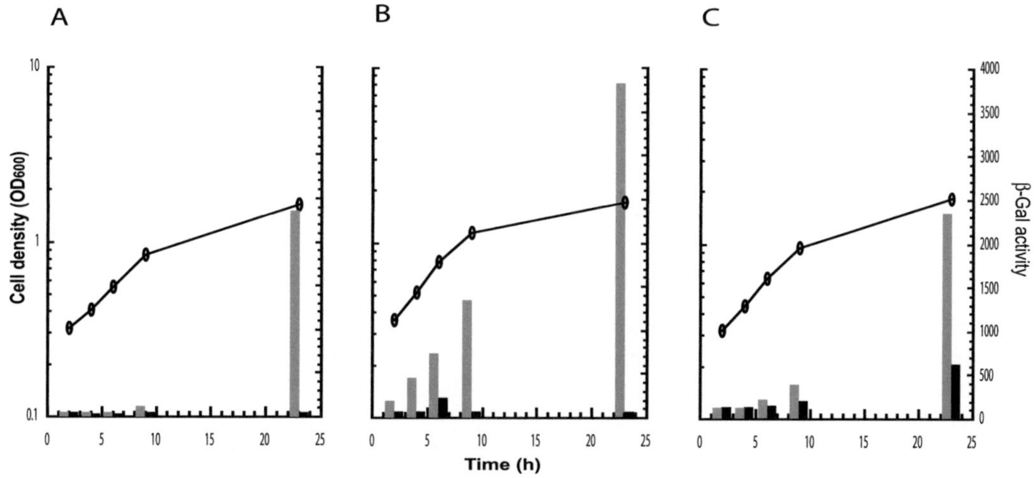

Fig. 1. Effect of iron concentration on *dhbCEBA* transcription. β-Galactosidase activity (Miller units) was determined from *B. abortus* 2308 derivatives growing in MG (gray bars) or in MG supplemented with 50 μM iron citrate (black bars). (**A**) *B. abortus* 2308 *dhbC,* (**B**) 2308 *bfr dhbC,* and (**C**) 2308 *fur dhbC*. Growth curves in MG were determined by measurment of OD_{600} (lines). Data are average of duplicates, standard deviation were less than 5%.

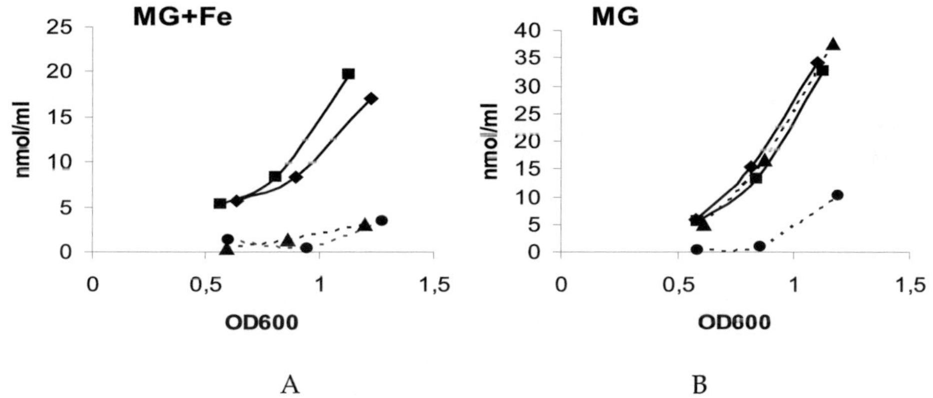

Fig. 2. *B. abortus* siderophore secretion in response to external iron concentration. Concentration of siderophores related to cell density from *B. abortus* 2308 (..●..), 2308 *fur* (-■-), 2308 *fur bfr* (-♦-), and 2308 *bfr* (..▲..).Values of catechol concentration (determined by the Arnow assay) are expressed from duplicates at three different time points during incubation. Results are representative of three independent experiments.

in *Brucella abortus* under iron sufficient conditions. Further studies are needed to determine the promoter region that interacts with Fur-Fe complexes.

There is a previous report showing that a *fur* mutant was producing less β-galactosidase activities than the wild type in MG. No differences were observed in the presence of iron. It should be noted that the data were obtained from a plasmid-borned *dhbC-lacZ* fusion expressed either in the wild-type *B. abortus* or in the isogenic *fur* mutant (Roop, et al., 2004).

Because the extracellular iron concentration does not represent the *Brucella* iron content, the experimental conditions used to test the *dhbC*-lacZ fusion, sometimes in a plasmid and others in the chromosome causing a mutation in the *dhbC* gene, do not result trivial, especially with Fur that needs intracellular free-iron to bind DNA near the promoter region of a gene. Thus, it should be important to determine the transcriptional level of the *dhbCEBA* operon relative to the internal iron content in *Brucella* strains in order to get comparable results and to better understand iron homeostasis in this pathogen.

2.1.4 Production of outer-membrane vesicles under iron limitation

The dogma that bacteria induce virulence factors under iron limitation and the possibility to find them concentrated in outer-membrane vesicles, as described for other pathogens, led us to isolate *B. abortus* membrane vesicles from cells grown in iron rich (2xYT) and iron-depleted (2xYT treated with 150 μM DIP) media at 37 °C for 1 week in a CO_2 incubator. Cells were collected in saline solution and heated at 60 °C for 30 minutes. Cells were discarded by centrifugation at 13,000 x g. Supernatants were centrifuged at 18,500 rpm for 30 min in the 70Ti Beckman-rotor. A second centrifugation of the supernatant was done at 43,500 rpm for 3 h in the same rotor for further purification. The pellet was suspended in PBS and tested under transmission-electron microscopy for the presence of pure vesicles. Samples of equal volume were subjected to electrophoresis in polyacrylamide gels and stained with Coomassie blue for protein detection. Proteins were detected only from cultures grown with iron limitation.

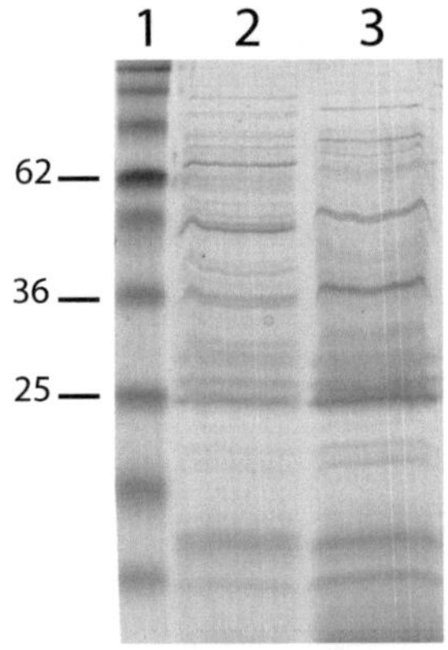

Fig. 3. Outer-membrane vesicles from *B. abortus* in response to iron limitation. 15% SDS-PAGE analysis of proteins obtained from outer-membrane vesicles preparations of *B. abortus* grown under iron limitation at 5 (line 2) and 15 days (line 3). Molecular mass standards (line1); kilodaltons are indicated on the left.

As shown in Figure 3, similar patterns were observed from cultures incubated between 5 and 15 days under the conditions mentioned before. Interestingly, it was also observed in samples prepared from *B. abortus irr* and *bfr* mutants.

The peptides obtained from the 36 KDa (adaivaxepeaveyv and ntvaednaxggiv) and the 25 KDa bands (enxgyv and adaivaqpateid) identified after trypsin digestion followed by HPLC-MS, led us to identify the porin Omp2b and OmpW as the major proteins expressed in *brucella* vesicles produced under iron limitation.

The bacterial liberation to the culture media of outer-membrane vesicles represents a phenomenon that has been described for many bacteria including *Brucella* (Gamazo et al., 1987; 1989). The origin of these bacterial structures and their function are still under investigation. So far, there is no genetic evidence supporting the idea that bacteria can regulate its production. In terms of function, it has been hypothesized that they can contribute to bacterial virulence by evading the immunological host-defense mechanisms and by redirecting or preserving the virulence factors accumulated in their lumen. In this regard, further studies are needed to understand whether the presence of these proteins in the *brucella* vesicles has a meaning in the virulence of this pathogen.

2.2 Intracellular growth

The growth- deficient phenotype of the B. *abortus bfr* observed under iron limitation *in vitro* was not reproduced when cells were growing intracellularly (Almiron & Ugalde, 2010). Nonetheless, we investigated whether siderophores were assisting *B. abortus bfr* for intracellular replication. The gentamicin protection assay was done in HeLa cells with the parental strain and the isogenic *bfr* and *bfr dhbC* mutants. Similar results were obtained for all strains (Figure 4) indicating that siderophores are not involved in *B. abortus bfr* intracellular survival.

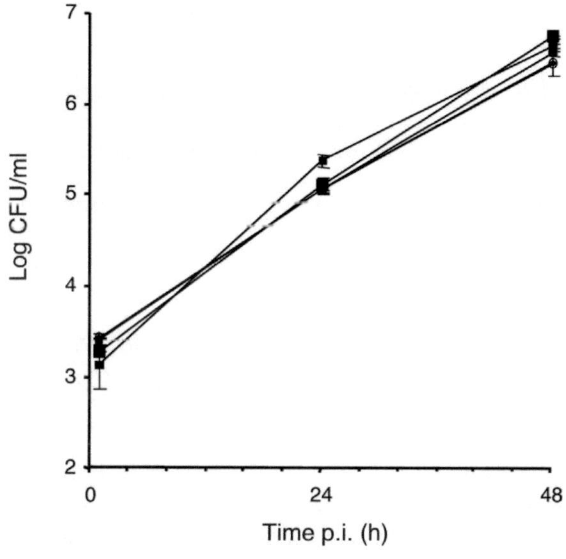

Fig. 4. Intracellular survival of *B. abortus* strains in HeLa cells. Monolayers of HeLa (10^5 cells/well) were infected with wild-type 2308 (■), 2308 *bfr* (•), 2308*dhbC* (Δ) and 2308 *bfr dhbC* (▲). At different times p.i. cells were lysed to determine the number of viable intracellular bacteria (CFU/ml). Data are expressed as means and standard deviations from one experiment performed in triplicate. They are representative of three independent experiments.

B. abortus mutants unable to produce 2,3-DHBA and brucebactin (*B. abortus dhbC* and *entF*) presented a wild-type behavior when infecting murine macrophages (Bellaire et al., 1999; Jain et al., 2011).

The role of *exbB*, *dstC* and *dugA* in the intracellular replication of *Brucella* were tested in bovine macrophages and in HeLa cells. None of these mutants showed attenuation in comparison to the wild type (Danese et al., 2004). These results are in agreement with those obtained with mutants that do not produce 2,3-DHBA.

A proteomic analysis of intracellular *B. abortus* recovered at different times after infection of murine macrophages revealed that proteins related to iron and haem transport were reduced during the first hours post-infection (p.i.) and interestingly, were induced after 20 or 44 h p.i (Lamontagne et al., 2009). These results suggest that once in the endoplasmic reticulum-related vacuole *Brucella* could get access to iron-sources facilitating the intracellular replication. In general, when *Brucella* infects a professional phagocytic cell-line, there is about one log reduction in the intracellular number of colony-forming units after 12 h p.i. Thus, it can not be discarded that the iron source encountered by *Brucella* latter in times have bacterial origin. The ferritins Bfr and Dps were reported to remain uninduced after 3 h of infection.

2.3 In animals

B. abortus dhbC was as virulent as wild type in the murine model using Balb/C mice, though this strain showed attenuation in pregnant cattle (Bellaire et al., 1999; 2003b). The author attributed the difference to the presence of erythritol in the bovine placental trophoblast which is absent in mice.

The *B. melitensis exbB*, *dstC* and *dugA* mutants were also tested for virulence in Balb/C mice. According to the bacterial counts obtained from mouse spleens at 1 and 4 weeks p.i., no difference was observed between wild type and mutants (Danese et al., 2004).

According to these data, the iron acquisition systems do not seem to be involved in *Brucella* pathogenicity when tested in a mouse model. The significance in the natural host requires further experimentation.

3. Involvement of haem in the replication of *B. abortus*

Whilst pathogenic bacteria possess different mechanisms for extracellular haem incorporation, their own biosynthesis is considered to be the main haem source.

The haem biosynthetic pathway in alpha-proteobacteria is similar to that in animal and yeast mitochondria. It starts with the action of the ALA synthase and finishes with the ferrochelatase. The last step, corresponding to the incorporation of a ferrous iron into protoporphyring IX, can be affected by the availability of intracellular iron, a condition usually faced by bacteria during infection. The oxidative characteristic of the chelated iron allows haem to participate as a cofactor in oxidative reactions. This type of reactions plays an important role in electron transfer for metabolism or energy generation (O'Brian & Thony-Meyer, 2002) and can also be employed in signal transduction systems. It has been described that haem participates in the sensing of diatomic gases and in the transcriptional and post-transcriptional regulation of several genes (Genco & Dixon, 2001).

Bacteria can produce cell lysis to gain access to the intracellular haem by secreting cellular proteases or haemolysins, or via complement. Also, bacteria can get extracellular haem through haemophores that will compete with haem-containing molecules for the haem group. Once haem is accessible, it is transported across the outer membrane via a TonB-dependent process. Because haem is hydrophobic and tends to aggregate at physiological pH it needs a recognition molecule at the bacteria surface and carrier proteins to be translocated to the cytoplasm. Then, haem can be used as an iron source after the action of haemoxigenases or incorporated to proteins (Lee et al, 1995; Wandersman & Delepelaire, 2004).

The synthesis of haem in *B. abortus* was reported to be altered by mutations in the *hemH* as an indication that *Brucella* is able to synthesize its own haem (Almirón et al, 2001). The protophorphyrin accumulation together with the decreased number of β-galactosidase units obtained from a plasmid-borne *hemB-lacZ* fusion expressed in the *irr* mutant under iron limitation, in contrast to the wild type, suggest that Irr down-regulates the haem biosynthesis. This kind of Irr regulation at the level of *hemB* has been described in *Bradyrhizobium japonicum* and in *Rhizobium leguminosarum* (Hamza et al., 1998; Wexler et al., 2003). Thus, it can be concluded that *B. abortus* has a haem biosynthetic pathway regulated by Irr.

Additionally, *B. abortus* can acquire haem from the environment for metabolic use (Almirón et al, 2001). The BhuA was shown to be involved in the internalization of haem during the stationary phase of *B. abortus* growth, under iron limitation. This outer-membrane protein is an homologue of Ton-B dependent haem transporters already characterized for other Gram-negative bacteria such as *Shigella dysenteriae, Yersinia pestis,* and *Bradyrhizobium japonicum* (Paulley et al., 2007).

The genome of *Brucella* possesses sequences coding for putative haemolysins. However no expression of such DNA has been described yet.

3.1 Extracellular survival

The auxothrophy of the *B. abortus hemH* mutant was restored only by the addition of haemin indicating the presence of some mechanisms in *Brucella* that allow the internalization and utilization of exogenous hemin as described for other bacteria (Almiron et al., 2001). Iron salts or hemoproteins did not revert the auxothorophy.

As predicted, a *B. abortus bhuA* mutant cannot use haem as an iron source. When this mutant and the parental strain were cultured in the low iron medium MG, no differences were observed during the logarithmic and the stationary phases of growth. However, the death phase of the mutant culture started earlier than the wild type. Since the addition of external iron salts prevented the loss of viability, the authors have suggested that BhuA plays a role in stationary-phase iron acquisition in *B. abortus*. It is hard not to relate iron with haem. In that sense, another data interpretation might suggest that iron allowed the cells to resume haem biosynthesis or instead, no more haem was used as an iron source thus, preserving this molecule. Is it haem or iron what *Brucella* needs to survive extracellularly under iron limitation or stationary phase? The growth capability of *B. abortus hemH* was not restored by the addition of iron salts, even under iron-sufficient conditions. This indicates that haem is essential for *B. abortus* to live as a free microorganism.

The transcription of *bhuA* is under the positive regulation of Irr in *B. abortus* (Anderson et al., 2011). Although this regulation was observed during the stationary phase, it should be considered that iron limitation occurs in *Brucella* when the internal iron content reaches a threshold, independently of the external iron concentration. This situation could be achieved by cells after several hours of incubation under iron-limited conditions. That is the stationary phase.

Interestingly, a mutation in the *B. abortus irr* has rendered an increase in haem content due to a derepression of the haem biosynthesis (Martinez et al., 2005; 2006). This phenotype assists *brucella* to survive under the oxidative stress produced by exposition to hydrogen peroxide. On the other hand, another mutation in the *B. abortus irr* prevented iron acquisition through siderophores, as previously reported, and haem internalization via the haem transporter BhuA (Anderson et al, 2011). Consequently, if a *Brucella irr* mutant is grown for several hours under iron limitation, it is expected that this mutant will not survive even if haem is added to the media. The iron depletion imposed does not support its own haem biosynthesis and the mutant is unable to internalize haem. But, if iron is added to the media, the *irr* mutant can resume the haem biosynthesis and survive. This hypothesis has been supported by the experimental data reported by Anderson. These data indicate that, besides the supply of iron that haem carries, haem itself is essential for *in vitro Brucella* growth.

3.2 Intracellular survival

Irr desregulation in *B. abortus* caused by a mutation in *irr* enables the microorganism with a better performance inside eukaryotic cells (Martinez et al., 2006). Thus, while wild type experienced a decrease in the number of intracellular bacteria during the first 24 h p.i. in HeLa or J774 cell lines, the *irr* mutant showed an increment in the bacterial count. Even though the invasion was not affected for the mutation, it is evident that it led *Brucella* to be better equipped than wild type for the survival strategy under iron limitation. Catalase as other haem-containing molecules can be considered as part of that equipment since the *irr* mutant showed higher intracellular haem content, catalase activity and resistance to hydrogen peroxide than the wild type. Paradoxically, the iron-acquisition system through siderophores was deficient in this mutant. This data is in agreement with those that indicate that siderophores are not involved in the intracellular replication of *Brucella*.

The *hemH* mutant was assayed for *in vitro* survival inside HeLa cells and J774 murine macrophages. This mutant was completely attenuated in both cell lines in comparison with the wild type. It was impaired in both invasion capability and intracellular survival. The mechanism that failed in this mutant remains unknown. Considering that haem is present in different kinds of molecules, it is possible to speculate that, with an outer-membrane haemoprotein deficiency, it could be involved in cell invasion. Once inside the cell, it is more likely that a synergistic effect from different haemoproteins leads to the unsuccessful survival.

Furthermore, the *B. abortus bhuA* mutant was attenuated in cultured murine macrophages compared to wild type (Paulley et al., 2007).

3.3 In animals

When Balb/C mice were infected with the *Brucella hemH* mutant it was interesting to note that as early as 2 weeks p.i. neither spleen nor liver colonization were observed in comparison with the wild type or the *hem*H mutant complemented with the wild-type *hemH*. In spite of this, the histological examination of the spleens revealed the same granulomatous reaction in mice infected with all three strains at 2 and 4 weeks p.i. Hyperplasia occurred to a lesser degree in mice inoculated with the *hemH* mutant.

Interestingly, mutations in *B. abortus* genes that affect the haem acquisition system, like *bhuA* or *irr*, were shown to be attenuated in C57BL6 mice at 4 weeks p.i. (Anderson et al., 2011; Paulley et al., 2007). When a different *B. abortus irr* mutant was previously tested in Balb/C mice, at 7 and 21 days after inoculation, neither the increment in catalase activity and haem content, nor the decline in siderophores biosynthesis affected the wild type virulence (Martinez et al., 2006). Although a different mice strain was used, the attenuation in the *brucella* virulence observed after 4 weeks p.i. could be an indication that *Brucella* suffers from iron limitation after one month of infection. Most importantly, it can be a clear indication that cells have access to haem but not to free iron at this stage in the infected animal.

4. Conclusion

It is as much impossible to dissociate free iron from haem as it is difficult to know whether bacteria incorporate haem in response to a real demand for this molecule or it just represents an iron source. Nonetheless, if we analyze the data presented here, there is a line of evidence that suggests the preferred value of haem over non-haem iron in the survival of *B. abortus* during its life cycle as a free organism or as an intracellular pathogen.

First of all, the transcriptional regulation as the protein stability of the major iron responsive regulator in *Brucella abortus* depends on haem. The *irr* gene is transcribed independently of the external iron concentration but it is autoregulated under low iron conditions. The Irr protein is able to bind haem in vitro and this situation probably contributes to the formation of dimers. Intracellularly, Irr is degraded when bacteria do not sense iron limitation. In this condition, bacteria are provided with both non-haem iron and haem.

In general, as it has been proved, the inability to acquire iron through siderophores does not alter the intracellular replication and the capacity to infect mice. On the contrary, the inability to synthesize its own haem or to acquire this molecule from the media affects both the *B. abortus* intracellular replication and the possibility to establish a normal infection in the mouse model.

5. Perspectives

Future research in haem biosynthesis under conditions that result more representative of those faced by *brucellae* during infection might help to increase our knowledge about the survival and pathogenesis of *B. abortus*.

6. Acknowledgment

This work was supported by grants from the Agencia Nacional de Promoción Científica y Tecnológica de la República Argentina PICT 6580 and PICT 651; and by Grant PIP 5463 obtained from the Consejo Nacional de Investigaciones Científicas y Técnicas de la Argentina (CONICET).

7. References

Almiron M, Link AJ, Furlong D, Kolter R (1992) A novel DNA-binding protein with regulatory and protective roles in starved *Escherichia coli*. *Genes Dev*, Vol.6, No.12B, pp. 2646-2654, ISSN 0890-9369

Almiron, M., Martinez, M., Sanjuan, N. & Ugalde, R.A. (2001) Ferrochelatase is present in *Brucella abortus* and is critical for its intracellular survival and virulence. *Infect Immun*, Vol. 69, No.10, pp. 6225-6230, ISSN 0019-9567

Almiron, M.A. & Ugalde, R.A. (2010) Iron homeostasis in *Brucella abortus*: the role of bacterioferritin. *J Microbiol* , Vol.48, No.5, pp. 668-673, ISSN 1976-3794

Anderson ES, Paulley JT, Roop RM, 2nd (2008) The AraC-like transcriptional regulator DhbR is required for maximum expression of the 2,3-dihydroxybenzoic acid biosynthesis genes in *Brucella abortus* 2308 in response to iron deprivation. *J Bacteriol* , Vol.190, No.5, pp.1838-1842, ISSN 1098-5530

Anderson, E.S., Paulley, J.T., Martinson, D.A., Gaines, J.M., Steele, K.H., et al. (2011) The iron responsive regulator Irr is required for wild-type expression of the gene encoding the heme transporter BhuA in *Brucella abortus* 2308. *J Bacteriol.*, Vol.193, No19, pp.5359-5364, ISSN 1098-5530

Anderson JD, Smith H (1965) The Metabolism of Erythritol by *Brucella Abortus*. *J Gen Microbiol*, Vol. 38, pp.109-124, ISSN 0022-1287

Andrews SC, Robinson AK, Rodriguez-Quinones F (2003) Bacterial iron homeostasis. *FEMS Microbiol Rev*, Vol. 27, No.2-3, pp. 215-237, ISSN 0168-6445

Bellaire BH, Elzer PH, Baldwin CL, Roop RM, 2nd (1999) The siderophore 2,3-dihydroxybenzoic acid is not required for virulence of *Brucella abortus* in BALB/c mice. *Infect Immun*, Vol.67, No.5, pp. 2615-2618, ISSN 0019-9567

Bellaire BH, Elzer PH, Baldwin CL, Roop RM, 2nd (2003) Production of the siderophore 2,3-dihydroxybenzoic acid is required for wild-type growth of *Brucella abortus* in the presence of erythritol under low-iron conditions in vitro. *Infect Immun*, Vol.71, No.5, pp. 2927-2832, ISSN 0019-9567

Bellaire BH, Elzer PH, Hagius S, Walker J, Baldwin CL, et al. (2003) Genetic organization and iron-responsive regulation of the *Brucella abortus* 2,3-dihydroxybenzoic acid biosynthesis operon, a cluster of genes required for wild-type virulence in pregnant cattle. *Infect Immun*, Vol.71, No. 4, pp. 1794-1803, ISSN 0019-9567

Burkhardt S, Jimenez de Bagues MP, Liautard JP, Kohler S (2005) Analysis of the behavior of *eryC* mutants of *Brucella suis* attenuated in macrophages. *Infect Immun*, Vol.73, No.10, pp. 6782-6790, ISSN 0019-9567

Danese I, Haine V, Delrue RM, Tibor A, Lestrate P, et al. (2004) The Ton system, an ABC transporter, and a universally conserved GTPase are involved in iron utilization by *Brucella melitensis* 16M. *Infect Immun*, Vol. 72, No.10, pp. 5783-5790, ISSN 0019-9567

Gamazo C, Moriyon I (1987) Release of outer membrane fragments by exponentially growing Brucella melitensis cells. *Infect Immun*, Vo.55, No.3, pp. 609-615, ISSN 0019-9567

Gamazo C, Winter AJ, Moriyon I, Riezu-Boj JI, Blasco JM, et al. (1989) Comparative analyses of proteins extracted by hot saline or released spontaneously into outer membrane blebs from field strains of *Brucella ovis* and *Brucella melitensis*. *Infect Immun*, Vol.57, No.5, pp. 1419-1426, ISSN 0019-9567

Garcia-Lobo JM, Sangari Garcia FJ (2004) Erythritol Metabolism and Virulence in *Brucella*. In: Lopez-Goni I, Moriyon I, editors. *Brucella*: Molecular and Cellular Biology. Norfolk: horizon bioscience. pp. 231-242.

Gerhardt P (1958) The nutrition of *brucellae*. *Bacteriol Rev*, Vol. 22, No.2, pp:81-98, ISSN 0005-3678

Genco CA, Dixon DW (2001) Emerging strategies in microbial haem capture. *Mol Microbiol* Vol.39, No.1, pp. 1-11, ISSN 0950-382X

Gonzalez Carrero MI, Sangari FJ, Aguero J, Garcia Lobo JM (2002) *Brucella abortus* strain 2308 produces brucebactin, a highly efficient catecholic siderophore. *Microbiology*, Vol.148, No.Pt2, pp. 353-360, ISSN 1350-0872

Hamza I, Chauhan S, Hassett R, O'Brian MR (1998) The bacterial irr protein is required for coordination of heme biosynthesis with iron availability. *J Biol Chem*, Vol.273. No.34, pp.21669-21674, ISSN 0021-9258

Her M, Cho DH, Kang SI, Cho YS, Hwang IY, et al. (2010) The development of a selective medium for the *Brucella abortus* strains and its comparison with the currently recommended and used medium. Diagn Microbiol *Infect Dis*, Vol. 67, No.1, pp. 15-21, ISSN 1879-0070

Hoffmann T, Schutz A, Brosius M, Volker A, Volker U, et al. (2002) High-salinity-induced iron limitation in *Bacillus subtilis*. *J Bacteriol*, Vol. 184, No.3, pp. 718-727, ISSN 0021-9193

Jain N, Rodriguez AC, Kimsawatde G, Seleem MN, Boyle SM, et al. (2011) Effect of entF deletion on iron acquisition and erythritol metabolism by *Brucella abortus* 2308. *FEMS Microbiol Lett* , Vol.316, No.1, pp. 1-6, ISSN 1574-6968

Johnston AW, Todd JD, Curson AR, Lei S, Nikolaidou-Katsaridou N, et al. (2007) Living without Fur: the subtlety and complexity of iron-responsive gene regulation in the symbiotic bacterium *Rhizobium* and other alpha-proteobacteria. *Biometals*, Vol. 20, No.3-4, pp. 501-511, ISSN 0966-0844

Lamontagne J, Forest A, Marazzo E, Denis F, Butler H, et al. (2009) Intracellular adaptation of *Brucella abortus*. *J Proteome Res*, Vol. 8, No.3,pp.1594-1609, ISSN 1535-3893

Lee BC (1995) Quelling the red menace: haem capture by bacteria. *Mol Microbiol*, Vol.18, No.3, pp. 383-390, ISSN 0950-382X

Lopez-Goni I, Moriyon I, Neilands JB (1992) Identification of 2,3-dihydroxybenzoic acid as a *Brucella abortus* siderophore. *Infect Immun* , Vol.60, No.11, pp. 4496-4503, ISSN 0019-9567

Martinez M, Ugalde RA, Almiron M (2005) Dimeric *Brucella abortus* Irr protein controls its own expression and binds haem. *Microbiology* Vol.151, No.Pt10, pp.3427-3433, ISSN 1350-0872

Martinez M, Ugalde RA, Almiron M (2006) Irr regulates brucebactin and 2,3-dihydroxybenzoic acid biosynthesis, and is implicated in the oxidative stress resistance and intracellular survival of *Brucella abortus*. *Microbiology*, Vol.152, No.Pt9, pp. 2591-2598, ISSN 1350-0872

O'Brian MR, Thony-Meyer L (2002) Biochemistry, regulation and genomics of haem biosynthesis in prokaryotes. *Adv Microb Physiol* , Vol.46, pp. 257-318, ISSN 0065-2911

Parent MA, Bellaire BH, Murphy EA, Roop RM, 2nd, Elzer PH, et al. (2002) *Brucella abortus* siderophore 2,3-dihydroxybenzoic acid (DHBA) facilitates intracellular survival of the bacteria. *Microb Pathog*, Vol.32, No.5, pp. 239-248, ISSN 0882-4010

Paulley JT, Anderson ES, Roop RM, 2nd (2007) *Brucella abortus* requires the heme transporter BhuA for maintenance of chronic infection in BALB/c mice. *Infect Immun*, Vol. 75, No.11, pp. 5248-5254, ISSN 0019-9567

Rodionov DA, Gelfand MS, Todd JD, Curson AR, Johnston AW (2006) Computational reconstruction of iron- and manganese-responsive transcriptional networks in alpha-proteobacteria. *PLoS Comput Biol* 2: e163.

Roop RM, Bellaire BH, Anderson E, Paulley JT (2004) Iron Metabolism in *Brucella*. In: Lopez-Goni I, Moriyon I, editors. *Brucella*: Molecular and Cellular Biology. Norfolk: Horizon Bioscience.

Schaible UE, Kaufmann SH (2004) Iron and microbial infection. *Nat Rev Microbiol*, Vol.2, No.12, pp. 946-953, ISSN 1740-1526

Smith H, Williams AE, Pearce JH, Keppie J, Harris-Smith PW, et al. (1962) Foetal erythritol: a cause of the localization of *Brucella abortus* in bovine contagious abortion. *Nature*, Vol. 193, pp.47-49, ISSN 0028-0836

Wandersman C, Delepelaire P (2004) Bacterial iron sources: from siderophores to hemophores. *Annu Rev Microbiol* , Vol.58, pp.611-647, ISSN 0066-4227

Wexler M, Todd JD, Kolade O, Bellini D, Hemmings AM, et al. (2003) Fur is not the global regulator of iron uptake genes in *Rhizobium leguminosarum*. *Microbiology*, Vol. 149, No. Pt5, pp. 1357-1365, ISSN 1350-0872